REPRODUCTIVE MEDICINE SECRETS

Peter T. K. Chan, M.D.
Director of Male Reproductive Medicine
Department of Urology
Department of Obstetrics and Gynecology
McGill University Health Center
Montreal, Canada

Marc Goldstein, M.D.
Professor of Reproductive Medicine and Urology
Department of Urology
Cornell Institute for Reproductive Medicine
Weill Medical College of Cornell University
New York, New York

Zev Rosenwaks, M.D.
Director, Center for Reproductive Medicine and Infertility
Professor of Obsetrics and Gynecology and Reproductive Medicine
Weill Medical College of Cornell University
New York Presbyterian Hospital
New York, New York

HANLEY & BELFUS, INC.
An Imprint of Elsevier

HANLEY & BELFUS, INC.
An Imprint of Elsevier

The Curtis Center
Independence Square West
Philadelphia, Pennsylvania 19106

Note to the reader: Although the techniques, ideas, and information in this book have been carefully reviewed for correctness, the authors, editors, and publisher cannot accept any legal responsibility for any errors or omissions that may be made. Neither the publisher nor the editors make any guarantee, expressed or implied, with respect to the material contained herein.

Library of Congress Control Number: 2004103673

REPRODUCTIVE MEDICINE SECRETS   ISBN 1-56053-588-1

Printed in the United States of America

Last digit is the print number: 9 8 7 6 5 4 3 2 1

REPRODUCTIVE MEDICINE SECRETS

TABLE OF CONTENTS

CONTRIBUTORS

Shumyle Alan
University of Illinois, Chicago, Illinois

Dania H. Al-Jaroudi, M.D.
Obstetrics and Gynaecology, McGill University, McGill University Health Centre, Montreal, Quebec, Canada

Linda D. Applegarth, Ed.D.
Assistant Professor of Psychology in Obstetrics and Gynecology and Reproductive Medicine, Weill Medical College of Cornell University, The New York Presbyterian Hospital Institute for Reproductive Medicine, New York, New York

Melissa B. Brisman, J.D.
Montvale, New Jersey

William M. Buckett, M.D.
Assistant Professor, Obstetrics and Gynaecology, McGill University, Sub-specialist in Reproductive Endocrinology and Infertility, Royal Victoria Hospital, Montreal, Quebec, Canada

Erkan Buyuk
Weill Medical College of Cornell University, New York, New York

Peter T. K. Chan, M.D.
Director of Male Reproductive Medicine, Department of Urology, Department of Obstetrics and Gynaecology, McGill University Health Centre, Royal Victoria Hospital, Montreal, Quebec, Canada

Janet Choi, M.D.
Assistant Professor, Obstetrics and Gynecology, Division of Reproductive Endocrinology and Infertility, Columbia University College of Physicians and Surgeons, New York Presbyterian Hospital, Columbia Presbyterian Medical Center, New York, New York

Ina N. Cholst, M.D.
Associate Professor of Clinical Obstetrics and Gynecology and Reproductive Medicine, Weill Medical College of Cornell University, New York Presbyterian Hospital, New York, New York

Weber W. Chuang, M.D.
Baylor College of Medicine, Houston, Texas

Pak H. Chung, M.D.
Associate Professor, Obstetrics and Gynecology, Division of Reproductive Endocrinology and Infertility, Weill Medical College of Cornell University, New York Presbyterian Hospital, New York, New York

Jessica Davis, MD
Codirector, Division of Human Genetics; Associate Professor of Clinical Pediatrics, Weill College of Medicine of Cornell University, New York, New York

Owen Davis, M.D.
Associate Professor, Associate Director of IVF, Reproductive Medicine, Obstetrics and Gynecology, Weill Medical College of Cornell University, New York Presbyterian Hospital, New York, New York

Kate Dragesic, M.D.
Department of Obstetrics and Gynecology, Center for Reproductive Medicine and Infertility, Weill Medical College of Cornell University, New York, New York

Sarah K. Girardi, M.D.
Clinical Assistant Professor of Urology, Department of Urology, Weill Cornell Medical Center, New York, New York; Attending Urologist, North Shore University Medical Hospital, Manhasset, New York

Dan Goldschlag, M.D.
Obstetrics and Gynecology and Reproductive Medicine, Cornell University, New York Presbyterian Hospital, New York, New York

Marc Goldstein, M.D.
Professor of Reproductive Medicine and Urology, Department of Urology, Cornell Institute for Reproductive Medicine, Weill Medical College of Cornell University, New York, New York

Elizabeth A. Grill, Psy.D.
Instructor of Psychology in Obstetrics and Gynecology and Reproductive Medicine, Center for Reproductive Medicine and Infertility, Weill Medical College of Cornell University, New York Presbyterian Hospital, New York, New York

Matthew P. Hardy, M.D.
Senior Scientist, Center for Biomedical Research, Population Council, New York, New York

Louis Hemo, Ph.D.
Professor, Anatomy and Cell Biology, McGill University, Montreal, Quebec, Canada

Keith Jarvi, M.D.
Associate Professor, Surgery, University of Toronto, Mount Sinai Hospital, Toronto, Ontario, Canada

Laura Josephs, M.D.
Clinical Assistant Professor of Psychology in Psychiatry, Center for Reproductive Medicine and Infertility, Weill Medical College of Cornell University, New York Presbyterian Hospital, New York, New York

Isaac Kligman, M.D.
Center for Reproductive Medicine, Weill Medical College of Cornell University, New York, New York

Dolores J. Lamb, Ph.D.
Professor, Scott Department of Urology, Associate Professor, Molecular and Cellular Biology, Urology, Baylor College of Medicine, Houston, Texas

Joanne Libraro, R.N., B.S.N.
IVF Team Leader, Center for Reproductive Medicine and Infertility, Weill Medical College of Cornell University, New York Presbyterian Hospital, New York, New York

Kirk C. Lo, M.D., C.M.
Fellow in Male Reproductive Medicine & Surgery, Scott Department of Urology, Baylor College of Medicine, Houston, Texas

Anne F. Malavé, Ph.D.
Private Practice, Clinical Psychologist and Psychoanalyst Specializing in Infertility and Adoption, New York, New York

Joel L. Marmar, M.D.
Professor of Surgery and Urology, Robert Wood Johnson Medical School at Camden, Head, Division of Urology, Cooper University Hospital, Camden, New Jersey

Gerald J. Matthews, M.D., F.A.C.S.
Assistant Professor, Department of Urology, New York Medical College, Director of Male Reproductive Medicine, Westchester Medical Center, Valhalla, New York; Chief of Urology, Metropolitan Hospital Center, New York, New York; Chief of Urology, Our Lady of Mercy Medical Center, Bronx, New York

Craig S. Niederberger, M.D.
Associate Professor, Urology, University of Illinois at Chicago, University of Illinois at Chicago Hospital, Chicago, Illinois

Robert S. Oates, M.D.
Associate Professor of Urology, Urology, Boston Medical Center, Boston, Massachusetts

Dana Ohl, M.D.
Head, Division of Andrology and Microsurgery, Department of Urology, University of Michigan, Ann Arbor, Michigan

Kutluk Otkay, M.D.
Associate Professor of Reproductive Medicine, Obstetrics and Gynecology, Center for Reproductive Medicine and Infertility, Weill Medical College of Cornell University, New York; Director, Brooklyn Hospital, Brooklyn, New York

Gianpiero Palermo, M.D.
Center for Reproductive Medicine and Infertility, Weill Medical College of Cornell University, New York

Susanne A. Quallich, C.N.P., Cu.N.P.
Nurse Practitioner, Division of Andrology and Microsurgery, Department of Urology, University of Michigan, Ann Arbor, Michigan

G. Durga Rao, M.D., M.R.C.O.G
Fellow in Reproductive Endocrinology and Infertility, Obstetrics and Gynaecology, McGill University, Royal Victoria Hospital, Montreal, Quebec, Canada

Bernard Robaire, M.D.
James McGill Professor, Pharmacology Therapeutics and Obstetrics and Gynaecology, McGill University, Medical Scientist, McGill University Hospital Centre, Montreal, Quebec, Canada

Zev Rosenwaks, M.D.
Director, Center for Reproductive Medicine and Infertility; Professor of Obsetrics and Gyencology and Reproductive Medicine, Weill Medical College of Cornell University; Attending Physician, New York Presbyterian Hospital, New York, New York

Jay I. Sandlow, M.D.
Associate Professor, Urology, Medical College of Wisconsin, Froedtert Medical Center, Milwaukee, Wisconsin

Glenn L. Schattman, M.D., F.A.C.O.G.
Associate Professor, Reproductive Endocrinology and Infertility, Weill Medical College of Cornell University, New York Presbyterian Hospital, New York, New York

Peter N. Schlegel, M.D., F.A.C.S.
Chairman, Department of Urology, Weill Medical College of Cornell University, Urologist in Chief, New York Presbyterian Hospital, New York, New York

Yefim R. Sheynkin, M.D., F.A.C.S.
Associate Professor of Clinical Urology, Director, Male Infertility and Microsurgery, Department of Urology, State University of New York at Stony Brook, Stony Brook University Hospital, Stony Brook, New York

Jens Sonksen, M.D., Ph.D., D.M.Sc.
Head, Section of Male Infertility and Microsurgery, Department of Urology, University of Copenhagen, Herlev Hospital, Copenhagen, Denmark

Steven D. Spandorger, M.D.
Center for Reproductive Medicine and Infertility, Weill Medical College of Cornell University, New York

Robert J. Straub, M.D.
Reproductive Biology Associates, Northside Hospital, Atlanta, Georgia

Andrea Lynn Stuart, M.D.
Resident, Urology, University of Illinois at Chicago, University of Illinois Hospital, Chicago, Illinois

Seang Lin Tan, M.B.B.S., F.R.C.O.G., F.R.C.S.C., M.Med (O&G), M.B.A.
James Edmund Dodds Professor and Chairman, Obstetrics and Gynaecology, McGill University, Obstetrician and Gynaecologist in Chief, McGill University Health Centre, Montreal, Quebec, Canada

Togas Tulandi, M.D., F.R.C.S.C., F.A.C.O.G.
Professor of Obstetrics and Gynaecology, The Milton Leong Chair in Reproductive Medicine, McGill University, McGill University Health Centre and The Jewish General Hospital, Montreal, Quebec, Canada

Lucinda L. Veeck, M.L.T., hD.Sc.
Assistant Professor of Embryology in Obstetrics and Gynecology and Reproductive Medicine, Cornell Institute for Reproductive Medicine, Weill Medical College of Cornell University, New York, New York

Steven S. Witkin, Ph.D.
Professor, Obstetrics and Gynecology, Weill Medical College of Cornell University, New York, New York

Kangpu Xu, Ph.D.
Associate Professor, Center for Reproductive Medicine and Infertility, Weill Medical College of Cornell University, New York, New York

Armand Zini, M.D.
Associate Professor, Surgery, University of Toronto, Mount Sinai Hospital, Toronto, Ontario, Canada

PREFACE

The dramatic advances in reproductive medicine we have witnessed in recent years have allowed successful treatment of previously hopeless cases of male and female reproductive disorders. These advances are largely dependent on a multi-disciplinary approach involving reproductive endocrinologists, urologists, genetic counselors, embryologists, molecular geneticists, psychologists, reproductive nurses, ethicists and legal representatives. For this approach to be effective, besides a thorough knowledge of their own fields, team members must have a basic understanding of the other specialties. Effective information flow among multidisciplinary team members — a concept known as "knowledge translation" — is crucial to providing quality care to patients.

In preparing the *Reproductive Medicine Secrets,* we have gathered a multidisciplinary team of specialists — all of whom are authorities in their corresponding fields – to provide updated and concise "secrets" over a broad range of topics in Reproductive Medicine. This book is not intended to be comprehensive textbook on the subject. Rather, we have attempted to highlight the key concepts in each field.

In addition to providing healthcare professionals in practice an overview of patient management approaches of specialists from other disciplines, this book will serve as a practical introduction for medical students and residents-in-training to reproductive medicine.

Patients undergoing fertility evaluation or treatment tend to be young, educated and highly motivated to seek detailed information about the care/treatment they are to receive. Information in this book, which is presented in a question-and-answer format in an informal tone, provides a basic reference for them to improve their understanding of their fertility problems and the treatments involved.

Lastly, it is our hope that the materials presented here will provide a strong foundation for providing the highest quality of care to our patients.

Peter T.K. Chan, M.D.
Marc Goldstein, M.D.
Zev Rosenwaks, M.D.

ACKNOWLEDGEMENT

The editors would like to thank *A1 Intellectual Media* for providing original illustrations for many chapters in this book.

To all the couples
we are privileged to care for.

I. Evaluation of Male Reproductive Disorders

1. ANATOMY OF THE MALE REPRODUCTIVE SYSTEM

Peter T.K. Chan, M.D., and Louis Hermo, Ph.D.

1. What are the essential components of the male reproductive system?

The three essential components are (1) the testis, (2) the male excurrent ductal system, and (3) male accessory glands.

2. What composes the male excurrent ductal system?

The male excurrent ductal system consists of seminiferous tubules of the testis, the rete testis, efferent ductules, the epididymis (subdivided into distinct segments: the initial segment, caput, corpus, cauda), the convoluted and straight portions of the vas deferens (Fig. 1), the ampulla of the vas deferens, and the ejaculatory ducts.

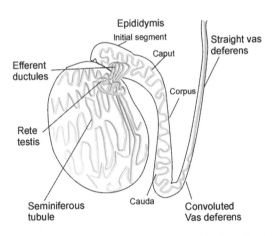

FIGURE 1. Part of the male excurrent ductal system: the testis, epididymis, and vas deferens.

3. What are the male accessory glands?

In addition to the testes, where sperm is produced, the accessory glands of the male reproductive tract contribute various components to the semen. Accessory glands include the seminal vesicles, prostate, and bulbourethral (Cowper's) glands. The semen consists of spermatozoa and secretions of the accessory glands.

4. Summarize the functions of the secretions of the male accessory glands.

In addition to serving as a lubrication or medium for transporting spermatozoa to the female reproductive tract, many of the biochemical components in seminal fluid from the male accessory glands have specific functional roles:

- The secretion of seminal vesicles allows the semen to coagulate, which may help maintain semen within the female reproductive tract.

1

- Prostate-specific antigen, a protease from the prostate, liquefies semen to allow passive flow and facilitate contact between the ovum and sperm.
- Fructose from the seminal vesicles provides the energy source for ejaculated sperm.
- In addition, various anti-oxidative enzymes (e.g., glutathione peroxidase, superoxide dismutase, and catalase) and anti-oxidative molecules (taurine, hypotaurine, and tyrosine) are present at high concentrations in semen to protect the spermatozoa from oxidative and free radical damage.

5. **Specify the embryonic origin of the various components of the male reproductive tract.**
- **Testis:** gonadal ridges (coelomic epithelium and underlying mesenchyme)
- **Germ cells:** primordial germ cells (endoderm) in the wall of the yolk sac along the dorsal mesentery (close to the allantois).
- **Seminiferous tubules:** primitive sex cords formed by proliferation of coelomic epithelium (toward the mesenchyme) on the gonadal ridges
- **Rete testis:** primitive sex cords formed by proliferation of coelomic epithelium (toward the mesenchyme) on the gonadal ridges
- **Efferent duct:** epigential tubules, which are remnants of the excretory tubules of the mesonephros
- **Appendix testis:** paramesonephric (müllerian) ductal remnants
- **Appendix epididymis:** mesonephric (wolffian) ductal remnantl
- **Epididymis:** mesonephric (wolffian) duct
- **Vas deferens:** mesonephric (wolffian) duct
- **Seminal vesicles:** distal outbudding of mesonephric (wolffian) ducts
- **Ejaculatory duct:** distal mesonephric (wolffian) duct
- **Prostate:** epithelium—outbudding of urethra (endoderm)
- **Prostatic utricle:** distal paramesonephric (mullerian) ductal remnants
- **Bulbourethral glands:** epithelium—outbudding of urethra (endoderm)
- **Paraurethral glands:** epithelium—outbudding of urethra (endoderm)

6. **What are the layers of tissues covering the testicles?**
From outside to inside:
- Scrotal skin
- Dartos muscle
- Colles' fascia (an extension of Scarpa's fascia)
- External spermatic fascia (an extension of external oblique aponeurosis)
- Cremasteric muscle (an extension of internal oblique muscle)
- Internal spermatic fascia (an extension of transversalis fascia)
- Parietal layer of tunica vaginalis (an extension of parietal peritoneum)
- Visceral layer of tunica vaginalis (an extension of visceral peritoneum)
- Tunica albuginea
- Innermost tunica vasculosa.

7. **Describe the arterial supply to the testis.** (Fig. 2)
    1. **Internal spermatic artery** (ISA), which arises directly from the abdominal aorta.
    2. **Deferential artery** (DA), which is derived either directly from the hypogastric (internal iliac) artery or the superior vesicle artery (also a branch of the hypogastric).
    3. **External spermatic/cremasteric artery** (CA), which is derived from the inferior epigastric artery.

8. **How are blood vessels distributed in the tunica albuginea of the testis?**
    With an imaginary equator on the testicle, arterial distribution in the tunica albuginea is denser in the upper anterior, lower anterior, lower lateral, and lower medial areas. In other words, there are fewer arteries on the upper medial and upper lateral surfaces, which are safer for inci-

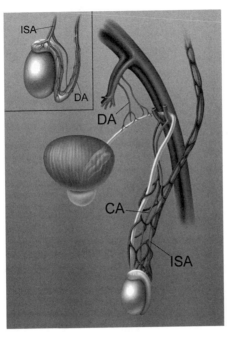

FIGURE 2. Arterial supply to part of the excurrent ductal system. CA = cremasteric artery, DA = deferential artery, ISA = internal spermatic artery. Inset: arterial supply to the epididymis (see question 37).

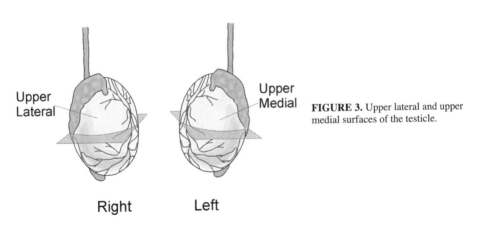

FIGURE 3. Upper lateral and upper medial surfaces of the testicle.

sion and suture placement (Fig. 3). However, because of individual variation, careful inspection, preferably with optical magnification if necessary, is crucial in the area where the incision is to be made to avoid damaging arteries.

9. Describe the venous drainage of the testis.

Venous drainage of the testis, consists of three major routes (Fig. 4):

1. **Internal spermatic veins,** which run within the internal spermatic fascia of the spermatic cord and drain into the internal gonadal veins.

2. **External spermatic and cremasteric veins,** which run outside the internal spermatic fascia.

3. **Deferential veins,** which run along the vasa deferentia within the spermatic cord.

Varicocele most commonly involves the internal spermatic veins, followed by cremasteric and external spermatic veins. The deferential veins rarely play a significant role in the development of varicoceles. Other minor venous drainage routes of the testis that may be of clinical significance in varicocele include the **gubernacular veins** (Fig. 5), which run toward the gubernaculum, an attachment from the inner scrotal wall to the inferior part of the testes. The gubernacular veins are completely outside the spermatic cord.

10. What are venae commitante?

Venae commitante (Latin for "accompanying veins") are small veins that "entangle" muscular arteries. The testicular arteries in the inguinal canal have venae commitante. The significance of the venae commitante is twofold:

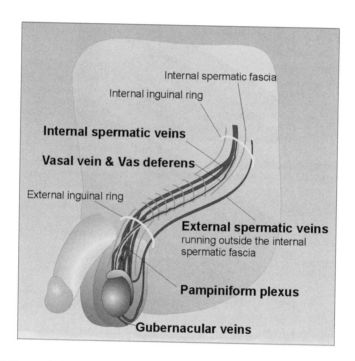

FIGURE 4. Three major routes of venous drainage of the testis.

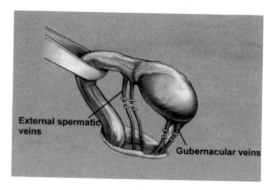

FIGURE 5. The gubernacular veins of the testis.

1. During varicocelectomy, the typical appearance of the side branches of veins (Fig. 6) helps facilitate the identification and preservation of testicular artery, which is directly below the venae commitante.

2. During varicocelectomy the venae commitante become dilated and serve as a venous drainage system, leading to recurrent varicoceles. Without the use of microsurgery, these venae are impossible to separate from the artery during procedures for ligation. Hence, in order to reduce the chance of varicocele recurrence, some surgeons ligate these veins along with the artery. Although this practice reduces the varicocele recurrent rate, it jeopardizes the arterial supply to the testis.

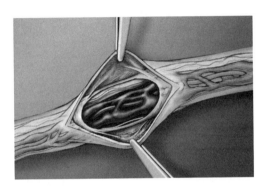

FIGURE 6. The side branches of the venae commitante facilitate identification of the testicular artery.

11. What is found within the testis parenchyma?

The testis parenchyma in humans is grossly divided into compartments or lobes separated by connective tissue septa. Within each lobe are seminiferous tubules and the interstitial tissue (Fig. 7). The seminiferous tubules consist of an epithelium containing differentiating germ cells and supporting Sertoli cells. In addition, smooth muscle-like cells called myoid cells envelop each tubule. These myoid cells contract and help move the sperm from the seminiferous tubular lumen into the lumen of the efferent ductules and hence epididymis. The interstitial tissue is comprised of Leydig cells, mast cells, fibrocytes, and macrophages as well as nerves and blood and lymphatic vessels. In humans, the interstitial tissue makes up 20–30% of the total testicular volume.

12. How many seminiferous tubules are found in each testis?

Anatomic studies have estimated that human males have approximately 600–1200 seminiferous tubules per testis.

13. How long is each seminiferous tubule?

Seminiferous tubules are arranged in a horizontal U-shaped orientation with their ends facing the mediastinum testis posteriorly, where they join into the rete testis. Each tubule has a stretched length of about 1 meter.

14. What are Leydig cells? Who was Leydig?

Leydig cells are interstitial cells of the testes. They contain masses of smooth endoplasmic reticulum and are involved in the production of testosterone. Leydig cells interact with macrophages of the interstitial space. The Leydig cells monitor macrophage numbers, and the macrophages affect testosterone production. Leydig cells are named after Franz von Leydig (1821–1908), a German zoologist and comparative anatomist.

15. What are Sertoli cells? Who was Sertoli?

Sertoli cells are stellate-shaped cells enveloping the germ cells of the seminiferous tubules. They are named after Enrico Sertoli (1842–1910), an Italian physiologist and histologist. Functions of the Sertoli cells include the following:

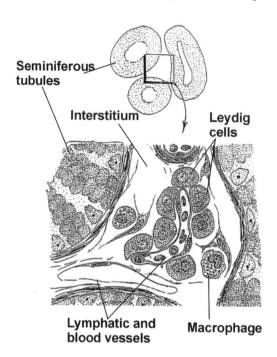

FIGURE 7. Contents of each lobe of the testis parenchyma.

- They support male germ cell development during spermatogenesis until spermatozoa are formed.
- They secrete numerous proteins that assist germ cell development, some of which also move into the lumen of the efferent ductules and epididymis, where they play important functions.
- They are active endocytic cells, taking up substances from the lumen as well as blood-borne substances arriving at the base of the epithelium.
- They form the blood-testis barrier. Adjacent Sertoli cells at the base of the epithelium contain tight junctions that prevent the entry of substances into the seminiferous tubular lumen.
- They move elongating spermatids at various levels of the epithelium, phagocytose residual bodies, and form adhesion sites with spermatids, referred to as the ectoplasmic specializations.

16. How many sperm are produced in humans on a daily basis?

It has been estimated that adult men produce from 27 million to 374 million sperm per day, with an average of 123 million.

17. Define spermatogenesis and spermiogenesis.

First described in rats by Leblond and Clermont in 1952 and then in humans by Clermont in 1963, **spermatogenesis** is defined as the complete series of events involving spermatogonia and their evolution into spermatozoa. It is the process of proliferation and differentiation of male germ cells within the testicular seminiferous tubules. This process involves (1) mitotic division of spermatogonia, (2) meiotic divisions of primary and secondary spermatocytes, and (3) metamorphosis of spermatids into spermatozoa.

Spermiogenesis, a subdivision of spermatogenesis, involves only the differentiation of spermatids into spermatozoa (see below).

18. At what age does spermatogenesis begin?

During infancy, the seminiferous epithelium consists of immature Sertoli cells and fetal spermatogonia. From age 4 onward, the pale (Ap) and dark (Ad) type A and B spermatogonia are evident. Primary spermatocytes appear at the beginning of puberty but undergo degeneration or progress to abnormal spermatids, which in turn degenerate, probably due to the lack of adequate testosterone and the lack of Sertoli cell functions. Thus active spermatogenesis begins only after puberty.

19. What hormone is required to initiate and maintain spermatogenesis?

Testosterone alone can initiate and maintain spermatogenesis. However, this process is only achieved qualitatively (i.e., with the presence of spermatozoa) and not quantitatively (i.e. the number of spermatozoa is below normal). Although follicle-stimulating hormone (FSH) is not required to initiate spermatogenesis in men with hypogonadotropic hypogonadism, optimal quantitative and qualitative spermatogenesis requires FSH in conjunction with the presence of testosterone.

20. What are the various germ cells?

From the least to the most differentiated (Fig. 8):

- Spermatogonia: dark type A spermatogonia (Ad), pale type A spermatogonia (Ap), type B spermatogonia (B)
- Primary spermatocytes: preleptotene (Pl), leptotene (L), zygotene (Z), pachytene (early [EP], middle [MP], late [LP])
- Secondary spermatocytes (II)
- Spermatids: early, round and late, elongated

21. How do germ cells propagate themselves?

The **pale type A** (Ap) spermatogonia divide to renew themselves and give rise to more differentiated cells. Thus, there is a constant supply of Ap spermatogonia. The Ap constitutes the renewing population of stem cells. The **dark type A** (Ad) spermatogonia do not appear to divide under normal conditions and act as a reserve population of stem cells. Such cells may become mitotically active after adverse conditions affect the testis.

22. What is a generation of germ cells?

A generation is a group of germ cells all at the same stage of development. In a given cross-sectional profile of a seminiferous tubule, 4–5 generations may be present, dependent on the stage of the cycle of the seminiferous epithelium. Although these generations evolve into one another with time, at any given moment the seminiferous epithelium appears to be identical, despite the fact that the different generations continue to evolve in the epithelium. An analogy can be drawn with a school. The class of each year contains a group of students at the same step of development. However, four generations of students are present at the school during any given year. When the fourth-year students eventually graduate, a new crop of students arrive in the first year to replace them. In this way, there are always four ongoing years, with students forming distinct groups at each year. In the seminiferous epithelium, despite the active mitosis and differentiation of germ cells and the eventual release of sperm, each tubular cross-section appears to be static, with either 4 or 5 generations of germ cells, dependent on the stage of the cycle.

23. What is a stage of the cycle of the seminiferous epithelium?

In any given cross-section of a seminiferous tubule, several generations of germ cells exist hand in hand with one another. Such a cellular association constitutes what is called a stage of the cycle of the seminiferous epithelium. At a given stage the various generations are constant, and one generation seen at a given stage never appears at a different stage. Thus, the cellular associations are constant for each stage. In addition, each stage has a fixed duration of time, after which the successive cellular association or stage appears in that given area of the tubule.

24. How many recognizable stages are involved in spermatogenesis?

Due to the complexity of the seminiferous epithelium, it has been noted that in humans six different cellular associations or stages can be defined. As the different generations of germ cells

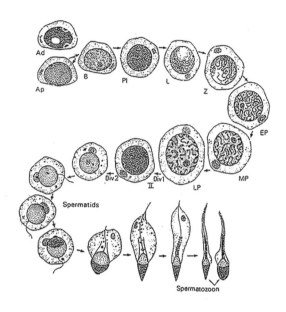

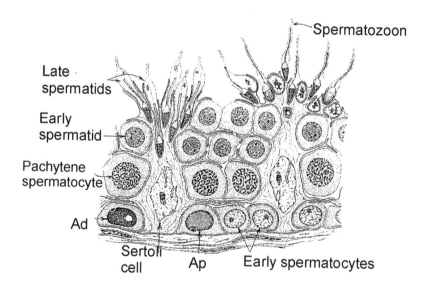

FIGURE 8. Types of germ cells.

become more mature, they change their location from the base of the seminiferous epithelium, where spermatogonia are present, to the lumen of the tubule, where maturing spermatids are predominant. At a given area of the seminiferous tubule, the composition of the specific generations of germ cells is typical for each stage of spermatogenesis. In addition, the six stages of spermatogenesis are cyclical; i.e., in a specific area of the seminiferous tubule, one stage evolves into the next until all six stages appear in that one given area of the tubule.

25. Which cell types constitute the six stages of spermatogenesis in humans?

Each stage of the cycle contains specific generations of germ cells. At all stages Sertoli cells are constantly present, but in adults these cells do not undergo mitosis. In addition, there are generations of spermatogonia, spermatocytes, and spermatids, according to their step of development. In the case of spermatids (Fig. 9):

Stage I is characterized by the presence of early, round spermatids and older, elongated spermatids.

Stage II is characterized by the presence of maturing spermatids prior to their release into the lumen.

Stage III includes only one generation of spermatids, with the mature spermatids having been released into the tubular lumen.

Stage IV is characterized by spermatids with nuclei showing the initial signs of elongation.

Stage V shows one generation of maturing, elongating spermatids.

Stage VI is characterized by the primary and secondary spermatocytes undergoing the first and second meiotic division and also by the presence of secondary spermatocytes at interphase.

26. Describe the cycle of the seminiferous epithelium. How long is it in humans?

The cycle is defined as the successive passage of the six stages in a given area of the seminiferous tubule. In other words, if we were to watch in a given area of a seminiferous tubule the successive progression of the various generations of germ cells beginning at stage I and how each generation evolved into stage II and them follow them through stages III, IV, V, and VI until we returned to the generations at stage I, we would have gone through all six stages. This progressive succession of the various generations of germ cells comprising the six stages in one given area of the seminiferous tubule is defined as the cycle of the seminiferous epithelium. In human, spermatogenesis, the process whereby a spermatogonium differentiates into spermatozoa is estimated to be approximately 64 days.

27. Which cells proliferate most rapidly?

Spermatogonia.

28. What cells undergo meiosis?

Primary and secondary spermatocytes.

29. Which germ cells are tetraploid (4n) in their nuclear genetic material?

Primary spermatocytes.

30. Which germ cells become haploid?

Spermatids.

31. When do mitosis and meiosis occur during spermatogenesis?

In addition to differentiation, spermatogonia undergo mitosis and give rise to more of their numbers. Spermatogonia differentiate into primary spermatocytes, with the chromsome number increasing from 2n (diploid) to 4n (tetraploid). At or shortly before puberty, primary spermatocytes begin to divide by meiosis, which consists of two divisions. During the first meiotic division, the primary spermatocytes become secondary spermatocyte with 2n number of chromosomes. During the second meiotic division, secondary spermatocytes divide into spermatids with 1n (haploid).

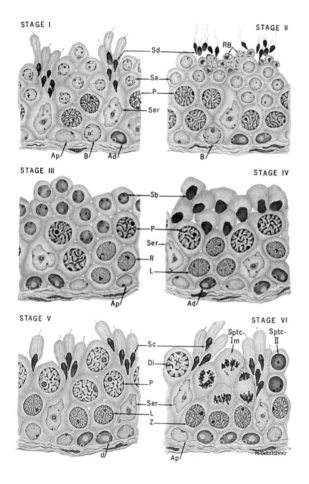

FIGURE 9. The six cellular associations or stages of spermatogenesis. Ser = Sertoli nuclei; Ap and Ad = pale and dark type A spermatognoia; B = type B spermatogonia; R = resting primary spermatocytes; L = leptotene primary spermatocytes; Z = zygotene primary spermatocytes; P = pachytene primary spermatocytes; Di == diplotene primary spermatocytes; Sa, Sb, Sc, Sd = spermatids at various steps of spermatogenesis; RB = residual bodies.

32. What events occur during spermiogenesis?

Spermiogenesis is the metamorphosis of round spermatids into elongating maturing sperm. No cell division occurs during spermiogenesis. In humans there are 12 steps of spermiogenesis. Various morphologic changes occur during spermiogenesis, such as extensive changes in nuclear shape, condensation of chromatin, loss of cytoplasm, and formation of the flagellum and acrosome.

33. In humans does more than one stage appear in a given tubular cross section?

In rodents, a given seminiferous tubule-cross section reveals cellular associations or stages at the same step of development (i.e., only one stage occupies a given cross-section). In humans, however, several stages appear in one given cross-sectional tubular profile. It has been suggested that an orderly sequence of stages occurs in oblique orientation, which implies a helical arrangement of the stages of the cycle in humans.

34. What are the various components of a spermatozoon? (Fig. 10).

Sperm head: The oval-shaped sperm head, measuring 4.5 μm in length and 3 μm in diameter in humans, contains a nucleus that is covered by a membrane-bound organelle called the **acrosome.** The acrosome contains various enzymes allowing sperm to penetrate the zona pellucida and eventually bind to the ovum to initiate fertilization.

Sperm tail: The sperm head, via the connecting piece, is attached to the middle piece of the tail, which consists of a long segment of helically arranged mitochondria surrounding a set of cy-

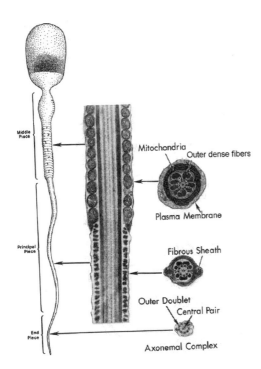

Mitochondria
Outer dense fibers

Plasma Membrane

Fibrous Sheath

Outer Doublet
Central Pair

Axonemal Complex

Figure 10. The components of a spermatozoon.

toskeletal elements called the **outer dense fibers** (9 in number). In the center of the tail is the **axoneme**, which consists of the characteristic $9+2$ microtubular doublets. The middle piece is connected to the principal piece of the sperm tail. The principal piece is covered by another cytoskeleton called **fibrous sheath,** replacing two of the outer dense fibers. Thus seven outer dense fibers and the axoneme are present in the principal piece. The principal piece of the tail is connected to the very last part of the tail called the **end-piece.** At that level, the outer dense fibers terminate, leaving the axoneme as the primary structure.

   Plasma membrane: With the exception of the end-piece of the tail, the entire sperm is covered by a highly specialized plasma membrane that regulates the transmembrane movement of ions and other molecules. In addition, various proteins on the plasma membrane, especially those at the areas covering the sperm head, are undergoing modification during sperm maturation. Many of these proteins have a role in zona pellucida interaction during fertilization.

35. Explain the function of the rete testis and efferent ducts.

   The **rete testis** is an anastomotic network lined by a cuboidal epithelium that serves to endocytose proteins from the lumen. From the rete testis arise the 6–12 ductuli efferentes (efferent ductules), which act as conduits to carry testicular fluid and spermatozoa into the initial segment of the epididymis.

   The **efferent ducts** are lined by a columnar epithelium where ciliated and nonciliated cells form the epithelium. Major functions of the efferent ducts are to endocytose proteins from the lumen in addition to transporting water from the lumen into the interstitial space. The latter serves to concentrate sperm in the initial segment of the epididymis, which has the narrowest luminal diameter of the entire duct. In this way, sperm can have more effective interactions with the secretory products of the epithelial cells lining this segment of the duct, as they pursue their quest for maturation. Estrogens regulate several functions of the efferent ducts, such as water removal.

36. List the major functions of the epididymis.

   1. Storage of spermatozoa. On average, 150–200 million spermatozoa are stored in each epi-

didymis, with approximately one-fourth in the caput, one-fourth in the corpus, and the remaining one-half in the cauda epididymidis.

2. Transport of sperm through the epididymis. Myoid cells envelop the epididymal tubules, which contract to move sperm through the duct.

3. Protection of sperm. The epithelial cells produce various anti-oxidants that serve to remove harmful free radicals and electrophiles.

4. Secretion of proteins and ions into the lumen, endocytosis of proteins from the lumen, and maintenance of water balance in the lumen.

5. Sperm maturation. Motility and fertilizing capabilities of sperm are acquired during their epididymal transit due to interactions of the secretory products of the epididymal epithelial cells with the sperm surface.

6. Many epididymal functions are regulated by dihydrotestosterone, although testicular factors emanating from the lumen of the seminiferous tubules also appear to regulate some epididymal functions.

37. Describe the arterial supply to the epididymis.

At the caput epididymidis, the main arterial supply is derived from the testicular artery. At the cauda epididymidis, arterial supply is derived from the deferential arteries along the vas deferens (see Fig. 2 inset). The arteries from the caput and cauda epididymidis form anastomotic collateral networks in the corpus epididymidis.

38. How long is the epididymal tubule in human?

In humans, the epididymal tubule is estimated to be 3–5 meters in length. The 6–12 efferent ductules coalesce to form a single epididymal tubule, which is coiled and encapsulated within the epididymal tunica. Since the epididymis is composed of a single tubule, injury or obstruction at any point of the tubule will render the entire organ obstructed.

39. What is the luminal size of the epididymis?

The epididymal lumen is variable in size, depending on the segment of the epididymis. In the initial segment the diameter is smallest, whereas in the cauda epididymidis it is the largest ($> 300\ \mu$m)

40. How long does it take for sperm to transport through the epididymis in human?

Approximately 1 week. Although this transit time is independent of a man's age, it is shorter in men with high daily sperm production than in men with low daily sperm production. In addition, transit through the caudal segment of the epididymis, which usually accounts for half the transit time, is reduced significantly by frequent ejaculations. In the absence of ejaculation, spermatozoa are retained in the cauda epididymidis, where they may remain viable for weeks.

41. What is the proportion of motile sperm in the various segments of the epididymis?

Efferent ductules	0%
Caput	3%
Proximal corpus	12%
Distal corpus	30%
Cauda	60%.

42. Where do unejaculated sperm go?

Evidence suggests that in vasectomized men macrophages gain access to the epididymal lumen and, along with macrophages in the vasal ampullary region, phagocytose unejaculated sperm.

43. What is peculiar in the anatomic details of the vas deferens?

The length of the human vas is 30–35 cm. Histologically, the vas has (1) an outer adventitial connective tissue sheet containing blood vessels and a rich network of autonomic (mainly sympathetic adrenergic) nerve fibers; (2) a thick trilayer muscularis with an outer and inner layer of longitudinal muscle sandwiching a middle circular muscle; and (3) an innermost mucosal layer lining a lumen of 500 μm in diameter. The vas is the only tubular structure in the human body in which the thickness of the wall exceeds the luminal diameter.

44. Describe the blood supply for the vas.

The deferential artery, originating from the inferior vesicle artery, is the main arterial supply to the proximal portion of the vas. In addition, the inferior epididymal artery, derived from the testicular artery, supplies the distal portion of the vas.

45. What is the function of the vas?

The vas appears to be more than a passive conduit for sperm. Adrenergic stimulation of the thick vasal muscularis can facilitate seminal emission. The vas can act as a reservoir of sperm by storing approximately 130 million spermatozoa. In addition, the epithelial cells of the vasal mucosal are known to be active in secretion of various glycoproteins and ions, removal of water, and phagocytosis of old spermatozoa.

46. What are the residual body and cytoplasmic droplet?

The **residual body** is the detached cytoplasm of sperm prior to their release into the seminiferous tubular lumen (Fig. 11). It contains mitochondria not used in tail formation, endoplasmic reticulum, ribosomes and membranous profiles. The Sertoli cells phagocytose the residual body.

At the time of sperm release (spermiation), not all of the cytoplasmic organelles of the sperm will enter the residual body. A small bulge of cytoplasm will remain at the connecting piece of the tail, called the **cytoplasmic droplet.** Containing Golgi saccular elements, the droplet moves along the tail's middle piece and eventually is shed from the sperm as they descend the epididymis. The Golgi saccules of the droplet appear to modify the sperm's plasma membrane during epididymal transit and may play a role in sperm maturation.

47. In a mature spermatozoon, what is in the cytoplasm?

Other than cytoskeletal elements in the tail, upon shredding of cytoplasmic droplet, the cytoplasm of sperm contains no loose organelles such as endoplasmic reticulum, mitochrondria, or ribosomes. During fertilization, the human sperm contributes only the male genome (from the nu-

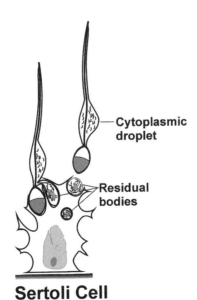

Cytoplasmic droplet

Residual bodies

Sertoli Cell

FIGURE 11. The residual body of sperm.

cleus) and the sperm centrosome, which is in the connecting piece of the sperm tail. The centrosome contributes to the formation of microtubules that are essential for pronuclear movement and thus for mitotic division of the embryo.

ACKNOWLEDGMENT

The authors thank Dr. Yves Clermont for kindly providing Figures 7, 8, 9, and 10.

BIBLIOGRAPHY

1. Amann RP, Howards SS: Daily spermatozoal production and epididymal spermatozoal reserves of the human male. J Urol 124:211–215, 1980.
2. Chan P: The cytoplasmic droplets of rat epididymal spermatozoa show diminution of glycosyl transferases during spermatozoa epididymal maturation. McGill J Med 1:13–31, 1995.
3. Clermont Y: The cycle of the seminiferous epithelium in man. Am J Anat 112:35–51, 1963.
4. Clermont Y: Renewal of spermatogonia in man. Am J Anat 118:509–524, 1966.
5. Leblond CP, Clermont Y: Definition of the stages of the cycle of the seminiferous epithelium in the rat. Ann N Y Acad Sci 55:548–573, 1952.
6. Oko R, Hermo L, Chan P, et al: The cytoplasmic droplet of rat epididymal spermatozoa contains saccular elements with Golgi characteristics. J Cell Biol 123:809–821, 1993.
7. Roosen-Runge ED, Holstein AF: The human rete testis. Cell Tissue Res 189:409–433, 1978.
8. Sertoli E: Dell'esistenza di particolari cellule ramificate nei canalicoli seminiferi del testicolo umano. Morgagni 7:31–40, 1865.
9. Setchell BP, Brooks DE: Anatomy, vasculature, innervation and fluids of the male reproductive tract. In Knobil E, Neill JD (eds): The Physiology of Reproduction, 2nd ed. New York, Raven Press, 1988, pp 753–836.
10. von Leydig F: Zur Anatomie der männlichen Geschlechtsorgane und Analdrüsen der Säugethiere. Zeitschrift für wissenschaftliche Zoologie. 2:1–57, 1850.

2. PHYSIOLOGY OF THE TESTIS AND EPIDIDYMIS

Bernard Robaire, M.D., and Matthew P. Hardy, M.D.

1. What is the normal range of serum total testosterone?

A wide range of serum total testosterone levels are considered "normal." In most centers in North America, the normal range is 10–38 nmol/L (S.I. unit) or 300–1100 ng/dl (conventional unit).

2. If the serum concentration of total testosterone is more than 10-fold above the dissociation constant of the androgen receptor, are the majority of androgen receptors constantly bound to testosterone?

The concentration of testosterone that is freely available to bind to the androgen receptor is typically lower (2–3% of total) than the total testosterone concentration in biologic fluids, including the seminiferous tubular fluid. Free testosterone levels in the testis may be close to the dissociation constant of the androgen receptor.

3. To what does testosterone bind when it is in the circulation?

Circulating testosterone is bound with various proteins. Approximately 55% of testosterone is bound to high-affinity testosterone-estradiol binding globulin (TEBG) (also known as sex hormone binding globulin [SHBG]). Approximately 40% is bound with low affinity to albumin.

4. What is bioavailable testosterone?

Bioavailable testosterone refers to the portion of testosterone that is either free (2–3%) or bound with low affinity to albumin (about 40%). The portion of the total testosterone that is bound with high affinity to SHBG is not considered bioavailable.

5. What is andropause?

With advancing age, a decrease in serum bioavailable testosterone leads to diminished muscle tone and libido along with a spectrum of clinical symptoms and signs collectively known as "andropause." Although sperm numbers do not change dramatically with advancing age, sperm quality declines, resulting in decreased fertility and possibly an increased incidence of genetic abnormalities in progeny. If andropause is defined as the cessation of androgen action, analogous to the definition of menopause as the cessation of menses, this condition clearly does not exist. However, partial androgen deficiency in the aging male (PADAM) is now recognized as a condition affecting a large proportion of aging men. Whether it should be treated with replacement therapy is currently highly controversial.

6. For aging men with androgen deficiency, what problems might arise from supplementing testosterone concentrations to maintain youthful testosterone levels?

The major concern in prescribing supplemental testosterone to older men is the potential for increased risk of benign prostatic hyperplasia and/or prostate cancer. Although testosterone has never been shown directly to cause prostate diseases, it is clear that it plays a permissive role for both conditions. Whether prolonged exposure of the prostate throughout aging to the higher levels of androgen found in younger men results in an increased risk of prostate disease has yet to be established. Of lesser concern are other side effects, such as polycythemia, sleep apnea, skin rashes associated with topical application of androgen in gel formulations and patches, and possible occurrences of acne.

7. The testis is a major site of androgen action. What specific androgen receptor-mediated changes in gene expression have been identified?

Androgen receptors are expressed in Leydig cells, peritubular myoid cells, and Sertoli cells. Very few genes that are transcriptionally regulated by androgen have been identified to date. Among them are PEM, a homeodomain protein expressed by Sertoli cells that is upregulated by androgen, and 17α-hydroxylase/lyase enzyme, which is expressed in the Leydig cells and is downregulated by androgen. Androgen action on Sertoli cells and peritubular myoid cells is expected because spermatogenesis is critically dependent on stimulation by androgen. Leydig cells secrete testosterone and a short-loop negative feedback effect of androgen may be one means of controlling intratesticular testosterone concentrations.

8. Virilization of the urogenital sinus and external genitalia involves further increase in the androgenic potency of testosterone. Which anatomic structures are involved? Describe the biochemical mechanism of the increase in testosterone potency.

Androgen action is mediated by androgen receptors that bind to testosterone and its metabolites with different affinities. The 5α-reduced metabolite of testosterone, dihydrotestosterone (DHT), has a comparatively higher affinity for the receptor and, therefore, a higher potency. DHT is synthesized from testosterone by 5α-reductase, which is abundantly expressed in the prostate. Portions of the urogenital sinus give rise to the prostate, whereas other wolffian duct derivatives, such as the vas deferens, epididymides, and seminal vesicles, lack 5α-reductase expression during embryonic development. The differentiation of wolffian-derived tissues is controlled by testosterone.

9. What is Sry?

Also known as the sex determining region of the Y chromosome, Sry is a gene locus on the Y chromosome that encodes müllerian-inhibiting substance (MIS).

10. Early in the development of the male embryo, at the indifferent gonad stage, the müllerian ducts, anlagen of the female reproductive system, are present but fail to develop. Why?

These structures atrophy in response to MIS.

11. By the same token, anlagen of the male reproductive tract (wolffian) are present in female embryos at the indifferent gonad stage. Why do these structures fail to develop further in female embryos?

The wolffian ducts require exposure to testosterone for the male reproductive tract to form.

12. In the early development of a male embryo, both Sry and testosterone are involved in differentiation of the male body plan. Which acts first?

Sry acts first, inducing MIS, which then suppresses development of müllerian ducts. Sry also elicits expression of steroidogenic factor-1, a nuclear transcription factor critical for onset of steroidogenesis and Leydig cell development. Testosterone is subsequently involved in the development of the wolffian duct system forming the male reproductive tract.

13. True or false: Anatomic remnants of the müllerian ducts are present in males after birth.

True. The appendix testis is a remnant of the müllerian duct.

14. Which hormones of the hypothalamic-pituitary-testicular axis are secreted in an episodic/pulsatile manner? What are the clinical implications of this method of secretion?

At all three levels of the hypothalamic-pituitary-testicular axis hormones are secreted in a pulsatile manner. Thus, gonadotropin-releasing hormone (GnRH), luteinizing hormone (LH), and testosterone are secreted episodically, and the serum profiles of LH and testosterone show a clear episodic pattern. Consequently, when a single blood sample is drawn, the resulting serum hormone concentrations can lie anywhere between the peak and the trough of the pulse. Most labs have wide ranges of values for what is considered "normal" for these two hormones. Ideally, although it may not always be practical, a more accurate way to obtain a "truer" reflection of serum hormones is to take three samples, 20 minutes apart, and assay the samples either individually or as a pooled sample.

15. Why is testosterone considered a prohormone?

Although testosterone can act on its own by binding to the androgen receptor, it is considered to be a prohormone because at least two of its metabolites have hormonal activities that are more potent than those of the parent compound. Testosterone is converted to dihydrotestosterone (DHT) by one of the two isoforms of 5α-reductase; DHT binds with greater affinity to the androgen receptor than does testosterone. Testosterone can also be converted to 17β-estradiol by the enzyme cytochrome P450 aromatase.

16. Other than testosterone, what other molecules have been shown to play a role in intragonadal communication?

A wide range of molecules have been shown to be present in the testis and postulated to play a role as intragonadal messengers, including estradiol, GnRH-like peptide, PModS, insulinlike growth factor 1 (IGF1), transforming growth factor alpha (TGFα), and oxytocin. However, the specific roles of most of these molecules remain elusive. Obtaining information about their specific functions may provide important leads for the development of male contraceptives or treating certain types of male infertility.

17. How does the role of follicle-stimulating hormone (FSH) differ in the initiation and maintenance of spermatogenesis?

The role of FSH in the *initiation* of spermatogenesis is well established: it induces development of the spermatogonia and growth in pre-Sertoli cells. Sertoli cells retain receptors for FSH during adulthood. The role of FSH in spermatogenesis *maintenance* is not fully understood but may involve preventing spermatogenetic arrest.

18. What is the nature of the effects of anabolic steroids on muscle? When taken by male athletes, do these compounds have potential consequences for the reproductive system?

Testosterone and other anabolic steroids increase muscle mass by stimulating cell growth and differentiation (hypertrophy) but not proliferation (hyperplasia). Testosterone acts as the active androgen in this tissue due to the absence of 5α-reductase activity. Because of the negative feedback effects of androgen, administration of anabolic steroids suppresses pituitary release of gonadotrophin, mainly LH, and thereby inhibits secretion of testosterone in the testes. The result is a reduction in spermatogenesis (smaller, flaccid testes) and a potential reduction in fertility.

19. Do estrogens normally play a role in male reproductive physiology?

Yes. Studies of estrogen receptor alpha and aromatase knockout mice (ERαKO and ArKO, respectively) have revealed effects of estrogen on the male reproductive system. Adult males that are deficient in estrogen action eventually become sterile. This effect is thought to result from abnormal fluid reuptake in the rete testis, which leads to back pressure atrophy on the seminiferous epithelium. Estrogen receptors are also localized elsewhere in the male tract, including the testis, epididymis, and prostate. ArKO mice have impaired sexual behaviour and an age-dependent disruption of spermatogenesis. This spermatogenic diruption block occurs during early spermiogenesis and is likely due to increased number of apoptotic round spermatids.

20. How does testosterone, a lipophilic molecule, get out of Leydig cells?

Testosterone is not packaged into vesicles, nor is there an active transport carrier to take it out of Leydig cells. Testosterone leaves Leydig cells by a process of facilitated passive transport. Although the exact mechanism has not been fully resolved, it appears that testosterone and other lipophilic steroids exit the Leydig cell down a concentration gradient across cell membranes into the blood stream, lymphatics, and seminiferous tubule fluid, where both high affinity-low capacity proteins (SHBG/ABP) and low affinity-high capacity proteins (albumin) bind androgens and carry them away from Leydig cells.

21. Which cells make inhibin? What hormone controls its synthesis? Describe the limitations of trying to administer inhibin as a male contraceptive.

Sertoli cells synthesize and secrete inhibin, a protein made up of two subunits, in response to FSH. The secretion of inhibin is regulated by a negative feedback mechanism. Although FSH plays a role in supporting spermatogenesis, overproduction of inhibin does not cause a complete arrest of spermatogenesis, and, in most animal models, fertility can be maintained when FSH is ablated. Hence, although attractive, this approach to male contraception has not been fruitful.

22. What is the blood-testis barrier?

It has been observed that many substances injected into the blood stream rapidly appear in the testicular lymph but not in rete testis fluid. This observation led to the concept of a "blood-testis barrier." The blood-testis barrier is made by projections from adjacent Sertoli cells and is highly selective in creating an intraluminal environment necessary for spermatogenesis.

23. How can spermatocytes migrate from the basal to the adluminal compartments of the seminiferous tubules when small organic molecules and proteins are excluded?

The blood-testis barrier is not a static but a highly dynamic structure. Spermatocytes are moved by Sertoli cells upward from the basal to the adluminal compartment. Sertoli cells form new projections below the rising spermatocytes and break the ones above. This process is analogous to a zipper effect.

24. What is the outlook for future male contraceptives?

An ideal male contraceptive has been sought for over 35 years. Some hormonal methods have been developed most extensively and are expected to reach the state of commercialization. However, even though these hormonal methods are effective, they are unlikely to provide instant birth control.

Spermatogenesis is a staggered cyclic process that, once initiated, does not end. It is a process that continues throughout adulthood unless a chemical or physical insult alters production of hormones responsible for spermatogenesis. In men, spermatogenesis takes 64 days and epididymal transit takes up to 1 week. The hormonal methods that have been developed most extensively suppress androgen production, causing a termination of the initiation of spermatogenesis within days, but the sperm that have been initiated usually complete their differentiation. Once sperm are formed in the testes, they are released into the epididymis, where they are matured and stored. Therefore, over 2 months must pass to be sure that stored sperm are cleared from the epididymal stores.

25. How do intratesticular and blood serum concentrations of testosterone differ? Can we take advantage of this difference for developing male contraceptives? How?

In men, the intratesticular concentration of testosterone is approximately 100-fold greater than that in the circulation. By giving exogenous testosterone at a dose that results in maintaining serum testosterone (after an initial spike), it is possible to dramatically reduce serum LH via negative feedback, leading to a decline in endogenous production of intratesticular testosterone. This decline, in turn, can result in a partial or complete arrest of spermatogenesis, since the intratesticular concentration necessary to maintain normal spermatogenesis is higher (about 10-fold) than that found in the circulation.

26. If a drug were to selectively block the initiation of spermatogenesis (first spermatogonial division), how long would it take before a man would become infertile?

Even if the initiation of spermatogenesis is stopped immediately, one assumes that the cells that have already started will complete the process and undergo maturation. Clermont and

Heller have shown that this process takes 70 days in humans (64 days spermatogenesis and about 1 week for epididymal transit). Thus, after the initiation of the drug, infertility is not achieved until azoospermia is demonstrated twice, or at least 20–25 ejaculations and the passage of 3 months.

27. After vasectomy, the rate of spermatogenesis is not significantly affected. What happens to these sperm?

In some species, such as the rat, sperm are retained within the male reproductive tract and granulomas are formed after vasectomy. The size of these granulomas is proportional to the time since vasectomy. In men, the fate of all of these sperm has not yet been resolved totally, although the above mechanism may be involved in their elimination. In addition, macrophage phagocytosis of aged sperm occurs in the epididymal lumen. The positive pressure in the excurrent ductal lumen can cause a disruption of the blood-epididymis/vas deferens barrier. This disruption results in the release of sperm or sperm antigens into the extratesticular compartment, and an immune response ensues. Since sperm are viewed by the body as foreign cells, formation of antisperm antibodies will occur after vasectomy.

28. Do any drugs accelerate or slow the process of spermatogenesis?

No. Many drugs partially or completely block spermatogenesis, but the complex process of spermatogenesis cannot be made to proceed at different rates.

29. Is frequency of ejaculation associated with altered rates of spermatogenesis?

No. The rate of spermatogenesis is constant and proceeds independently of the rate of ejaculation. The number of spermatozoa in the first part of the epididymis (head or caput) is also constant over time; however the number of sperm in the tail (cauda) of the epididymis, where sperm are stored, is highly variable with the frequency of ejaculation.

30. What are the advantages and disadvantages of using spermatogonia as stem-cell agents for gene therapy?

The most obvious advantage is that this process would ensure incorporation of the inserted gene into the germ line and subsequent transmittal to progeny. Another positive aspect is that germ-cell nuclei are highly competent to initiate and sustain embryonic development, relative to those of somatic cells. Under this scenario, men with heritable diseases, once treated with gene therapy, would be able to father healthy children. Methodologically, the testes of the affected male could provide the source of the spermatogonia, which could then be amplified in number by culture in vitro. Germ cells remaining in the testes would then be removed by irradiation and/or chemical treatment. After insertion of the normal gene, the corrected spermatogonia would be injected into the testes to recolonize the denuded seminiferous epithelium. Many barriers to the realization of this technical feat exist, however. To date, it has proved difficult to maintain long-term cultures of spermatogonia, setting back efforts to obtain cell fractions in which the gene is stably incorporated. There are also problems with preparing the testis for reception of altered spermatogonia, including permanent sterility and Leydig cell tumors.

31. True or false: Rat spermatogonia can colonize the mouse seminiferous epithelium, resulting in complete rat spermatogenesis.

True. The drive for the formation of a species-specific germ cell lies in the germ cell itself and not in the environment that nourishes it.

32. How may it be possible to produce sperm heterospecifically without provoking an immune response?

The germ cells would have to be placed in an immuno-privileged site such as the testis, which is separated by the blood-testis barrier from the immune cells that would otherwise recognize and destroy germ cells. The barrier is formed by tight junctions between Sertoli cells and prevents the cells on opposite sides of the barrier from coming into contact.

33. Since spermatozoa synthesize proteins that are seen to be different from self, can we take advantage of this fact for developing antisperm vaccines as a male contraceptive?

An immunocontraceptive, typically based on a vaccine that would induce antisperm antibodies (preventing sperm motility or sperm-egg binding), has been a topic of intensive research. To date, however, no promising products are based on this approach. Although immunocontraception has the obvious advantage of specifically targeting sperm antigens, there are many hurdles to product development. First, there is no guarantee that the binding between the antibodies to sperm can result in a contraceptive effect, because the proposed methods usually call for the antibodies to interfere with fertilization in the female tract. In the male, the antigenic load is high due to the presence of a large quantity of sperm and individual immune responses are variable. The access of the antibodies to the seminiferous tubules, due to the presence of the blood-testis barrier, and epididymal lumen is highly restricted for immunoglobulins. Moreover, there is the risk of inducing autoimmune orchitis. Therefore, the focus has been on immunocontraceptive development for women, in large part because of the smaller antigenic burden. Clinical trials using this approach have not resulted in a greater than 70% effectiveness.

34. In which stages of spermatogenesis are sperm particularly sensitive to damage by drugs and environmental chemicals?

During mitosis and meiosis, drugs that affect cell division (e.g., anticancer drugs) often target dividing sperm. Drugs that block androgen action act either on the initiation of spermatogenesis or at the time germ cells are released (spermiation). Drugs that cause alkylation or other damage to chromatin often are seen to target more selectively germ cells that have completed their divisions and are in the process of differentiation (spermiogenesis). The reason is that germ cells lose the enzyme machinery involved in DNA repair as they undergo nuclear condensation.

35. Is intracyctoplasmic sperm injection (ICSI) a cure for male infertility? Does it completely replicate the natural process of fertilization?

No. ICSI simply bypasses the normal fertilization process. The consequences of such a bypass are still not clear. With ICSI, the membrane fusion events associated with natural fertilization do not occur. After ICSI, the sperm acrosome and perinuclear structures are retained. In contrast, during normal fertilization these structures are typically removed at the oolemma. This process may affect sperm decondensation, although, assuming that it does, whether this effect has developmental implications has not been established.

36. Would a genetic predisposition to male factor infertility be more or less probable in male progeny of pregnancies resulting from ICSI?

The likelihood for inheriting a predisposition would be higher in the event that the father has a fertility problem.

37. In humans there are 23 paired chromosomes (22 pairs of autosomes and 1 pair of sex chromosomes). Unlike the 22 autosome pairs, the sex chromosomes are unequal in size, with the Y chromosome being smaller. How did evolution of the sex chromosomes produce a smaller Y chromosome?

The Y chromosome has lost more than 1,000 genes in the course of its evolution. It is thought that when sex chromosomes synapse to form bivalents during prophase I of meiosis, the proto-Y, due to differences in size and configuration, did not recombine with the X to the same extent as the somatic chromosome bivalents. Instead, cross-over events occurred internally along the arms of the Y chromosome, resulting in the progressive and permanent loss of DNA throughout evolution.

38. Does microgravity (i.e., weightlessness) have an effect on male reproductive function?

No adverse consequences have been observed for male fertility, but zero gravity does lower circulating testosterone levels. It is unclear whether this finding is a mild stressor effect or due to changes in temperature and/or blood flow.

39. Why is the temperature of the testis generally a few degrees below core body temperature? What are the potential consequences of hot baths, tight underwear, and protracted driving times (e.g., truck drivers)?

In most mammals, core temperature is 3–6 °C higher than scrotal temperature. Bringing testes to core temperature causes an arrest of spermatogenesis during meiotic division. The higher core body temperature damages germ cells and results in vacuolation of the seminiferous tubule. The heat shock protein 90 is normally expressed at high levels in the testis and prevents necrosis but, with higher temperatures, the defense mechanism is overcome and germ cells die. Frequent hot baths, tight underwear, and protracted driving can cause a smaller sperm count and increase frequency of abnormal sperm morphology.

40. Are there animal species in which the temperatures of the testes and core body do not differ? How is this explained in light of the answer to question 39?

There are instances of warm-blooded animals with internal testes. Cetaceans (whales and dolphins) have internal testes but have evolved a vascular heat exchanger system that cools the arterial blood leading into the testes through close contact with venous blood returning from the fins. In birds, however, the testes appear to be at core body temperature. Birds are able to counteract the deleterious effect of temperature on spermatogenesis by having a higher expression of heat shock proteins in germ cells than that found in mammalian species.

41. What changes take place in a sperm nucleus to allow the haploid chromatin to be packaged at least six times more tightly than that of somatic cells?

In sperm nuclei, the group of histone proteins that lie within the DNA grooves of the double helix are replaced by transition proteins that are highly basic and cysteine-rich. These transition proteins are called protamines. They form large numbers of disulfide protein-protein bonds that result in tightly packaged, highly stable chromatin.

42. How does human sperm production compare with other species?

Men produces fewer sperm on a gram-testis basis and sperm of worse quality (motility and morphology) than nearly any other species. This finding may be in part due to the fact that the normal mechanisms for regulating decreased testicular and epididymal temperature are circumvented in men in two ways: standing erect (often sitting down) and wearing clothes. Mild increases in scrotal temperature are associated with lower sperm count, decreased motility, and an increased incidence of abnormal sperm.

43. When released from seminiferous tubules, spermatozoa do not have the ability to swim or fertilize eggs. Where are these functions acquired?

Spermatozoa acquire motility and the ability to fertilize eggs in the epididymis.

44. What are the major structural and biochemical changes that take place in spermatozoa during this epididymal maturation process?

During epididymal sperm maturation, a few structural changes occur: loss of the cytoplasmic droplet, reshaping of the acrosome, increased cross-linking of chromatin, and change in the membrane surface charge. In addition, the sperm plasma membrane undergoes major changes in protein and lipid composition. Among the changes are addition and subtraction of sperm-surface antigens, sperm-surface carbohydrates, and lipid content. The appearance of surface proteins that can recognize egg elements probably results from the addition of proteins secreted by the epididymal epithelium.

45. What is sperm capacitation?

Unlike sperm maturation, which takes place over several days in the epididymis, sperm capacitation is completed in most mammals in only minutes to hours and normally takes place in the female reproductive tract (uterus and Fallopian tubes). Capacitation consists of a series of biochemical transformations that spermatozoa undergo after entering the female reproductive tract. The triggering event for capacitation appears to be an increase in intracellular calcium that results in increased production of cyclic adenosine monophosphate (cAMP). In addition, several changes in membrane proteins and lipids cause reorientation of sperm membrane elements to allow them to interact with the zona pellucida.

46. What is the sperm acrosomal reaction?

The binding of capacitated sperm to the zona pellucida causes further activation of cAMP/PKA and protein kinase C, which leads to a depletion of calcium in the acrosome resulting in membrane fusion and the acrosome reaction. The acrosome reaction is an exocytotic event that involves the rupture of the acrosomal membrane and the release of several enzymes that cleave proteins and sugars in the layers surrounding the oocyte enabling sperm to penetrate.

BIBLIOGRAPHY

1. Anwalt BD, Merriam GR: Neuroendocrine aging in men. Andropause and somatopause. Endocrinol Metab Clin North Am 30:647–669, 2001.
2. Bonde JP, Storgaard L: How work-place conditions, environmental toxicants and lifestyle affect male reproductive function. Int J Androl 25:262–268, 2002.
3. Brinster RL: Germline stem cell transplantation and transgenesis. Science 296:2174–2176, 2002.
4. Heinlein CA, Chang C: Androgen receptor (AR) coregulators: an overview. Endocr Rev 23:175–200, 2002.
5. Jarow JP, Chen H, Rosner TW, et al: Assessment of the androgen environment within the human testis: minimally invasive method to obtain intratesticular fluid. J Androl 22:640–645, 2001.
6. Muyata Y, Robertson KM, Jones ME, Simpson ER: Effect of estrogen deficiency in the male: the ArKO mouse model. Mol Cell Endocrinol 193:7–12, 2002.
7. Owaga T, Ohmura M, Yumura Y, et al: Expansion of murine spermatogonial stem cells through serial transplantation. Biol Reprod 68:316–322, 2003.
8. Pabst D, Rommel S, McLellan W, et al: Thermoregulation of the intra-abdominal testes of the bottlenose dolphin (Tursiops truncatus) during exercise. J Exp Biol 198:221–226, 1995.
9. Robaire B, Hinton BT: The Epididymis: From Molecules to Clinical Practice: A Comprehensive Survey of the Efferent Ducts, the Epididymis and the Vas Deferens. Kluwer Academic/Plenum Publishers, New York, 2002.
10. Turner K, McIntyre B, Phillips S, et al: Altered gene expression during rat wolffian duct development in response to in utero exposure to the antiandrogen linuron. Toxicol Sci 74:114–128, 2003.
11. Waites GM: Development of methods of male contraception: Impact of the World Health Organization Task Force. Fertil Steril. 80:1–15, 2003.

3. EVALUATION OF MALE REPRODUCTIVE DISORDERS

Jay I. Sandlow, M.D.

HISTORY

1. How common is infertility? When should an evaluation be performed?

Up to 15% of all couples attempting conception are unsuccessful within the first year. However, this number increases with the age of the couple. Thus, infertility evaluation should be pursued on request by the couple rather than waiting until a full year has elapsed.

2. What is secondary infertility? What are the common causes in men?

Secondary infertility does not refer to the cause of the problem but rather to the history of a previous conception by either partner. Common causes of secondary infertility in men include previous sterilization, varicocele, infection, and gonadotoxin exposure.

3. Who is more likely to have a problem—the man or woman?

Although traditionally considered a female problem, infertility is typically multifactorial and may involve both partners. Approximately 40% of cases involve a female factor; 30%, a male factor; and 20%, combined male and female factors. Approximately 10–15% of cases remain unexplained. Therefore, in 50% of infertile couples a male factor is involved.

4. Why should the man be evaluated?

1. In 50% of infertile couples, a significant male factor is involved.

2. Many of the causes of male infertility are treatable, thus allowing the couple to conceive naturally.

3. A small but significant number of causes of male infertility represent serious underlying health problems (testis cancer, pituitary tumor, diabetes, hormonal abnormalities).

4. One would not consider putting a woman through advanced reproductive techniques without an evaluation; therefore, it makes sense to treat the man in a similar fashion.

5. What is the most common cause of male infertility?

Although there are many causes of male infertility, varicocele is the most common. A clinically significant varicocele can be identified in nearly 40% of men with primary infertility and up to 80% of men with secondary infertility.

6. How do varicoceles cause infertility?

Varicoceles disrupt the countercurrent heat exchange that keeps the testes cooler than body temperature. This pooling of the warm blood surrounding the testis creates an insulating effect.

7. If the varicocele is only on one side, why does it cause a problem with both testes?

Because the affected testis is constantly being heated, this heat is conducted to the unaffected side, thus raising the temperature of both testes.

8. Which is better, boxers or briefs?

Numerous studies have demonstrated that the type of underwear has no significant effect on sperm counts, motility, or pregnancy rates. Despite these studies, however, many people, including physicians, still subscribe to this fallacy.

9. What are the effects of various sexual practices (frequency, position, masturbation) on male fertility?

If the frequency of intercourse is too high, such as every day, the testes are not able to keep up with sperm production, and sperm counts can go down. Frequency of ejaculation overall, including intercourse and masturbation, may contribute to lower sperm counts. There is no evidence that the position during intercourse affects conception, although positions that do not allow full penetration may make delivery of the seminal bolus to the cervix more difficult.

10. Explain the optimal timing of intercourse for conception.

Timing of intercourse should be centered on the woman's day of ovulation, preferably every day, beginning 2–3 days before ovulation. Once a woman has ovulated, it is too late. Ovulation can be predicted in various ways, including ovulation prediction kits and basal body temperature charts, although these methods tend to be cumbersome and time-consuming. The likelihood of conception increases as intercourse occurs closer to the day of ovulation, peaks on the day of ovulation, and decreases after the day of ovulation.

11. Explain the relationship between sexual dysfunction and male infertility.

It is important to determine whether sexual dysfunction affects either the man or the woman. Male problems include erectile dysfunction and ejaculatory dysfunction, both of which may affect the frequency or timing of intercourse.

12. Which lubricants are toxic to sperm? Which ones are not?

Many common lubricants have demonstrated in vitro toxicity to sperm, including KY Jelly, hand lotion, and saliva. However, some lubricants, both natural and available over the counter, are not toxic to sperm. Examples include vegetable oil, glycerin, egg whites, and specific vaginal lubricants that are marked "nonspermicidal."

13. What is the most common sexually transmitted disease? How can it cause fertility problems?

The most common sexually transmitted disease is due to *Chlamydia trachomatis*. This infection tends to be relatively asymptomatic in women; however, infected men typically suffer from urethritis and/or epididymitis. Either has the potential to result in scarring, particularly in the epididymis, thus causing obstruction. In the case of bilateral epididymitis, a bilateral obstruction can result in azoospermia. Other sexually transmitted diseases that may play an important role in male infertility include gonorrhea and urinary tract infections, which may cause epididymo-orchitis and/or prostatitis.

14. What medical conditions may be associated with infertility? How?

Many medical conditions have effects on male fertility. Overall, poor health can cause a decrease in sperm production. However, some specific conditions have specific effects. Diabetes mellitus typically causes ejaculatory dysfunction, usually through sympathetic dysfunction. It may also cause erectile dysfunction through parasympathetic dysfunction. Diabetics often give a history of decreased amount of ejaculate and occasionally report that no fluid accompanies ejaculation. Neurologic problems, including spinal cord injury, multiple sclerosis, and other associated conditions, can also cause ejaculatory dysfunction. Any medical condition that requires chemotherapy or radiation therapy certainly affects male fertility.

15. What is the fertility potential of a man with a history of unilateral cryptorchidism? Bilateral cryptorchidism?

Men with unilateral cryptorchidism typically have near-normal fertility potential; studies have indicated paternity rates ranging from 80% to 90%. However, men with unilateral cryptorchidism tend to have lower sperm counts, although they are able to achieve paternity. Men with bilateral cryptorchidism typically have markedly decreased sperm counts, and their fertility potential is significantly less than that of unaffected men. Some studies quote paternity rates as low as 25–30%, although other sources say that the paternity rate may be as high as 50%.

16. Does the timing of orchidopexy for cryptorchidism affect fertility? What other factors are important?

To date, the timing of orchidopexy has not been shown to affect fertility potential In the past, many cryptorchid testes were not brought down into the scrotum until the child was as old as 7 or 8 years. Over the years, orchidopexy has been performed earlier and earlier, and now many advocate performing the procedure in the first year after birth. Some evidence suggests that early orchidopexy may improve fertility potential, although other factors, such as the location and gross appearance of the testis, may play a role in future fertility.

17. What types of surgery are more likely to be associated with infertility? Why?

Several different kinds of surgery can affect fertility by various mechanisms. Surgeries in the pelvis and retroperitoneal area can affect the nerves that control erection and ejaculation, thus interfering with the delivery of sperm to the female. Inguinal surgery can damage either the blood supply to the testes (e.g., inguinal varicocele ligation) or the vas deferens (e.g., pediatric hernia repair). Typically, vasal damage during inguinal surgery is related to ischemia rather than direct damage to the vas deferens and therefore may not be recognized at the time of surgery. Furthermore, with the recent use of Marlex mesh in hernia repairs, late scarring from the dense inflammatory reaction can also cause vasal obstruction. Finally, any kind of scrotal surgery can cause epididymal and/or vasal obstruction secondary to direct damage to the structures or scarring. Therefore, it is recommended that most patients of reproductive age not undergo scrotal surgeries such as hydrocelectomies or spermatocelectomies unless absolutely indicated.

18. What medications are typically associated with infertility?

Many medications can have an effect on sperm production, and several medications are well-known gonadotoxins. Examples include cimetidine, which increases aromatase activity, thus causing hyperestrogenemia; sulfasalazine, which is used in inflammatory bowel disease; and many antibiotics. Certainly any kind of chemotherapy can affect fertility, but chemotherapy associated with testicular cancer and lymphoma tends to cause significant spermatogenic damage that, in up to 25% of patients, is irreversible.

19. Describe the effect of alcohol and tobacco on male reproduction.

Although no definitive evidence establishes that alcohol and tobacco play a significant role in male infertility, heavy exposure to either can certainly have a negative impact. Most studies examining alcohol use have found that heavy use can cause reversible spermatogenic problems. But it is unknown whether there is a threshold above which alcohol use causes infertility. The data about tobacco use are also unclear, although it appears that significant exposure to cigarette smoke can cause motility problems.

20. What other gonadotoxins or exposures can cause male infertility?

Illicit drugs, such as marijuana, androgenic steroids, and cocaine, have been implicated in male infertility, sometimes in an irreversible fashion. Androgenic steroids shut down the normal hypothalamic-pituitary-gonadal axis and often result in sterility. Marijuana tends to upset this axis as well, but the effect is usually reversible, although there may be a dose-dependent response above which damage is irreversible. Finally, thermal exposure (e.g., hot tubs), radiation exposure, and chemical exposure (e.g., pesticides) can all play a role in male infertility.

21. What family history is significant in the evaluation of male infertility?

The most common genetic disorder that may be identified in the family history is cystic fibrosis. The carrier frequency in the Caucasian population approaches 1:20, and the female carrier is phenotypically silent. Although most male carriers for the mutations of the CFTR gene are infertile themselves, there are certainly fertile men who pass the mutation to their offspring. A good family history should uncover this problem. Other less common familial disorders, such as androgen receptor deficiencies, polycystic kidney disease, and intersex conditions, may provide clues to the cause of male reproductive problems.

22. With what cause of male infertility is lack of smell (anosmia) typically associated? Discuss its etiology and embryology.

Anosmia is typically associated with Kallman's syndrome, which is a specific genetic variant of hypogonadotrophic hypogonadism. The neural crest cells that migrate during embryogenesis to form both the hypothalamus and the olfactory bulb do not reach their final destination; therefore, there is a lack of sense of smell as well as a lack of gonadotropin-releasing hormone (GnRH) production. This syndrome is an autosomal recessive disorder due to a single gene mutation (KAL-1) on the X chromosome.

23. What is the significance of galactorrhea and/or visual changes in the infertility evaluation?

Both symptoms can be signs of a pituitary tumor, such as a prolactinoma or other mass lesions of the pituitary. The increased prolactin can cause gynecomastia and galactorrhea, whereas visual changes may be due to direct pressure of the pituitary mass on the optic chiasm. Although infertility is a rare presentation for these disorders, the possibility once again underlines the importance of performing a thorough history and physical exam in the evaluation of the infertile male.

24. How much evaluation should be performed for the female partner? What questions should be asked?

Fertility is a two-person process; therefore, the female partner cannot be ignored. At the very least, one should ascertain the age of the woman, previous pregnancies, either with the present partner or previous partners, and outcome of these pregnancies. It is important to know whether the woman cycles on a regular basis and how long these cycles last as well as whether this pattern has changed at all in the recent past. Contraceptive use, both present and past, should be ascertained, and any work-up that has already been done on the woman should be noted. When in doubt, a referral to a female infertility specialist may be in order.

25. What is the significance of ejaculatory problems, such as pain or hematospermia?

Problems with ejaculation may represent disorders of the prostate and/or seminal vesicles. Typically, they are due to inflammatory conditions; however, congenital anomalies may also produce these symptoms. Therefore, in a male of reproductive age who has intractable ejaculatory pain or hematospermia, transrectal ultrasound may be indicated to rule out abnormalities such as ejaculatory duct stones, prostatic cysts, or mullerian remnants.

26. What is the significance of orchalgia?

Orchalgia, although frustrating, is most often due to a benign, albeit idiopathic, condition. Although orchalgia itself is not typically a cause of infertility, it may be associated with an underlying disorder, such as a varicocele or testicular tumor, that causes the fertility problem. Therefore, men with orchalgia must undergo a complete history and physical exam to rule out any potentially treatable and, more importantly, medically significant causes. Scrotal ultrasound is a relatively inexpensive, noninvasive test that can rule out most intratesticular lesions, whereas a good physical exam rules out infection, inflammation, or varicocele. Postvasectomy orchalgia, which is a broad category, may be caused by congestive epididymitis due to the obstruction itself, and open-ended vasectomy or, in rare instances, vasectomy reversal may be the appropriate treatment.

PHYSICAL EXAM

27. What parts of the general physical exam are important for the infertility evaluation? Why?

The general physical exam is an important part in the evaluation of the subfertile male for several reasons. Overall general health can affect sperm production and male fertility and therefore needs to be evaluated. Specifically, diseases that affect the entire body, such as diabetes, can play a role in male infertility, and often signs and symptoms can be picked up on a thorough physical exam. Furthermore, it is important to examine the man for general body habitus and hair distribution, which may give clues to endocrinopathy, such as hypogonadism. Finally, serious medical problems, such as testicular cancer, can present with infertility, and signs of metastatic disease, such as lymphadenopathy, can be picked up on a thorough physical exam.

28. What is the significance of gynecomastia in a male?

Gynecomastia in a male is typically secondary to hyperestrogenemia, which can be caused by several factors, such as a hormone-producing tumor, exogenous testosterone with conversion to estradiol, or significant weight gain. Because of the suggestion of hyperestrogenemia, gynecomastia should be a clue to check serum hormonal studies, including both testosterone and estradiol. Hyperprolactinemia can also cause gynecomastia; serum estrogen and prolactin levels should be measured.

29. Which penile abnormalities can be associated with infertility?

Any abnormalities that inhibit deposition of the seminal bolus in the correct location can cause infertility. Therefore, hypospadias, particularly more severe forms such as penile or penoscrotal hypospadias, can result in poor sperm deposition. Phimosis of the foreskin can also inhibit deposition of the ejaculatory bolus and severe Peyronie's disease with subsequent deformity of the penile shaft can inhibit normal function as well. Therefore, the penile exam should rule out all of these disorders.

30. What is normal testicular size? Volume? How should they be measured?

Although normal testicular size varies greatly among men from various backgrounds, it has been well established that testicular size is positively correlated with sperm production. Therefore, accurate measurement, using either an orchidometer or ultrasound, should be performed on all patients undergoing evaluation for infertility. A testicular length greater than 3.5 cm or a volume of 18 ml or greater is typically indicative of normal testicular size. However, relative testicular size as measured within the same patient is often of great importance. Significant discrepancy in testicular size should be investigated; it can be due to several factors, such as testicular atrophy secondary to varicocele, previous trauma, or infection, or an underlying problem, such as testicular tumor.

31. What is the best method for evaluating patients for a varicocele?

Examination of a patient for a varicocele is extremely operator-dependent. However, several steps can be taken to optimize the diagnostic yield. First, the patient should be placed in a warm, comfortable room for the exam. He should remain standing several minutes before the exam to allow blood to pool in the varicocele. Next, the examiner should grasp the spermatic cord with both hands to palpate all associated structures, including the epididymis and vas deferens, before having the patient perform a Valsalva maneuver. If there is any question whether the patient truly has a varicocele, he can be placed in a spine position and the cord reexamined, both with and without a Valsalva maneuver. Typically, the Valsalva maneuver results in an increase in size and distention of the spermatic cord in patients with varicoceles, producing an impulse that can be felt in both supine and standing positions.

32. What is the significance of a unilateral right-sided varicocele? What further testing, if any, should be performed?

Typically, varicoceles are found on the left side, with up to 30% being bilateral; less than 2% of unilateral varicoceles are on the right side. Unilateral right-sided varicocele can be seen in rare cases, such as sitis inversus. However, unilateral right-sided varicoceles typically should raise the examiner's awareness of underlying pathology, including a retroperitoneal process causing obstruction. Also important in the history is the rapidity of the onset of the varicocele; a relatively new-onset varicocele again should suggest a retroperitoneal process. Ultrasound or CT scan of the abdomen and pelvis can make the diagnosis of any significant pathology, and both are relatively inexpensive and noninvasive.

33. How can obstructive vs. nonobstructive azoospermia be differentiated on physical exam?

Because of its positive correlation with sperm production, testicular size and consistency are among the most predictive factors of obstructive vs. nonobstructive azoospermia. Typically, patients with nonobstructive azoospermia have smaller testes, whereas those with obstructive azoospermia typically have normal-sized testes. Also of importance is examination of the epididymis and vas deferens. The epididymides of men with obstructive azoospermia typically are distended and/or indurated, whereas in men with nonobstructive azoospermia the epididymides tend to be flat. Finally, the presence or absence of the vas deferens can help make the diagnosis as well.

34. What is the significance of a nonpalpable vas deferens on one side? Both sides?

Unilateral absence of the vas deferens is typically associated with ipsilateral renal agenesis. This condition is due to a defect in mesonephric duct development during weeks 6–8 of embryogenesis. Because the ureter and excurrent ductal system of the male originate from the same embryologic source, any early insult will affect both. However, a percentage of men who have unilateral absence of the vas deferens may be carriers for the cystic fibrosis transmembrane receptor (CFTR) mutation and, therefore, must be tested in the event that no renal anomalies are present. In contrast, congenital bilateral absence of the vas deferens (CBAVD) is highly associated with mutations of the CFTR and rarely seen with renal anomalies. This condition is due to a different pathophysiologic mechanism, in which the vas deferens and associated excurrent ductal structures are formed during embryogenesis and subsequently involute over time. Such men typically have normal kidneys bilaterally but are carriers for the CFTR gene mutation.

35. What abnormalities on rectal exam may be associated with infertility?

Typically, the rectal exam reveals little, if any, useful information in the evaluation of the subfertile male. However, in certain instances, such as men with symptomatic prostatitis, the disease process can cause fertility problems as well. In addition, obstructed seminal vesicles may be palpable on a rectal exam. Furthermore, the semen analysis yields clues that may prompt a transrectal ultrasound, which is a much more sensitive indicator of seminal vesicle obstruction.

36. What are the general effects of androgen deficiency before puberty? Are they different from those seen after puberty?

The classic eunuchoid appearance is associated with androgen deficiency before the onset of puberty. This condition leads to delayed epiphyseal closure, resulting in tall stature, arm span exceeding body length, and legs that are longer than the trunk. This is the classic description of the Klinefelter's patient, although many men with Klinefelter's syndrome do not demonstrate such changes, and many men with similar body proportions do not have Klinefelter's syndrome. However, if the androgen deficiency occurs after puberty, the body proportions do not change; instead, the muscle and fat distribution may be altered.

LABORATORY TESTING

37. How should a semen analysis be collected?

Typically, a semen analysis should be collected after 2–5 days of ejaculatory abstinence. The specimen is best collected via masturbation into a clean, wide-mouthed cup to ensure complete collection. The sample should be processed and evaluated as soon as possible, within 1–2 hours of collection; if it must be transported to the lab, the sample should be kept as close to body temperature as possible. Typically, at least 2–3 semen analyses over a 3- to 4-week period should be collected to determine the true baseline seminal parameters.

38. What are the indications for postejaculate urinalysis? Fructose testing?

Postejaculate urinalysis typically should be performed for low-volume ejaculate or anejaculation as well as azoospermia. Small amounts of sperm in the postejaculate urine with the majority of the sperm in the antegrade portion typically represent residual semen within the urethra and are not clinically significant. The utility of fructose testing is controversial. Many andrologists believe that volume and pH of semen are the best indicators for presence or absence of seminal vesicle contributions to the semen. Fructose, which is produced only in the seminal vesicles, can confirm the presence or absence of seminal vesicle secretions. However, this is a qualitative test and, therefore, open to interpretation. In the author's opinion, fructose testing should be a confirmatory test at best in the case of low-volume azoospermia.

39. What are the minimal standards of adequacy for the semen analysis?

The World Health Organization has set minimal standards of adequacy, but they do not translate into prognosis for fertility. These standards include an ejaculate volume of 1.5–5 ml, with a sperm density greater than 20 million sperm per ml; motility greater than 60%, with a forward progression of greater than 2 on a scale of 1–4; and normal morphology of at least 30% normal forms. Furthermore, there should be no significant sperm agglutination, pyospermia, or hyperviscosity.

40. Is there a threshold for sperm count and/or motility that can predict fertility?

No. Many studies have demonstrated a wide variation of both sperm count and total motile count with fertility. One recent study has shown that men with sperm counts less than 13.5 million/ml and less than 32% motility are more likely to be in the subfertile range, whereas men with greater than 48 million/ml and 63% motility are more likely to be in the fertile range. However, there was great overlap between both groups as well as an area of indeterminate fertility.

41. Does a "normal" semen analysis predict fertility? Why or why not?

Despite various studies demonstrating the typical semen analysis results for fertile men, there is no way to predict fertility based on semen analysis. This lack of predictive value is due to several factors, including the fact that fertility is a two-person process. Therefore, some men may be able to achieve pregnancy with subnormal numbers due to their partner's fertility status, whereas other men with "normal numbers" may not be able to achieve pregnancy. Furthermore, semen analysis is a poor indicator of sperm function and therefore cannot predict fertilization capability in vivo.

42. What hormones should be tested? When should hormonal testing be performed? Why?

Typically, hormonal testing in the infertile male consists of testosterone and follicle-stimulating hormone (FSH) determinations. However, men with sperm counts greater than 10 million/ml rarely have significant hormonal abnormalities; therefore, testosterone determination is unlikely to be of any benefit. FSH values can be predictive for prognostic outcome of any type of fertility treatment, including hormonal manipulation and/or varicocele repair. Therefore, FSH determination may be beneficial in all men before undergoing any therapy, but testosterone determination probably should be reserved for men who have severe oligoasthenospermia and/or signs of hypogonadism, including small testicular size and/or symptoms of hypogonadism. In the case of a low testosterone level, it is important to look at other hormones that may affect testosterone production, including prolactin, estradiol, luteinizing hormone (LH) and FSH. These hormones are typically best measured early in the morning or with a pooled sample over several hours, because most of them are secreted in a cyclic fashion throughout the day.

43. What genetic testing should be performed? What are the indications?

Several genetic and chromosomal tests can be performed. In the azoospermic male, testing for the CFTR mutations as well as Y chromosome microdeletions and karyotype can yield useful information. Typically, CFTR mutations are seen in men with CBAVD. However, there are instances of idiopathic epididymal obstruction due to an intact excurrent ductal obstruction, but the patient may be a carrier of the CFTR mutation or its poly-T variant. Y-chromosome microdeletion and karyotype are typically performed in men suspected of having nonobstructive azoospermia or severe oligospermia. Andrologists use various cutoffs, ranging from less than 5 million/ml to less than 1 million/ml for genetic testing. Whatever the cutoff, the couple should be counseled before genetic testing about its utility and how it may affect future decisions.

44. What is the role of transrectal ultrasound in the evaluation of infertile men?

Transrectal ultrasound is a sensitive tool for the imaging of the prostate and seminal vesicles. However, this test should be reserved for men who are azoospermic with low-volume ejaculate, because men with normal-volume azoospermia, particularly if it is fructose-positive, do not have seminal vesicle obstruction and, therefore, do not need to undergo transrectal ultrasound. Furthermore, men with oligospermia, by definition, cannot have complete ejaculatory duct obstruction; therefore, transrectal ultrasound is likely to be of little use. In select cases, transrectal ultrasound may reveal partial ejaculatory duct obstruction in which the seminal vesicles may be enlarged. However, this condition is rare and difficult to diagnose.

45. What is the role of scrotal ultrasound in the evaluation of infertile men?

Scrotal ultrasound is an inexpensive and noninvasive test that may yield significant information. Any significant discrepancy in testicular size or any palpable abnormalities should be evaluated with a scrotal ultrasound, as should any intrascrotal masses, including hydroceles and spermatoceles in young men. However, scrotal ultrasound is not recommended for the diagnosis of varicoceles, because the repair of subclinical varicoceles does not yield significant improvement in pregnancy rates.

46. In assessing response to any fertility treatment in men, how long must one wait? Why?

The spermatogenic cycle typically takes about 70 days from the spermatogonia to the development of mature spermatozoa. Another 18–20 days is required for transit time through the epididymis and vas deferens. Therefore, typically 3 months are needed to assess response to treatment. Often, treatments can take up to 6 months or even longer to exhibit full effect. Therefore, most men are evaluated every 3 months for a 6- to 12-month period to determine response to treatment. The same holds true for any attempt to eliminate factors that may be responsible for infertility, such as heavy alcohol use, gonadotoxin exposure, or medications.

BIBLIOGRAPHY

1. Anguiano A, Oates RD, Amos JA, et al: Congenital bilateral absence of the vas deferens. A primarily genital form of cystic fibrosis. JAMA 267:1794–1797, 1992.
2. Behre HM, Yeung CH, Nieschlag E: Diagnosis of male infertility and hypogonadism. In Nieschlag E, Behre HM (eds): Andrology: Male Reproductive Health and Dysfunction. Berlin, Springer, 1997, pp 88–104
3. Guzick Ds, Overstreet JW, Factor-Livak P, et al: Sperm morphology, motility, and concentration in fertile and infertile men. N Engl J Med 345:1388–1393. 2001.
4. Jarow JP: Life-threatening conditions associated with male infertility. Urol Clin North Am 21:409–415. 1994.
5. Kolettis PN, Sandlow JI: Clinical and genetic features of patients with congenital unilateral absence of the vas deferens. Urology 601073–1076. 2002.
6. Miller KD, Coughlin MT, Lee PA: Fertility after unilateral cryptorchidism. Paternity, time to conception, pretreatment testicular location and size, hormone and sperm parameters. Horm Res 55(5):249–253, 2001.
7. Pryor JL, Kent-First M, Muallem A, et al: Microdeletions in the Y chrommosome of infertile men. N Engl J Med 336:534–539, 1997.
8. Sandlow JI, Sparks AET: Evaluation of the male in couples seeking reproductive assistance: Going beyond the seminal fluid analysis. Assist Reprod Rev 8:36–39, 1998.
9. Sigman M, Jarow JP: Endocrine evaluation of infertile men. Urology 50:659–664, 1997.
10. Sigman M, Lipshultz LI, Howards SS: Evaluation of the subfertile male. In Lipshultz LI, Howards SS (eds): Infertility in the Male. St. Louis, Mosby, 1997, pp 173–193.
11. Woodhouse CR: Prospects for fertility in patients born with genitourinary anomalies. J Urol 165 (Pt 2):2354–2360, 2001.
12. World Health Organization: WHO Laboratory Manual for the Examination of Human Semen and Sperm-Cervical Mucus Interaction, 3rd ed. WHO, Cambridge, 1992, p 44.

4. SEMEN ANALYSIS

Shumyle Alam, M.D., and Craig Niederberger M.D., FACS

1. What is necessary for the appropriate collection of a semen sample?

Concerning the collection device, a clean (not necessarily sterile) wide-mouthed container should be used. A masturbated sample is preferred, and the entire ejaculated volume must be collected. The physician's office should provide the appropriate collection device and detailed instructions for collection. A period of abstinence of at least 2 days but no longer than 1 week before sample collection is necessary for accurate comparison of repeat samples. Use of chemically laden lubricants and contact with vaginal secretion during procurement of the sample should be avoided.

2. How do you address patient embarrassment or inability to masturbate in the office?

Home collection may be more comfortable for some patients. Specimens can be obtained away from the office but should be transported to the laboratory within 1–2 hours and be kept warm during transport. Recent literature suggests that the location of semen collection has no significant effect on the quality of samples.

3. What if a patient has religious beliefs that prohibit him from producing a sample?

Patients should be instructed to consult their rabbi, priest, or spiritual leader about this issue. Many religious laws have been rewritten to address the conundrum about masturbating for clinical purposes. A Mylex condom allows collection of the sample during intercourse. Couples who do not believe in contraception have reconciled the problem by placing a small pinhole at the tip of the condom. Latex condoms and lubricants are harmful to the sample and must be avoided.

4. Can any one parameter of the semen analysis reliably and accurately make the diagnosis of infertility or subfertility?

Although the finding of azoospermia defines infertility, the semen analysis cannot definitively separate patients into sterile or fertile groups. If the semen parameters decrease in quality, the chance of subfertility and subsequent infertility rises but does not preclude further diagnostic work-up.

5. What are the minimal standards of adequacy for the semen analysis?

The components of the semen analysis were defined by the World Health Organization (WHO) in 1999. Minimal standards include the following:

1. Volume: 2.0 ml or more
2. pH: 7.2 or greater
3. Sperm concentration: 20×10^6 or more sperm/ml
4. Total sperm number: 40×10^6 or more spermatozoa per ejaculate
5. Motility: 50% or more with grade A + B motility or 25% or more with grade A motility
   - A: Rapid progressive motility
   - B: Slow progressive motility
   - C: Nonprogressive motility
   - D: No motility
6. Morphology: 30% or more
7. Viability: 75% or more of sperm viable
8. White blood cells: less than 1 million/ml

6. Given the components of the WHO criteria for the semen analysis, what is the sensitivity of the test? Is semen analysis an accurate solitary test for infertility?

The sensitivity of any test depends on the thresholds that the clinician or consensus group sets as normal. The eight WHO criteria ultimately miss many infertile patients. For example, the sensitivity of sperm density at 20 million/ml is only 17%.

The threshold of 20 million/ml for sperm density originated in the work of MacLeod and was extended by WHO. MacLeod divided male subjects into two groups, fertile and infertile, and found that only 5% of the fertile men in his study population had sperm counts less that 20 million/cc, while 17% of the infertile men had counts below that range. Thus the sensitivity of sperm density at 20 million/cc is only 17%, while the specificity is 95%. This single parameter will miss 83% of infertile men. After more than half a century of studying the semen analysis there still does not exist one single parameter that will distinguish fertility from infertility, and the semen analysis remains a poor solitary test to distinguish males with abnormal reproductive potential.

7. What does the presence of white blood cells (WBCs) in the semen analysis mean?

Greater than 1 million WBC/ml is abnormal and suggests either infection or inflammation. However, under the microscope immature germ cells and white blood cells appear similar. Cells should be stained to make this differentiation. Although an experienced technician may be able to differentiate white blood cells from immature germ cells by standard stains (for example, hematoxylin and eosin) stains based on antibodies to immunologica cell types yield the most specific diagnosis. If WBCs are present, the patient should be evaluated for a genital tract infection.

8. When is semen culture necessary? What is the limitation of semen culture?

In the presence of pyospermia and symptoms of a genital tract infection, a culture can be performed. However, contamination from urine, the distal urethra, and the genital skin can decrease the sensitivity of the test. Special cultures are required for mycoplasmal and chlamydial organisms.

9. How many tests are necessary for accurate results in the work-up of the infertile patient?

A least two separate semen analyses should be obtained with adequate abstinence for each (2-day minimum). Patients should maintain the same period of abstinence before providing each sample to ensure reliable comparison. If the two tests vary greatly, additional samples can be obtained. If clinically feasible, the analyses may be performed over a period of 2–3 months, which allows at least one life cycle of the sperm.

10. Can a semen analysis alone differentiate between hypospermatogenesis and obstruction?

No. Both diagnoses can yield azoospermia or severe oligospermia. It is critical to centrifuge the semen in azoospermic males, because many are proved to have sperm by this technique and thus are placed in the diagnostic category of severe oligospermia.

The volume of the sample may provide information for the diagnosis of distal (ejaculatory ductal) obstruction, assuming no technical errors in sample collection. With the exception of bilateral congenital absence of the vas deferens, seminal volume is normal in proximal (vasal, epididymal, and rete testis) obstruction and low in distal (ejaculatory ductal) obstruction. This finding is due to the relatively small contribution of the testis to the ejaculate (approximately 0.5 ml). The low seminal volumes seen in bilateral congenital absence of the vas deferens are generally due to concomitant hypoplasia of the seminal vesicles, a distal effect.

The difference between aspermia and azoospermia is important to note. Aspermia is the absence of seminal fluid, whereas azoospermia is the absence of sperm from the ejaculate.

11. What physical and laboratory findings lead one to suspect obstruction?

If the long axis of the testis is greater than 4.5 cm and the level of follicle-stimulating hormone (FSH) is less than 7.6 mIU/ml, 96% of men are expected to harbor obstruction. Conversely, if the long axis of the testis is less than 4.5 cm, and the FSH level is greater than 7.6 mIU/ml, 89% of men are expected to have hypospermatogenesis or some other testicular abnormality in the seminiferous epithelium that explains their azoospermia. Often, small, soft testes clue the physician that testicular failure is the cause, whereas large, firm testes indicate obstruction.

12. What is the normal volume of a properly collected semen sample?

As defined by the WHO criteria, the normal value for ejaculate volume is greater than or equal to 2 ml. A low volume does not necessarily indicate pathology. One must first rule out improper collection and/or failure to remain abstinent before the sample was obtained. A volume of less than 1.5 ml should prompt investigation.

13. What are the indications for postejaculate urinalysis?

A postejaculatory urinalysis is mandated in patients with semen volumes < 1.0 ml to evaluate the possibility of retrograde ejaculation. Persistently low seminal volumes (< 1.5 ml on repeat evaluations) also serves as an indication for postejaculate urinalysis.

14. What is the role of fructose testing in determining the cause of low ejaculate volume?

Because the seminal vesicles account for the majority of the ejaculate volume, their contribution is in question when a low volume is found on semen analysis. Fructose is produced in the seminal vesicles, and the normal semen fructose concentration ranges from 120 to 450 mg/dl. Low fructose in the semen may suggest an inflammation of the seminal vesicles, androgen deficiency, or partial obstruction of the ejaculatory ducts. Complete lack of fructose suggests an absence of the seminal vesicles, or complete ejaculatory ductal obstruction. The modality of choice for the diagnosis of absence or obstruction of the seminal vesicles is transrectal ultrasound.

15. What are the sources of the total volume of the semen sample?

The volume of the ejaculate is derived approximately as follows:
- Cowper's glands: 0.1–0.2 ml,
- Prostatic secretions: 0.5 ml
- Seminal vesicles: 1.5–2.0 ml.
- Testes: 0.5 ml

The distal epididymis provides the majority of the ejaculated sperm. The ampulla of the vas is a small reservoir of sperm.

16. What are antisperm antibodies? Explain their significance.

Antisperm antibodies result from a disruption of the blood-testis barrier. This is a significant finding when all other parameters of the semen analysis are normal or in cases or sperm agglutination or impaired motility on semen analysis. Effects include the impairment of penetration of cervical mucous as well as premature induction of the acrosome reaction, inhibition of capacitation, and impairment of zona binding or actual fertilization. Risk factors for development of antisperm antibodies include vasectomy, congenital bilateral absence of the vas deferens, epididymitis, cryptorchidism, and trauma.

17. What is a viability test?

A viability test is performed to determine whether the spermatozoon is alive and to assess the integrity of the plasma membrane. The sperm are stained with dye, commonly eosin. Only viable sperm are able to exclude the pigment and remain unstained.

18. When is a viability test performed?

Asthenospermia, or defects in sperm movement, signifies an impairment of the forward progression of the sperm. A viability test should be performed when sperm motility is completely absent or motility is less than 5%. Occasionally the patient may have a congenital abnormality, such as immotile cilia syndrome, in which there are ultrastructural abnormalities of the cilia. Such patients may also have a history of upper respiratory infections. One should be suspicious of this entity if there is a high percentage of viable sperm in a sample with low motility. Electron microscopy is necessary for the diagnosis. Prolonged periods of abstinence or exposure of the sample to contaminants can also alter motility.

19. What special preparation, if any, is necessary for the semen sample in an HIV discordant couple undergoing intrauterine insemination (IUI)?
Investigators have suggested that semen can be processed to remove viral particles, but the safety of this procedure has not been proved.

20. What parameter of the semen analysis is most significantly affected by varicocelectomy?
After varicocelectomy, the most consistently improved parameter is motility.

21. What is the significance of sperm head defects?
Many different head defects have been observed, such as pin heads, tapered heads, round heads, and others. Sperm are pleomorphic by nature, and a multitude of different head types, although often bizarre in appearance, does not necessarily infer a reproductive defect. However, a consistent defect, such as all sperm with pin heads, indicates a likely genetic defect. A consistent appearance of round-headed sperm implies absence of the acrosomal cap, which results in disrupted capacitation and the inability of the sperm to fertilize the ovum. This defect also precludes the use of IUI as treatment.

22. Is sperm morphology an accurate predictor of fertility?
The nonspecific nature of the WHO definition of morphology prompted Kruger to propose "strict criteria" that delineate specific metrics by which to describe a normal sperm. Any abnormal metric identifies the counted sperm as abnormal. However, the great variability among laboratories in reporting strict criteria outcomes and a lack of consistent broadly reported data correlating strict criteria outcomes to reproductive outcomes, such as fertilization by in vitro fertilization, have limited the utility of strict criteria.

23. Summarize Kruger's strict criteria for sperm morphology.
Kruger's strict criteria, published in 1986, include the following:
- Smooth oval head 3–5 mm in length and 2–3 mm in width
- Well-defined acrosome, making up at least 40–70% of the head
- Absence of defects of the neck, midpiece, or tail
- Absence of cytoplasmic droplets larger than half the size of the head

These criteria, however, cannot uniformly predict the success of IVF

24. What factors alter sperm morphology?
Trauma, exposure to heat (whirlpool, fever, sauna use), and congenital abnormalities such as a varicocele have been reported to affect morphology.

25. What is the most reliable predictor of fertility on semen analysis?
A normal sperm count is most reliably associated with positive reproductive outcomes.

26. Does the semen analysis alone contain enough information to proceed with medical treatment?
It is necessary to perform a thorough history and physical exam (and if the sperm density is less than 10 million/ml, a hormonal analysis) to exclude potentially life-threatening concomitant medical conditions. Neither medical nor surgical treatment can be based on the semen analysis alone.

27. Does oligospermia always signify a spermatogenic deficit?
Oligospermia means that the sperm density is less than 20 million/ml. The cause may be idiopathic, or the condition may be due to abnormal spermatogenesis, androgen deficiency, varico-

cele, medication use, childhood conditions such as cryptorchidism, orchitis, or external conditions such as heat toxicity. It may also occur in a male with adequate reproductive potential.

28. In which of the following scenarios are you likely to identify an abnormality on semen analysis? What type of abnormality is likely to be present?

Prepubertal mumps: generally has little effect on fertility or semen analysis.

Postpubertal mumps: infertility in approximately 13% of patients with bilateral testicular effects. Semen analysis may reveal oligospermia.

Unilateral testis secondary to trauma: generally normal parameters.

Unilateral cryptorchidism repaired at age 2: generally normal parameters. However, sperm concentrations below 12–20 million/ml have been found in up to 25% of males with unilateral cryptorchidism.

Unilateral testis secondary to germ-cell tumor: generally normal volume with depressed-to-normal sperm count.

Bilateral cryptorchidism repaired with Fowler-Stephens orchiopexy at age 2 for prune belly syndrome: azoospermia with low-volume ejaculate. Patients also have prostate hypoplasia.

29. What congenital abnormality results in a normal semen analysis but inability to conceive with a normal female partner?

Distal shaft hypospadias can cause this phenomenon and may be associated with a genetic abnormality. Proximal or mid-shaft hypospadias are often corrected, but occasionally the distal shaft or coronal hypospadias is missed or never repaired.

30. What further test(s) will reveal the cause of the problem in the previous question?

Postcoital testing is useful to look for the presence of sperm at the level of the cervix.

31. If a patient has two completely normal semen analyses and normal laboratory profiles, what further testing is required?

Athorough history and physical examination of the patient and a thorough evaluation of his partner are necessary. Postcoital testing and assay for the presence of antisperm antibodies may also be indicated.

32. How is sperm motility determined?

Sperm motility is calculated as the percentage of sperm that demonstrate flagellar motion. This analysis should be performed within 1–2 hours after the sample is obtained and the sample should be at room or body temperature. Sperm motility of at least 50% with forward progression (higher than grade 2 on a scale of 0–4; 0 = no movement and 4 = excellent motion) is considered normal. In practice, due to operator variability, grading systems are seldom used.

33. A 30-year-old type I diabetic presents for primary infertility work-up. The serum FSH and LH are within the normal range, as is serum testosterone. Physical exam is unremarkable, and the female partner's work-up is unrevealing. Semen analysis reveals:

- Volume = 0.4 ml
- Concentration = 7.3 million/ml
- Motility = 4%
- pH = 5.5

What is the next step?

The patient needs a postejaculate urinalysis. The low volume and presence of diabetes raise the suspicion of retrograde ejaculation.

34. A 28-year-old man recently underwent left radical orchiectomy for stage I seminoma. He did not receive radiation to the abdomen postoperatively and now presents for an infertility work-up after two previous semen analyses 1 week postoperatively revealed volumes

of 2.3 and 2.6 ml, concentrations of 6.3 and 8.1 million/ml, and motilities of 38% and 41%. What is the likely diagnosis?

A repeat semen analysis should be performed before invasive work-up is considered. Subfertility has been observed in such patients in the immediate postoperative period.

35. A 31-year-old weightlifter presents for evaluation. His past history is otherwise unremarkable. On exam his testicular volume is 15 ml bilaterally. You suspect anabolic steroid use. What would you expect to find on the semen analysis? Is a testis biopsy necessary, assuming that steroid abuse is the cause?

Semen analysis will reveal marked oligospermia or even azoospermia. The patient will have high circulating androgen levels from an exogenous cause and therefore will have decreased spermatogenesis secondary to feedback inhibition and the induction of a hypogonadal state within the testis. Testicular biopsy is not necessary to make the diagnosis. The history and frank questioning of the patient's habits will provide the answer. The actual incidence of steroid abuse has been shown to be between 30% and 75% of professional body builders. Semen parameters should return to the baseline levels months after discontinuing the steroids. Administration of intramuscular hCG may be of benefit in selected cases.

36. A tall, thin 32-year-old man presents for infertility work-up after a previous semen analysis revealed azoospermia. On examination testicular volume is 4 ml bilaterally. There is no history of trauma, infection or cryptorchidism. What is the likely diagnosis?

The presentation is suspicious for Klinefelter's syndrome. Patients are azoospermic, but testicular sperm extraction for intracytoplasmic sperm injection (ICSI) has been successful in some patients.

BIBLIOGRAPHY

1. Burrows B, Schrepferman C, Lipshultz L: Comprehensive office evaluation in the new millennium. Urol Clin North Am 29:873–894, 2002.
2. Dulioust E, Du A, et al: Semen alterations in HIV-1 infected men. Hum Reprod 17:2112–2118, 2002.
3. Gillenwater J, Grayhack J, Howards S, Mitchell M: Male infertility. In Gillenwater J, Grayhack J, Howards S, Mitchell M (eds): Adult and Pediatric Urology, 4th ed. Philadelphia, Lippincott Williams & Wilkins, 2002, pp 1683–1757.
4. Leruez-Ville M, de Almeida M, et al: Assisted reproduction in HIV-1 serodifferent couples: The need for viral validation of processed semen. AIDS 16:2267–2273, 2002.
5. Niederberger C: Understanding the epidemiology of fertility treatments. Urol Clin North Am 29:829–840, 2002.
6. Menkveld R, Wong W, et al: Semen parameters, including WHO and strict criteria morphology, in a fertile and subfertile population: An effort towards standardization of in vivo thresholds. Hum Reprod 16:1165–1171, 2001.
7. Nudell D, Mara M, Lipshultz L: Common medications and drugs: How they affect male fertility. Urol Clin North Am 29:965–973, 2002.
8. Saidi J, Chang D, Goluboff E: Declining sperm counts in the United States: A critical review. J Urology 161:460–462, 1999.
9. Schoor RA, Elhanbly S, Niederberger CS, Ross LS: The role of testicular biopsy in the modern management of male infertility. J Urol 167:197–200, 2002.
10. World Health Organization: WHO Laboratory Manual for the Examination of Human Semen and Sperm-Cervical Mucous Interaction, 4th ed. Cambridge, Cambridge University Press, 1999.

5. ENDOCRINE DISORDERS

Sarah K. Girardi, MD

1. What constitutes the standard hormone profile for the evaluation of infertile men?
The hormone profile should evaluate the hypothalamic-pituitary-testis axis. It should therefore include follicle stimulating hormone (FSH) and luteinizing hormone (LH) levels as well as total testosterone level. A prolactin level is obtained when LH and FSH are suppressed, and an estradiol level can be helpful when testosterone is low.

2. What is the single most important hormone level in the evaluation of infertile men?
FSH is the most important hormone level. It is indirectly related to sperm concentration and therefore can be helpful in determining whether lack of sperm production or obstruction is responsible for a low sperm concentration.

3. What is hypogonadism?
Hypogonadism is defined biochemically by a low serum testosterone level and physically by less-than-normal testicular volume. Hypogonadism is further classified as either primary or secondary, depending on the serum levels of pituitary hormones, LH and FSH. **Primary hypogonadism** is defined as a low serum testosterone level with normal or elevated LH and FSH levels. An example of primary hypogonadism is Klinefelter's syndrome. **Secondary hypogonadism** is defined as a low serum testosterone level associated with low FSH and LH levels. Examples include Kallman's syndrome and hypopituitarism.

4. Which is more accurate—total or free testosterone?
Testosterone exists in the serum in two forms, bound and free. Approximately 98% of testosterone is bound to either albumin or sex hormone-binding globulin (SHBG). The remaining 2% is free or biologically active.
    In most cases free and total testosterone levels correlate well, and therefore the measurement of total testosterone suffices. Any condition that results in an increase or decrease in SHBG, however, can lead to a discrepancy in free and total testosterone levels, and in such conditions both should be measured. Examples include hyperthyroidism, epilepsy, and obesity. Hyperthyroidism and the use of antiepilepsy medications result in an increase in SHBG. Total testosterone is elevated, without an increase in biologically active or free testosterone. The opposite occurs in obesity, in which SHBG is decreased. Total testosterone level is low, but free testosterone level is normal.

5. Does the time of day influence hormone level results in men?
Yes. Testosterone, like most hormones, has diurnal variation. Levels peak in the morning and decrease toward evening. Morning values can be as much as 20% higher than evening values. It is therefore recommended that blood levels be drawn in the early morning for evaluation of male infertility. If this schedule cannot be arranged, the time of day should be taken into account in interpreting results.

6. Is it necessary to repeat testosterone levels?
In general, no. Several factors, however, can influence the result. Brief and intensive physical exercise can increase serum testosterone levels, whereas prolonged exhaustive training can lower serum levels. Chronic illness as well as certain medications (e.g., ketoconazole) can lower the levels. In such situations it may be worthwhile to repeat the test.

7. If the testosterone level is low, how should testosterone be replaced?
The answer depends on the cause of the hypogonadism and the goal of testosterone therapy. This discussion is restricted to testosterone replacement for treatment of subfertility rather than

erectile dysfunction, andropause, or other symptoms of hypoandrogenism. This distinction is essential in selecting the type of testosterone replacement.

In men trying to improve or restore fertility, a distinction between primary and secondary hypogonadism is important. In **secondary hypogonadism** (hypogonadotropic hypogonadism), the testosterone level can be restored by replacing gonadotropin-releasing hormone (GnRH) or gonadotropins. GnRH must be restored using a GnRH pump, which administers a small bolus of GnRH every 2 hours. Alternatively, the gonadotropins can be replaced with LH in the form of human chorionic gonadotropin (hCG; 75 IU intramuscularly 3 times/week) and FSH in the form of human menopausal gonadotropin (hMG) or one of the newer recombinant preparations (1500 IU intramuscularly 3 times/week). The induction of spermatogenesis requires both gonadotropins. Once spermatogenesis has been restored, it can be maintained with hCG alone.

In **primary hypogonadism,** such as Klinefelter's syndrome, FSH and LH levels are already elevated, and there is little Leydig cell reserve. The testes are small and firm, and spermatogenesis is rare. Such men are generally considered sterile, and therefore testosterone therapy is aimed solely at treating hypogonadism and avoiding the long-term consequences of androgen deprivation, including osteoporosis, anemia, muscular weakness, and impotence. Testosterone injections (testosterone cypionate or enanthate, 200 mg every 2 weeks), patches (Androderm) or gel (Androgel, 5–10 gm daily) are all acceptable forms of replacement.

More recently, pregnancies have been achieved through in vitro fertilization in men with nonmosaic Klinefelter's syndrome by using sperm retrieved from the testes. In such men, testosterone should be avoided because it will suppress spermatogenesis. It is preferable to discontinue all exogenous testosterone while pregnancies are trying to be achieved or to use an alternative such as an aromatase inhibitor, which will raise testosterone levels by inhibiting the conversion of testosterone to estradiol.

8. How do you replace testosterone in infertile men with a low normal testosterone level?

If the patient has idiopathic hypogonadism, a slightly low or low normal testosterone level, and a normal estradiol level, clomiphene citrate may be helpful. Clomiphene citrate blocks estrogen receptors. At the pituitary level, this blockade has the effect of increasing FSH and LH levels, which should improve testosterone production in the testis and optimize sperm production. In these same men with mild hypogonadism, if the estradiol (E_2) level is elevated in conjunction with a low serum testosterone (T) level (T/E_2 ratio < 10), an aromatase inhibitor such as testolactone (50–100 mg 2 times/day) or anastrozole (Arimidex; 1 mg daily) can be used.

9. Describe the effect of anabolic steroids on fertility.

Anabolic steroids should be thought of as contraceptives. The use of exogenous steroids suppresses gonadotropin release by the pituitary, and consequently suppresses testosterone and sperm production by the testes. Such patients often present with severe oligospermia and even azoospermia. Blood tests reveal negligible levels of gonadotropins. Patients should be instructed to discontinue all androgen supplements. In the vast majority of cases, testosterone production and normal spermatogenesis return within 1 or 2 years.

10. Explain the clinical usefulness of the FSH level.

FSH is an indirect indicator of how well sperm are being produced. When spermatogenesis is normal, Sertoli cells in the testis elaborate inhibin B, which acts on pituitary receptors to inhibit FSH production. A low FSH level, therefore, is indicative of normal sperm production. When spermatogenesis is impaired, inhibin B is not elaborated at normal levels and FSH levels increase. An elevated FSH level indicates impaired spermatogenesis.

11. Is it necessary to repeat the FSH level?

No. FSH levels remain stable.

12. Why do you obtain a prolactin level?

Prolactin, a hormone secreted by the anterior pituitary, is responsible for lactation in women. It serves no physiologic role in men. The serum level of prolactin should remain very low in men (less than 18 ng/dl). An elevated serum level has the effect of suppressing LH and FSH, thereby suppressing testosterone production and spermatogenesis.

13. What do you do if the prolactin level is elevated?

If the elevation is mild, repeat the blood test. Often the prolactin level normalizes on repeat testing. If the level remains mildly elevated, check for contributing factors. The most common are medications (e.g., phenothiazines, imipramine, methyldopa, reserpine) and physiologic or psychological stress.

The most common cause of more significant elevations in serum prolactin levels is a prolactin-secreting adenoma in the pituitary gland. These lesions are classified as micro- or macroadenomas. A brain MRI is diagnostic. In most cases, medical treatment of hyperprolactinemia (cabergoline [Dostinex], bromocriptine) normalizes prolactin levels as well as LH and FSH levels.

14. What lab findings are consistent with a prolactin-secreting tumor of the pituitary?

Elevated prolactin, low LH and FSH, low testosterone, and low sperm concentration.

15. What are the clinical symptoms of a prolactin-secreting tumor?

Symptoms are variable. In some cases there are no symptoms at all. In some men infertility is the only symptom. Other associated symptoms are depressed libido, galactorrhea, headache, fatigue, and erectile dysfunction.

16. Explain the usefulness of an estradiol level in the evaluation of male infertility.

An elevated estradiol level results in a disturbance in testosterone/estradiol ratios and may contribute to infertility. The ratio of testosterone to estradiol should be 10:1. A lower ratio may warrant treatment aimed at correcting the imbalance. This goal is achieved most directly with an aromatase inhibitor such as testolactone or anastrozole.

17. What do you do if estradiol is elevated?

First, repeat the measurement. If elevation is confirmed, determine whether the patient is symptomatic—that is, has infertility, poor libido, fatigue, or erectile dysfunction. If so, treat as above.

18. What chemistries need to be obtained while a man is on testosterone replacement?

Because testosterone is metabolized by the liver, liver function studies must be followed. Testosterone is also associated with granulocytosis; therefore, a complete blood count should be obtained or therapy. If the indication for testosterone is a depressed testosterone level or an abnormal testosterone-to-estradiol ratio, these values should be followed periodically as well. If the man is over age 40, a prostate-specific antigen level should also be obtained.

19. What is the association between thyroid disease and infertility?

Both hyper- and hypothyroidism are associated with subfertility. Hyperthyroidism results in an increase in circulating SHBG, and hypothyroidism results in a decrease. In the case of hyperthyroidism, increased SHBG levels results in an increased total testosterone level and a decrease in free testosterone. Gynecomastia can develop. Thyrotoxicosis has been associated with decreased spermatogenesis.

20. When are thyroid function studies indicated?

Thyroid function studies should be obtained in any man with clinical signs of hyper- or hypothyroidism. In addition, thyroid-stimulating hormone (TSH) should be measured in any man with depressed levels of gonadotropins in whom a diagnosis of hypopituitarism is being considered.

21. When is it necessary to involve an endocrinologist in the evaluation or treatment of infertile men?

Whenever infertility is associated with other endocrinologic disorders (e.g., diabetes mellitus, thyroid disease, hypercortisolism) or long-term replacement with gonadotropins (hypogonadotropic hypogonadism) is required, it is wise to involve the endocrinologist to assist with the management of the associated condition.

22. True or false: Luteinizing hormone is produced by the anterior pituitary.

True.

23. True or false: Follicle-stimulating hormone is produced by the posterior pituitary.

False. FSH is produced by the anterior pituitary.

24. True or false: Luteinizing hormone stimulates Sertoli cells of the testis to produce testosterone.

False. LH stimulates the Leydig cells of the testis to produce testosterone.

25. True or false: Sertoli cells of the testis provide negative feedback to the pituitary gland via a hormone called inhibin B.

True.

26. True or false: Testosterone provides negative feedback to the pituitary and hypothalamus.

True.

BIBLIOGRAPHY

1. Depenbusch M, von Eckardstein S, Simoni M, Nieschlag E: Maintenance of spermatogenesis in hypogonadotropic hypogonadal men with human chorionic gonadotropin alone. Eur J Endocrinol 147:617–624, 2002.
2. Jarow P, Sharlip I, Belker AM, et al: Best practice policies for male infertility. J Urol 167:2138–2144, 2002.
3. Nieschlag E, Behre HM (eds.): Andrology: Male Reproductive health and dysfunction. New York, Springer-Verlag, 1997.
4. Palermo GD, Schlegel PN, Sills ES, et al: Births after intracytoplasmic injection of sperm obtained by testicular extraction from men with non-mosaic Klinefelter's syndrome. N Engl J Med 338:588–590, 1998.
5. Pavlovich CP, King P, Goldstein M, Schlegel PN: Evidence of a treatable endocrinopathy in infertile men. J Urol 165:837–841, 2001.
6. Raman JD, Schlegel PN: Aromatase inhibitors for male infertility. J Urol 167:624–629, 2002.
7. Turek PJ, Williams RH, Gilbaugh JH III, Lipshultz LI: The reversibility of anabolic steroid-induced azoospermia. J Urol 153:1628–1630, 1995.

6. ANTISPERM ANTIBODIES IN INFERTILITY

Steven S. Witkin, PhD

1. How can antisperm antibodies interfere with fertility?

Antibodies that bind to the surface of living motile spermatozoa can interfere with fertility in several different ways:

1. Antibodies, especially IgM antibodies, can bind to more than one spermatozoa and cause the sperm to agglutinate. Agglutinated sperm no longer are capable of progressive motility and so cannot reach the ovum.

2. Antibodies that react with the sperm tail interfere with the motility of the spermatozoa and prevent it from reaching the ovum.

3. Cervical mucus has a high affinity for the constant (Fc) region of antibodies. Therefore, if antibodies are bound to any region of the spermatozoa, the antibodies will also react with cervical mucus and prevent the passage of sperm through the cervix. The observation of "shaking sperm" on a postcoital test is due to the interaction between sperm-bound antibodies and cervical mucus.

4. Phagocytic cells, such as macrophages and polymorphonuclear leukocytes, have receptors on their surface for the Fc region of antibodies. Therefore, these phagocytic cells recognize, engulf, and digest sperm that have antibodies on their surface. Cell-surface antibodies also activate the complement system, resulting in the deposition of complement components on the sperm surface. Phagocytic cells also have receptors for complement and engulf sperm with bound complement. Complement activation at the sperm surface can also result in damage to the sperm membrane and result in a loss of motility. All complement components are present in the female genital tract, although at a lower level than in the peripheral circulation.

5. The binding of antibodies to the sperm head can, by steric hindrance, interfere with sperm-ovum interaction and prevent sperm penetration of the ovum. Large antibodies, such as secretory IgA and IgM, are especially effective in blocking these sites.

2. Who should be tested for antisperm antibodies?

Antisperm antibody testing is indicated for a couple if:

1. Semen analysis shows the presence of agglutinated or nonmotile or abnormally shaped spermatozoa. Antisperm antibodies are a major cause of this problem. The female partners of males with abnormal sperm or sperm with bound antibodies need to be tested for antisperm antibodies.

2. Semen analysis shows that the sperm count is low or that no sperm are present. If the sperm count is low due to a obstruction of the male excurrent ductal system, antisperm antibodies will be present. In fact, in men with no sperm (azoospermic) the presence of antisperm antibodies is diagnostic for a blockage.

3. Sperm recovered from the cervix 6–12 hours after coitus (postcoital test) are shaking or nonmotile. Although a poor result on a postcoital test is highly suggestive of antisperm antibodies, it should be emphasized that a normal postcoital test result, especially if the sperm have been examined less than 6 hours after coitus, does not rule out the presence of antisperm antibodies.

4. The cause of the couples infertility is unexplained.

5. The male partner has had a vasectomy reversal (vasovasostomy) and failed to achieve a natural pregnancy in the female partner. Most men develop antisperm antibodies as a consequence of a vasectomy. These antibodies may remain for a prolong period after the reversal.

6. The female partner is scheduled to undergo invasive testing. All noninvasive tests should be performed prior to any invasive procedures.

7. The couple is undergoing in vitro fertilization (IVF). Antibodies on the surface of the male partner's spermatozoa or in the female partner's serum that is used as part of the fertilization in-

cubation medium can block fertilization. If the presence of antisperm antibodies is known prior to IVF, the protocol can be modified to overcome this problem. The wasted expense and emotional trauma of a failed IVF cycle due to the presence of antisperm antibodies is completely avoidable.

3. What test should be used to detect antisperm antibodies?

The only valid antisperm antibody tests are those that measure the binding of antibodies to the surface of living motile spermatozoa. Two tests, the immunobead binding assay and the mixed antiglobulin reaction (MAR) test, meet these criteria. The use of nonviable sperm for testing is unacceptable since antibodies will adhere nonspecifically to dead sperm, yielding false-positive results. Similarly, the use of assays that employ sperm lysates or sperm antigens should be avoided due to the problems of nonspecific antibody binding and the likelihood of false-negative and false-positive results.

4. What are the differences in the various antibody tests on the market?

Both the immunobead binding assay and the MAR test measure antibodies on the surface of living motile spermatozoa. The immunobead binding assay employs beads that are coated with antibodies against the various immunoglobulin isotypes—IgG, IgA, and IgM.

To detect antibodies on ejaculated sperm, a fresh semen sample is washed several times to remove the seminal fluid, and the spermatozoa are then incubated with the various antibody-coated beads. Antibodies on the beads bind to antisperm antibodies on sperm. After several minutes the sample is placed on a glass slide and examined under a microscope. A total of 100 motile sperm are examined for the presence of beads that are bound to the sperm surface—either the head, midpiece, or tail. The number of motile sperm with bead binding at each sperm location is noted for each antibody isotype.

To test for antisperm antibodies in serum or cervical mucus, spermatozoa from the male partner (preferable) or from a sperm donor of proven fertility, tested and found negative for antisperm antibodies on the sperm surface, is incubated with a dilution of serum or cervical mucus at 37°C for 60 minutes. The spermatozoa are then exhaustively washed to remove any unbound antibodies, and the deposition of antibodies from the serum or cervical mucus onto the sperm surface is measured by bead binding, as described above.

For the MAR test, unwashed fresh semen is mixed on a microscope slide with IgG-coated or IgA-coated sheep red blood cells. Latex particles are sometimes used instead of sheep cells. Antibodies to human IgG or IgA are then mixed into the solution, which is observed under the microscope. If antibodies are present on the spermatozoa, red blood cells are seen adhering to the sperm. Eventually, large aggregates of sperm will be seen if antisperm antibodies are present. The MAR test can also be used to test for antibodies in serum by incubating antibody-free sperm with serum, as described for the immunobead binding assay, and then testing for antibody-bound sperm.

Both the immunobead binding assay and the MAR test can be modified to test for antisperm antibodies in cervical mucus. The cervical mucus must first be liquefied by incubation in bromelin for a short period. The sample is centrifuged and the supernatant tested for antisperm antibodies by the indirect immunobead or MAR assays.

The cost of the immunobead binding assay and MAR test is roughly equivalent, ranging from $50–$150 per sample.

5. What fluid compartment should be tested for antibodies?

Antisperm antibodies can be present in serum, semen, and cervical mucus. Therefore, in the ideal situation all three compartments should be assayed. However, in the overwhelming majority of women with antisperm antibodies in cervical mucus, the serum sample will also be antisperm antibody-positive. This is not true, however, for semen. A man may have antisperm antibodies on his ejaculated sperm but be negative for antisperm antibodies in his serum. It is imperative, therefore, to test men for antisperm antibodies on the surface of ejaculated spermatozoa.

6. Does the distribution of antibodies on ejaculated sperm or in different fluid compartments have any significance?

Because antibodies binding to the sperm surface can interfere with sperm passage through the cervical mucus and serve as targets for engulfment by phagocytic cells, any antisperm antibody—whether on ejaculated sperm, in serum, or in the cervical mucus—is relevant to infertility. Knowledge of the distribution of antisperm antibodies between among these three compartments is of some clinical value. Antisperm antibodies in the serum of an azoospermic man indicate a blockage in the male genital tract. In couples undergoing in vitro fertilization, knowledge of the distribution of antisperm antibodies determines the specific protocol to be followed.

7. Is there any value to testing azoospermic patients for antibodies?

In azoospermic men, the presence of antisperm antibodies in serum indicates that the outflow of sperm is blocked within the male reproductive tract and that further evaluation and possibly surgical reconstruction to correct the blockage may be indicated.

8. Does the antibody isotype have any significance?

Antisperm antibodies may be IgG, IgA or IgM. The antibodies on the surface of ejaculated sperm are exclusively IgG or secretory IgA. Either isotype is important in interfering with sperm migration in the female genital tract to reach the ovum. The secretory IgA antibodies are more of a problem than the IgG antibodies when the sperm are used in IVF. The larger size of the secretory IgA makes it more likely to interfere with sperm penetration of the ovum. Antisperm antibodies in cervical mucus are typically secretory IgA, reflecting their production in the endocervix as part of the mucosal immune system. Serum antibodies may be IgG, monomeric IgA, or IgM.

9. Does the titre of antibody have any significance?

Generally, in both the immunobead binding assay and the MAR test, the greater the percentage of sperm with bound antibodies or the greater the number of spermatozoa that acquire antibodies following incubation with serum or cervical mucus, the lower the probability of fertility without some form of intervention. Since, in most cases, not every spermatozoa is coated with antibodies, couples with antisperm antibodies can, on occasion, conceive with no intervention. However, the odds of conception, compared with couples with no antisperm antibodies, are greatly reduced. Similarly, the higher the percentage of sperm that do not acquire antibodies, the greater the odds of success.

10. Does the titer change with time in the same person? Is one test enough?

With couples in monogamous relationships, with no chance of acquiring a genital tract infection, antisperm antibody levels typically remain constant. The only situation in which antisperm antibodies may disappear is when the antibodies are not directed against a sperm component but instead are specific for a microorganism adhering to the sperm. In this case, treatment of the infection leads to the elimination of what appeared to be antibody binding to sperm.

11. At what stage in the infertility work-up should antisperm antibody testing be performed?

Since antisperm antibodies are a well-recognized cause of infertility and the test is relatively inexpensive and noninvasive, it should be performed before any invasive testing.

12. What causes antisperm antibody formation in men?

Spermatozoa are not produced until puberty—long after the time for development of tolerance to self antigens. Therefore, sperm-specific antigens are viewed as foreign by the male's immune system. However, because the male genital tract is basically a closed tube, spermatozoa are sequestered from the immune system. Any disruption in the integrity of the male genital tract that allows leakage of spermatozoa out of the tract or immunologically competent cells into the tract can lead to antisperm antibody formation. Such leakage may result from:

- Trauma to the testicles
- Congenitally weak epididymal or vas deferens
- Genital tract infection
- Deliberate severing of the vas deferens (vasectomy)
- Deposition of spermatozoa outside the genital tract, as when a homosexual or bisexual man engages in anal intercourse, also leads to antisperm antibody formation.

13. What causes antisperm antibody formation in women?

Unlike in men, the female genital tract is accessible to cells of the immune system. The reason that not every sexually active woman has antisperm antibodies is the immunosuppressive properties of the seminal fluid portion of the ejaculate. Seminal fluid contains a variety of components that inhibit all aspects of the immune response. Antisperm antibodies can arise in a woman if:

1. She has a genital tract infection that overrides the immunosuppressive properties of seminal fluid.

2. The male partner's seminal fluid is defective in providing a sufficient level of immunosuppression.

3. The male partner has sperm with abnormal morphology or sperm that is coated with microorganisms. Either case induces a proinflammatory immune response in the female genital tract.

4. The male partner has antisperm antibodies on his ejaculated sperm. Sperm with bound antibodies also are efficient inducers of proinflammatory immunity.

14. What is the relation between postcoital test results and antisperm antibodies?

To be a valid test for the presence of antisperm antibodies either on the surface of motile sperm or in the cervical mucus, the sperm should be retrieved from the cervix and examined at least 6 hours after coitus and before 16 hours. The presence of nonmotile sperm or shaking sperm, under conditions in which the sperm in the ejaculate exhibited normal motility, is highly indicative of antisperm antibodies. Postcoital tests performed earlier than 6 hours after intercourse may yield false-negative results, and testing after 16 hours may yield false-positive results.

15. Should couples with secondary infertility be tested for antisperm antibodies?

Because it is possible for couples with antisperm antibodies occasionally to beat the odds and become pregnant, couples with secondary infertility in which no other cause can be found should be tested for antisperm antibodies. In addition, acquisition of a genital tract infection following the initial pregnancy can lead to the subsequent development of antisperm antibodies.

16. Should couples undergoing in vitro fertilization be tested for antisperm antibodies?

All couples undergoing IVF should first be tested for antisperm antibodies. Antibodies on the surface of ejaculated spermatozoa inhibit the sperm from penetrating and fertilizing the egg. Serum from the female partner is frequently used as a component of the medium in which the unfertilized egg and sperm are incubated. If the woman's serum contains antisperm antibodies, they can bind to the sperm and inhibit fertilization. If the presence of antisperm antibodies on the ejaculated sperm is detected, the problem be totally avoided by performing intracytoplasmic sperm injection (ICSI). When the sperm is injected into the egg, the presence of antibodies on its surface is irrelevant to fertilization. If antisperm antibodies in the woman's serum are noted, it is a simple matter to substitute another solution for her serum in the incubation medium.

To fail an IVF cycle due to the presence of antisperm antibodies, when prior testing and modification of the IVF protocol can easily avoid this outcome, is unwarranted.

17. What are the effective treatments for antisperm antibodies in men and women?

Several options are available:

1. If not all spermatozoa in the ejaculate are coated with antibodies, intrauterine insemination with washed sperm may be successful. This technique bypasses the problem of sperm ad-

hering to cervical mucus and also greatly increases the numbers of spermatozoa that normally reach the uterus. The greater the numbers of spermatozoa in the uterus, the greater the probability that one will reach and fertilize the oocyte. Combining intrauterine insemination with induced ovulation further increases the probability of success. This treatment is also sometimes beneficial for women with antisperm antibodies in their serum and/or cervix.

2. Steroids such as prednisone or methylprednisolone increase the rate of antibody degradation and inhibit the production of new antibodies. Although controversial, steroids apparently have been a successful treatment for antisperm antibodies in some men and women. The success rate varies because of individual differences in steroid metabolism and the kinetics of antibody degradation and synthesis. In general, antibodies are at their lowest level about 2 weeks after steroid administration. Cases of sterile necrosis of various joints after steroid use for antisperm antibodies have been reported.

3. In vitro fertilization bypasses the problem of sperm migration through the female genital tract. The spermatozoa are placed in direct contact with the egg in a dish outside the woman's body. This technique eliminates the effects of the female's immune system on sperm with bound antibodies. If the antisperm antibodies are present only in the woman's serum or cervical mucus, IVF completely eliminates this impediment to fertility, provided that the serum is omitted from the in vitro incubation medium.

4. Intracytoplasmic sperm insemination (ICSI) is an assisted reproduction procedure in which a single spermatozoan is injected directly into an oocyte. It has been amply demonstrated that the presence of antisperm antibodies on the sperm surface is irrelevant for the success of ICSI. In men with antisperm antibodies on the majority of their spermatozoa, ICSI appears to be the most effective, albeit expensive, option.

5. It must be mentioned that antisperm antibodies reduce but do not completely eliminate the probability of conception. Successful natural fertilization does occur with no treatment in a proportion of antisperm antibody-positive individuals after a variable period of attempted conception.

18. Compare the effectiveness of IUI, IVF, and ICSI in managing infertility due to antibodies.

Intrauterine insemination (IUI), combined with induced ovulation, is the least expensive option for couples with antisperm antibodies. The success rate is inversely proportional to the level of antisperm antibodies, i.e., the lower the antisperm antibody level, the greater the success rate. However, as with all biological procedures, there are wide individual variations; some couples with high antisperm antibody levels successfully conceive after IUI.

In vitro fertilization (IVF) has a higher success rate than IUI and is independent of the antisperm antibody concentration. It is recommended when the woman has antisperm antibodies in her serum and/or cervix or when the proportion of spermatozoa with bound antibodies in the ejaculate is relatively low ($\leq$ 50%). If the woman has antisperm antibodies, her serum must not be used in the in vitro incubation solution. The success rate for IVF for couples with antisperm antibodies is the same as for couples without these antibodies.

Intracytoplasmic sperm injection (ICSI) has the highest success rate of any treatment for men with antisperm antibodies on ejaculated sperm. The direct injection of spermatozoa into the egg completely bypasses this antibody problem.

19. Can antibiotics be used to treat someone with antisperm antibodies?

Although an infection might have been the precipitating cause of antisperm antibody production, the infecting microorganism is long gone. Treatment with antibiotics does not reduce or eliminate antisperm antibodies.

20. Is condom therapy (use of a condom) an effective treatment for eliminating antisperm antibodies?

No. Once an antibody response is induced, memory cells are generated that rapidly produce antibodies on any subsequent exposure to the eliciting antigen. This is the principal of vaccination. In women with antisperm antibodies, a period of nonexposure to spermatozoa by condom use during sexual intercourse will have no effect on the memory cells. Subsequent exposure to spermatozoa will again rapidly lead to antisperm antibody production.

21. Can a person develop antisperm antibodies as a result of oral sex?

Ingestion of spermatozoa has not been shown to lead to antisperm antibody formation. In fact, there have been a few intriguing suggestions that oral sperm ingestion might lead to tolerance, i.e., nonrecognition of sperm as foreign antigens. Oral sex, however, is not a recommended therapy for antisperm antibodies.

22. Can a person develop antisperm antibodies from anal intercourse?

Homosexual men who engage in receptive anal intercourse have a very high incidence of antisperm antibodies. Antisperm antibodies were also induced in laboratory animals by anal insemination of semen. It thus appears that rectal semen deposition can lead to production of antisperm antibodies.

23. What is the relation between vasectomy and antisperm antibody formation?

In vasectomy, the vas deferens is cut and then ligated. This procedure blocks the release of spermatozoa from the male genital tract. However, sperm production does not cease, leading to a build-up of spermatozoa with the tract. Subsequent leakage of spermatozoa out of the genital tract leads to antisperm antibody formation. Most men who undergo a vasectomy develop antisperm antibodies within a few months.

24. Can antisperm antibodies interfere with the success of a vasovasostomy (vasectomy reversal)?

Although the blockage due to a vasectomy can be reversed surgically (vasovasostomy), antisperm antibody production is often not similarly reversed. Antisperm antibodies on ejaculated spermatozoa can be a major problem, interfering with the ability of vasovasostomy to lead to resumption of fertility.

25. Do antisperm antibodies have any medical consequences besides a reduction in fertility?

In the early 1980s, experiments in nonhuman primates linked vasectomy to an increased risk of atherosclerosis. This finding was thought to be due to the induction of antisperm antibodies. Subsequent exhaustive studies failed to establish a linkage between vasectomy and cardiac problems in humans. At present there is no credible evidence that antisperm antibodies are of any medical consequence besides interfering with fertility.

QUESTIONS FREQUENTLY ASKED BY PATIENTS

26. Can a woman have antisperm antibodies against the sperm of one partner but not against the sperm of other men?

In the great majority of cases, a woman's antisperm antibodies react with the spermatozoa from all men. An exception is when the antibodies are directed against a microorganism adhering to the sperm. In this case, the antibodies that bind to sperm will be partner-specific. If the male partner has an atypical sperm surface component, it also may lead to partner-specific antisperm antibody production.

27. Was I born with antisperm antibodies?

No one is born with antisperm antibodies. Women who were never exposed to semen do not have antisperm antibodies.

28. Are antisperm antibodies like an allergy? Am I allergic to my husband's sperm?

Antisperm antibodies are more like an immunization than an allergic reaction. Spermatozoa do not make a woman sneeze. The immune system has learned to recognize spermatozoa as foreign, similar to an infection, and produces antibodies to eliminate them from the body. In almost every case, these antibodies recognize spermatozoa from all men and are not partner-specific.

29. Will I have to undergo treatment again if I want to have more children?

Sperm antibody treatments are not permanent. The antibodies remain even after a successful conception and birth. Repeated treatment is required for further conceptions.

30. How can a man have antibodies to his own sperm?

Spermatozoa are first produced in the testes during puberty, which is long after the immune system learns to discriminate self from nonself. Therefore, sperm-specific antigens are viewed as foreign, similar to an infection, by the male immune system. Under conditions in which the immune system comes into contact with spermatozoa, antisperm antibodies will be produced.

31. What percentage of couples has antisperm antibodies?

It has been estimated that about 5% of infertility is related to antisperm antibodies. The percentage is about equal for men and women.

32. Why is fresh semen needed for antisperm antibody testing?

The only valid assays for antisperm antibodies are those that measure antibodies that react with living, motile spermatozoa. If the semen sample is not fresh, the spermatozoa are no longer motile. In addition, degradation of the sperm membrane leads to the reactivity of antibodies with sperm components that are not accessible on living sperm. This process leads to false-positive results.

33. Do I have to refrain from eating prior to antisperm antibody testing?

The sperm antibody test can be performed any time during the day and is independent of eating patterns.

34. Does the stage of the menstrual cycle matter when a woman is tested for antisperm antibodies?

Antibodies in cervical mucus can vary with the menstrual cycle, and mid-cycle mucus is usually obtained for antisperm antibody testing. A woman's serum can be tested at any time during the menstrual cycle.

35. Are antisperm antibodies contagious?

Antisperm antibodies are not contagious. However, there is a statistical association between the titre of antisperm antibodies on ejaculated sperm and the titire of antisperm antibodies in the female partner's serum. This finding may be the result of a genital tract infection that triggered antisperm antibody formation in both partners. Alternatively, antisperm antibodies on ejaculated sperm activate the immune system in the female genital tract and thereby increase the likelihood of antisperm antibody induction.

36. How can you tell if antisperm antibodies are present from a blood test? Don't you need to test a mucus sample?

In the overwhelming majority of cases in which antisperm antibodies are detected in cervical mucus, these antibodies are also present in blood.

37. My doctor told me that antisperm antibody testing is not necessary. Is he correct?

The use of inaccurate tests for antisperm antibody testing, plus the observation that couples with antisperm antibodies occasionally conceive, has led some clinicians to the erroneous conclusion that antisperm antibody testing of couples seeking treatment for infertility is unnecessary. It is unambiguous, however, that an accurate antisperm antibody test identifies couples with compromised fertility potential that can be improved by established protocols.

38. If antisperm antibody testing is a noninvasive procedure, why was I not tested before undergoing invasive surgery?

Unfortunately, some clinicians are not familiar with immunologic mechanisms of infertility and/or have had unsatisfactory experiences with the use of inaccurate antisperm antibody testing. It is important for the patient to become a knowledgeable advocate for the correct treatment sequence.

39. If antisperm antibodies interfered with the success of my in vitro fertilization (IVF) cycle, why was I not tested before undergoing this expensive procedure?

Some gynecologists and infertility specialists are not well versed in immunology and/or lack familiarity with the value of an appropriate antisperm antibody test. Additionally, since IVF is so expensive, some clinicians seek to minimize non-IVF costs by omitting antisperm antibody testing in the belief that this testing will most likely be negative. The IVF patient and her partner should be knowledgeable about the financial and emotional risks involved in not being tested for antisperm antibodies prior to an IVF cycle and must be so informed by the clinician.

40. If I do become pregnant, can antisperm antibodies harm my baby?

Some studies in experimental animals have suggested that antisperm antibodies might be involved in early-stage pregnancy loss. However, no evidence suggests that this finding applies to humans. Women with antisperm antibodies who conceive by in vitro fertilization or intracytoplasmic sperm injection have the same chance of having a healthy term infant as women who do not have antisperm antibodies.

BIBLIOGRAPHY

1. Bronson RA. Antisperm antibodies: a critical evaluation and clinical guidelines. J Reprod Immunol 45:159–183, 1999.
2. Hjort T. Do autoantibodies to sperm reduce fecundity? A mini-review in historical perspective. Am J Reprod Immunol 40:215–222, 1998.
3. Kelly R, Critchley HOD. Immunomodulation by human seminal plasma: a benefit for spermatozoon and pathogen? Human Reprod 12:2200–2207, 1997.
4. Lombardi F, Gandini L, Dondero F, Lenzi A. Antisperm immunity in natural and assisted reproduction. Hum Reprod Update 7:450–456, 2001.
5. Mclachlan RI. Basis, diagnosis and treatment of immunological infertility in men. J Reprod Immunol 57:35–45, 2002.
6. Witkin SS. Production of interferon gamma by lymphocytes exposed to antibody-coated spermatozoa: a mechanism for sperm antibody production in females. Fertil Steril 50:498–502, 1998.
7. Witkin SS. Mechanisms of active suppression of the immune response to spermatozoa. Am J Reprod Immunol Microbiol 17:61–64, 1998.
8. Witkin SS, Chaudhry A. Relationship between circulating antisperm antibodies in women and autoantibodies on the ejaculated sperm of their partners. Am J Obstet Gynecol 161:900–903, 1989.
9. Witkin SS, David SS. Effect of sperm antibodies on pregnancy outcome in a subfertile population. Am J Obstet Gynecol 158:59–62, 1988.
10. Witkin SS, Viti D, David SS, Stangel J, Rosenwaks Z. Relation between antisperm antibodies and the rate of fertilization of human oocytes in vitro. J Assist Reprod Genetics 9:9–13, 1992.

7. SEXUALLY TRANSMITTED DISEASES

Gerald J. Matthews, M.D.

1. What is the incidence of sexually transmitted diseases (STDs) in the U.S. population?

It is estimated that up to 50% of the U.S. population will acquire an STD by age 35. In 1998, 2 million STDs were self-reported to the Centers for Disease Control and Prevention (CDC). Population studies suggest that reporting accuracy is less than 40% of actual cases. Estimates for new cases of gonorrhea exceed 600,000 per year, with over 4 million new cases per year for chlamydial infection. An estimated 31 million people are infected with genital herpes simplex virus (HSV) and 24 million with human papillomavirus (HPV).

2. What is the most common mechanism by which STDs in men contribute to infertility?

The greatest infertility risk for men with an STD is transmission to the female partner with subsequent development of pelvic inflammatory disease (PID) and tubal obstruction. Up to 90% of women who are partners of infected men have an STD. A single episode of PID carries a 15% risk of infertility; the risk rises to 35% with the second episode and to 75% with the third. A woman with a single episode of PID has a 25% likelihood of having a second episode.

3. What is the incidence of STDS among couples with male factor infertility?

A large multicenter study of 2871 subfertile couples reported a 1.6% incidence of male genital tract infection as the most proximal cause of fertility abnormalities. In up to 35–40% of couples with unexplained infertility, chlamydial DNA is found in the semen of the male partner.

4. By what mechanisms do STDs impair male fertility?

STDs may affect male fertility at multiple levels. Urethritis causes pyospermia. The presence of white blood cells in the semen has been documented to impair sperm quality and function. Urethritis may progress to epididymitis with epididymal obstruction or epididymo-orchitis with subsequent testis atrophy. Other STDS, such as hepatitis and HIV, and their treatment may lead to systemic disease.

5. Which STDs cause urethritis in men?

Numerous sexually transmitted organisms are known to cause urethritis in men. Bacterial pathogens include *Neisseria gonorrhoeae, Chlamydia trachomatis, Ureaplasma urealyticum,* and *Mycoplasma hominis.* Viral agents include HSV and HPV. Other organisms include the protozoan *Trichomonas vaginalis.*

6. Can more than one pathogen be documented for any episode of STD-related urethritis?

A second organism is documented in up to 60% of patients with a confirmed STD. Up to 40% of men with gonorrheal urethritis are found to have accompanying chlamydial infection.

7. How does urethritis directly affect male fertility?

Demonstration of a direct bacterial or viral effect on sperm quality and function has been controversial. However, an inflammatory response and the presence of white blood cells typically accompany urethritis. The presence of white blood cells in the semen is associated with impaired sperm morphology and function. Leukocytes are the source of reactive oxygen species (ROS) and are associated with elevated seminal levels of ROS. ROS are known to cause lipid peroxidation of sperm membranes and have been demonstrated to alter sperm quality and function.

8. What are the symptoms of gonococcal urethritis (GU) and nongonococcal urethritis (NGU)?

GU typically produces a heavy purulent discharge. The urethral discharge with chlamydial urethritis (NGU) tends to be scant. Both are associated with dysuria. Up to 60% of known contacts of partners GU may harbor an asymptomatic infection. Up to 25% of men infected with chlamydia may be asymptomatic.

9. How is urethritis diagnosed?

Urethritis is suggested by the presence of more than 5 white blood cells (WBCs) per high-power field (HPF) of a urethral swab or more than 10 WBCs per HPF and the presence of leukocyte esterase from a first morning void.

For GU, in experienced hands, a Gram stain of a urethral swab demonstrating intracellular gram-negative diplococci approaches 99% specificity and 95% sensitivity. GC culture is also highly sensitive when modified Thayer-Martin or New York media are ued. DNA probes employing a polymerase chain reaction (PCR) are highly reliable and accurate.

Culture is considered an unreliable means of chlamydial detection. From 30% to 40% of properly collected and handled specimens have a false-negative culture. Antigen detection techniques, such as enzyme immunosorbant assays (EIA) and direct fluorescent antibody assays (DFA), offer increased sensitivity and specificity over culture for chlamydial infection. (Culture is more sensitive for GC). However, the CDC recommends use of a PCR assay for the laboratory confirmation of chlamydial infection.

10. What are the recommended treatment protocols for GU and NGU?

GU: ceftriaxone, 125 mg intramuscularly once plus either azithromycin, 1 gm orally once, or doxycycline, 100 mg orally twice daily bid for 7 days.

NGU: azithromycin, 1gm orally once, or doxycycline, 100 mg orally twice daily for 7 days.

11. Is retesting required after treatment?

Retesting for cure of asymptomatic patients is not required, provided that they have followed the prescribed treatment course and their partner(s) is (are) known to be free from disease. For this reason, many advocate concurrent treatment of all sexual partners. Diagnostic assays should be repeated for all men with persistent symptoms. To avoid the possibility of a false-negative assay, one should wait at least 48 hours after the completion of treatment for gonorrhea and up to 3 weeks after completion of treatment for chlamydial infection.

12. What is Reiter's syndrome?

Reiter's syndrome follows approximately 1–4% of cases of NGU. It has also been reported after GU and bacterial gastroenteritis. It consists of a triad of urethritis, uveitis, and arthritis. It is believed to represent an abnormal immune response to infection. Symptoms are usually self-limited, but arthritic complaints can last up to 6 months and may relapse.

13. What are *Ureaplasma urealyticum* and *Mycoplasma hominis*?

Both are mycoplasmal organisms distinguished by the ability to split urea. They are believed to be causal organisms in chlamydia-negative NGU. Culture systems for these organisms are not generally available, and their diagnosis largely rests on clinical suspicion. Treatment recommendations include tetracyclines, which are also included in chlamydial protocols (doxycycline). Approximately 10% of ureaplasmal and mycoplasmal oganisms are resistant to tetracycline. An alternative protocol for tetracycline-resistant strains calls for erythromycin, 500 mg 4 times/day for 7 days.

14. What is *Trichomonas vaginalis*? How is it diagnosed?

Trichomonads are flagellated protozoans. Along with *Ureaplasma* and *Mycoplasma* species, they are believed to cause chlamydia-negative NGU. Trichomonal urethritis is best diagnosed by saline wet mount microscopy. In expert hands the sensitivity of microscopic diagnosis is no more than 70%. Culture systems are accurate but largely unavailable.

Treatment calls for metronidazole, 2 gm orally once. Because of high reinfection rates, simultaneous treatment of sexual partners is recommended.

15. Does herpes simplex virus cause urethritis?

The primary infection with HSV can often lead to urethritis in men. Up to 44% of men with a first infection with HSV report dysuria, and 27% report a urethral discharge. HSV can be isolated from the urethra in most of these men. A primary infection with HSV may cause urethritis in the absence of any external lesions. Recurrent HSV infections are less likely to present with urethritis. Less than 2% of recurrent HSV infections are accompanied by urethritis.

16. How is HSV diagnosed and treated?

The HSV produces a characteristic eruption of grouped vesicles on an erythematous base. Virus isolation by tissue culture of noncrusted vesicles is a highly sensitive and reliable means of diagnosis. DNA probes employing PCR technology are the most reliable and sensitive method of diagnosis.

Treatment protocols for HSV call for either acyclovir (400 mg orally 3 times/day) or famcyclovir (250 mg orally 3 times/day) for 7–10 days. Approximately 80% of men with HSV have recurrent infections. Men with more than six recurrences per year should be offered suppressive therapy with either acyclovir (400 mg orally twice daily), famcyclovir (250 mg orally twice daily), or valacyclovir (500–1000 mg /day orally).

17. What is HPV?

HPV is the pathogen for venereal warts or condyloma acuminatum. More than 75 different HPV viral genotypes have been identified to date. HPV genotypes 6 and 11 are most commonly identified with the typical exophytic wart as well as low-grade cervical dysplasia. Infections with other HPV genotypes carry an increased risk of cervical, penile, anal, and urethral cancers. These include genotypes 31, 33, 35, 45, 51, 52, and 56, which have an intermediate cancer risk, and genotypes 16 and 18, which are associated with a high risk for malignancy.

18. What is the likelihood of urethral infection with HPV?

The presence of venereal warts near the urethral meatus should raise suspicion of intraurethral disease. Eight percent of men with lesions near the meatus have intraurethral lesions. Most are distal and located in the fossa navicularis. They are often visualized by careful inspection of the meatus and fossa. Cystoscopy should be performed to rule out any more proximal urethral lesion.

19. How is HPV diagnosed and treated?

HPV should be diagnosed by direct visualization of an external lesion or endoscopic visualization of a urethral lesion. Patients with perianal disease should undergo anoscopic evaluation. Uses of acetic acid detection methods are neither sensitive nor specific.

Treatment is based on eradicating visible disease. Low-volume external disease can be treated on an outpatient basis with self-administered topical agents (podofilox, 0.5% solution or gel). More extensive disease may require cryotherapy, laser ablation, or surgical excision. Intraurethral lesions located close to the meatus may be treated with self-administered 5% 5-fluorouracil solution. Other more proximal lesions or distal lesions not responding to topical agents require ablative therapy.

20. What are subclinical HPV infections? How should they be managed?

Subclinical HPV infection typically refers to the "uninfected" partner of a patient with documented HPV. These patients have no visible lesions and should be counseled, as should all patients and partners with HPV, about the infective nature of the disease and the use of condoms to reduce disease transmission.

21. Discuss the potential complications of an STD-related urethritis.

Acute complications of urethritis include ascending infection and epididymitis or epididymo-orchitis. Epididymitis is most often associated with either chlamydial or gonorrheal urethritis. Sexually active men under 35 years of age presenting with signs and symptoms of epididymitis should be suspected of having an STD. Postepididymitis sequelae may include epididymal obstruction and azoospermia. Epididymitis progressing to epididymo-orchitis can result in atrophy and diminished sperm production in the affected testis. Infection of other genitourinary organs, such as the prostate, has been described after STD-related urethritis. The long-term risk of urethral stricture disease after gonococcal urethritis has been well documented.

22. How is epididymitis diagnosed and treated?

Men presenting with signs and symptoms of epididymitis should undergo a complete history and physical examination. Torsion should be excluded from the diagnosis. A scrotal sonogram may be helpful.

Urinalysis frequently reveals pyuria. Urethral swab and culture are diagnostic for *N. gonorrhoeae*. A PCR-based DNA probe of a urethral swab is equally effective for *N. gonorrhoeae* and the diagnostic method of choice for *C. trachomatis*. Therapy should include ceftriaxone (250 mg intramuscularly once) and doxycycline (100 mg orally twice daily for 10 days). Scrotal elevation and nonsteroidal anti-inflammatory agents are helpful. Men presenting with fever and a high white blood cell count may require hospitalization, although the majority of cases can be managed on an outpatient basis.

Men failing to respond to therapy and men with persistent scrotal pain should have scrotal imaging to rule out abscess formation.

23. Does HIV infection have a direct effect on fertility?

HIV-positive men have been shown to have lower sperm counts and sperm motility compared with fertile non-HIV controls. Histologic studies have demonstrated a higher incidence of impaired spermatogenesis, maturation arrest and testis atrophy in HIV-positive men. Autopsy studies have demonstrated that up to 39% of patients with AIDS have opportunistic infections of the testes. Long-term HIV-positive men have a 50-fold greater risk of developing testis cancer than the general population.

24. What fertility options exist for HIV-discordant couples with an HIV+ male partner who desire children?

Numerous studies have reported use of sperm washing and assisted reproduction (in vitro fertilization with intracytoplasmic sperm injection) to safely achieve pregnancies and live births without seroconversion among mothers or children.

25. What about the other STDs?

Other common STDs, such as syphilis, lymphogranuloma venereum, chancroid, and granuloma inguinale, although of great clinical interest, have not been demonstrated in and of themselves to be directly related or causative of male factor infertility. Because these STDs are often found concurrently with other pathogens, one should always have a high index of suspicion for the presence of polymicrobial infection.

BIBLIOGRAPHY

1. Burnman MS, Ramuthaga TN, Mahomed MF, et al: Chlamydial infection in asymptomatic men attending an andrology clinic. Arch Androl 41:203–208, 1998.
2. Chan PTK, Schlegel PN: Inflammatory conditions of the male excurrent ductal system. Part II. J Androl 23:461–469, 2002.
3. Crittendon JA, Handelsman DJ, Stevant GJ: Semen analysis in HIV infection. Fertil Steril 56:1294–1299, 1992.
4. Gillenwater JY, Grayhack JT, Howards SS, Duckett JW (eds): Adult and Pediatric Urology, 3rd ed. St. Louis, Mosby, 1996.

5. Gilling-Smith C: Assisted reproduction in HIV discordant couples. AIDS Read 10:581–587, 2000.
6. Granato PA, Schneible-Smith C, Weiner WB: Use of New York City media for improved recovery of *N. gonorrhoeae* from clinical specimens. J Clin Microbiol 13:963, 1981.
7. Greenberg SH: Nongonococcal urethritis. Arch Androl 3:321, 1979.
8. John J, Donald WH: Asymptomatic gonorrhea in men. Br J Vener Dis 54:322, 1978.
9. Kassopoulou E, Tomlinson MJ, Banet CLR, et al: Origin of reactive oxygen species in semen; spermatozoa or leukocytes. J Reprod Fertil 94:463–470, 1992.
10. Liebovich LI, Goldwasser B: The spectrum of AIDS-associated testicular disorder. Urology 44:818–824, 1994.
11. Menkveld K, Kruger TF: Sperm morphology and male urogenital infection. Andrology 30(Suppl):49–53, 1998.
12. Moskowitz MO, Mellinger BC: Sexually transmitted disease and their relation to male infertility. Urol Clin North Am 19:35–46, 1992.
13. Muller CH, Coombs RW, Krieger JN: Effects of clinical stage and immunological states on semen analysis in HIV type-1 seropositive men. Andrology 30(Suppl 1):15–22, 1998.
14. Ness RB, Markovic N, Carlson CL, Coughlin MT: Do men become infertile after having sexually transmitted urethritis? An epidemiologic examination. Fertil Steril 68:205–213, 1997.
15. Pinto PA, Mellinger BC: HPV in the male patient. Urol Clin North Am 26:797–808, 1999.
16. Sauer MV, Chang PL: Establishing a clinical program for HIV-1 seropositive men to father seronegative children by means of IVF-ICSI. Am J Obstet Gynecol 186:627–633, 2002.
17. Sharma RK, Agarwal A: Role of reactive oxygen species in male infertility. Urology 48:835–850, 1996.
18. Skekarriz NM, Sharma RK, Thomas AJ Agarwal A: Positive myeloperoxidase staining (Endtz test) as an indicator of excessive reactive oxygen species formation in semen. J Assist Reprod Genet 12:70–74, 1995.
19. Siegel JF, Mellinger BC: Human papillomavirus in the male patient. . Urol Clin North Am 19:83–92, 1992.
20. Walsh PC, Retik AB, Vaughan ED, Wein AJ (eds): Campbells Urology , 8th ed. Philadelphia, W.B. Saunders, 2002.
21. Wein AJ, Elder JS: The AUA Annual Review Course. Houston, American Urological Association Office of Education, 2000.
22. Wentworth BB, Bonin P, Holmes KK, et al: Isolation of virus, bacteria and other organisms from venereal disease clinic patients: Methodology and problems associated with multiple isolates. Health Lab Sci 10:75, 1973.
23. Wilson TW, Frankel F, Vultch F, et al: Testicular tumors in men with HIV. J Urol 147:1038–1040, 1992.
24. Witkin SS, Jerimias J, Grifi JA, Ledger WJ: Detection of *Chlamydia trachomatis* in semen by the polymerase chain reaction in male members of infertile couples. Am J Obstet Gynecol 168:1957–1962, 1993.
25. Wolff H: The biologic significance of WBC's in semen. Fertil Steril 63:1143–1157, 1995.
26. Zenilman JM: Update on bacterial sexually transmitted disease. Urol Clin North Am 19:25–34, 1992.

8. OBSTRUCTION AZOOSPERMIA

Joel L. Marmar, M.D.

1. When azoospermia is reported on a semen analysis, what should the clinician do with the specimen or with additional specimens?

1. **Check the semen volume.** According to the World Health Organization (WHO), the normal semen volume should be 2.0 ml or more. In cases of azoospermia, a low semen volume may be associated with retrograde ejaculation, ejaculatory duct obstruction, or absence of the seminal vesicles and vas deferens. Historically, most cases of retrograde ejaculation are related to alterations of normal bladder neck closure resulting from transurethral resection of the bladder neck, Y-V plasty of the bladder neck, or medical conditions such as diabetic neuropathy and/or treatment with antihypertensive medication. In the laboratory, postejaculatory urine should be examined for sperm in patients with a low semen volume. On physical examination, a careful palpation of the scrotal contents is necessary to document the possible absence of the vas deferens. For imaging, transrectal ultrasound of the prostate or a CT scan of the pelvis may document the presence or absence of the seminal vesicle and the condition of the ejaculatory duct (normal or dilated/obstructed).

2. **Measure fructose.** The seminal plasma contains the sugar fructose that originates from the seminal vesicles. A simple office procedure can evaluate the presence or absence of fructose using a colorimetric technique. An aliquot of 0.25 ml seminal plasma and 0.25 ml of 0.1% resorcinol in ethenol can be mixed in a test tube. After the addition of 1 ml of water to each tube, the solution is heated over the flame for approximately 7 minutes. The observation of red coloration confirms the presence of fructose. However, some men with bilateral congenital absence of the vas deferens (BCAVD) have only remnants of the seminal vesicles. In such cases, the red coloration is pale. In other cases of complete ejaculatory duct obstruction, the color of the fluid remains clear (no red color) because of the absence of fructose secondary to complete obstruction. Transrectal ultrasound of the prostate may demonstrate dilation of the ejaculatory duct, which may be amenable to transurethral resection to relieve the obstruction.

3. **Consider the need for spinning down the sample to look for "virtual azoospermia" or cryptospermia.** In cases of azoospermia, several investigators have advocated extended sperm preparation (ESP) in the search for sperm. The semen specimens from azoospermic men were centrifuged, droplets from the pellet were examined, and in some cases sperm that may be useful for ICSI were identified. This procedure may eliminate the need for testicular biopsy and epididymal aspiration.

4. **Consider the need for repeating the test.** At least three semen samples should be observed within 6 months to avoid misleading interpretation of transient results, because even fertile donors occasionally produce a sample with no sperm in the ejaculate.

2. How frequently is male infertility due to obstruction of the excurrent ductal system?

According to 1997 WHO survery, causes of infertility include disturbances in both partners (26%), disturbances in the female partner (39%), and disturbances in the male partner (20%). No identifiable cause was found in 15% of cases. Of these diagnoses, 1.5% were attributed to obstruction of the excurrent duct system.

3. Can obstruction present as secondary infertility?

Secondary infertility can result from (1) intermittent or permanent obstruction to the ejaculatory duct, (2) obstruction to the epididymis due to associated epididymitis, and (3) iatrogenic obstruction of the vas due to a prior vasectomy or hernia surgery. The detection of secondary infertility due to obstruction can be suggested by a careful history and physical examination. Specific types of obstruction are considered below.

4. What clues suggest obstruction of the ejaculatory duct/seminal vesicles?

A history of pain with ejaculation or pressure in the perineum at the time of ejaculation may suggest obstruction of the ejaculatory duct and the cause of azoospermia. These findings suggest the use of transrectal ultrasonography (TRUS) to evaluate the prostate, seminal vesicles, and ejaculatory duct.

5. What measurements by TRUS suggest obstruction of the ejaculatory duct and dilation of the seminal vesicles?

The normal seminal vesicle width is 0.4–1.4 cm, the normal seminal vesicle length is 1.9–4.1 cm, the ejaculatory duct is 0.04–0.08 cm in diameter, and the normal vas deferens diameter is 0.26–0.4 cm. Several investigators suggest that a seminal vesicle width greater than 1.5 cm represents obstruction of the ejaculatory duct.

6. Discuss the value of MRI in the evaluation of obstruction of the ejaculatory duct/ seminal vesicles.

Although MRI imaging is more expensive then TRUS, it is capable of providing multiplanar images with greater sensitivity to differentiate tissue substances. The initial MRI of a the seminal vesicles, prostate, and ejaculatory duct may be performed with standard body coils, but endorectal coils and fast spin-echo MRI imaging have been used to provide details of the excretory duct system. In general, T1-weighted spin-echo images show fat as the principal tissue; it appears bright, whereas water appears dark. In the T2-weighted images the reverse is true. In T1-weighted images, the seminal vesicles have a signal intensity equal to or greater than that of skeletal muscle and always greater than that of urine. When T2-weighted images are used, the signal intensity depends on the age and androgen status of the patient. The signal intensity is usually equal to or less than that of fat in prepubertal patients and men older than 70 years. Postpubertal men have signal intensities equal to or greater than those of fat, but there may be exceptions in various clinical conditions. The convolutions of the seminal vesicles are best documented with a low signal intensity on a T2-weighted image or T1-weighted images with contrast enhancement.

7. What clues suggest epididymal obstruction?

A history of testicular pain or testicular swelling, especially in association with a urinary tract infection, may suggest epididymitis leading to epididymal obstruction. A history of orchiditis secondary to *Neisseria gonorrhoeae, Chlamydia trachomatis,* or species of *Enterobacter* may lead to epididymal involvement. Physical examination may reveal distinct epididymal thickening, which can be documented by scrotal ultrasound.

Occasionally, direct trauma to the testis and epididymis, such as penetrating wounds or gun shot wounds, may be the source of epididymal obstruction. Orchidopexy of the contralateral side following torsion of the testicle may cause epididymal obstruction by the placement of the pexing suture through the epididymis.

8. What clues suggest vasal obstruction?

The history may identify the source of vasal obstruction, such as prior elective vasectomy or bilateral inguinal surgery (e.g., hernia repair). The physical examination may document bilateral congenital absence of the vas, which is another source of obstructive azoospermia.

9. What is the value of a vasogram in the evaluation of vasal obstruction?

Vasograms have been used less often in clinical practice, but they have a role for the workup of selected cases. Vasograms may be needed, along with testicular biopsy (see question 14), in men with prior inguinal hernia surgery to document obstruction and to determine whether surgical reconstruction is feasible. Recently, newer microsurgical techniques have been proposed for vasography to avoid iatrogenic damage to the vas during the study. The vas may be punctured with microscopic guidance, using a 30-gauge lymph angiogram needle. Alternatively, a micro vasotomy can be performed with a 1.5-mm microblade along the length of the vas and placement of a 24-gauge angiocath in the direction toward the prostate. Following vasography, the opening in the vas is closed with microtechnique using 9–0 nylon sutures.

10. How is a fluoroscopy or x-ray vasogram performed?

A vasogram with contrast must be done carefully. The contrast should be diluted 1:1 with saline to avoid irritation to the vas mucosa. Only a small volume of contrast is injected initially (0.2–0.5 ml) to avoid rupture. If the vas proves to be patent, larger volumes of contrast may be used to gently fill the ejaculatory duct and seminal vesicals.

11. Is fluoroscopy or x-ray always needed to document obstruction of the vas during vasography?

As an alternative, a 2–0 Prolene suture may be used as a probe and measure obstruction by advancement of the suture through the vasostomy to the point of blockage. The length of suture documents the anatomic location of the blockage and may be helpful for choosing the site of the incision for reconstructive microsurgery. In addition, methylene blue or indigo carmine dyes may be injected into the angiocatheter after a Foley is placed into the bladder. If blue dye appears in the urine of the Foley drainage, the vas is patent.

12. Can partial obstruction of the vas be treated by vasography?

Sequential irrigation of the vas may flush through a partial obstruction. This technique is accomplished by using increasing larger syringes filled with saline (1 ml tuberculin, 3-ml syringe, 5-ml syringe, and 10-ml syringe). The saline-filled syringes may be injected through an angiocath inserted into the vas lumen after microvasotomy. By irrigating with the increasing volumes of fluid and syringes, the operator can feel resistance to the irrigation and report the specific syringe and volume that demonstrate the first feeling of complete resistance. The operator must limit the irrigation at this point to avoid rupture of the ejaculator duct or seminal vesicle. However, in cases with a partial obstruction, the feeling of resistance will disappear during the sequential irrigation. Once the vas lumen feels patent and the irrigation flows freely, diluted methylene blue or indigo carmine can be flushed through the angiocatheter. The color will appear in the Foley catheter after compression over the urinary bladder. A carefully done procedure of this type with microscopic closure can be repeated in the event that a partial ejaculatory duct obstruction becomes closed at a later date. This technique may relieve partial ejaculatory duct obstruction and lead to pregnancies in 30–40% of these specific cases.

13. Discuss the value of hormone assays in the evaluation of azoospermia.

In clinical practice, it is important to distinguish the hormonal status of patients with oligospermia and azoospermia. Most men will have normal hormonal assays, but some may have hormonal imbalances that include low serum testosterone and low serum levels of follicle-stimulating hormones (FSH) and luteinizing hormone (LH) (i.e., hypogonadotrophic hypogonadism, or Kallman's syndrome). This group may be treatable with hormone replacement therapy.

Some men with azoospermia may have end-organ failure. They demonstrate elevated FSH (hypergonadotrophic hypogonadism) associated with reduced testicular function and internal scarring of the seminiferous tubules. The testes may be small by measurement. In the past, this group was considered untreatable, but recently some of these men have been candidates for sperm aspiration and ICSI. An elevated FSH does not exclude the patient from therapy, but the hormone assays are an important part of the work-up. Men with elevated FSH values may be considered for microsurgical testicular explorations for sperm retrieval, and in some cases pockets of sperm may be found even among men with the predominant histology of Sertoli cell only and maturation arrest. These sperm may be used for ICSI.

14. What is the value of testicular biopsy in the evaluation of nonobstructive and obstructive infertility?

The histology of the testis biopsy distinguishes between nonobstructive and obstructive infertility. In cases of **nonobstructive azoospermia** (NOA), the histology distinguishes among hypospermatogenesis, maturation arrest, and Sertoli cell only The presence of late spermatids or spermatozoa in the biopsy may foretell the ability to retrieve sperm from testis tissue at the time of ICSI with standard percutaneous or open biopsies. Furthermore, excess biopsy material may be cryopreserved and stored for future use in fertility management.

The author performs a limited percutaneous diagnostic biopsy on azoospermic men so that they have a full understanding of their chances of having sperm available for ICSI. If no spermatozoa are seen in the limited biopsy, the patient may be offered the option of microsurgical testicular sperm retrieval. With this approach, some patients without sperm on the diagnostic biopsy choose to proceed with sperm retrieval, with donor sperm as a backup for ICSI. Others decline surgery and choose insemination of the female partner with donor sperm.

In **obstructive azoospermia,** the testicular biopsy generally demonstrates 15–20 spermatids per round tubule. In cases of congenital absence of the vas deferens, diagnostic biopsies are probably no longer necessary because other reports indicate that these men usually have normal spermatogenesis within the seminiferous tubules. However, simplified percutaneous testis aspiration biopsies enable the urologist to obtain seminiferous tissue with minimal trauma and thereby establish the diagnosis.

15. What is the incidence of antisperm antibodies in evaluation of obstructed infertility?

Clinically, antisperm antibodies are found in 3–12% of men who undergo an evaluation for infertility compared to 0–1% of the general population. Immunologic infertility may be suggested by poor postcoital tests as well as the appearance of "shaking" motion or a clumping on semen analysis. Antisperm antibodies are found in three locations: serum, seminal plasma, and sperm surface. Two specific antibodies are thought to be clinically relevant. IgG antibodies is thought to be derived from transudation of the bloodstream, and IgA is thought to be locally derived from prostatic secretions.

Among men with prior vasectomies, antibodies are detected in the blood stream in about 50% of the cases, but after reconstructive microsurgery (vasovasostomies) antibodies appear in the semen in only about 10–12% of cases. The antibodies may be detected in the laboratory by means of immunobeads on both serum and seminal sperm. The motile sperm attract anti-IgG and IgA antibody beads to their surface. Such patients usually experience infertility when high titers of antibodies cover the sperm head or sperm tail. In the former cases, the sperm have difficulty penetrating through the cervical mucous. In the latter cases, the tail antibodies limit motility, and semen analysis shows clumping.

16. What therapies are available for sperm antibodies?

Sperm washing and IUI may be carried out among patients with limited titers of sperm antibodies; the pregnancy rate has been reported at about 30%. Most recently, ICSI has been used even among patients with greater than 80% antibody titers, resulting in pregnancy rates of 35–40% and implantation rates of 20–23%. The use of steroids has diminished in recent years because of the reported complications associated with aseptic necrosis of the femoral head.

17. What are the treatment modalities for obstruction of the ejaculatory ducts?

The obstruction may be amendable to surgical treatment that relieves the obstruction so that sperm return to ejaculate. This surgery can generally be performed transurethrally (transurethral resection of the ejaculatory ducts) or endoscopically. Alternatively, sperm can be retrieved from testis, epididymis, or other parts of the excurrent ductal system for assisted reproduction.

18. Is transurethral resection of the ejaculatory duct (TURED) a reasonable procedure?

When ejaculatory duct obstruction is documented, some clinicians resect the verumontanum to expose the ejaculatory duct. The author prefers resection proximal to the verumontanum but distal to the bladder neck to avoid retrograde ejaculation. A small 24- French, one-handed resectoscope is used. An O'Connor drape allows the prostate to be elevated during the resection to provide control of depth for the resecting loop. A small loop and reduced power are used for the electrocautery device. When the resection is completed, the dilated ejaculatory ducts become observable in the area of resection.

19. What complications may be seen after TURED?

Long-term reflux of urine into the vas and seminal vesicles may cause postvoid dribbling and infection. Furthermore, long-term urinary reflux may affect the epididymis, leading to epididymitis or epididymal obstruction. In the presence of epididymal obstruction, no sperm appear in the ejaculate despite successful TURED, as documented by vasography or opacification of the seminal vesicle by direct injection of ultrasonic guidance. Such men may require scrotal exploration and vasoepididymostomy.

20. Discuss the value of cystoscopy in the evaluation of recurrent ejaculatory duct obstruction.

After resection of the ejaculatory duct, excessive postoperative scarring may cause restenosis. During cystoscopy, the recurrent scar can be observed by direct vision. In some of these cases, the strictures may be reopened cystoscopically with a guide wire passed into the ejaculatory duct. A balloon dilator is placed over the guide wire to reopen the ejaculatory duct. This procedure can be performed repetitively on different occasions.

21. Can an ejaculatory duct obstruction be managed by percutaneous puncture and ultrasonic guidance?

As an alternative to TURED, a minimally invasive procedure has been developed that uses transrectal puncture of the seminal vesicle by ultrasonic guidance and antegrade balloon dilation of the ejaculatory duct with fluoroscopy. Initially, the seminal vesicle is aspirated with a 35-cm long, 21-gauge needle. In cases of complete and partial ejaculatory duct obstruction, the aspirated fluid usually contains sperm. In contrast, fluid from the nonobstructive seminal vesicles usually has no sperm. When obstruction is documented and treatment is indicated, a small amount of contrast is injected through the 21-gauge needle into the seminal vesicle with fluoroscopic guidance. An angiographic guide wire is advanced through the needle into the seminal vesicle, and the needle is withdrawn. A 5-French angiocatheter is advanced over the guide wire and then manipulated into the ejaculatory duct. An 0.035 heavy-duty straight guide wire is passed through the catheter and through the ejaculatory duct into the urethra. It is retrieved with a grasper during cystoscopy. A 5-mm angiographic balloon dilation catheter is advanced in retrograde fashion through the urethra and over the guide wire and positioned in the ejaculatory duct. The position of the balloon is confirmed by cystoscopic observation and fluoroscopy before it is maximally inflated to complete the dilation of the ejaculatory duct. This technique avoids direct puncture of the vas lumen and the need for vasography; it also avoids any resection of the prostate gland.

22. What are the treatment options for obstructive azoospermia versus nonobstructive azoospermia?

In cases of **obstructive azoospermia,** the patient has two therapeutic options. He may choose reconstructive microsurgery or sperm aspiration from the epididymis and testis for ICSI. Many decisions are based on the economic realities of the case. Some insurance companies cover vasectomy reversal and reconstruction of the epididymis, but they may fail to cover advanced assisted reproductive techniques such as IVF or ICSI. Recently, many states have mandated insurance coverage for IVF/ICSI. Thus, both reconstructive microsurgery and sperm aspiration are available. The results of reconstructive microsurgery are discussed in a later chapters.

Men with **nonobstructive azoospermia** and detection of sperm on the diagnostic biopsy are candidates for ICSI with fresh or frozen testis tissue. If sperm are absent from the seminiferous tubules on biopsy, they are still potential candidates for microsurgical testicular sperm retrieval in search of pockets of sperm in connection with ICSI. Sperm may be retrieved in 20–30% of such cases.

23. What options are available to retrieve epididymal sperm secondary to obstruction?

The first pregnancies with epididymal sperm and in vitro fertilization (IVF) occurred in 1985 following open dissection of the epididymis under general anesthesia. Until 1994, most urologists continued to perform open dissection of the epididymis to retrieve sperm. In 1995, less traumatic percutaneous procedures were developed to acquire sperm. The epididymis was punctured with a 21- to 23-gauge butterfly needle with tubing attached to a 20-ml syringe and a pistol grip. After vacuum was applied, only droplets were accumulated in the tubing; a hemostat was clamped to the tubing above the droplets to secure the specimen. These droplets represent the specimen and contain 1–5 million sperm per ml. Presently, in cases of obstructive azoospermia, epididymal sperm aspiration is performed along with testis aspiration biopsy as long as the epididymis is easily palpable. The embryologist may choose the sperm for ICSI, but most embryologists prefer the epididymal sperm because these spermatozoa are already in a fluid medium. The testis tissue generally requires some dissection to free the sperm, and some embryologists are uncomfortable with this type of specimen.

24. What are the treatment options for obstruction of the vas?

When couples are counseled, the outcomes of vasectomy reversal surgery must be discussed in terms consistent with the clinical situation that applies to their specific condition. For example, in a large series that studied the outcome of vasovasostomy (VV) in 1762 patients from all categories, the rate of delivered infants after VV was 76% when the obstructed interval was less than 3 years, 53% when the interval was 3–8 years, 44% when the interval was 9–14 years, and 30% when the intervals were greater than 15 years. More recently, the results of vasectomy reversals among men with obstructed intervals greater than 15 years was reported. About 60% of these men required unilateral or bilateral vasoepididymostomies, and the reported rate of delivered infants was 38%. Another study reviewed birth rates with microsurgical vasectomy reversal specifically for couples with female partners greater than 37 years of age. They reported a live birth rate of 17% among 23 couples followed for more than 1 year. Thus, it seems important for urologists to counsel patients about specific outcomes related to the interval of obstruction and the female partner's age.

25. What are the operative treatments for obstruction of the epididymis?

A vasoepididymostomy is a more difficult surgical procedure, but with the use of specific tubule anastomosis the rates of delivered infants range from 25% to 42%. However, the time to pregnancy may be lengthy, with a range of 9–30 months. Recently, new methods for VE have used the invagination of a single epididymal tubule into the vas lumen. After invagination, the epididymal tubule seems to incorporate into the mucosa of the vas lumen. The first appearance of sperm with these techniques seemed shorter compared with conventional anastomoses and the outcome may lead to earlier pregnancies, but more data are needed to evaluate such methods.

26. When should IVF/ICSI be considered as a treatment option in obstructive azoospermia?

Couples considering vasectomy reversals vs. sperm aspiration and ICSI must be fully informed of the implications of each procedure so that they may select the option that best suits their specific chances for success. Sperm aspiration and ICSI have the advantage of being less invasive for the male but expose the female to one or more cycles of hormone stimulation and needle aspiration of the ovaries. Sperm aspiration and ICSI offer the opportunity to establish a pregnancy during the first cycle, but the rate of delivered infants on the first cycle is between 25% and 27% with female partners under 37 years of age. As a result, about 75% of the couples are candidates for repeat cycles. When the female partners were older than 37 years, the rate of delivered infants with sperm aspiration and ICSI is only about 15%. Over time, the results with reconstructive microsurgery might be more economical and lead to more delivered infants. The cost of a newborn after vasectomy reversal is about $28,530. In contrast, with sperm aspiration and ICSI, the estimated cost per newborn for female partners less than 37 years of age was $48,200, and for female partners older than 37 years of age the cost was estimated at $99,940 per newborn. In addition, the rate of multiple births with low-birth-weight babies ranges between 25% and 30% with ICSI. All of the facts concerning clinical outcome and economics should be discussed with the couple at the time of their initial office appointment so that they can intelligently chose the treatment options that best suit their needs.

BIBLIOGRAPHY

1. Marmar JL: The emergence of specialized procedures for the acquisition, processing and cryopreservation of epididymal and testicular sperm in connection with intra cytoplasmic sperm injection. J Androl 19:517–562, 1998.
2. Marmar JL: The diagnosis and treatment of male infertility in the new millennium. Int J Fertil Womens Med 46(3):116–136, 2001.
3. Marmar JL, Seligman ES: Seminal vesicularography and vasography. In Pollack HM, McClennon BL (eds): Clinical Urography. Philadelphia, W.B. Saunders, 2000, pp 378–387.
4. Nieschlag E, Behre HM (eds): Andrology. Male Reproductive Health and Dysfunction. Berlin, Springer-Verlag, 1997
5. Seligman ES, Marmar JL: Pathophysiology, treatment and imaging of male infertility. In Pollack HM, McClennon BL (eds): Clinical Urography. Philadelphia, W.B. Saunders, 2000, pp 3013–3029.
6. World Health Organization Manual for the Examination of Human Semen and Sperm-Cervical Mucus Interaction, 4th ed. Cambridge, Cambridge University Press, 1999.

9. NONOBSTRUCTIVE AZOOSPERMIA

Robert Oates, M.D.

1. What is nonobstructive azoospermia (NOA)?

Azoospermia, or the absence of spermatozoa in ejaculate, can be due either to obstruction of the excurrent ductal system (obstructive azoospermia) or to a problem with sperm production. The latter form of azoospermia is termed nonobstructive azoospermia. Other terms that have been used to describe the condition include testicular failure or spermatogenic failure. NOA represents the most severe form of male infertility, and its management poses significant challenges to andrologists.

2. What are the semen analysis findings in men with NOA?

By definition, the semen specimen is azoospermic. The volume is > 1 ml, and the pH is alkaline. In men with NOA, the problem lies in testicular spermatogenesis, not with patency or anomalies of the excurrent ductal system. The seminal vesicles contribute 70% of the fluid to the ejaculate, the prostate about 20%, and the vasa 10%. The seminal vesicles empty their alkaline contents through the ejaculatory ducts (along with the vasal fluids) into the prostatic urethra during the emission phase of the ejaculatory sequence. This volume overwhelms the small amount of acidic prostatic secretions; the typical ejaculate is, therefore, alkaline (pH > 7.0).

Because the vasa, seminal vesicles, ejaculatory ducts, and prostate are normal in men with NOA, so are semen volume (> 1 ml) and pH (> 7.0). Conversely, in men with congenital bilateral absence of the vas deferens (CBAVD, in which the distal vasa and seminal vesicles are atrophic, aplastic, or dysfunctional) or with complete ejaculatory duct obstruction (blockage of the ejaculatory ducts prevents the seminal vesicles and vasa from emptying their contents into the prostatic urethra), the ejaculate represents only prostatic fluid and is typically < 1 ml in volume and has a pH < 7.0. Hence, the volume and pH are important parameters of the azoospermic semen specimen because a preliminary differential diagnosis is easily based on these two factors.

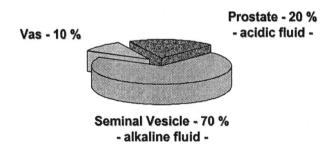

Vas - 10 %

Prostate - 20 %
- acidic fluid -

Seminal Vesicle - 70 %
- alkaline fluid -

Contributory sources to normal ejaculate.

3. Is semen fructose helpful as a measurement in men with NOA?

No. Semen fructose does not need to be measured in men with NOA if they have normal semen volume and pH, indicating that the seminal vesicles contribute to the ejaculate. Because fructose is a component of the secretions of the seminal vesicles, attention to the volume and pH obviates the need for a fructose assay. Conversely, if the volume and pH are low, indicating the presence only of prostatic fluid, there is no need to measure seminal fructose, because a diagnosis of CBAVD or ejaculatory duct obstruction with no contribution to the ejaculate from the seminal vesicles is already obvious.

4. What is cryptospermia?

In men with cryptospermia or cryptozoospermia, sperm are found only in a centrifuged semen sample. If any motile sperm are seen in a centrifuged pellet, they may potentially be used as the sperm source for intracytoplasmic sperm injection (ICSI); thus, the need for surgical sperm harvesting is avoided.

5. Can a patient with of NOA ever have sperm in his ejaculate?

Yes. Patients with NOA may occasionally have some sperm in the ejaculate. Centrifugation and examination of the pellet are necessary to determine that the specimen is completely azoospermic. When spermatogenesis is severely compromised, the patient may have severe oligospermia, virtual azoospermia (a few sperm seen in the ejaculate on occasion), cryptospermia, or complete azoospermia (the level of sperm production within the testis is so low that no individual sperm can be detected in the semen).

6. Is one azoospermic specimen sufficient for a diagnosis?

No. Sperm counts fluctuate around a baseline in all men. If the baseline is exceedingly low, on most days the ejaculate will be azoospermic, but occasionally it may demonstrate some sperm. These sperm may be useable (see above). If any sperm are seen, the diagnoses of CBAVD, complete bilateral ejaculatory duct obstruction, or other forms of complete obstruction of the excurrent ductal system are unlikely.

7. What items in the history are important in helping to make the diagnosis of NOA?

Obvious clues that lead to suspicion of NOA that suggest or predict spermatogenic compromise:

- A long duration of primary infertility with no evident female factors implies a significant male factor.
- Cryptorchidism, especially if bilateral, occurs when the prenatal testis is not able to direct its own descent into the scrotum. This unspecified "abnormality of function" may present in adulthood as compromised sperm production. Whether early orchidopexy, as now practiced, will reverse these later effects is not yet clearly known.
- Chemotherapeutic agents used for both benign and malignant disease have a profound immediate effect on spermatogenesis. Most postpubertal males become azoospermic shortly after chemotherapy initiation. Depending on the medication and the duration of treatment (alkylating agents are the most spermatotoxic), permanent azoospermia may result. Parenthetically, in about 60% of postchemotherapy men with NOA sperm can be retrieved from testis tissue (see below).
- Testicular trauma, torsion, or tumor may hint at resultant spermatogenic compromise.
- Sparse beard growth, inability to build muscle and gain strength, or decreased libido may be indications that the androgenic axis has failed; as a consequence, spermatogenesis is most often adversely affected as well.
- In practice, however, most men with NOA have no history that would forecast spermatogenic inefficiency.

8. What physical examination findings may be present in men with NOA?

In general, there are no signature phenotypic manifestations of NOA. Because the bulk of each testis is composed of the seminiferous tubules, a reduction in tubular diameter or mass leads to a smaller, softer testis. The ductal structures are palpably normal as there is no obstructive process present. However, if a specific etiology underlies the NOA, certain physical signs may be detectable. For example, a male with Klinefelter syndrome (KS) may also be hypogonadal due to a compromised androgenic axis (Leydig cells are also dysfunctional in KS) and demonstrate eunichoid body proportions as well as decreased beard growth and muscle mass. The testes are most often quite atrophic and have a firm consistency. A male with idiopathic hypogonadotropic hypogonadism (IHH) is also poorly virilized secondary to lack of hypothalamic/pituitary function with consequent failure of stimulation of both the androgenic and spermatogenic axes of the testes. Certain major chromosomal abnormalities involving the Y chromosome, such as ring Y, may have other phenotypic expressions (e.g., short stature).

9. Are imaging studies necessary in the diagnosis of NOA?

Because NOA is due to failure of optimal spermatogenesis and not to ductal blockage, no imaging studies are worthwhile. Semen volume and pH are normal because the seminal vesicles and vasa ampullae are able to deliver their contents through the ejaculatory ducts into the prostatic urethra. Therefore, transrectal ultrasonography, which images these structures, is not helpful. Scrotal ultrasonography is not helpful if the vasa are palpable, the epididymis is nondistended, and the testes are either of adequate or small size. Scrotal ultrasound adds nothing beyond the findings of a careful physical examination.

10. What endocrine studies are important in the diagnosis of NOA?

The hypothalamus secretes gonadotropin-releasing hormone (GnRH), which stimulates production of follicle-stimulating hormone (FSH) and luteinizing hormone (LH) by the pituitary. FSH targets the Sertoli cell and is required, at the very least, for initiation of spermatogenesis. Inhibin is released from the Sertoli cell and regulates, via a negative feedback, the elaboration of FSH. LH directs the Leydig cell to produce testosterone, which has both local paracrine-like actions necessary for spermatogenesis and a distal feedback function regulating LH release. If a primary abnormality of the germ cells results in depressed spermatogenesis, inhibin levels are lower and FSH secretion increases in a compensatory manner. Therefore, in general, serum FSH values rise as spermatogenesis decreases and are a valuable, although indirect, indicator of spermatogenic capability. If the androgenic axis is also affected by whatever pathologic process limits sperm production, testosterone levels may be low while its feedback-loop partner LH may be higher than typically seen. Hence, FSH, LH, and testosterone measurements are helpful in the azoospermic patient to secure the diagnosis of NOA and to pinpoint the etiology.

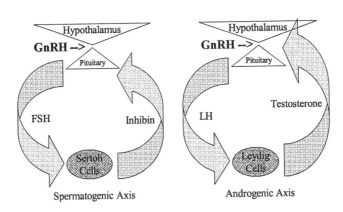

The hypothalamic-pituitary-gonadal axis.

11. What patterns of FSH, LH, and testosterone may be seen in various causes of NOA?

If we view FSH as a reflection of the spermatogenic axis and LH/testosterone as a mirror of the androgenic axis, a diagnosis of whether the cause lies at the hypothalamic/pituitary or testicular level can generally be made quite easily.

1. If FSH is elevated while LH and testosterone are totally normal, the hypothalamus and pituitary are functioning normally and the Leydig cells are producing testosterone without difficulty. The elevated FSH indicates that spermatogenesis is deficient at the germ-cell level. This deficiency may be due to microdeletions in the AZFc region (see Chapters 12 and 13) or other genetic aberrations of germ-cell mitosis or meiosis.

2. If FSH and LH are elevated and testosterone is low, both the spermatogenic and androgenic axes of the testes are deficient while the hypothalamus and pituitary are responding appro-

priately and trying their best to provide compensatory stimulation. Such a pattern is often seen in men with 47, XXY Klinefelter syndrome.

3. If FSH, LH, and testosterone are all exceedingly low, the hypothalamic-pituitary team is not releasing the necessary stimulatory hormones for both spermatogenesis and androgen production. In these cases of hypogonadotropic hypogonadism, the testicle may have a normal potential that is not being realized secondary to lack of stimulation. Cases of idiopathic hypogonadotropic hypogonadism (IHH) may be X-linked, autosomal dominant, or autosomal recessive in their transmission pattern. For example, Kallmann syndrome (IHH coupled with anosmia) is X-linked.

4. If the testosterone level is adequate or high while FSH and LH are markedly suppressed, the testosterone is likely exogenous in origin. Often the patient is a body builder or weight lifter and uses supplemental anabolic steroids of various types, dosages, and routes of administration; physical appearance is usually an obvious sign. Because testosterone must be produced by the Leydig cells for spermatogenesis to occur, an exogenous testosterone supply leads to feedback inhibition of GnRH/LH release and consequent lack of Leydig-cell stimulation.

FSH	LH	TESTOSTERONE	DIAGNOSIS	EXAMPLE
Elevated	Normal	Normal	Spermatogenic failure	AZFc microdeletion
Elevated	Elevated	Low	Testicular failure	Klinefelter syndrome
Extremely low	Extremely low	Extremely low	Hypogonadotropic hypogonadism	Kallmann syndrome
Extremely low	Extremely low	Normal/high	Exogenous testosterone	Body builder

12. What is a "normal" FSH level?

The reference range published for each assay on the report sheet is not equivalent in concept to the normal range in regard to FSH. Pituitary output of FSH increases steadily as spermatogenesis decreases (less inhibin is released from the Sertoli cells). Therefore, there is no absolute level of serum FSH below which spermatogenesis is "normal" and above which spermatogenesis is "abnormal." The serum FSH value must be interpreted in the context of the clinical situation. For example, if the reference range happens to be 2–20 mIU/ml for a particular assay and the measured FSH is 10 mIU/ml in the context of prior chemotherapy, small, soft testes, normal semen volume and pH, and azoospermia, the FSH level represents compensatory output by the pituitary secondary to poor spermatogenesis. This FSH level fits the circumstance nicely; it is not to be interpreted as "normal" with a conclusion that, since it is "normal," spermatogenesis is adequate and the implied cause of the azoospermia is an obstructive process.

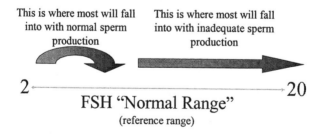

FSH: what is normal?

13. Is a diagnostic testis biopsy necessary in azoospermic patients?

No. A testis biopsy is not required to make the diagnosis of either obstructive or nonobstructive azoospermia.

1. If the semen volume and pH are low, the testis size is adequate and the patient has no palpable vasa deferentia, the diagnosis is easily established as congenital absence of the vas deferens. No further diagnostic steps are necessary.

2. If the semen volume and pH are low, the testis size is adequate, and the patient has palpable vasa deferentia that feel full and firm, transrectal ultrasonography will most likely image an ejaculatory duct obstruction (e.g., midline prostatic cyst, dilated ejaculatory ducts, dilated seminal vesicles). No testis biopsy is necessary. No vasogram is necessary.

3. If the semen volume and pH are normal, the testis size is adequate, and the patient has palpable vasa deferentia, full and firm epididymides are indicative of obstruction at the level of the epididymis or vasal/epididymal junction. No testis biopsy and no vasogram are necessary prior to definitive reconstruction. A vasogram will only confirm distal ductal patency, which is already known since semen volume and pH are normal and will lead to scarring at the site of the intervention, possibly compromising reconstructive success.

4. If the semen volume and pH are normal, the testes are small and soft, the vasa and epididymides are palpable and not distended, and the serum FSH is above the lower aspects of the reference range, the diagnosis of NOA is straightforward. No preliminary testis biopsy is necessary. A histologic specimen can be sent at the time of formal testis sperm extraction (TESE).

14. What genetic evaluation is necessary in men with NOA?

If there is no obvious etiology for the NOA (e.g., prior chemotherapy, prior bilateral mumps orchitis), two tests should be performed before contemplating TESE: karyotype analysis and Y chromosomal microdeletion assay. These tests provide information on (1) the prognosis of sperm presence/absence during TESE, (2) genetic information for counseling the couple about the genetic risks to future offspring, and (3) health issues related to the genetic anomalies diagnosed.

15. Explain the value of karyotype analyis.

A karyotype assesses the structure and number of chromosomes in the cell. Anomalies that can be diagnosed with a karyotype analysis include balanced translocation and aneuploidy. A **balanced translocation** (pieces of different chromosomes flip-flop) is found in approximately 3% of men with NOA. The translocation is "balanced"; hence his cells contain all of the genetic material (although not in the normal arrangement) required for optimal function and the patient is generally healthy. However, the process of sperm production (most likely meiosis) requires proper arrangement of all of the chromosomal material; if a translocation is present, spermatogenesis may be quantitatively reduced. In addition, individual spermatozoa may carry an unbalanced chromosomal complement and lead to a less-than-ideal outcome for an embryo or fetus.

Aneuploidy occurs when the total number of chromosomes is abnormal (either more or less than 46,XY in men). The most common chromosomal abnormality in azoospermic men is Klinefelter syndrome (47,XXY), which is present in 10% of such men. The androgenic axis must be carefully assessed before TESE is done because these men often have coexisting hypogonadism. Other less common but well-known aberrations in chromosomal number or structure include 46,XX male syndrome, isodicentric Y chromosomes, and ring Y chromosomes. Certainly, 46,XX males are missing all of the AZF regions (see below) and do not possess spermatozoa in their testis tissue. TESE does not yield sperm. Hence a karyotype can provide prognostic information.

16. Explain the value of the Y chromosomal microdeletion assay.

This polymerase chain reaction (PCR)-based blood test assesses the AZF regions on the long arm of the Y chromosome (Yq). These regions contain genes that are important in the process of spermatogenesis. In approximately 13% of men with NOA, the AZFc region is absent due to microdeletion of this segment of the chromosome. Spermatogenesis is severely compromised but may not be absent altogether. Any spermatozoa retrieved are capable of initiating pregnancy in an ICSI setting. All male offspring will have AZFc-deletions and are predicted to be infertile/sterile on reaching sexual maturity. The prognosis of sperm presence is abysmal if the AZFa region, the AZFb region, or a combination of AZFb and AZFc is found to be deleted.

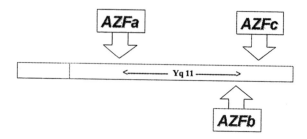

AZF regions on he long arm of the Y chromosome.

17. What is TESE?

Testis sperm extraction (TESE) is not to be confused with a testis biopsy. During a testis biopsy a small (3-mm) piece of testis tissue is sent in a fixative to the pathology department for histologic analysis. The pathologist fixes and stains the specimen and determines the "pattern" of spermatogenesis within the seminiferous tubules as well as any abnormalities in the interstitium (e.g., Leydig cell hyperplasia).

During TESE, the extracted tissue is minced and searched for the presence of whole spermatozoa. No fixation, no staining, and no pattern of spermatogenesis are described. The goal is simply to visualize complete sperm. The sperm may come from the 1 in 5, the 1 in 10, or the 1 in 1000 seminiferous tubules that are able to complete the spermatogenic process. They can be used on the same day in conjunction with ICSI, or the tissue can be cryopreserved for later use in conjunction with ICSI.

18. Should I bill for TESE using a testis biopsy code (CPT 54505)?

No. TESE is not a testis biopsy as defined for CPT use. In addition, TESE is a therapeutic rather than a diagnostic maneuver. Each insurance situation should be individually checked before the procedure.

19. Does the result of a testis biopsy predict the result of TESE?

The result of a testis biopsy does not absolutely predict whether sperm will be found upon TESE. Spermatozoa are more likely to be retrieved if hypospermatogenesis is seen on a previous biopsy than if only Sertoli cells are visualized, but no strict prediction can be made for an individual patient. Sperm may still be found in up to 30% of men with a prior biopsy that indicated Sertoli cell-only syndrome. The apparent discrepancy exists because the histologic assessment is done on only a few tubules, whereas TESE looks only for spermatozoa that may have come from any of a number of tubules in the tissue that will be minced and searched. Therefore, if the diagnosis of NOA is clearcut from history, physical examination, and laboratory data, a preliminary biopsy is not necessary before TESE.

20. Does the result of the genetic analysis predict the result of TESE?

Certain findings on karyotype or Y-chromosomal microdeletion assay predict the absence of sperm in the testis tissue during TESE. For this reason alone, both tests should be performed before any surgical intervention. For example, a 46,XX male is missing almost all of the Y chromosome and will have no sperm on TESE. The most distal aspect of Yp with the important sex-determining region (SRY) is typically translocated to one of the X chromosomes, but the entirety of the long arm, including the three AZF regions, is absent. Therefore, the result of karyotypic analysis is prognostic and spares the patient unnecessary testicular surgery. If the approach for the couple is to perform TESE in conjunction with a simultaneous ICSI cycle, the prior knowledge and certainty that TESE will be unsuccessful also spares the female partner an unnecessary ICSI stimulation. It is likely that AZFa microdeletions, AZFb microdeletions, combinations of AZFb and AZFc microdeletions, ring Y chromosomes, and many types of isodicentric Y chromosomes also forecast an absence of sperm in the seminiferous epithelium.

21. Does the result of the hormonal analysis predict the result of TESE?

No. Although generally serum FSH values rise as spermatogenesis decreases quantitatively, there is no specific FSH value below which sperm will always be found and above which no sperm will ever be found. FSH is a poor predictor of sperm presence/absence during TESE. In general, the same limitation applies to LH and testosterone. However, if testosterone output is exceedingly low while the LH level is high, indicating severe Leydig cell dysfunction, as may occur in some end-stage testes, the probability of finding sperm is lower.

22. Will sperm be found during TESE in men who have undergone prior chemotherapy?

It is certainly possible that sperm will be found in the testis tissue during TESE in men who have been left permanently azoospermic as a result of prior cytotoxic therapy. Approximately 60–70% of such men will have sperm that, when used as the source for ICSI, can indeed effect fertilization, embryo development, and term pregnancy of healthy offspring. Only with continued accumulation of patients will more accurate predictions be able to be made for an individual based on tumor type, regimen used, and exact agents. In general, alkylating agents have the most spermatotoxic affect, in both the short and the long term.

23. If the patient has a history of bilateral orchidopexy as a child, will sperm be found during TESE?

Yes. TESE may be successful where the underlying etiology is bilateral cryptorchidism. If unilateral cryptorchidism is present, repaired or not, the opposite, descended testis may have such poor spermatogenesis that azoospermia results. TESE may be successful in such cases.

24. If the man has CBAVD, might he also have deficient spermatogenesis?

Almost all men with CBAVD have perfectly adequate spermatogenesis. However, if the testes are small in size or soft in inconsistency, there may also be a problem with sperm production and a work-up, as detailed above, is indicated. This combination, however, is rare.

25. In summary, what steps should be taken in evaluation and treatment of azoospermic men?

- Record semen volume and pH, and formulate a set of possible differential diagnoses.
- Record history and note facts predictive of NOA or obstructive processes.
- Carefully examine the testes for size and consistency.
- Carefully examine the vasa and epididymides for presence/absence and obstruction.
- When azoospermia is not clearly due to obstruction, obtain FSH, LH, and testosterone levels as the initial hormonal evaluation.
- When NOA is probable, obtain genetic testing (karyotype and Y-chromosomal microdeletion assay).
- Discuss results of genetic analyses prior to TESE.
- Proceed to TESE if appropriate—either simultaneously with ICSI or as a preliminary event with cryopreservation.

BIBLIOGRAPHY

1. Damani M, Master V, Meng MV, et al: Post-chemotherapy azoospermia: Fatherhood with sperm from testis tissue using intracytoplasmic sperm injection" J Clin Oncol 2:930–936, 2002.
2. Damani M, Mittal R, Oates RD: Testicular tissue extraction in a young male with 47, XXY Klinefelter syndrome: Potential strategy for preservation of fertility. Fertil Steril 76:1054–1056, 2001.
3. Hopps CV, Goldstein M, Schlegel PN: The diagnosis and treatment of the azoospermic patient in the age of intracytoplasmic sperm injection. Urol Clin North Am 29:895–911, 2002.
4. Kuroda-Kawaguchi T, Skaletsky H, Brown LG, et al: The human Y chromosome's AZFc region features massive palindromes, uniform recurrent deletions, and testis gene families Nature Genet 29, 279–286, 2001.
5. Mulhall J, Burgess CM, Cunningham D, et al: Presence of mature sperm in testicular parenchyma of men with non-obstructive azoospermia: Prevelence and predictive factors. Urology 49: 91–96, 1997.

6. Mulhall J, Reijo R, Alagappan R, et al: Azoospermic men with deletion of the DAZ gene cluster are capable of completing spermatogenesis: Fertilization, normal embryonic development and pregnancy when retrieved testicular spermatozoa are used for intracytoplasmic sperm injection. Hum Reprod 12:503–508, 1997.

7. Oates RD: Genetic considerations in the treatment of male infertility. Infertil Reprod Med Clin North Am 13:551–585, 2002.

8. Oates RD: The azoospermic male: Diagnostic and therapeutic options. Serono Symposia USA Reproductive Health Online Continuing Medical Education Program, March, 2002.

9. Oates RD, Brown L, Silber SJ, Page D: Clinical characterization of 42 oligospermic or azoospermic men with microdeletion of the AZFc region of the Y chromosome, and of 18 children conceived via intracytoplasmic sperm injection. Hum Reprod 17:2813–2824, 2002.

10. Oates RD, Mulhall J, Burgess C, et al: Fertilization and pregnancy using intentionally cryopreserved testicular tissue as the sperm source for intracytoplasmic sperm injection in 10 men with non-obstructive azoospermia. Hum Reprod 12:734–739, 1997.

11. Sun C, Skaletsky H, Rozen R, et al:Deletion of AZFa (azoospermia factor a) region of human Y chromosome caused by recombination between HERV15 proviruses. Hum Molec Genet 9:2291–2296, 2000.

12. Vernaeve V, Tournaye H, Osmanagaoglu K, et al: Intracytoplasmic sperm injection with testicular spermatozoa is less successful in men with non-obstructive azoospermia than in men with obstructive azoospermia. Fertil Steril 79:529–533, 2003.

10. PEDIATRIC ISSUES IN MALE INFERTILITY
Yefim R. Sheynkin, M.D., FACS

1. What is the incidence of varicocele in the pediatric population?

Varicocele is present in about 15% of the adult male population, but it is uncommon to identify varicocele in boys younger than 9 years. In children below the age of 5, varicocele may be the presenting findings of a neoplasm (e.g. Wilms' tumor), which often causes ipsilateral renal vein obstruction. The incidence of varicocele detection gradually increases between 10 and 15 years to a reported incidence of 13.7–16.2% and remains constant thereafter.

2. What is special about varicoceles in the pediatric population compared with the adult population?

Presentation. Adult men with varicoceles in an infertility clinic often are "asymptomatic"; the only sign is impaired semen parameters. On the other hand, pediatric varicoceles presented to medical attention generally have significant clinical findings unrelated to infertility. The presentations may include pain, decrease in testicular size, and abnormal scrotal appearance due to the typical "bag-of-worms" appearance in high-grade varicoceles.

Treatment controversy. Since treatment of varicoceles generally requires surgery, the indication and timing of treatment in pediatric population have been topics of debate, especially in those who are asymptomatic with no sign of testicular atrophy (see question 11).

Follow-up issues. Semen analysis and improvement in fertility are usually not the outcome variables for evaluation of treatment benefits in the pediatric population. Instead, reduction of pain and increase in testicular volume (catch-up growth) are are more relevant outcome measurements in the pediatric population.

Recurrence rate. The recurrence rates of varicoceles are significantly higher in the pediatric population than in adults. Factors such as surgical techniques, smaller size of veins that are not identified and ligated (persistent varicocele), longer and closer follow-up, and growth of small veins that eventually become significant varicoceles may contribute to a higher recurrence rate.

3. What is the favored explanation of testicular damage by varicocele?

To date, heat stress due to elevation of scrotal temperature via reflux of warm blood through incompetent venous valves remains the favored explanation.

4. How does elevated temperature potentially affect testicular function?

DNA polymerase activity and the enzymes of DNA recombination in germ cells are temperature-sensitive, with optimal activity at 33°C, and protein synthesis in round spermatids has been shown to be optimal at 34°C. With the increase in temperature in patients with a varicocele, spermatogonial numbers have been reduced. It is also thought that an increase in testicular temperature is associated with increased apoptosis of germ cells and potential oxidative stress.

5. Describe the other theories of varicocele effect on testicular function.

Testicular damage with varicocele has been attributed to altered blood flow and venous stasis, increased hydrostatic pressure of the internal spermatic veins, adrenal reflux, endocrine imbalances, testicular paracrine imbalances, hypoxia, and enhancement of noxious effect of certain gonadotoxins.

6. Are histologic changes in the testis different in adults vs. adolescents with varicocele?

The histologic changes in the varicocele-affected adolescent testis are similar to those seen in adults but not as severe. The histology of the varicocele-affected testis indicates that all cell types and compartments can be involved. Degeneration and sloughing of germ cells into the lumen of the tubule or of germ cells in various stages of maturation arrest are commonly present. Sertoli cells also display ultra-structural changes and appear to slough portions of the adluminal cytoplasm. The basement membrane of the seminiferous tubule is often thickened.

7. What is the hallmark of clinical presentation in pediatric varicocele?

The hallmark of testicular damage in adolescents with varicocele is a discrepancy in testicular size. Testicular volume during preadolescence is relatively constant. Prospective randomized studies have shown that in boys with varicocele testicular volume either decreases or fails to increase. It becomes clinically significant during rapid growth of the testes between 11 and 16 years of age. As many as 75% of adolescents with varicocele demonstrate ipsilateral testicular hypotrophy, with 10% having a left testis one-fourth the size of the right.

8. Do pediatric varicoceles have a different grading scale from adult varicoceles ?

The grading system for varicoceles is the same in both adult and pediatric populations:

Grade I: a small variocele is palpable when the patients performs a Valsalva maneuver.

Grade II: a medium variocele with venous dilatation and tortuosity is palpable when the patient stands.

Grade III: a large varicocele is visible through the scrotal skin.

9. How is the testicular size measured?

Since in the management of pediatric varicoceles change in the size of the testicle is a key follow-up parameter, objective and reliable measurement of testicular size is important. The most common methods used to measure the testicular size are comparative assessment with an orchidometer and ultrasound evaluation. Orchidometer measurements are simple but not as accurate or reproducible as those determined by ultrasound. False-negative size discrepancies may occur in up to 24% of orchidometer measurements.

10. What are the benefits of varicocele repair in the pediatric population?

The necessity for treating varicocele during adolescence, when growth in the testes is greatest, is no longer questioned. However, identifying patients with varicocele that will ultimately have fertility problems is more complicated. Thus, the benefits of surgery include (1) catch-up growth in hypotrophic testis, (2) potential improvement in semen parameters, and (3) the ability to eliminate "continued patient" status that may lead to primary or secondary infertility in adulthood.

11. What are the indications for varicocele repair in adolescents?

Ultimately, not every adolescent with varicocele will be infertile if left untreated; therefore, routine prophylactic varicocelectomy is not a current practice. Of the current clinical parameters (testicular size, varicocele size, semen analysis, hormonal stimulation test), only ipsilateral testicular growth retardation remains an unequivocal indication for repair. Varicocelectomy is recommended for a greater than 2 ml difference in testicular volume as noted by ultrasound evaluation or a two-standard deviation decrease in testicular size based on normal testicular growth curves, regardless of varicocele size. Another indisputable indication for surgery is varicocele-related pain

12. Describe follow-up of adolescents with varicocele.

Unlike in the adult population, semen analysis is not always necessary or useful in following pediatric patients with varicoceles. If no testicular volume discrepancy or pain is identified in pediatric patients, careful follow-up with scrotal ultrasound every 6–12 months and earliest possible semen analysis are indicated. If regular follow-up is problematic, earlier surgical treatment may be considered. A recent study indicated that up to 50% of patients who did not have surgery were dropouts from follow-up. The potential for progressive testicular dysfunction and infertility later in life has to be carefully discussed.

13. What are the benefits of microsurgical varicocelectomy in pediatric varicoceles?

As in adult varicoceles, benefits of varicocelectomy performed microsurgically include clear identification and preservation of the testicular arteries and lymphatics. In addition, it is easier to identify the small venous collaterals, particularly the cremasteric veins, periarterial venous plexus, and extraspermatic and gubernacular collaterals, which, if missed, may lead to recurrence of varicocele.

14. What is the incidence of varicocele recurrence in the pediatric population? What are the main causes?

The overall incidence of varicocele recurrence in adolescents is higher than that observed in adults; reported rates vary from 9% to 16%. The major cause of recurrence/persistence of varicocele results from small internal spermatic veins accompanying the internal spermatic (testicular) artery. The outcome of varicocelectomy in children has not been as favorable as results reported in adults due to technical difficulties in identifying and ligating the tiny periarterial veins. If left behind, they subsequently become dilated, leading to recurrence. Less commonly, failure is due to unrecognized parallel communicating internal spermatic veins or distal cremasteric, deferential, gubernacular, suprapubic and retropubic crossover veins.

15. What are the recommended surgical techniques for varicocele correction in pre- and postpubertal boys?

Ideally, the least morbid procedure with the best results should be performed. Varicoceles in children potentially pose an even more difficult problem because of the reduced size of the veins and lymphatics and arteries with a diminished arterial pulse. In prepubertal boys, because the artery is so small, a microsurgical inguinal approach is recommended. In postpubertal adolescents, as in adults, a subinguinal microsurgical approach can be used.

16. Is ligation of the testicular artery recommended during varicocelectomy?

The issues of occult residual veins along the internal spermatic artery and maintaining integrity of the internal spermatic artery remain controversial. The risk of testicular atrophy secondary to spermatic artery transection/ligation has been widely debated. Studies failed to reveal testicular atrophy postoperatively. Intentional ligation of the testicular artery is associated with lower rate of recurrence, which strongly confirms the persistence of periarterial venae comitantes as an important cause of recurrence. The major objection to arterial ligation is the unknown long-term effect on spermatogenesis. Although the testis receives additional blood supply from vasal (deferential) and cremasteric arteries, the testicular (internal spermatic artery) artery is the major arterial supply to the testis. It is inarguable that ligation of testicular artery will not enhance testicular function.

17. If the testicular artery has been ligated, what procedure must the patient be cautioned about in the future?

Boys in whom the internal spermatic artery has been ligated have to be cautioned about vasectomy later in life because it may be associated with transection of the deferential artery, which may significantly decrease testicular blood supply and result in atrophy.

18. What is the major cause of postoperative hydrocele after varicocelectomy?

As in adults, the most common postvaricocelectomy complication is hydrocele, which is caused by inadvertent ligation of lymphatics.

19. How does testicular torsion affect fertility?

The first cell population lost during the initial period of testicular ischemia is the germ cells, following by Sertoli cells and, finally, Leydig cells. It is believed that unilateral testicular torsion can have a negative effect on bilateral testicular function and fertility. However, the pathogenesis of contralateral testicular damage remains poorly understood. Clinical information is limited by small study populations and lack of long-term follow-up. Abnormal semen analyses have been noted in 40–60% of patients with surgically treated unilateral testicular torsion. Limited evaluation of paternity indicates successful conception in about 15–17% of patients with a history of treated unilateral torsion

20. Is fertility protected by early orchidopexy in patients with torsion?

Early surgical detorsion with unilateral or bilateral orchiopexy can salvage the torsed testis but does not protect against contralateral testicular damage regardless of patient age and degree of torsion. In addition, no reliable data confirm that early orchidopexy preserves or protects ipsilateral spermatogenesis. Until further data from large-scale prospective studies are available, cautious follow-up of surgically treated patients with testicular torsion is indicated. Patients and parents have to be counseled about potential fertility problems

21. What is the most common cause of iatrogenic injuries to the vas deferens?

Vasal injuries have been reported after pelvic surgery, hydrocelectomy, orchiopexy, and varicocelectomy, but herniorrhaphy remains the most common cause of iatrogenic vasal obstruction and testicular atrophy due to compromised blood supply. The estimated incidence of injury to the vas deferens in pediatric inguinal surgery is 0.8–2%.

22. What are the consequences of iatrogenic injuries to the vas deferens in children?

Among children who have undergone bilateral hernia repair, 2% subsequently developed azoospermia. In addition, the incidence of unilateral vas deferens obstruction in subfertile males after pediatric inguinal hernia repair is reported to be 26.7%. The vasal obstruction is commonly inguinal or retroperitoneal and associated with severe scarring. Longstanding vasal obstruction from early childhood increases the likelihood of secondary epididymal obstruction and testicular atrophy. Therefore, treatment of iatrogenic injuries is complicated and requires complex microsurgical reconstructive procedures.

23. Is it possible to prevent and treat iatrogenic injuries to the vas deferens in children?

Meticulous surgical technique with early identification as well as minimal handling of the vas deferens and spermatic vessels is the key to prevention of the iatrogenic injuries. Despite the small size of the vas deferens in early childhood, repair is possible with microsurgery and should be attempted immediately if injury is recognized.

24. Are boys with prune belly syndrome fertile?

No. They are infertile, and there are no documented cases of natural conception

25. Does active spermatogenesis occur in the testes of patients with prune belly syndrome?

Spermatogonia in fetuses with prune belly syndrome were found in a significantly reduced number relative to the normal control group. However, active spermatogenesis was documented in a small number of patients who underwent sperm retrieval.

26. Describe factors affecting fertility in patients with imperforate anus.

Infertility in patients with imperforate anus often is a direct result of iatrogenic injuries. Surgical correction and extensive pelvic dissection can damage the ejaculatory ducts, vasa deferentia or sympathetic fibers, causing excurrent ductal obstruction and/or ejaculatory dysfunction. Recurrent and severe epididymitis is a fairly common complication, especially in patients with rectourethral fistula. Other genitourinary malformations, which often coexist with imperforate anus and require separate treatment (e.g. ureteral reimplantation, orchiopexy), may also decrease fertility potential. Ejaculatory dysfunction was found in 30% and obstructive azoospermia in 55% of these patients.

27. What are the treatment options for infertile patients with imperforate anus?

Treatment options in adults include microsurgical reconstructive procedures (ipsilateral or transscrotal vasovasostomies, vasoepididymostomies), electroejaculation, and sperm retrieval for assisted reproductive technologies.

28. Describe factors affecting fertility in patients with posterior urethral valves.

The most common finding (40%) is slow ejaculation (when the ejaculation lacks force). In adults treated for posterior urethral valve, the posterior urethra remains widely dilated. Sterility due to retention of the ejaculate in the posterior urethra has been reported. The ejaculatory failure may also result from inability to generate adequate pressure in the prostatic urethra. In 50% of the evaluated men, semen analysis was grossly abnormal with high viscosity, high pH, and low motility. Sperm concentration widely varied between 5 and 30×10^6 /ml. Finally, cryptorchidism, a commonly associated presentation (12%) in these patients, may also contribute to impaired fertility

29. How is fertility affected in patients with myelomeningocele?

The fertility problems are thought to depend on neurogenic ejaculatory (and erectile) dysfunction. Natural pregnancies have been reported. However, azoospermia was also documented with the Sertoli cell-only pattern on testicular biopsy. Therefore, a more complex fertility problem may be seen in patients with a history of myelomeningocele. Finally, a high risk of transmission of neural tube defects to the offspring remains a serious problem

30. What is the major cause of infertility in patients with bladder extrophy?

Infertility may be secondary to (1) recurrent and chronic urinary tract infection, (2) epididymitis, and (3) iatrogenic injuries to the genital tract as a result of cystectomy or multiple reconstructive procedures. However, ejaculatory dysfunction remains the major cause of failure to conceive. The emission is slow and may continue over several hours after orgasm. Normal pregnancies have been achieved with the ejaculated sperm (with intrauterine insemination) and vasal sperm retrieval with in vitro fertilization (IVF).

31. What are retractile testes? How do they affect fertility?

A retractile testis is a normally descended gonad (unilateral or bilateral) that is retracted upward toward the superficial inguinal pouch after active cremasteric reflex. It is likely that retractile testis experience the deleterious effects of a nonscrotal environment, particularly higher temperature. The temperature increase lasts for rather a short time but, repeated for years, can be an important factor in abnormal testicular morphology and impaired spermatogenesis. Limited studies have addressed fertility issues in boys with retractile testes. Although early questionnaire-based studies revealed normal fertility in adult men with the history of retractile testis during childhood, lower testicular volume, reduced sperm count, and infertility has been associated with this condition.

32. What is spermarche?

Spermarche is characterized by the first appearance of spermatozoa in the ejaculate. It occurs on average at the age of 13 years.

33. Is it possible to preserve fertility in postpubertal boys treated for pediatric cancer?

Recovery of spermatogenesis after cytotoxic treatment of pediatric cancer is possible but unpredictable. It largely depends on the type and dose of treatment received. Sperm cryopreservation for pubertal and postpubertal boys with cancer is now an available modality. It is essential to assess the developmental stage of puberty. Only boys in Tanner 3 stage or more are considered able to deliver a semen sample. In the majority of sexually mature patients, semen is obtained by masturbation. In younger pubertal boys with no masturbation experience, the use of vibratory stimulation or electroejaculation has been reported. These procedures should be carefully discussed with patient and parents and performed only if both strongly wish to proceed with the treatment.

34. Is it possible to preserve fertility in prepubertal boys treated for pediatric cancer?

Prepubertal boys do not have haploid gametes (spermatozoa and spermatids) in the testis. In this group, attention has turned toward cryopreservation of the gonadal tissue and germ-cell transplantation. These options are presently experimental.

35. How does cryptorchidism affect fertility?

The effect of cryptorchidism on testicular development and subsequent fertility has been extensively evaluated. Prevalence of cryptorchidism in the infertile population (9.4%) is significantly higher than in the fertile population (1–3%). Both bilateral and unilateral forms are well-known causes of altered spermatogenesis. Infertility was documented in 50–70% of patients with untreated unilateral cryptorchidism and in almost all patients with untreated bilateral cryptorchidism. Impaired fertility in patients with cryptorchidism frequently is attributed to intratesticular histologic abnormalities and hormonal deficiencies.

36. Describe the effect of bilateral and unilateral cryptorchidism on fertility.

Paternity is considerably compromised after bilateral cryptorchidism. Lack of paternity is almost 10 times as frequent among men with former bilateral cryptorchidism. Published reports of paternity after bilateral cryptorchidism indicated that only 13–62% of married men were able to father children. The mean time to conception in formerly bilaterally cryptorchid men was found to be significantly longer than in control groups. Paternity in patients with unilateral cryptorchidism decreased to a level that is barely statistically significant. The formerly unilateral cryptorchid group had a 10.5% rate of failed attempts at paternity vs. 5.4% rate in the control group. The time to conception in this group was found to be slightly longer than in control group or similar in both groups.

37. What is the most reliable predictive factor for future fertility in boys undergoing treatment for cryptorchidism?

Multiple studies attempted to predict future fertility based on different factors such as age at surgery, testicular location, laterality of the undescended testes, use of hormonal treatment, testicular biopsy at the time of orchidopexy, and size of the cryptorchid testis. It is clear that the potential for spermatogenesis among cryptorchid testes varies considerably. Above all, it seems that the most important factor for both sperm quality and paternity is whether cryptorchidism is bilateral or unilateral. High abdominal location of the cryptorchid testis considered to have a borderline significance with regard to future fertility.

38. How significant is a childhood mumps infection for future fertility?

Prepubertal mumps does not affect the testes. If the disease occurs postpubertally (after the ages of 11–12), unilateral mumps orchitis may develop in 30% and bilateral orchitis in 10%. The testicular damage may be severe and result in testicular atrophy.

BIBLIOGRAPHY

1. Chan P, Goldstein M: Varicocele: Options for management. AUA News 6:1–5, 2001.
2. Ciftci AO, Muftuoglu S, Cakar N, Tanyel FC: Histological evidence of decreased contralateral testicular blood flow during ipsilateral testicular torsion. Br J Urol 80:783–786, 1997.
3. Cortes D: Cryptorchidism: Aspects of pathogenesis, histology and treatment. Scand J Urol Nephrol 32(Suppl):9–54, 1998.
4. Costabile RA, Skoog SJ, Radowich M: Testicular volume assessment in the adolescent with varicocele. J Urol 147:1348–1350, 1992.
5. Hadziselimovic F, Geneto R. Emmons LR: Increased apoptosis in the contralateral testes of patients with testicular torsion as a factor for fertility. J Urol 160:1158–1160, 1998.
6. Hadziselimovic F, Herzog B, Liebundgut B, et al: Testicular and vascular changes in children and adults with varicocele. J Urol 142:583, 1989.
7. Holt B, Pryor JP, Hendry WF: Male Infertility after surgery for imperforate anus. J Pediatr Surg 30:1677–1679, 1995.

8. Huff DS, Coughlin MT, Bellinger MF, et al:.The undescended testis: An update. Dialog Pediatr Urol 22:1–8, 1999.
9. Jarow JP: Effect of varicocele on male fertility. Hum Reprod Update; 7:59–64, 2001.
10. Laor E, Fitsch H, Tannenbaum S, et al: Unilateral testicular torsion: Abnormal histological findings in the contralateral testis—cause or effect. Br J Urol 65:520–523, 1990.
11. Lee PA, Coughlin MT: Fertility after bilateral cryptorchidism. Horm Res 56:28–32, 2001.
12. Lee PA, O'Leary LA, Songer NJ, et al: Paternity after unilateral cryptorchidism: A controlled study. Pediatrics 98:676, 1996.
13. Lemack GE, Uzzo RG, Schlegel PN, Goldstein M: Microsurgical repair of adolescent varicocele. J Urol 160:179–181, 1998.
14. Leissner J, Filipas D, Wolf HK, Fisch M: The undescended testis: Considerations and impact on fertility. BJU Int 83:885–892, 1999.
15. Levitt GA, Jenney ME: The reproductive system after childhood cancer. Br J Obst Gynecol 105:946–953, 1998.
16. Okuyama A., Nakamura M, Takeyama M, et al: Surgical repair of varicocele at puberty: Preventive treatment for fertility improvement. J Urol 139:562, 1988.
17. Paduch D, Niedzielski J: Repair versus observation in adolescent varicocele: A prospective study. J Urol 158:1128–1132, 1997.
18. Relander T, Cavalin-Stahl E, Garwics S, et al: Gonadal and sexual function in men treated for childhood cancer. Med Pediatr Oncol 35:52–63, 2000.
19. Sheynkin YR, Hendin BN, Schlegel PN, Goldstein M: Microsurgical repair of iatrogenic injury to the vas deferens. J Urol 159:139–141, 1998.
20. Sigman M, Howards SS: Male infertility. In Walsh PC, Retik AB, Vaughan EDJ, et al (eds): Campbell's Urology. W.B.Saunders, Philadelphia, 1998, pp 1287–1330.
21. Waring AB, Wallace WHB: Subfertility following treatment for childhood cancer. Hosp Med 61:550–557, 2000.
22. Woodhouse CRJ, Snyder HM III: Testicular and sexual function in adults with prune belly syndrome. J Urol 133:607–609, 1985.
23. Woodhouse CRJ, Reilly JM, Bahadur G: Sexual function and fertility in patients treated for posterior urethral valves. J Urol 142:586–588, 1989.

11. GENETIC BASIS OF MALE INFERTILITY

Weber W. Chuang, M.D., Kirk C. Lo, M.D., and Dolores J. Lamb, Ph.D.

1. What is idiopathic infertility?

In patients with idiopathic infertility no specific cause can be identified. Currently the basic genetic/molecular mechanisms regulating sexual motivation, production of sperm, transport and maturation of sperm in the genital tracts of males and females, fertilization, and early embryonic development are not clearly understood. Thus we are unable to properly diagnose (and perhaps treat) many cases of male infertility. Presumably many idiopathic cases may have a genetic basis.

2. Are most cases of idiopathic infertility due to genetic causes?

Approximately one-third of cases of unexplained male infertility have been found to have a genetic etiology.

3. What methods can be used to detect genetic defects?

Karyotyping detects abnormalities in chromosome number (such as aneuploidy) or gross structure (such as translocations) with a resolution of 2–3 Mb using standard Giemsa staining.

Fluorescence in situ hybridization (FISH) detects a DNA sequence by hybridizing the sample with a fluorescent marker bound to a nucleotide strand probe, thereby improving resolution to about 1 kb. M-FISH employs probes of different color to examine more than one chromosome at once.

High-resolution (HR) banding cytogenetics is an improvement on the standard karyotype analysis, involving methods that enhance chromosome preparation and separation and increase the resolution or number of bands seen on each chromosome. The International Standing Committee on Human Cytogenetic Nomenclature (ICSN) in 1995 established guidelines for resolution: grade 1 = 150 bands; grade 2 = 400 bands; grade 3 = 550 bands; and grade 4 = 850 bands.

Spectral karyotyping (SKY) uses sophisticated equipment such as a Sagnac interferometer and a CCD camera as well as dedicated computer software to enhance the detection and discrimination of the fluorescent probes.

Chromosome painting labels the entire length of a chromosome with a collection of probes of a single color to detect the structural abnormalities resulting from the exchange of chromosomal material.

Polymerase chain reaction (PCR) employs short nucleotide sequences or sequence-tagged sites (STSs) that flank a specific DNA region and amplifies it, thus detecting the presence of short DNA deletions.

4. What are the common chromosomal abnormalities in infertile men?

Abnormalities of chromosome number seen in infertile males include Klinefelter syndrome, trisomy 21, mixed gonadal dysgenesis, and XYY genotype. Abnormalities of chromosome structure include robertsonian translocations and reciprocal translocations.

5. What is a balanced translocation?

A balanced translocation occurs when parts of two chromosomes are exchanged without the loss of chromosome material. Such an exchange causes no problems for mitosis but may result in unequal distribution of chromosomes during meiosis. A robertsonian translocation occurs when acrocentric chromosomes exchange entire arms with the loss of the resulting smaller arms; usually the short arms do not contain any unique genetic sequences. Unequal segregation of chromosomes occurs during meiosis.

6. How is a karyotype analysis performed?

Lymphocytes are isolated from a peripheral blood sample and induced to divide in culture with a mitogen, most commonly phytohaemagglutinin. When the majority of lymphocytes are in metaphase, the cells are harvested and fixed on a slide. Then the chromosomes are stained with one of several banding techniques, the most common being Giemsa banding, in which the slides are treated with the protease trypsin or are incubated in a hot saline-citrate solution before staining with Giemsa solution. The dark bands correlate with A+T-rich DNA and contain few active genes.

7. Does a normal karyotype rule out the possibility of genetic defects?

No. Karyotyping examines chromosomes for numerical or gross structural abnormalities, such as hyperploidy or translocations. Some fairly large microdeletions can be observed by cytogenetics; nevertheless, most specific gene deletions or abnormalities cannot be detected by karyotyping.

8. Can karyotyping detect a Y-microdeletion?

The original report of Y chromosome microdeletions in azoospermic men was published by Tiepolo and Zuffardi. The authors demonstrated that small regions of the distal portion of the Y chromosome were missing on cytogenetic analysis and that these deletions were visible microscopically. Karyotyping has a resolution of about 3 MB; thus deletions smaller than 3 MB are difficult or impossible to see with a karyotype. FISH can improve the resolution to 1 MB. Smaller deletions (such as Y-microdeletion) require the use of PCR and specific STSs that span the Y chromosome.

9. What are the limitations of karyotype analysis?

Karyotyping examines chromosomes for numerical or gross structural abnormalities, such as hyperploidy or translocations or deletions of relatively large portions of the chromosome. Genetic deletions less than 3 MB are at the limit of optical resolution and are difficult or impossible to see with Giemsa staining. The use of FISH may enhance the detection resolution.

In addition, in genetic disorders that can present as a mosaic karyotype, in which some somatic cells have a certain karyotype and others have a different one, karyotype analysis may be subject to sampling error, depending on the number of cells evaluated. An example of such a genetic disorder is Klinefelter's syndrome, the most common chromosomal abnormality in male infertility. A mosaic pattern, most commonly 47XXY/46XY, can occur.

10. In the absence of abnormalities in the genetic work-up, what genetic concerns are relevant to the use of in vitro fertilization (IVF) and intracytoplasmic sperm injection (ICSI) for infertile couples?

The procedure-related genetic risks of ICSI are a little over 2% in the published literature, a rate not higher than that found in newborns in the general population. There is also an increased risk of sex chromosome anomalies of about 1%. These risks must be presented with several qualifications, the first being that the total number of children examined thus far may not be sufficient to detect a small increase in mutation rates. In addition, only major congenital malformations and developmental defects have been examined. In many cases, the cause of infertility is unknown; thus it is not certain what the outcome in the offspring may be. Finally, given that ICSI is a relatively new technique, little long-term follow-up data are available about these children. Recent studies suggest that there may be up to a two-fold increased risk of major birth defects in both IVF and ICSI births. These data must also be offered with the above qualifications. With the current state of knowledge, couples undergoing IVF/ICSI should be counseled that the possibility of birth defects exists, albeit small.

11. Describe the anatomy of the Y-chromosome.

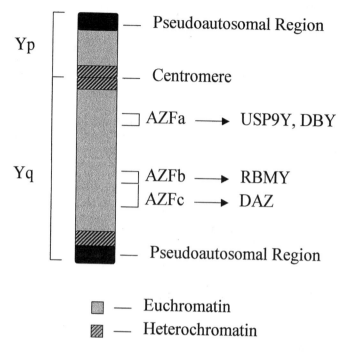

Representation of the Y chromosome. Yp = short arm; Yq = long arm.

The pseudoautosomal regions (PAR) are located at the ends of the Y chromosome with PAR1 on the short end (Yp) and PAR2 on the long end (Yq). These portions of the Y chromosome pair up and exchange material with the X chromosome during meiosis. The nonrecombining Y (NRY) consists of the area between PAR1 and PAR2 and comprises the short-arm paracentric region, the centromere, the long-arm paracentric region, the heterochromatic region, and the euchromatic region.

12. How many genes are located on the Y chromosome?

Relative to other human chromosomes, the Y chromosome has a small number of genes (about 34). These genes can be divided into those that are expressed only in the testes and exist in multiple copies and those that are expressed elsewhere and have X homologs.

13. How is Y microdeletion detected?

A peripheral blood sample is obtained, and genomic DNA is extracted from white blood cells. The genomic DNA is then scanned for the presence of certain relevant genetic sequences on the Y chromosome using PCR and several STSs. STSs are specific oligonucleotide markers that can identify a matching sequence of DNA and are used to detect a missing genetic sequence or deletion. Genetic sequences that are present will be amplified and appear as a band on an electrophoresis gel. Thus, men with a segment of Y chromosome deleted have missing STS bands on the gel, allowing the detection of a Y microdeletion.

14. Are more STSs better?

The more STSs used, the finer the resolution in detecting Y microdeletions; in other words, the more STSs that are used, the smaller the deletion that can be detected. That said, several specific regions of the Y chromosome are thought to be implicated in male fertility; analysis of other regions that have unknown clinical utility should be considered a research tool until clinical relevance is established.

15. How common are chromosomal abnormalities in infertile males?
Chromosomal abnormalities are more common in infertile men with an incidence of about 5% compared with 0.5% in the general population. The number increases to 16% in azoospermic patients.

16. How common are sex chromosomal vs. autosomal chromosomal abnormalities in infertile males?
Sex chromosomal abnormalities are more common in infertile males at 4.2% compared with 1.5% for autosomal chromosomal abnormalities.

17. Do any mutations cause abnormalities in the gonadotropins luteinizing hormone (LH) and follicle-stimulating hormone (FSH) and their receptors?
The gonadotropins LH and FSH are dimeric molecules that share a common α-subunit and have unique β-subunits. Abnormalities in these subunits lead to biologically inactive hormones. LH mutations have been identified in some infertile males. Variable phenotypes ranging from complete failure of virilization to less severe forms of hypogonadism have been observed, but suboptimal Leydig-cell stimulation and absence of spermatogenesis are the characteristic features. Rarely, deficiencies in FSH have been reported in subfertile males. The genetic causes of these abnormalities have yet to be identified, but β-subunit mutations have been hypothesized.

The integrity of the LH and FSH receptors plays a critical role in maintaining the hypothalamic-pituitary-gonadal axis. Constitutive activation of the LH receptor leads to male precocious pseudopuberty, whereas pseudohermaphroditism and Leydig-cell agenesis are the clinical phenotypes of LH resistance. On the other hand, less is known about the FSH receptors; one mutation causing gain of function has been reported in a hypophysectomized man who maintained fertility.

18. What is a repeat CAG sequence ?
A repeat CAG sequence is a microsatellite or a region of DNA with the same code (mono-, di-, tri-, and tetra-nucleotide) repeated many times in a row. These types of sequences are found on all chromosomes. Expansion of some of these repeats is associated with genetic diseases and, in some cases, infertility. For example, the DNA sequence of the androgen receptor gene contains a polymorphic CAG repeat sequence in the exon 1. The CAG trinucleotide encodes for the amino acid glutamine, and in the androgen receptor gene the repeat CAG sequence encodes for a polyglutamine tract in the transactivation domain of the protein. The length of this repeat has been shown to be inversely correlated to the transactivation activity of the androgen receptor. The abnormal increase in CAG tandem repeats in the androgen receptor gene is associated with azospermia.

In addition, the abnormal increase in the CAG tandem repeats is associated with a group of **polyglutamine neurodegenerative diseases.** Among them, Kennedy disease (also known as X-linked spinal and bulbar muscular atrophy) is associated with expansion of the polyglutamine tract within the androgen receptor protein domain; signs and symptoms include gynecomastia, testicular atrophy, and male infertility. This rare motor neuron disease (< 1:50,000) is caused by a unique mutation in exon 1 of the androgen receptor gene. The syndrome ranges in severity from mild muscular weakness and tremor to severe disabling weakness and death by aspiration. These neurodegenerative diseases also follow an inheritance pattern called genetic anticipation, and the expansion of CAG alleles occurs regardless of whether the mutation is transmitted through the male or female germ line.

19. What is genetic anticipation?

In this unique pattern of inheritance of genetic disorders, the succeeding generations acquire a greater extent of gene mutation (such as an increase in the CAG repeat tandem in the androgen receptor gene), resulting in greater severity and/or an earlier age of onset of the disease. For example, Kennedy disease is transmitted by expansion of the normal parental genotype (CAG_{13-30}) to the disease genotype (CAG_{40-62}) range of tandem repeats. The onset of the disease is earlier in the affected offspring. This phenomenon raises a serious issue in the genetic counseling of couples with Kennedy disease who wish to conceive.

20. Are any genes known to cause congenital genital urinary tract abnormalities and gonadal dysgenesis?

Several genes have been identified as causing congenital abnormalities of the genital urinary tract.

ABNORMALITY	GENES	CHROMOSOMAL LOCATION
Pseudohermaphroditism	NR5A1	9q33
Sex reversal	SOX9	17q24.3-q25.1
	SRY	Yp11.3
	NR0B1	Xp21.3–21.2
Denys-Drash syndrome	WT1	11p13
Pseudovaginal	SRD5A	5p15
perineoscrotal	SRD5A2	2p23
hypospadias		
Cryptorchidism	HOXA10	7p15-p14.2
	INSL3	19p13.2
	GREAT	13q12-q13
Congenital bilateral absence of vas deferent	CFTR	7q31.2
Persistent müllerian duct syndrome	AMH	19p13.3-p13.2
	AMHR	12q13

21. What is a microarray/DNA chip?

DNA chips, or DNA microarray, are made by high-speed robotics, generally on glass or nylon substrates, for which tens of thousands of "probes" with known identity are used to determine complementary binding. In contrast to the traditional "one gene in one experiment" method, this technology allows researchers to have a better picture of the interactions among thousands of genes simultaneously. Current applications include the following:

1. For expression analysis, this approach facilitates the measurement of RNA levels for the complete set of transcripts of an organism.

2. For genotyping, it can determine alleles at hundreds of thousands of loci from hundreds of DNA samples.

3. This approach also allows the possibility of whole genome association studies to determine the genetic contribution to complex genetic disorders.

A collection of articles describing the history, technique, and current and future applications of DNA chips can be found in Nature Genetics 21(Suppl):1–60.

22. What are the limitations of a microarray?

As with most great advances, there are certain limitations to the current technology of the DNA microarray chip:

1. Difficulties in reliable detection of the most rarely expressed genes due to the dilution effect of highly abundant transcripts on low abundant transcripts. In addition, tissue samples used for probe synthesis contain different cell types that can prevent the detection of transcripts expressed in a small proportion of the tissue sample.

2. Errors related to sample tracking that lead to a wrong identity of the spotted DNA and the possibility of cross-contamination of the DNA samples.

3. Cross hybridization between closely related transcripts, either between gene family members or genes that possess short but highly conserved domains. Understanding these limitations will allow more careful approach to this powerful technology with cautious optimism.

23. How is the human genome project helping us understand genetic disorders?

Coinciding with the 50th anniversary of the landmark publication by Watson and Crick about the double helix structure of the DNA, the International Human Genome Sequencing Consortium announced the successful completion of the Human Genome Project. The Human Genome Project was launched in 1990 and was considered by many to be one of the most ambitious scientific undertakings of all time.

The finished sequence contains 3 billion DNA letters covering about 99% of the human genome's gene-containing regions, and it has been sequenced to an accuracy of 99.99%. Genome, gene, and cDNA sequences are continuously being deposited into public databases (for example, the National Center for Biotechnology Information (NCBI; http://www.ncbi.nlm.nih.gov) or the Wellcome Trust Sanger Institute (http://www.sanger.ac.uk) with amazing speed.

Functional expression and sequence data are also being collated into collections, such as the Ovarian Kaleidoscope database (http://ovary.stanford.edu) the Male Reproductive Genetics database (http://mrg.genetics.washington.edu/home.html) and the GermOnline database (http://germonline.igh.cnrs.fr).

With the use of microarrays for expression analysis of reproductive tissues, these 'bits' of data will increase exponentially. With this wealth of expanding knowledge, there is an urgent need for bioinformatics advances to facilitate compiling and sorting through this information for future clinical applications.

24. Explain the cytogenetic mechanism leading to Klinefelter's syndrome.

Nondisjunction of the paternal and/or maternal sex chromosome during meiotic reduction division is believed to be the cause of Klinefelter's syndrome (KS), which is characterized by the presence of 47XXY karyotype in somatic cells. However, Huang et al. detected a significantly greater incidence of sex-chromosome aneuploidy in the germ cells of infertile man using FISH, suggesting that a possible mitotic nondisjunction at the spermotogonial stage can also contribute to the cytogenesis of 47XXY offspring.

Controversies remain as to whether 47XXY spermatogonia do indeed undergo meiosis, producing "hyperhaploid" round spermatids (24XY, 24XX), or are simply eliminated from the testis. Some investigators believe the latter. Mroz et al. conclude that the small proportions of disomic spermatids (24XY, 24XX) are results of errors in the 46XY germ-cell segregation during meiosis I and II only. This belief is further supported by the observation of Yamamoto et al. that no spermatids are found in testicular biopsies from patients with nonmosaic KS whose germ cells are exclusively 47, XXY. The same authors also reported the presence of spermatids in 12 of 24 men with nonmosaic KS, who have mixed 47XXY and 46XY spermatogonia in the testis biopsy. The spermatids are predominately euploid (51.9% 23X and 41.6% 23Y) with only 2.83%, 1.04%, and 0.37% of 24XY, 24XX, and 24YY spermatids, respectively. The fact that there is a higher percentage of 23X and 24 XY spermatids suggests the possibility of a few 47XXY germ cells that can undergo meiosis.

25. Is natural fertility possible in men with KS?

In mosaic KS (47XXY/46XY), sperm can be found in the ejaculate, thus making natural fertility possible. The majority of men with nonmosaic KS have no natural fertility, but two cases of naturally conceived offspring of proven paternity have reported by Laron et al. and Terzoli et al.

Sterility in males with KS is thought to be due to loss of germ cells during testicular development. However, rare breakthrough patches of spermatogenesis in the testis of males with KS and occasional spermatozoa in the ejaculate have been reported by Tournaye et al. Therefore, testicular sperm extraction (TESE), followed by intracytoplasmic sperm injection (ICSI), is required. To date, Yamamoto et al. have reported 14 healthy neonates following ICSI with sperm from men with nonmosaic KS. Ron-El et al., however, reported one case in which the karyotype analysis of the fetus from a patient with nonmosaic KS revealed a 47, XXY chromosome pattern; subsequently, the fetus was reduced at 14 weeks of gestation. With the potentially increased risk of chromosomal abnormality in the offspring, preimplantation evaluation of the embryo from patients with KS is recommended.

BIBLIOGRAPHY

1. Benn PA, Tantravahi U: Chromosome staining and banding techniques. In Rooney DE, Czepulkowski BH (eds): Human Cytogenetics: Constitutional Analysis, A Practical Approach. Oxford, Oxford University Press, 2001, pp 99–128.
2. Bonuelle M, et al: Prospective follow-up study of 877 children born after intracytoplasmic sperm injection (ICSI) with ejaculated epididymal and testicular spermatozoa and after replacement of cryopreserved embryos obtained after ICSI. Hum Reprod 11(Suppl 4):31–155, 1996.
3. Clouston HJ: Lymphocyte culture. In Rooney DE, Czepulkowski BH (eds): Human Cytogenetics: Constitutional Analysis, A Practical Approach. Oxford, Oxford University Press, 2001, pp 33–54.
4. Collins FS, Green ED, Guttmacher AE, Guyer MS: A vision for the future of genomics research. Nature Apr 24: 835, 2003.
5. Cross I, Wolstenholme J: An introduction to human chromosomes and their analysis. In Rooney DE, Czepulkowski BH (eds): Human Cytogenetics: Constitutional Analysis, A Practical Approach. Oxford, Oxford University Press, 2001, pp 1–32.
6. Dohle GR, et al: Genetic risk factors in infertile men with severe oligospermia and azoospermia. Hum Reprod 17:13–16, 2002.
7. Gromoll J, Simoni M, Nieschlag E: An activating mutation of the follicle-stimulating hormone receptor autonomously sustains spermatogenesis in a hypophysectomized man. J Clin Endocrinol Metab 81:1367–1370, 1996.
8. Hansen M, Kurinczuk JJ, Bower C, Webb S: The risk of major birth defects after intracytoplasmic sperm injection and in vitro fertilization. N Engl J Med 346:725–730, 2002.
9. Huang WJ, Lamb DJ, Kim ED, et al: Germ-cell nondisjunction in testes biopsies of men with idiopathic infertility. Am J Hum Genet 64:1638–1645, 1999.
10. Johnson MD: Genetic risks of intracytoplasmic sperm injection in the treatment of male infertility: Recommendations for genetic counseling and screening. Fertil Steril 20:23–33, 1998.
11. Kearny L, Buckle VJ: The application of fluorescence in situ hybridization to chromosomal analysis. In Rooney DE and Czepulkowski BH (eds): Human Cytogenetics: Constitutional Analysis, A Practical Approach. Oxford, Oxford University Press, 2001, pp 33–54.
12. Kurinczuk JJ: Safety issues in assisted reproduction technology. Hum Reprod 18: 925–931, 2003.
13. Laron Z, Dikerman Z, Zamir R, Galatzer A: Paternity in Klinefelter's syndrome—a case report. Arch Androl 8:149–151, 1982.
14. LaSpada AR, Wilson EM, Lubahn DB, et al: Androgen receptor gene mutations in X-linked spinal and bulbar muscular atrophy. Nature 352:77–79, 1991.
15. MacLean HE, Warne GL, Zajac JD: Defect of androgen receptor function: From sex reversal to motor neurone disease. Mol Cell Endocrinol 112:133–141, 1995.
16. Matthews CH, Borgato S, Beck-Peccoz P, et al: Primary amenorrhoea and infertility due to a mutation in the beta- subunit of follicle-stimulating hormone. Nat Genet 5: 83–86, 1993.
17. Matzuk MM, Lamb DJ: Genetic dissection of mammalian fertility pathways. Nature Cell Biol Nature Med Suppl: s41-s49, 2002. Available at <www.nature.com/fertility>.
18. Mroz K, Hassold TJ, Hunt PA: Meiotic aneuploidy in the XXY mouse: Evidence that a compromised testicular environment increases the incidence of meiotic errors. Ham Reprod 14:1151–1156, 1998.
19. Palermo GD, et al: Evolution of pregnancies and initial follow-up of newborns delivered after intracytoplasmic sperm injection. JAMA 276:1893–1897, 1996.
20. Quintana-Murci L et al : The human Y chromosome: The biological role of a "functional wasteland." J Biomed Biotechnol 1(1):18–24, 2001.
21. Ron-El R, Strassburger D, Gelman-Kohan S: A 47, XXY fetus conceived after ICSI of spermatozoa from a patient with non-mosaic Klinefelter's syndrome. Hum Reprod 15:1804–1806, 2000.
22. Schieve LA, Meikle SJ, Ferre C, et al: Low and very low birth weight in infants conceived with use of assisted reproductive technology. N Engl J Med 346:731–737, 2002.

23. Terzoli G, Lalatta F, Lobbiani A, et al: Fertility in a 47, XXY patient: Assessment of biological paternity by deoxyribonucleic acid fingerprinting. Fertile Steril 58:821–822, 1992.
24. Tournaye H, Staessen C, Liebaers I, et al: Testicular sperm recovery in nine 47, XXY Klinefelter patients. Hum Reprod 11:1644–1649, 1996.
25. Wisanto A, et al: Obstetric outcome of 904 pregnancies after intracytoplasmic sperm injection. Hum Reprod 11(Suppl 4):121–130, 1996.
26. Wolstenholme J, Burn J: The application of cytogenetic investigations to clinical practice. In Rooney DE, Czepulkowski BH (eds): Human Cytogenetics: Constitutional Analysis, A Practical Approach. Oxford, Oxford University Press, 2001, pp 129–174.
27. Wu SM, Leschek EW, Rennert OM and Chan WY: Luteinizing hormone receptor mutations in disorders of sexual development and cancer. Front Biosci 5: D343-D345, 2000.
28. Yamamoto Y, Sofikitis M, Mio Y, et al: Morphometric and cytogenetic characteristics of testicular germ cells and Sertoli cell secretory function in men with non-mosaic Klinefelter's syndrome. Hum Reprod 17:886–896, 2002.

12. GENETIC DISORDERS

Andrea Stuart, M.D., and Craig Niederberger, M.D., FACS

1. What percentage of fertile men are affected by chromosomal abnormalities? Of subfertile men?

The incidence of chromosomal abnormalities in fertile men is approximately 0.5%, whereas it is estimated that 5.8% of infertile men have chromosome abnormalities. This estimate was based on a survey of 9,766 infertile males. Of these men, 4.2% had abnormalities of the sex chromosomes and 1.5% had autosomal anomalies.

2. Why should men in couples undergoing infertility treatment be counseled before assisted reproductive techniques (ARTs) are used?

There is a 7–13% chance of abnormal karyotypes for men with idiopathic infertility. Pregnancies after intracytoplasmic sperm injection (ICSI) have higher-than-normal rates of chromosomal abnormalities.

3. What gene is involved in testis determination?

The SRY (sex-determining region Y) gene located on the short arm of the Y chromosome.

4. In the 1970s, structural changes of the Y chromosome were found to play an instrumental role in male factor infertility. Which arm of the Y chromosome is required for spermatogenesis?

The long arm of the Y chromosome (Yq) has three distinct loci: AZFa, AZFb, and AZFc. Proposed genes in these loci include USP9Y (ubiquitin-specific protease 9 on Y) and DBY (dead box on Y) in the AZFa locus; RBMY (RNA binding motif on Y) in AZFb; and DAZ (deleted in azoospermia) in the AZFc locus.

5. What is the most commonly identified microdeletion of the Y chromosome in azoospermic and severely oligospermic men?

The most common microdeletion often involves the DAZ gene in the AZFc locus. The incidence of Y microdeletions is approximately 8–18% in infertile men.

6. What histology is more likely to be found in patients with large deletions involving more than one AZF region?

In patients with larger deletions that may affect more than one AZF locus, the histology commonly seen is Sertoli-cell only. This finding is associated with lower sperm retrieval.

7. What gene, identified on the Y chromosome, is required for the completion of normal spermatogenesis?

The DAZ gene, identified in 1995.

8. Are men with DAZ mutations always azoospermic?

Men with DAZ mutations may be azoospermic or oligospermic.

9. When patients with Y microdeletions undergo ARTs, how should they be counseled?

All patients undergoing infertility treatments should be counseled about the potential for passing their genetic abnormalities to their offspring. Such counseling is especially important in men with Y microdeletions, which they may pass to their male offspring.

10. What is the proposed translocation in an XX male? Are sperm present?

An XX male occurs in approximately 1/20,000 live births. The proposed mechanism includes translocation of a fragment of the Y chromosome from the testis/sex-determining region (SRY) to a homologous locus on the X chromosome. Such patients are azoospermic. In fact, there has been no documented case of successful surgical sperm retrieval for in vitro fertilization (IVF) or ICSI in XX males.

11. What are the characteristics of an XYY male? What spermatogenic impairments are seen?

XYY males are phenotypically normal but may have increased height. They may also have decreased intelligence, antisocial behavior, and increased incidence of leukemia. Spermatogenic impairments include spermatogenic failure maturation arrest or Sertoli cell-only syndrome. Not all men with XXY have spermatogenic failure, however. Offspring produced by XYY males are at increased risk of having an extra sex chromosome.

12. Describe the karyotype and typical presentation of a patient with Klinefelter's syndrome. What percentage of men with azoospermia have Klinefelter's syndrome?

Approximately 90% of males with Klinefelter's syndrome have 47XXY; 10% have a mosaic of 46XY/47XXY. These patients typically are taller than normal. They may also have lower extremity varicosities, obesity, diabetes mellitus, nonseminomatous extragonadal germ-cell tumors, and infertility. Patients typically present with small, firm testes, increased levels of follicle-stmiulating hormone (FSH), and normal or low testosterone. Approximately 14% of patients treated for azoospermia have Klinefelter's syndrome.

13. What is the most common X-linked disorder in an infertility practice? How do patients present?

Kallman's syndrome, with an incidence of 1/10,000 to 60,000 live births, is the most common X-linked disorder in an infertility practice. Some men have an isolated gonadotropin deficiency, whereas others may note delayed puberty, tall stature, small testes and penis, anosmia, cryptorchidism, cerebellar dysfunction, or cleft palate.

14. What is the most prevalent genetic mutation in Kallman's syndrome?

The most prevalent genetic mutation is in KAL-1 (which may encode a neural cell adhesion molecule). This mutation results in decreased secretion of gonadotropin-releasing hormone (GnRH) from the hypothalamus.

15. In patients treated for Kallman's syndrome with exogenous testosterone, what happens to intratesticular testosterone?

Treatment with continuous exogenous androgens results in decreased intratesticular testosterone.

16. What is Kennedy disease? What should be done before patients receive infertility treatment?

Kennedy disease is an X-linked recessive disorder that causes spinal and bulbar muscular atrophy. It is caused by expansion of the CAG tract, which increases with each paternal transmission. Each increase is accompanied by an increase in severity and a decrease in age of onset of the disease. Patients suffer with progressive proximal spinal and bulbar muscle weakness. Before any infertility treatment, patients must undergo genetic counseling because female offspring will be carriers of the disease.

17. What syndrome is characterized by facial dysmorphism, webbed neck, short stature, and pulmonary and cardiac defects? What are the causes of infertility in these patients?

Patients with Noonan's syndrome have a phenotypic appearance similar to that of patients with Turner's syndrome, but chromosome analysis reveals 46XY genotype. Although the exact genetic mutation is still under investigation, familial cases have linked a gene to chromosome 12. Patients have impaired spermatogenesis with elevated gonadotropins and testicular atrophy. They may also have cryptorchidism.

18. What are the predominant features in patients with Prader-Willi syndrome?
Predominant features include obesity, mild or moderate mental retardation, infantile hypotonia, and hypogonadotrophic hypogonadism.

19. What is the chromosomal abnormality in Prader-Willi syndrome?
Mutations or deletions of a locus on the paternal chromosome 15 are the more common cause. Less frequently, maternal uniparental disomy occurs at this locus.

20. Myotonic dystrophy is an autosomal dominant disease in which patients may have myotonia, subcapsular cataracts, cardiac conduction defects, premature frontal baldness, and mental retardation. What percent of patients will develop testicular atrophy during adulthood?
Almost 80% of patients with myotonic dystrophy develop testicular atrophy and have infertility secondary to seminiferous tubule damage.

21. What is the most common genetic cause of obstructive azoospermia in patients who have not undergone elective sterilization? With what genetic disorder can it be associated?
Congenital bilateral absence of the vas deferens (CBAVD) occurs in approximately 1–2% of infertile men. It may be associated with cystic fibrosis, which is autosomal recessive. Patients often have hypoplastic and nonfunctional seminal vesicles. Spermatogenesis may not be impaired, but because of its association with CF, genetic testing and counseling should be performed before infertility treatments are initiated.

22. What other genitourinary anomalies can be found in patients with CBAVD?
Patients may have unilateral renal agenesis, but this finding is more common in patients with unilateral vasal agenesis.

23. Androgen insensitivity can be partial (resulting in ambiguous genitalia or infertility) or complete. Testicular feminization, a form of complete androgen insensitivity, results in what phenotype?
Patients with complete androgen insensitivity are phenotypically female with intra-abdominal testes.

24. What are the characteristics of a man with Young's syndrome?
Patients with Young's syndrome usually have chronic sinusitis, bronchiectasis, and obstructive azoospermia. The obstruction can be reversed by microsurgery; however, patients may have motion deficiencies, possibly secondary to abnormal cilia function.

25. What are the characteristics of patients with Kartagener's syndrome? What is the cause of their infertility?
Patients with Kartagener's syndrome have primary ciliary dyskinesia and suffer from chronic sinusitis, bronchiectasis, and situs inversus. Sperm motility is the major cause of infertility; spermatogenesis is usually not affected. This syndrome has an autosomal recessive pattern of inheritance, and patients should undergo genetic counseling.

26. What is the microsomal tubule organization found in immotile cilia syndrome?
The standard 9+2 microsomal tubule organization is defective with abnormal numbers of their microtubles and their associated elements. This affects both the sperm and respiratory cilia. When this is combined with situs inversus, the patient has Kartagener's syndrome.

27. In patients with Sertoli cell-only syndrome, what histology is found on biopsy? How do the levels of FSH, luteinizing hormone (LH), and testosterone compare with those in a normal male?

Sertoli cell-only syndrome is a histologic diagnosis with Sertoli cells lining seminiferous tubules and complete absence of germ cells and normal interstitium. FSH is frequently but not always elevated. LH and testosterone levels are normal.

28. In what percent of males with Sertoli cell-only syndrome can spermatozoa be recovered by testicular sperm extraction (TESE)?

Even though germ cells appear to be absent, spermatozoa are recovered in 24–81% of patients undergoing TESE. Recovery of spermatozoa depends on whether the tissue is *predominantly* or *purely* Sertoli cell-only.

29. In males with deficiencies in 5α-reductase, what are the typical findings?

Males that do not have this enzyme, which converts testosterone to dihydrotestosterone, have infertility resulting from underdeveloped external genitalia and are unable to deliver sperm effectively.

BIBLIOGRAPHY

1. Jaffe TM: Genetic disorders affecting male infertility. In Book MT (ed): Advances in Urology, vol. 9 Chicago, Year Book Medical Publishers, 1996, pp 363–405.
2. Jiang MC, Lien YR, Chen SU, et al: Transmission of de novo mutations of the deleted in azoospermia genes from a severely oligozoospermic male to a son via intracytoplasmic sperm injection. Fertil Steril 71:1029–1032, 1999.
3. Johnson MD: Genetic risks of intracytoplasmic sperm injection in the treatment of male infertility: Recommendations for genetic counseling and screening. Fertil Steril, 70:397–411, 1998.
4. Lim AST, Fong Y, Yu SL: Analysis of the sex chromosome constitution of sperm in men with a 47,XYY mosaic karyotype by fluorescence in situ hybridization. Fertil Steril, 72: 121–123, 1999.
5. Maduro MR, Lamb DJ: Understanding the new genetics of male infertility. J Urol 168:2197–2205, 2002.
6. Sigman M, Jarow JP: Male infertility. In Walsch PC, Retik AB, Vaughan ED, Jr, Wein AJ: Campbell's Urology, vol. 2, 8th ed. Philadelphia, W.B. Saunders, 2002, pp 1475–1531.
7. Su LM, Palermo GD, Goldstein M, et al: Testicular sperm extraction with intracytoplasmic sperm injection for nonobstructive azoospermia: Testicular histology can predict success of sperm retrieval. J Urol 161: 112–116, 1999.
8. Vogt PH, Edelmann A, Kirsch S, et al: Human Y chromosome azoospermia factors (AZF) mapped to different subregions in Yq11. Hum Mol Genet 5: 933–943, 1996.
9. Yokota T, Ohno N, Tamura K, et al: Ultrastructure and function of cilia and spermatozoa flagella in a patient with Kartagener's syndrome. Intern Med 32: 593–597, 1993.

13. CONGENITAL BILATERAL ABSENCE OF VAS DEFERENS

Keith Jarvi, M.D., and Peter T.K. Chan, M.D.

1. What is congenital bilateral absence of the vas deferens (CBAVD)?

CBAVD is a condition in which the vas deferens is found to be absent. It is often associated with absence of the distal portion of the epididymis and abnormalities (absence, cystic distension, atrophy) of the seminal vesicles. CBAVD usually affects only the structures derived from the wolffian duct (distal epididymis, vas deferens, seminal vesicle, and ejaculatory ducts); the other portions of the male reproductive tract are not affected. Typically, the testicles and prostate are of normal size and shape.

2. When should we suspect that a man might have CBAVD?

Most commonly a diagnosis of CBAVD is made in men undergoing investigation for infertility. All men with CBAVD are infertile. In men presenting for an infertility investigation, CBAVD should be suspected in those with low volume azoospermia (usually < 1.0 ml) and low seminal pH. Typically such men also have normal testicular volume and normal serum hormonal profile (normal levels of follicle-stimulating hormone and leutinizing hormone).

3. How is the diagnosis of CBAVD made?

In most cases, the diagnosis is made by a careful physical examination of the contents of the scrotal sac. The vas deferens is a firm, cordlike structure palpable from the tail of the epididymis all the way to the external inguinal ring. It is usually easily palpated in the posterior portion of the scrotum by rolling the contents of the cord (vas deferens, cremasteric fibres, blood vessels) between the examining fingers. It is important to palpate the vas deferens all the way from the tail of the epididymis to the upper scrotum.

4. What other modalities of investigation can be used to confirm a diagnosis of CBAVD?

Occasionally, the vas deferens may be difficult or impossible to palpate, as in men with a thick scrotum, previous surgery, or inflammation. In such settings, testing may be required to confirm the diagnosis of CBAVD. A transrectal ultrasound is often used to visualize the seminal vesicles and vas deferens close to the prostate. Occasionally an endorectal MRI may help delineate the course of the vas deferens close to the prostate. Only on rare occasions is surgery needed to confirm the diagnosis of CBAVD.

5. How often does CBAVD occur?

CBAVD is found in 1/500 men in the general population but is identified in 2–3% of men presenting with infertility.

6. What causes CBAVD?

CBAVD is a congenital condition. There are two theories about the mechanisms of development of CBAVD. The most widely accepted theory proposes that the vas deferens are initially formed and then atrophy. In this theory, the vas deferens are formed (usually by 8–12 weeks of development), then atrophy due to the presence of inspissated material obstructing the vas deferens. In a similar fashion, the inspissated material would obstruct the epididymis, seminal vesicles, and ejaculatory duct, leading to atrophy and alterations in these organs. The alternative hypothesis (agenesis hypothesis) is that the vas deferens and the other structures derived from the wolffian duct fail to develop normally.

In almost all cases of men with CBAVD there is an underlying genetic abnormality. In over 80% of men with CBAVD a cystic fibrosis (CF) gene mutation is identified. In the remaining 20% of men, it is suspected that another, as yet unidentified, genetic cause for CBAVD is a factor.

7. What is cystic fibrosis?

Cystic fibrosis (CF) is the most common autosomal recessive lethal condition in people of Northern European descent. The disease is found in approximately 1/2500 people of Northern European background with a carrier frequency of 1/25. Although there is a spectrum of disease, patients with classical CF have significant respiratory dysfunction (recurrent bronchial infections/inflammation, pneumonia) and may have pancreatic insufficiency, meconium ileus, malabsorption syndromes, sinusitis, nasal polyps, and male infertility secondary to CBAVD. Patients typically show a progressive decline in pulmonary function. Over the past 30 years there has been a dramatic increase in the expected lifespan of people with CF, mainly due to improved nutritional support, physiotherapy, and antibiotic therapy. Still, most patients with CF die before 30 years of age, usually due to an overwhelming respiratory infection.

CF is caused by an alteration in the function of a critical calcium-dependant transmembrane chloride channel. Mutations in the gene encoding this chloride channel (named the cystic fibrosis transmembrane conductance regulator gene [CFTR] lead to reduced or altered function of the chloride channel. This, in turn, leads to thick and viscous secretions in the lumen of structures in which CFTR is abundantly expressed. The resultant intraluminal obstruction (due to the thick inspissated material) contributes to the obstructive respiratory disease, pancreatic insufficiency, recurrent sinusitis, gut malabsorption, and male infertility, which are hallmarks of CF.

8. Are all men with CF infertile?

More than 95% of men with CF are azoospermic due to bilateral absence of the vas deferens and other structural defects of the excurrent ductal system (the wolffian duct system described above). However, such men generally have normal spermatogenesis and, with advanced assisted reproductive technologies such as intracytoplasmic sperm insertion (ICSI), they can father biologically related children.

9. When was the CFTR gene cloned?

The CFTR gene, located on chromosome 7q31.2, was positionally cloned in 1989.

10. How do you test for CF?

The classic test, which remains the gold standard to this day, is sweat chloride testing. A sample of sweat from a non-hair-bearing area is tested for chloride concentration. If two tests show high levels of sweat chloride, a diagnosis of CF is given.

A diagnosis of CF may also be based on the results of the genetic testing to look for mutation of the CFTR gene. If CFTR-causing mutations are identified on both CFTR alleles of the patient (since CF is an autosomal recessive disease) and the patient has clinical signs of CF, the diagnosis of CF may be given.

11. What are the genetic tests for CF?

As described above, genetic alterations in CFTR lead to CF. Over 1000 mutations have now been identified in the CFTR gene (CFTR Mutation Database at http://www.genet.sickkids.on.ca). There is no practical way to test for all of these mutations in routine practice; instead, assays for CF gene mutations use a panel of mutations representing the most common mutations found in patients with CF. These panels identify up to 85% of the CFTR mutations in patients with CBAVD.

12. Do all CFTR mutations present with similar phenotype?

No. A wide spectrum of disease is associated with cystic fibrosis mutations, varying from severe cystic fibrosis to milder CF with no or only mild clinical symptoms.

Patients with more severe CF typically have recurrent bronchial infections and pneumonia, usually leading to a progressive decline in pulmonary function. Death is usually due to an over-whelming respiratory infection. Such patients may also have pancreatic insufficiency, meconium ileus, malabsorption syndromes, diabetes, nasal polyps, recurrent sinusitis, and male infertility secondary to CBAVD.

Recently, milder forms of CF have been recognized and are now usually described as atypical CF. Conditions now associated with atypical CF include CBAVD, chronic pancreatitis, atypical asthma, sinusitis, and nasal polyps.

13. Are specific CFTR gene mutations associated with severe or mild CF?

Although there are approximately 1000 known mutations on the CFTR gene, only a small percentage are proven to cause classic severe CF. In a consensus statement, the Cystic Fibrosis Foundation identified 24 CFTR gene mutations that cause CF.

CFTR Gene Mutations That Cause Cystic Fibrosis

MUTATION	FREQUENCY (%)	MUTATION	FREQUENCY (%)	MUTATION	FREQUENCY (%)
ΔF508	66	R117H	0.3	A455E	0.1
G542X	2.4	R1162X	0.3	S549N	0.1
G551D	1.6	R347P	0.2	R560T	0.1
N1303K	1.3	Δ1507	0.2	1898+1G→T	0.1
W1282X	1.2	3849+10kbC→T	0.2	2184delA	0.1
R533X	0.7	G85E	0.2	2789+5G→A	0.1
621+1G→T	0.7	1078delT	0.1	3659delC	0.1
1717–1G→T	0.6	R334W	0.1	711+1G→T	0.1

Since cystic fibrosis is an autosomal recessive condition, a combination of any two of these CFTR gene mutations is likely to cause classic severe cystic fibrosis. Although less common, other CFTR gene mutations not in the above table may cause severe CF.

Milder or atypical forms of CF, such as atypical asthma, chronic pancreatitis, recurrent si-nusitis, and CBAVD in men, may result from either a compound heterozygote state (with two CFTR gene mutations, at least one of which is mild) or a single CFTR gene mutation (either mild or causing cystic fibrosis disease). Panels to screen for CFTR gene mutations usually include all of the above mutations. Many laboratories offer additional CFTR gene mutation assays.

14. Do all patients with CFTR gene mutations have cystic fibrosis?

No. Although most patients with two of the CF-causing mutations have severe cystic fibro-sis, the phenotype of patients with at least one mild mutation or a single mutation is variable. Such patients may have no clinical symptoms (probably the majority), may have an atypical form of CF, or, rarely, may have severe CF.

15. What is 5T polymorphism?

Intron 8 of the CFTR gene contains a thymidine (T) tract with 5, 7, or 9 Ts. The presence of a 5T allele, which is found in about 10% of the population, has been shown to cause skipping of exon 9 in about 60% of the CFTR transcripts, resulting in reduced concentration of normal chlo-ride channels. The presence of 5T allele alone generally does not lead to classical symptoms of CF, but it is important for two reasons:

1. The 5T allele is the most frequent mutation associated with absence of the vas deferens in men.

2. 5T acts to increase the severity of CF. In patients presenting with CFTR gene mutations, the presence of 5T on one allele may do any of the following:

- Increase the severity of the classical CF phenotype (e.g., may increase the severity of the lung dysfunction)

- Convert a phenotype from an atypical CF pattern to a severe CF pattern or
- Convert a patient from an asymptomatic to a pattern of atypical CF

16. What is the ethnic association of CFTR mutation?

The carrier frequency of CFTR mutation is the highest among the Ashkenazi Jewish and non-Hispanic Caucasian population (1/25). Hispanic Americans (1/46) and African Americans (1/65) have a lower carrier frequency. The carrier frequency among Asians is the lowest (1/90).

Although the recommended panel for a CFTR mutation screening is considered "panethnic," it is primarily based on mutation frequency in the Ashkenazi Jewish and other non-Hispanic Caucasian populations due to the high frequency of the disease and the availability of existing data. One should be aware of the variation in mutation frequencies as applied to the testing population when interpreting screening results for other ethnic groups.

17. Does a negative (normal) screen for the CFTR mutation rule out the risk that man with CBAVD is a carrier?

No. Close to 15% of the CFTR gene mutations in men with CBAVD are "missed" when a panel screening technique is used.

18. What other abnormalities are associated with CBAVD?

Two other major abnormalities are associated with CBAVD: renal anomalies and bronchial tract inflammation. Men with CBAVD have a high incidence of renal alterations (unilateral absence and malposition). Men with CBAVD who lack CF gene mutations are at particulary high risk of having a renal anomaly. Imaging of the upper urinary tract is appropriate for all men with a diagnosis of CBAVD.

Many men with CBAVD are found to have CF gene mutations and may have mild forms of CF. Up to 10% of men with CBAVD have clinically significant respiratory disease. Most commonly it presents as recurrent bronchitis and pneumonia. The sputum of such men is often colonized with bacterial pathogens. Features of long-term respiratory dysfunction, such as clubbing of the fingers, may also be detected. All men with significant respiratory disease should be referred to a respirologist, preferably one with expertise in the care of patients with CF.

In addition, men with CBAVD may have other features of mild CF, including nasal polyps and recurrent sinusitis.

19. Do men with CBAVD have CF?

Mutations in the CFTR gene may cause a wide spectrum of diseases. Men with severe mutations on both alleles generally have classic CF (see above), whereas those with other less severe mutations or with a severe mutation coupled with a mild or no detectable mutations may have mild or atypical CF.

Up to 80% of men with CBAVD have at least one CF gene mutation, and up to 56% have two CFTR mutations. In general, these mutations are milder than in patients with classic CF. If a severe mutation is identified, usually there is either no second mutation or the second mutation is mild. These milder mutations are not classified as causing CF disease.

Up to 25% of men with CBAVD have either a genetic diagnosis of CF (two CF disease-causing mutations) or sweat chloride abnormalities leading to a clinical diagnosis of CF. However, in only 10% are clinically significant symptoms identified.

20. What is CUAVD?

Congenital unilateral absence of vas deferens, a closely related condition that is found much less frequently in men with infertility. Its true prevalence in the population is unknown since affected men are generally asymptomatic. Fertile men with CUAVD may never be discovered unless a thorough physical examination is performed or during a vasectomy.

21. In CUAVD, which side is more frequently affected?

Left-sided CUAVD is twice as common as right-sided CUAVD.

22. How is CUAVD different from CBAVD ?

Aside from the fact that men with CUAVD have sperm in the ejaculate (unless spermatogenesis or patency of the excurrent ductal system is compromised for other reasons), CUAVD and CBAVD differ in the frequency with which CFTR mutation and associated anomalies are identified. In addition, men with CUAVD and a CFTR mutation generally do not have renal agenesis.

	CUAVD	CBAVD
Frequency of 1 CFTR mutation	40%	50–80%
Renal agenesis	25% (ipsilateral)	10%

23. How is infertility associated with CBAVD treated?

With present technology the only option that we can offer men with CBAVD is sperm retrieval coupled with intracytoplasmic sperm injection (ICSI). Men with CBAVD usually have normal sperm production, with sperm found in the testis and the residual portion of the epididymis. In most cases the proximal third of the epididymis is present, and sperm is often identified in this area. Sperm may be retrieved from either the testis or epididymis using either a percutaneous open or microsurgical approach. The sperm is then processed and either frozen or used immediately in a program of ICSI.

24. What are the pregnancy rates for this procedure among men with CBAVD?

Pregnancy rates for sperm from the ejaculation and sperm aspirated from the epididymis or testis are approximately the same. The major determinant of pregnancy rates is the age of the partner. Overall, for most good ICSI programs, one may expect pregnancy rates of approximately 21%.

25. Does the sperm from men with CBAVD have normal function?

Sperm from the men with CBAVD are capable of fertilizing oocytes and allowing term pregnancies. Some evidence suggests that the sperm from men with CBAVD who have CFTR mutations may be unable to adhere or penetrate oocytes. It is unclear what this defect is related to, but it is bypassed by the ICSI procedure and has become clinically unimportant.

26. Do any factors in men with CBAVD help to predict pregnancy rates using ICSI?

In general, no factors help predict pregnancy rates for men with CBAVD. Specifically, the presence of CF gene mutations, other signs of CF, and general health do not correlate with pregnancy rates. Most men with CBAVD have sperm in the testis and the epididymis. There are also reports of testicular dysfunction in men with CBAVD. Although this is an unusual situation, in men with small testis and elevated FSH a diagnostic biopsy may be required to confirm that sperm is present.

27. For men with CBAVD, what are the risks that their children will develop CF?

The children are at higher risk of developing CF than the general population. The carrier frequency of CFTR gene alterations in the population is 4% (allele frequency of 2%), whereas the allele frequency in men with CBAVD is as high as 70%. Based on this fact alone, one may estimate that the risk of having CF gene mutations in both CFTR alleles in the children is more than 35-fold higher than expected. The relative risk of developing classic CF is less but still significantly higher than in the general population. In addition, the children are at higher risk of developing mild or atypical CF. This risk is impossible to quantify.

28. For men with CBAVD, how do you better assess the children's risk of developing CF?

Before establishing a pregnancy, both the man with CBAVD and his partner should have CFTR mutation screening. If the partner is negative for CFTR gene mutations, the couples risk of having a child with classic CF is low (not zero, since there is a risk that the mutation was not identified). If both partners have CFTR gene mutations, detailed genetic counseling is recommended.

29. If one parent has two CFTR gene mutations and the other is a carrier of a significant CFTR gene mutation, what is the chance of each child having two mutations or being a carrier?

The chance of each child having two mutations is 50%, whereas the chance of each child being a carrier 100%. If these two mutations cause CF disease, the chance that the child will have CF is high.

30. If one parent has two CF mutations and the other is negative on CFTR mutation screening, what is the chance of each child having CF or being a carrier?

Because a negative test does not completely rule out the presence of rare forms of CFTR mutations, there remains a chance that the "negative" parent will have a CFTR mutation. Thus the chance of each child having two CF mutations is not zero, but low (generally < 1/800). Since most of the rarer mutations are less severe, the chance that the child will have severe CF is very low. The chance of the child being a carrier is 100%.

31. If both parents are carrier of a severe form of CFTR mutation, what is the chance of each child having CF or being a carrier?

The risk of each child being a carrier is at least 50%. The risk that the child will have severe CF is at least 25%.

32. What can be done if both the man and his partner have CF gene mutations?

Using either pre-implantation diagnosis or amniocentesis, embryos or fetuses with two CF gene mutations may be identified. With pre-implantation diagnosis, embryos are biopsied and the affected embryos may be identified and discarded. Alternatively, amniocentesis may be used to establish the CFTR mutation status of the fetus; if the fetus is affected, the pregnancy can be terminated.

BIBLIOGRAPHY

1. Chan PTK: Genetic risks associated with advanced reproductive technology. J Male Sex Reprod. Health 2(4):161–164, 2002.
2. Grody WW, Cutting GR, Klinger KW et al: Laboratory standards and guidelines for population-based cystic fibrosis carrier screening. Gen Med 3:149–154, 2001.
3. Kolettis PN, Sandlow JI: Clinical and genetic features of patients with congenital unilateral absence of the vas deferens. Urology 60:1073–1076, 2002.
4. Lyon A, Bilton D: Fertility issues in cystic fibrosis. Paediatr Resp Rev 3:236–240, 2002.
5. Richards CS, Bradley LA, Amos J et al: Standards and guidelines for CFTR mutation testing. Gen Med 4:379–391, 2002.
6. Rosenstein BJ. Cutting GR: The diagnosis of cystic fibrosis: A consensus statement. Cystic Fibrosis Foundation Consensus Panel. JPediatr 132:589–595, 1998.

II. Management of Male Reproductive Disorders

14. MEDICAL THERAPY FOR MALE INFERTILITY

Peter T.K. Chan, M.D., and Peter N. Schlegel, M.D.

1. What types of male factor infertility are amendable to specific medical therapy?

Many medical conditions can directly or indirectly lead to poor production or suboptimal quality of sperm (see table below), resulting in male infertility. Specific medical therapies targeted at these conditions can be used to treat the resulting male-factor infertility.

Medical Conditions That Can Cause Male Infertility

Gonadotropin-releasing hormone (GnRH) deficiencies
Luteinizing hormone (LH) and follicle-stimulating hormone (FSH) deficiencies
Hypogonadism
Hyperprolactinemia
Estrogen excess
Hyperthyroidism
Hypothyroidism
Growth hormone deficiency
Inflammation/infection of excurrent ductal system
Retrograde ejaculation
Neoplastic diseases
Systemic illness
Drug- or gonadotoxin-induced infertility
Steroid abuse

2. Explain the use of "empirical" therapies for male infertility.

Although specific medical conditions listed in question 1 may be the cause of infertility in a subset of men, most cases of male infertility are idiopathic. It has been speculated that most, if not all, cases of idiopathic male infertility have a genetic basis; thus, no specific therapy can be used to amend reproductive status. However, many empirical therapies have been used with various rates of success in treating idiopathic male infertility.

Typically these empirical therapies are based on sound physiologic principles. However, well-designed, randomized, placebo-controlled control trials proving the efficacy of these treatments are rarely available. For this reason, these treatments are considered empirical and could be associated with impaired sperm production.

3. Describe a prudent approach to initiating empirical therapy for male infertility.

The following principles should be followed in initiating empirical therapy for male infertility:

1. Only after ruling out all specific treatable or untreatable disorders (such as identifiable chromosomal or genetic abnormalities) should one embark on a potentially costly course of empirical therapy.

2. Since infertility is generally not a life-threatening condition, it is important to avoid toxicity or severe side effects in selecting and initiating an empirical therapy.

3. When counseling patients about empirical therapy, physicians must be realistic about the potential benefits. Generally, empirical therapy alone is unlikely to enable a man with azoospermia or severe oligospermia to achieve natural pregnancy within a reasonable period of treatment.

4. Finally, although many empirical therapies hold potential benefits, given the recent advances and success with assisted reproductive technologies, a treatment timeline and endpoints should be clearly defined before the initiation of empiric therapy to avoid unnecessary delay of fertility management with assisted reproduction.

SPECIFIC MEDICAL THERAPIES

4. What are the causes of hypogonadotropic hypogonadism?

Hypogonadotropic hypogonadism accounts for less than 1% of male infertility cases. These patients have low FSH and LH levels, resulting in low testosterone levels. Congenital causes of hypogonadotropic hypogonadism include Prader-Willi syndrome (obesity, hypotonic musculature, mental retardation, and small hands, feet, and statue), Laurence-Moon-Bardet-Biedl syndrome (retinitis pigmentosa, polydactyly, and hypomentia), or Kallmann's syndrome (delayed pubertal development and "mid-line" developmental defects such as anosmia). Acquired etiologies include radiotherapy, pituitary adenoma, and pituitary infarct.

5. How is hypogonadotropic hypogonadism treated?

Adult-onset hypogonadotropic hypogonadism due to GnRH deficiency can be treated with long-term GnRH replacement with successful restoration of fertility. Exogenous GnRH therapy requires frequent parenteral administration due to the hormone's short biologic half-life. Routes of GnRH administration include intranasal spray, subcutaneous injections, or the use of a portable pump for pulsatile infusion. Longer-acting preparations are available for both intranasal and subcutaneous administration.

6. What are exogenous gonadotropins?

Because of the difficulty in delivering GnRH, exogenous gonadotropins are typically used for treatment of GnRH deficiency. For men with infertility due to hypogonadotropic hypogonadism, various studies have reported the use of gonadotropins injection, with or without concomitant GnRH therapy, in improving fertility status. Exogenous gonadotrophins include human chorionic gonadotropin (hCG), human menopausal gonadotropin (hMG), and recombinant follicle-stimulating hormone (rFSH).

LH is available as Profasi (Serono, Norwell, MA) or Pregnal (Organon, West Orange, NJ); hCG functions physiologically like LH and stimulates the Leydig cell secretion of both testosterone and estradiol.

FSH is available as Pergonal (Serono, Norwell, MA) or Metrodin (Organon, West Orange, NJ); hMG has both FSH and LH activity. A dose that provides adequate FSH effect generally has too low an effect on LH to maintain Leydig cell function. Hence, a combination of hMG (for its FSH activity) and hCG (for its LH activity) is usually required to achieve fertility in men with hypogonadotropic hypogonadism. Exogenous FSH is available as purified urinary FSH or the recently introduced recombinant FSH (Gonal-F, Serono, Norwell, MA). Both have higher specific FSH activity than hMG.

7. What impact does hyperprolactinemia have on male infertility?

Elevated serum prolactin levels, via negative feedback, downregulate secretion of GnRH, leading to low secretion of LH and FSH. Causes of hyperprolactinemia include macrocytic or microcytic adenoma of the anterior pituitary gland, hypothyroidism, renal insufficiency, and hepatic dysfunction; hyperprolactinemia also may be idiopathic. In addition, certain medications, such as phenothiazines and tricyclic antidepressants, may lead to elevated levels of prolactin.

8. How is hyperprolactinemia managed?

Significantly elevated levels of prolactin suggest the presence of pituitary adenoma. Additionally, in advanced cases, visual changes (hemianopia) can suggest a pituitary tumor. Magnetic resonance imaging (MRI) of the brain should be performed with gadolinium contrast, and a neurosurgical evaluation may be indicated for possible surgical management of large tumors. In addition, because thyrotropin-releasing hormone stimulates prolactin secretion, hypothyroidism should be ruled out.

Although surgery and radiation therapy have been successful treatments of prolactin-secreting pituitary tumors, currently the vast majority of patients can be managed with medical therapy. The release of prolactin can be inhibited by the catecholamine, dopamine. Thus, the dopamine agonist cabergoline (0.5–1 mg/week) may be administered to restore normal gonadal function.

9. How does thyroid function affect fertility in men?

Both hypo- and hyperthyroidism in men can lead to infertility. Thyroid hormones are involved in differentiation, growth, and function of many organs, including the male reproductive organs. Hypothyroidism has been associated with reduced seminal volume and sperm motility. Of interest, hyperthyroidism has also been found to cause oligospermia, asthenospermia, and abnormal sperm morphology. Although the exact mechanism is unknown, infertility in hyperthyroidism may be due to increases in sex hormone-binding globulins, resulting in decreased levels of bioavailable testosterone. Screening of thyroid function in all infertile men is generally unnecessary, since significant fertility impairment from thyroid hormone deficiency or excess is rarely seen clinically. However, men with obvious clinical pictures of hypo- or hyperthyroidism should be further evaluated.

10. How does anabolic steroid abuse affect male fertility?

Anabolic steroid abuse may be seen in many athletes and body-builders. Anabolic steroids may produce hypogonadotropic hypogonadism by suppression of hypothalamic and pituitary stimulation of the testes, resulting in oligo- or azoospermia and even testicular hypotrophy or atrophy.

11. Describe the management of male infertility due to anabolic steroid abuse.

In the majority of cases, recovery of spermatogenesis and hormonal production occurs spontaneously with the cessation of steroid use; usually no additional treatment is required. However, recovery may take months. For men who do not respond with adequate endogenous levels of testosterone and spermatogenesis, gonadotropin replacement (with hCG) may be necessary. It should be noted that early use of exogenous gonadotropins continues to suppress pituitary production of gonadotropins, hence delaying spontaneous recovery of the pituitary-gonadal axis. FSH treatment may be added later if normal spermatogenesis does not return with hCG therapy alone.

12. How does growth hormone improve fertility?

Growth hormone is a pituitary hormone essential for normal pubertal testicular maturation. Growth hormone is also thought to stimulate the release of testicular insulin-like growth factor-1, which contributes to normal spermatogenesis as an autocrine/paracrine growth factor. Deficiency of growth hormone leads to a delay in the onset of puberty and impaired production of steroidal hormones. Studies have indicated that subfertile men have lower than normal levels of serum growth hormone. However, the role of growth hormone delivered via subcutaneous injection for improvement in male fertility remains to be established.

13. Discuss the significance of leukocytospermia.

According to the standard of the World Health Organization (WHO), the presence of over 1 $\times$ 10^6 white blood cell/ml indicates leukocytopsermia. Identification of "round cells" on semen analysis may not always reflect leukocytospermia, because immature germ cells, such as round spermatids, may appear similar to leukocytes on light microscopy. Special staining techniques, such as peroxidase stains, or immunohistochemistry, can be used to distinguish the two.

Leukocytes in semen can originate from any part of the excurrent ductal system, including the epididymis, prostate, seminal vesicles, and urethra. Particularly in men with genitourinary symptoms, a semen culture and a urethral swab for *Chlamydia, Ureaplasma,* and *Mycoplasma* species should be performed. However, even in the presence of significance leukocytospermia, a positive seminal culture is infrequently found, particularly in asymptomatic men.

14. How is leukocytospermia managed?

In the presence of inflammation of the exucrrent ductal system, semen quality can be severely impaired. Furthermore, active inflammation or infection can lead to scarring and obstruction of the excurrent ductal system. Treatment with antibiotics should be directed to the culture results. Common causes of infection in the male reproductive tract include *Chlamydia trachomatis* and *Neisseria gonorrhoeae*. Some investigators suggest daily ejaculation for more efficient clearance of microbes, although data supporting the efficacy of this management approach are lacking. The results of antimicrobial or anti-inflammatory therapy for leukocytospermia when cultures are negative are variable. If medical treatment fails to allow natural pregnancy to be achieved, sperm-washing techniques may be attempted to separate sperm from seminal plasma and cellular contaminants for artificial insemination.

15. How do antisperm antibodies affect male fertility?

Antisperm antibodies impair fertility by decreasing sperm motility and by interfering with sperm penetration of the zona pellucida of the oocyte. Antisperm antibodies may be caused by inflammation/infection and obstruction (partial or complete) of the excurrent ductal system. Not all antisperm antibodies interfere with fertility. Furthermore, the impact of antisperm antibodies depends on the antibody titre and the site of sperm binding. Generally, antisperm antibodies are most significant if detected on ejaculated sperm.

16. How is infertility due to antisperm antibodies managed?

Antimicrobial/anti-inflammatory medications may significantly decrease antibody titre. Microsurgical correction of ductal obstruction may be necessary to prevent further production of antisperm antibodies.

The use of a short course of low dose systemic corticosteroids (10–20 mg/day prednisone) may increase the chance of natural pregnancy. However, significant side effects, including peptic ulcer, mood changes, altered glucose metabolism, impairment of testicular function, and aseptic necrosis of the hip, may be experienced. Hence, the use of corticosteroids requires close follow-up and should not exceed 3–6 months.

Sperm washing for intrauterine insemination (IUI) should be considered early in treatment. In vitro fertilization with ICSI is a highly effective treatment for infertility due to antisperm antibodies.

17. Define retrograde ejaculation. What are the causes?

Retrograde ejaculation occurs when semen is propulsed backward from ejaculatory ducts in the urethra toward the bladder (instead of antegrade toward the exterior). The result is low volume or absence of ejaculate at orgasm. Any conditions that disrupt the closure of the bladder neck during ejaculation (via sympathetic control) can lead to retrograde ejaculation. Common causes include diabetes, bladder neck surgery, spinal cord injury, retroperitoneal lymph node dissection, and medications, including antipscyhotics, alpha blockers for prostatic hypertrophy, and certain antihypertensive medications.

18. How is retrograde ejaculation managed?

Various sympathomemmetics can be used over several days or several weeks to facilitate closure of the bladder neck during ejaculation:
- Pseudoephedrine, 60 mg 4 times/day
- Ephedrine, 25–50 mg 4 times/day
- Imipramine, 25 mg 3 times/day

Alternatively, an initial approach is to use a short-term course of a higher dose of pseudoephedrine (90 mg every 12 hours and 1 hour before ejaculation).

If these medications fail to achieve natural pregnancy, sperm may be collected from the bladder after ejaculation for use in intrauterine insemination. The patient should be instructed to avoid dehydration by drinking a large volume of fluid (> 2 liters for 24 hours), since high urine osmolality may impair spermatozoa. Alkalinzation of urine can be achieved by taking 5 ml of Polycitra at 12 hours and 1 hour before ejaculation. Alternatively, 5 doses of 1 gm of sodium bicarbonate or 250 mg of acetazolamide every 6 hours can be used. The patient is instructed to void immediately before attempting to produce a semen specimen to avoid a high urine volume in bladder. After ejaculation, sperm in the bladder can be obtained from voided urine and processed. Alternatively, the bladder can be catheterized and washed with appropriate buffered solution to collect sperm.

DIET SUPPLEMENTS FOR MALE INFERTILITY

19. What advice in terms of general lifestyle can be given to men for a better reproductive health?

Like the general health of an individual, overall reproductive health is highly sensitive to many negative lifestyle factors. These factors are important to identify because they are under the patient's direct control. Whereas subsequent medical treatments may not always overcome their adverse effects, avoidance of continued exposure may improve reproductive and general health.

1. **Tobacco use.** Cessation of smoking is a simple, specific step that may enhance the reproductive health of men. Studies have demonstrated that smokers have a decreased sperm concentration compared with nonsmokers. Elevated serum levels of prolactin and estradiol, both of which have been implicated as a contributing cause for subfertility, have been noted in smokers. Smoking has also been reported to exacerbate the effect of other causes of infertility, such as varicocele.

2. **Alcohol consumption.** Chronic alcoholism is associated with testicular atrophy, diminished serum testosterone levels, and subfertility. Moderate consumption of alcohol, however, has not been clearly shown to have deleterious effects on semen parameters.

3. **Stress.** Infertility is a condition that poses significant stress for the couple. Studies have demonstrated impairment of sperm count in men under chronic stress. One of the mechanisms of stress-induced subfertility may be disturbance of the hypothalamic-pituitary-gonaldal axis, resulting in gonadotropic dysfunction. For this reason, a team approach with social workers and psychologists is advisable to reduce the emotional stress of the couple.

4. **Exercise.** Although a moderate degree of regular exercise is an effective method of stress reduction, excessive endurance physical training (e.g., running over 100 miles/wk, cycling more than 50 miles/wk) can result in diminished sperm quantity and quality.

5. **Nutrition.** Although specific dietary factors that are important in the metabolic pathways involved with spermatogenesis or normal sperm development are not yet identified, it is always appropriate to recommend a healthy diet to all patients, particularly those whose are overweight or obese (body mass index > 25). Excessive fat in the body may enhance the peripheral conversion of testosterone to estrogens by aromatization, leading to subfertility.

6. **Heat exposure.** Some studies suggest that chronic exposure to excessive heat may have negative effects on semen parameters. Avoidance of the use of saunas, hot tubs, and tight pants is thus advisable for subfertile men.

7. **Gonadotoxins.** In addition to tobacco and alcohol, various recreational drugs (e.g., marijuana, cocaine, heroin), industrial solvents and chemicals (e.g., lead, ethylene bromide, mercury, carbon disulfide), and radiation can be detrimental to reproductive health.

20. Do vitamins and minerals help in male infertility?

Many over-the-counter diet supplements, including vitamins and minerals, have antioxidant activity. These supplements include vitamin E, vitamin C, and glutathione. Antioxidants are thought to be beneficial to sperm function by "neutralizing" the damaging effects of reactive oxygen species (ROS), which are a group of highly reactive oxygen radicals that can damage aerobic cellular systems. High levels of ROS have been identified in the semen of approximately 40% of infertile men and have been implicated as a cause of idiopathic infertility.

Some minerals may also be beneficial to sperm production/function. Zinc is thought to be important in testosterone metabolism and in sperm production and motility. Selenium, in addition to being an antioxidant, is also thought be important for sperm motility.

Finally, low serum levels of folic acid (vitamin B9) are thought to be associated with low sperm count and motility.

Unfortunately, no controlled studies have proved the effectiveness of these regimens.

21. What is arginine? Is it helpful for male reproduction?

Arginine is an amino acid. Anecdotal reports suggest that L-arginine supplements can improve fertility in men who have low sperm counts or poor sperm motility.

22. What is CoQ_{10}?

As an antioxidant as well as a cofactor for oxidation for energy production in sperm, coenzyme Q_{10} (CoQ_{10}) is thought to be important for sperm motility.

23. What is carnitine? Is it helpful for male reproduction?

L-carnitine and acetylcarnitine are highly polar, water-soluble amines. In addition to effects such as cellular membrane stabilization, they play an important role in intracellular energy metabolism. Uncontrolled studies have demonstrated that consumption of carnitine significantly increases sperm motility. Thus, some male infertility experts offer carnitine as a diet supplement for infertile men with primarily idiopathic asthenospermia.

24. Are these "diet-supplements" safe?

As mentioned previously many of these diet supplements, whether vitamins, amino acids, minerals or others, are not tested or proven to be effective in all men with idiopathic infertility. These supplements are generally available without a prescription and are generally safe at the recommended dosage. However, when counseling patients about these diet supplements, one must emphasize that they should not delay seeking more effective fertility treatment options, including in vitro fertilization.

OTHER EMPIRICAL THERAPIES FOR MALE INFERTILITY

25. Do nonsteroidal anti-inflammatory drugs (NSAIDs) work for male infertility?

In addition to treating inflammatory conditions, including antisperm antibodies, NSAIDs may improve sperm production and quality by suppressing the synthesis of prostaglandin, which may exert an inhibitory effect on testicular steroidogenesis or spermatogenesis and sperm motility. Although this treatment is inexpensive, chronic use of NSAIDs may have significant gastrointestinal side effects, such as gastritis, nausea, and diarrhea.

26. What is pentoxyphylline? What are its effects on male infertility?

Like caffeine and theophylline, pentoxyfylline is a derivative of methylxanthine. Pentoxyphylline is a phosphodiesterase inhibitor that inhibits the breakdown of cyclic adenosine monophosphate. Oral pentoxifylline has been demonstrated to enhance sperm motility, although its impact on pregnancy rates remains to be established.

27. How do alpha blockers improve male fertility?

The common medical uses of alpha blockers include blood pressure control or alleviation of urinary symptoms due to benign prostatic hyperplasia. Terazosin hydrocholoride, one of the alpha blockers, is a competitive and reversible alpha$_1$-adrenoreceptor antagonist. Studies have shown that it may improve spermatogenesis by causing a chemical sympathectomy, resulting in improved conditions for sperm transport and storage. On a theoretical basis, alpha blockers may relax the smooth muscle in the arterial walls, resulting in improved testis microcirculation and overall testis function. Although other alpha blockers may have side effects such as retrograde ejaculation, the common side effects of terazosin are hypotension, dizziness, and asthenia.

28. What is the significance of serum testosterone in male infertility?

Normal spermatogenesis requires a high level of intratesticular testosterone produced by the Leydig cells upon stimulation by LH from the pituitary gland. Low production of testosterone from the testis results in a low serum level of testosterone, or hypogonadism. Thus, a low serum testosterone suggests impairment of sperm production.

29. Can an exogenous testosterone supplement be used to restore fertility?

Although intuitively testosterone replacement therapy for men with low serum testosterone levels seems logical, in reality further impairment of semen parameter usually occurs. Exogenous testosterone in any form suppresses LH secretion from the pituitary via negative feedback; hence it shuts down the production of intratesticular testosterone and spermatogenesis. Although exogenous androgen may increase serum testosterone, suppression of intratesticular testosterone generally results in further impairment in fertility. Thus, continuous androgen administration has a contraceptive effect on men and should not be used in the treatment of infertility.

30. Explain testosterone "rebound" therapy.

Some investigators in the past have used androgen rebound therapy. A subfertile man is placed on a high dose of exogenous androgen for a certain period. Exogenous androgen is then discontinued abruptly in the hope that the system will rebound and improved spermatogenesis will result, usually within 4 months. Few studies in the literature confirm the benefit of this therapy.

31. What is the significance of serum estradiol levels in the male fertility work-up?

Estradiol, an estrogen, is the predominant downregulator for FSH secretion. Thus, excessive estradiol in men can suppress FSH production in the pituitary, leading to poor spermatogenesis.

32. What is the main source of estradiol in men?

Up to 90% of estrogens in men normally result from peripheral conversion of testosterone through aromatization. This process occurs in fatty tissue, where the enzyme aromatase is found in abundance. Since aromatization is an irreversible process, men with high fatty tissue mass are at risk for subfertility due to "hormonal imbalance," as signified by a low testosterone and high estradiol levels. In men with severe infertility excessive estrogens may be produced within the testes.

33. Explain the T/E ratio.

The T/E ratio is the ratio between serum total testosterone and estradiol levels. It is used to determine the presence of estrogen excess. A normal T/E ratio (T in ng/dl and E in pg/ml) should be above 10. (In S.I. units [T in nmol/dl and E in pmol/L], one may use the E/T ratio, which should normally be below 10).

34. In men with excessive estradiol levels, what medical therapy is available?

Excessive estradiol due to testosterone aromatization can be managed medically with aromatase inhibitors, which inhibit aromatase in estrogen-secreting tissues, thus limiting estrogen production with preservation of testosterone levels.

Testolactone is a steroidal aromatase inhibitor. The most significant side effect is hepatic dysfunction. Anastrazole is a nonsteroidal aromatase inhibitor with less severe hepatic side effects. Other side effects include musculoskeletal discomforts, headache, dizziness, hot flashes, and nausea.

35. Can anti-estrogen be used for male infertility?

Anti-estrogen is another form of empirical therapy for male idiopathic infertility. Clomiphene citrate and tamoxifen are examples of anti-estrogen medications that have been used for this purpose. They increase pituitary gonadotropin secretion by blocking feedback inhibition by estrogen, thus increasing serum FSH and LH levels as well as the testicular production of testosterone.

36. How is anti-estrogen administered?

Clomiphene citrate, available as Serophene (Serono, Norwell, MA) or Clomid (Aventis, Bridgewater, NJ), can be administered at dosages ranging from 15 to 50 mg daily. It is a nonsteroidal drug that is similar in structure to diethylstilbestrol. Although it has a mild estrogenic effect, its mechanism is predominantly as an antiestrogen. Clomiphene citrate binds competitively to estrogen receptors in the hypothalamus and pituitary and blocks the inhibitory effects of estrogens in men. suppression of this negative feedback leads to an increase in GnRH and, subsequently, FSH and LH—potentially leading to increased testosterone production and sperm production.

Some regimens have described a 5-day rest period each month, but there is no real rationale for this cycling dosage. The response to clomiphene citrate varies greatly from patient to patient. Ideally, serum FSH levels should be maximized without pushing testosterone levels above the normal range. Since men treated with clomiphene citrate consistently demonstrate an elevation in serum gonadotropins and testosterone, monthly follow-up of hormonal levels is recommended. A semen analysis should be checked about 3 months after initiation of therapy and regularly thereafter.

Tamoxifen citrate, an antiestrogenic compound commonly used in the treatment of breast cancer, functions similarly to clomiphene citrate but with less estrogenic effect. It can be administered orally in doses of 10–15 mg twice daily for 3–6 months. Uncontrolled studies indicate a positive effect on sperm density but not on motility or morphology. The follow-up regimen and side effect profile are similar to those for clomiphene citrate.

37. How successful is anti-estrogen therapy?

A pregnancy rate of up to 30% can to achieved with this therapy in idiopathic infertility. However, the success varies significantly depending on the pretreatment semen parameters. As with other empirical therapy, no well-controlled studies have established the efficacy of this treatment.

38. What is clonidine? How does it improve male fertility?

Clonidine is an alpha-adrenergic agonist that may stimulate growth hormone secretion. Oral clonidine has been demonstrated to improve sperm density in semen significantly. Side effects of oral clonidine therapy include mild hypotension and drowsiness.

39. Discuss the role of exogenous gonadotropins in treatment of idiopathic male infertility.

For men with idiopathic infertility (without a demonstrable hormonal abnormality), the use of exogenous gonadotropins has not been consistently proved to improve fertility status. Evidence indicates a potential benefit of exogenous gonadotropin in increasing testicular volumes and improving some semen parameters as well as ultrastructural morphology of sperm. However, the significance of these findings remains to be established. Such preliminary and circumstantial evidence of benefits can be considered reasons for further investigations into the physiologic and clinical role of exogenous gonadotropin in human spermatogenesis and treatment of male infertility. Keep in mind that administration of gonadotropins for a prolonged period is expensive. Thus, until the efficacy of this treatment is clearly established, gonadotropin therapy for idiopathic male infertility is best reserved for clinical trials.

40. Can GnRH be used for idiopathic oligospermia?

Based on the collective information from the current literature, the responses of idiopathic oligospermia to GnRH therapy are mixed. Although GnRH treatment is safe and well-tolerated, its high cost and lack of substantial evidence for its efficacy discourage its routine use for male infertility due to idiopathic oligospermia.

BIBLIOGRAPHY

1. Chan PTK: Azoospermia—evaluations and treatments. J. Male Sex. Reprod Health 2(3):113–118, 2002.
2. Chan PTK, Schlegel PN: Inflammatory conditions of the male excurrent ductal system. Part II. J. Androl 23:461–469, 2002.
3. Raman JD, Schlegel PN: Aromatase inhibitors for male infertility. J Urol. 167(2 Pt 1):624–629, 2002.
4. Siddiq FM, Sigman M: A new look at the medical management of infertility. Urol Clin North Am 29(4):949–963, 2002.

15. VARICOCELE

Armand Zini, M.D.

EPIDEMIOLOGY

1. What is a varicocele?

Varicocele is defined as the presence of dilated testicular veins in the scrotum and is due to reflux of blood into these veins. Variocele is the most common identifiable pathology in infertile men.

2. What is the prevalence of varicoceles in populations of fertile and infertile men?

The prevalence of varicoceles in the general adult male population is about 15%. The prevalence of varicoceles is 30–40% in men with primary infertility and 50–80% in men with secondary infertility.

3. When do varicoceles develop?

Varicoceles develop at puberty during growth of the testicle and associated blood vessels. Oster observed that no varicoceles were detected in boys 6–9 years of age, but they were detected with increasing prevalence in boys 10–14 years of age, suggesting that varicoceles develop at puberty. Recently, Akbay et al. reported on a large cohort of children and adolescents aged 2–19 (n = 4,052). They found that the prevalence of a varicocele in boys aged 2–10 was 0.9% vs. 11.0% in boys aged 11–19. Akbay et al. also found that the prevalence of varicocele-related testicular atrophy increased with age.

4. Which side is more likely to have varicoceles?

Although varicoceles are more common and almost always larger on the left side, the prevalence of bilateral varicoceles is up to 50%.

5. What should be suspected in a significant isolated right-sided varicocele?

The rare, isolated right-sided varicocele generally suggests that the right internal spermatic vein enters the right renal vein (the right internal spermatic vein normally enters the inferior vena cava). This finding should prompt further investigation because of its possible association with situs inversus or retroperitoneal tumors.

ETIOLOGY

6. What do we know about the etiology of varicoceles?

The etiology of varicoceles is probably multifactorial. The anatomic differences between the left and right internal spermatic vein, the absence or incompetence of venous valves resulting in reflux of venous blood, and increased hydrostatic pressure are among the most likely causes of varicocele. The left vein is about 8–10 cm longer than the right vein, and its greater length is believed to result in an increase in hydrostatic pressure. This pressure is transmitted to the internal spermatic vein at the level of the pampiniform plexus, causing dilatation of the veins. The report by Braedel et al. about the venographic patterns of 659 consecutive men with varicocele revealed that in the majority of cases (484/659) venous valves were absent. Compression of the left renal vein between the aorta and the superior mesenteric artery ("nutcracker effect") may also contribute to the increased internal spermatic venous pressure. A number of radiologic studies have documented relative distension of the proximal left renal vein, suggesting partial distal obstruction.

7. Why are varicoceles more common and usually larger on the left side?
As stated before, the anatomic differences between the left and right internal spermatic vein are the main explanation. The left vein is about 8–10 cm longer than the right vein, and this greater length is believed to result in an increase in hydrostatic pressure. In addition, the left vein enters the left renal vein, whereas the right vein enters the inferior vena cava.

8. Are there any predisposing factors in the development of varicoceles?
Scaramuzza et al. Recently demonstrated that the prevalence of varicoceles in young boys is directly associated with the level of sports-related activity (soccer playing), suggesting that varicoceles may develop as a result of increased intra-abdominal pressure during childhood and puberty.

PATHOPHYSIOLOGY

9. What is the most important mechanism to explain the pathophysiology of varicoceles?
Increased scrotal temperature has been demonstrated in humans with varicoceles and in animals with surgically induced varicoceles and is the mechanism most widely believed to be responsible for varicocele-induced pathology. The sensitivity of spermatogenesis to temperature elevations has been well documented. The meticulous work of Zorgniotti and McCleod revealed that men with varicocele have higher intrascrotal temperatures than controls. However, the observed elevation in intrascrotal temperatures in men with varicocele is probably nonspecific, since men with idiopathic infertility also often demonstrate elevated intrascrotal temperature readings. The observed decrease in testicular temperature after varicocelectomy supports the theory.

10. What mechanisms other than temperature effect may explain the pathophysiology of varicoceles?
The theory of adrenal and renal metabolite reflux stems from early anatomic radiographic studies documenting reflux of blood from the renal vein into the internal spermatic vein. Despite reports demonstrating correlations between increased concentrations of these metabolites in the internal spermatic vein and the presence of a varicocele, few of these metabolites have clearly been shown to be gonadotoxic. Increased hydrostatic pressure in the internal spermatic vein from renal vein reflux may represent an additional mechanism for varicocele-induced pathology.

11. Is a varicocele associated with any gross clinical findings?
Testicular atrophy has been well documented in men with varicocele. Lipschultz and Corriere demonstrated that left testicular size in men with a left varicocele was significantly decreased compared to controls without varicocele. The World Health Organization (WHO) presented similar results in a multicenter study that evaluated the physical findings and semen characteristics of men presenting for infertility. The WHO study reported that varicoceles (most of which were on the left side) were associated with relative left testicular atrophy compared with the contralateral testis. Using scrotal ultrasonography to accurately measure testicular volume, the author and his colleagues have shown that a left varicocele is associated with relative left testicular atrophy. In contrast, we have reported that right and left testicular volumes are not significantly different in men without varicocele.

12. Are testis histologic features specific to varicoceles?
A number of studies have attempted to characterize the changes in testicular histology associated with varicocele. Most of these studies have documented the bilateral nature of such changes. The histologic findings have ranged from normal spermatogenesis to Sertoli cell-only pattern, with most studies reporting varying degrees of hypospermatogenesis. In addition, histologic features that have been identified in a number of studies include premature sloughing of germ cells into the seminiferous tubule lumen and Leydig-cell hyperplasia.

13. Does a varicocele have any adverse effects on the endocrine function of the testis?

Leydig-cell dysfunction has been associated with varicocele. A WHO multicenter study of the influence of varicocele on fertility parameters demonstrated that the mean testosterone concentration of men with varicocele older than 30 years of age was significantly lower than that of younger patients with varicocele, whereas this trend was not observed in men without varicocele. Rajfer et al. demonstrated that in animals with surgically induced varicocele, the inhibition of testosterone synthesis is due primarily to a reduction in the activity of the enzyme 17,20-desmolase. Scholler et al. demonstrated that the early peak of testosterone and dehydrotestosterone (DHT) in response to human chorionic gonadotropin (hCG) is blunted in men with varicocele. Similarly, they suggested that this effect may be due to a block at the level of the steroidogenic enzyme 17,20-desmolase, based on the increase in 17α-hydroxyprogesterone levels.

14. Are any characteristic semen abnormalities associated with varicoceles?

Semen parameter abnormalities in infertile men with varicocele were first well described by Macleod in 1965. Macleod observed that the vast majority of semen samples, obtained from 200 infertile men with varicocele, were found to have an increased number of abnormal forms, decreased motility, and lower mean sperm counts. However, this "stress pattern," which is also characterized by an increased number of tapered forms and immature cells, may not be specific to varicocele. We recently found that varicocele is associated with the retention of residual cytoplasm along the midpiece of the sperm. This morphologic finding has been correlated with the excessive elaboration of reactive oxygen species in semen.

15. What is the likelihood that a varicocele is associated with testicular pain?

Varicoceles have been associated with scrotal and testicular pain, but this relationship has been less extensively studied than the association between varicocele and infertility. Peterson et al. estimated that the prevalence of pain in men with varicoceles is 2–10%. This pain has been described as a dull, throbbing pain, exacerbated by physical exertion with increased intra-abdominal pressure and alleviated by rest.

16. What is the likelihood that a varicocele is associated with infertility?

Although it has been reported that the majority of young men with varicocele appear to have abnormal semen parameters (nearly 70% in one study), abnormal semen parameters do not necessarily equate with infertility. It is estimated that 20–30% of men with varicocele are infertile. This estimate is based on the following observations:
- 5–10% of all men in their reproductive years suffer from infertility.
- 35–40% of infertile men (or about 3% of all men) have a varicocele.
- 10–15% of all men have a varicocele.

Jarow thus concluded that the majority of men with varicocele are fertile and that the prevalence of infertility in men with varicocele is only modestly greater than that in the general male population.

17. Do untreated varicoceles lead to progressive testicular damage?

Some evidence suggests that testicular function declines in men with untreated varicoceles, but this theory remains controversial. The evidence used to support this theory comes from studies demonstrating an increased prevalence of varicoceles in men with secondary infertility compared to men with primary infertility. Additional support comes from the study of Chevall and Purcell, which demonstrated declining semen parameters in a small group of men (n = 13) with untreated varicoceles. In contrast, Jarow et al. reported that the prevalence of varicoceles in men with secondary infertility is no greater than in men with primary infertility. More recently, Lund and Larsen found no decline in semen parameters in a group of men (n = 24) with untreated varicocele. Nonetheless, it may be prudent to monitor serial semen parameters (every 1–2 years) in men with untreated varicoceles and to consider intervention if semen parameters decline.

DIAGNOSIS

18. How is the diagnosis of a varicocele established?
The diagnosis of a varicocele is generally made on physical examination. A warm examining room, promoting relaxation of the scrotal dartos muscle, facilitates accurate evaluation for varicocele. Varicoceles are classified as grade I (palpable only with Valsalva maneuver), grade II (palpable without Valsalva maneuver), and grade III (visible).

19. Is there significant interphysician variation with respect to physical examination?
The diagnosis of a varicocele is best established by an experienced clinician. Although large varicoceles are easily diagnosed, small (grade 1) varicoceles are harder to detect, and the diagnosis is subject to interphysician variation. The evaluation of testicular volume by physical examination is also subject to significant interphysician variation and can often overestimate the true testicular volume.

20. Is ultrasound useful in the evaluation of varicoceles?
The availability, reproducibility, and noninvasiveness of scrotal ultrasonography have led to its increased use in the diagnosis of varicocele. However, because the significance of a subclinical varicocele (not clinically palpable) remains controversial, ultrasonography is not used to establish the diagnosis of a varicocele. Instead, ultrasonography may be used to aid in the diagnosis of a varicocele in men with a tight scrotum (often with a high-lying testicle).

21. Are all varicoceles benign?
All varicoceles are benign, but in rare cases they may be associated with an underlying malignancy. A large and tense varicocele (right or left sided) that does not reduce upon lying supine may be a sign of an underlying retroperitoneal tumor.

22. What is the significance of a subclinical varicocele?
A number of modalities have been used to diagnose varicoceles, including venography, Doppler stethoscope, radionuclide angiography, scrotal thermography, and scrotal ultrasonography. However, the significance of a subclinical varicocele (not clinically palpable) remains controversial. The lack of standardized criteria for diagnosis and the conflicting treatment outcome reports for subclinical varicocele raise questions about the existence and significance of this entity.

23. Are there any indications for treating a subclinical varicocele?
Although the clinical significance of a subclinical varicocele remains questionable, there may be certain circumstances under which a subclinical varicocele warrants treatment. In a man with a small, tight scrotum, it may be difficult to establish the diagnosis of a varicocele, and scrotal ultrasonography is useful in this setting. The outcome data on varicocelectomy for subclinical varicoceles suggest that a vein diameter greater than 3 mm (ultrasound-derived measurement) is clinically significant.

VARICOCELECTOMY

24. What are the common indications for adult varicocelectomy?
Varicocelectomy is indicated in men with a clinical varicocele, abnormal semen parameters, and couple infertility. This recommendation is based on the finding that varicocele is associated with impaired testicular function and that repair of varicocele can improve spermatogenesis. Varicocelectomy is also indicated in men with a clinical varicocele and testicular pain.

25. What are the indications for pediatric varicocelectomy?
Varicocelectomy is indicated in adolescents with a clinical varicocele and decreased ipsilateral testicular volume (greater than 2-ml difference between the right and left testis). This rec-

ommendation is based on outcome data suggesting that varicocelectomy in this setting is associated with catch-up growth of the testis and better semen parameters than in an untreated group of adolescents with varicocele. It may also be reasonable to consider varicocelectomy in the child with a large varicocele (grade 3) without associated testicular atrophy. Varicocelectomy is also indicated in the adolescent with a clinical varicocele and testicular pain.

26. What are the possible approaches to treating varicoceles?

A variety of surgical approaches have been advocated for varicocelectomy, including retroperitoneal and conventional inguinal open techniques, microsurgical inguinal and subinguinal approaches, laparoscopic repairs, and radiographic embolization. The importance of using a varicocelectomy technique that minimizes the risk of complications and recurrences cannot be overemphasized.

27. What are the advantages of the subinguinal microsurgical varicocelectomy?

The microsurgical varicocelectomy is regarded as the gold-standard technique. The advantage of the microsurgical varicocelectomy is that it enables the surgeon to easily identify the spermatic cord structures (arteries, veins, lymphatics, vas deferens) and, therefore, easily preserve the arteries and lymphatics. With delivery of the testis it is possible to identify and ligate the external spermatic and gubernacular veins. The subinguinal approach described by Marmar et al. obviates the need for opening any fascial layer and as a result is associated with less postoperative pain and a more rapid recovery. However, the microsurgical varicocelectomy is a technically challenging operation.

28. What technical modifications may help simplify the microsurgical varicocelectomy?

The use of intraoperative papaverine may aid in the identification of the testicular artery(ies) by enhancing the subtle pulsations. Intraoperative Doppler may also help identify the testicular artery. Dividing the spermatic cord package (separating the external spermatic fascia and vas deferens with its associated vessels from the internal spermatic vessels) may also aid in the dissection of the cord. This divide-and-conquer approach facilitates cord dissection. We have also observed that such a cord dissection reduces operating time without compromising the surgical outcomes.

29. What risks may be associated with simultaneous vasal reconstruction and varicocelectomy?

Simultaneous vasal reconstruction and varicocelectomy involve a theoretical risk of testicular atrophy. Vasectomy can often be associated with injury to or ligation of the vasal artery and vein(s). Microsurgical varicocelectomy leads to complete ligation of all internal spermatic veins (only the vasal veins are preserved). Therefore, with simultaneous interruption of the vasal and internal and external spermatic veins, testicular venous congestion and atrophy may result. However, in experienced hands, the actual risk of testicular atrophy is low.

TREATMENT OUTCOMES

30. Does varicocelectomy restore testicular endocrine function?

Evidence suggests that varicocelectomy can restore testicular endocrine function. Comhaire and Vermeulen evaluated 10 patients with decreased testosterone, impotence, and varicocele and observed that after varicocelectomy the serum testosterone increased in all cases and potency was restored in the majority of patients. Su et al. also observed a significant increase in mean testosterone levels after varicocelectomy in a group of 53 infertile men with varicocele.

31. Is varicocelectomy effective in treating varicocele-induced testicular pain?

Successful surgical treatment of painful varicoceles depends largely on proper patient selection (chronic, dull, nonradiating pain, exacerbated by physical exertion and alleviated by rest) and avoidance of complications such as hydrocele or varicocele recurrence. Overall, 50–90% of patients experience complete resolution of pain. In 1981, Biggers and Soderhal reported complete resolution of scrotal pain in 48% (24/50) of the men who underwent high ligation. More recently, Peterson et al. reported complete resolution of pain in 86% of patients who underwent inguinal or subinguinal nonmicrosurgical varicocelectomy. Yaman et al. similarly reported that 88% of their patients experienced complete resolution of pain after subinguinal microsurgical varico-celectomy.

32. Does varicocelectomy improve semen parameters?

A large number of studies have evaluated the effect of varicocelectomy on semen quality. Most of these studies have shown improved semen parameters (concentration, motility, mor-phology) in approximately 70% of men undergoing varicocelectomy. The magnitude of semen parameter improvement is generally proportional to the initial semen quality (i.e., men with low initial parameters have a modest improvement, whereas men with high initial semen parameters have a more substantial improvement). The obvious flaw with the majority of these studies is that they are uncontrolled or nonrandomized. As such, although the bulk of the literature supports a favorable effect of varicocelectomy on semen parameters, the true effect of varicocelectomy on testicular function remains unresolved.

33. Does varicocelectomy result in increased pregnancy rates?

A large number of studies (controlled and uncontrolled) have evaluated the effect of varico-celectomy on fertility. Most studies have reported pregnancy rates in the range of 20–50% after varicocelectomy. Controlled studies of varicocelectomy indicate that pregnancy rates after vari-cocelectomy are typically two-fold higher than in the control group (about 35% vs. 15–20%). Like studies of semen quality and varicocelectomy, studies of pregnancy outcome after varicocelec-tomy are flawed in that they are largely uncontrolled or nonrandomized. As such, the true effect of varicocelectomy on fertility remains unknown.

The randomized trials of varicocelectomy have shown variable results in terms of semen quality and pregnancy outcome. In 1979, Nilsson et al. reported lower pregnancy rates in men treated by varicocelectomy (n = 51) compared with 45 randomized controls. The major criti-cisms of this study are the wide standard deviations, the wide variations in serial semen analy-ses, and the remarkably low pregnancy rates reported by this group. Laven et al. evaluated the results of varicocelectomy in adolescents with varicoceles (n = 67) in a prospective, random-ized fashion. They demonstrated improved semen parameters in the surgically treated group but not in the control group. Unfortunately, due to the patient population, the authors could not as-sess the effect of varicocelectomy on fertility. Nieschlag et al. reported no significant difference in pregnancy rates between the control (n = 48) and treatment (n = 47) arms, although semen parameters improved significantly only in the treatment arm. The larger follow-up study of Ni-eschlag et al. reported similar results. The randomized, crossover study by Madgar et al. demon-strated significantly higher pregnancy rates in the early and delayed varicocelectomy groups compared with the nonoperated group. The major weakness of the Madgar study is the small sample size (total n = 45).

34. Does the initial sperm concentration predict pregnancy outcome after varicocelectomy?

In our report of close to 200 microsurgical operations, nearly 50% of couples were pregnant at 2-year follow-up, and the most important predictor of successful outcome was the initial sperm concentration. Pregnancy rates were 60% in couples in whom the man's initial sperm concentra-tion was greater than 5 million per ml and only 8% when the man's initial sperm concentration was less than or equal to 5 million per ml.

These data are in keeping with those reported more than 20 years ago by Dubin and Amelar. These investigators demonstrated that pregnancy rates and sperm quality improvement were sig-nificantly higher in couples in whom the man's preoperative sperm concentration was greater than 10 million sperm per ml compared to those with less than 10 million sperm per ml.

In contrast, Rodriguez-Rigau et al. demonstrated improved sperm counts in men with initial sperm concentration greater than 10 million sperm per ml but not in those with less than 10 million per ml despite observing equivalent pregnancy rates after varicocelectomy (about 45%) in both groups. However, the study is weakened by the fact that the group of men with low sperm counts (less than 10 million per ml) was small (n = 19) compared with the group of men with high sperm counts (n = 89). Matkov et al. recently reported that the initial total motile sperm count (TM) was predictive of outcome after varicocelectomy. In their study, varicocelectomy was the most cost-effective intervention in men with an initial TM greater than 5 million.

35. Does varicocele grade predict outcome after varicocelectomy?

Some evidence suggests that varicocele grade does influence outcome after varicocelectomy; however, this issue remains controversial. Steckel et al. and Jarow et al. have shown that although large varicoceles are associated with poorer semen parameters than small varicoceles, the relative improvement in semen parameters is greater after repair of large varicoceles. Dubin and Amelar reported that the magnitude of improvement in semen parameters after varicocelectomy was independent of varicocele grade.

36. Is there a role for varicocelectomy in men with azoospermia?

Recent studies by Matthews et al. and Kim et al. indicate that there may be some benefit in repairing varicoceles in infertile men with azoospermia and clinical varicocele. Although significant improvement in semen quality (appearance of sperm in the semen) is reported in approximately 50% of these men, a clinically significant outcome (with spontaneous pregnancy) is reported in less than 20%. Preoperative testicular biopsy is predictive of outcome in such cases. Only men with mature spermatids or spermatozoa on testicular biopsy had a good outcome (appearance of sperm in the semen). Men with maturation arrest or Sertoli cell-only pattern on testicular biopsy remained azoospermic post-operatively.

COMPLICATIONS OF VARICOCELE REPAIR

37. What are the common complications of varicocelectomy and how do they present?

Complications of varicocelectomy (hydrocele, varicocele recurrence, testis atrophy) are technique-specific. A hydrocele generally develops early after varicocelectomy. It presents as a painless scrotal swelling that persists long after the postoperative inflammation has subsided. Varicocele recurrence generally presents as a persistent varicocele after varicocelectomy. (In most cases, the varicocele never resolved.)

Testicular atrophy is not commonly reported after varicocelectomy. Patients may initially present with dull, chronic testicular pain that persists long after the acute postoperative inflammation has subsided. Associated swelling of the scrotum is hard to distinguish from the usual postoperative changes. Several weeks or months after the varicocelectomy, testicular atrophy becomes apparent. Occasionally the atrophy may be masked by a hydrocele. A scrotal ultrasound may help document atrophy and reduced arterial blood flow.

38. What are the treatment options for recurrent/persistent varicoceles?

Varicocele recurrence is a common complication after nonmicrosurgical varicocelectomy and generally results from incomplete ligation of collateral venous channels. Magnification of the spermatic cord with the use of the operating microscope reduces the potential for the development of such a complication. Microsurgical varicocelectomy is the preferred option for the management of recurrent varicoceles. With microsurgical varicocelectomy, complete dissection of the spermatic cord is possible (all of the internal spermatic veins are tied). Alternatively, for recurrent varicoceles after nonmicrosurgical varicocelectomy, percutaneous embolization is possible.

39. What causes a hydrocele to develop after varicocelectomy?

Hydrocele formation is a common complication of nonmicrosurgical varicocelectomy. The incidence varies from 3% to 33%, with an average incidence of about 7%. The difficulty in identifying and preserving lymphatics using nonmicrosurgical approaches (especially retroperitoneal) results in the development of this complication. Analysis of the hydrocele fluid clearly indicates that hydrocele formation after varicocelectomy is due to ligation of the lymphatics. The effect of hydrocele formation on sperm function and fertility is unknown. Use of magnification to identify and preserve lymphatics can virtually eliminate the development of hydrocele after varicocelectomy. In addition, radiographic embolization is not complicated by hydrocele formation.

ALTERNATIVES TO VARICOCELE REPAIR

40. What are the alternatives to varicocele repair?
Although varicocelectomy should be considered the treatment of choice for infertile men with varicocele because it has the potential to reverse the pathology and provide a permanent cure, assisted reproductive techniques (ARTs) may be considered as alternatives. Furthermore, varicocelectomy has been shown to be more cost-effective than advanced ARTs, and as discussed earlier, failure to treat a varicocele may result in a progressive deterioration in semen quality.

Intrauterine insemination (IUI) is indicated in infertile couples in whom the man has modestly reduced semen quality. In general, the minimum requirement for attempting IUI is 3–5 million motile sperm (post-wash). In men with poor semen quality (severe oligo-, astheno-, or teratospermia) or azoospermia (requiring surgical sperm retrieval), in vitro fertilization with intracytoplasmic sperm injection (IVF/ICSI) may be attempted.

41. What factors favor the use of assisted reproduction rather than varicocelectomy?
IVF or IVF/ICSI may be considered the treatment of choice for couples who have an independent requirement for such techniques to treat or bypass a female factor (e.g., tubal obstruction).

In men with very poor semen parameters, varicocelectomy is generally associated with a modest improvement in semen quality, and spontaneous pregnancy rates are in the range of 5–15%. In these couples, assisted reproduction (i.e., IVF/ICSI with pregnancy rates in the range of 20–40%) should be considered as an alternative to varicocelectomy. The potential health risks to the female partner and the long-term effects of IVF/ICSI on the offspring should be considered.

BIBLIOGRAPHY

1. Akbay E, Cayan S, Doruk E, et al: The prevalence of varicocele and varicocele-related testicular atrophy in Turkish children and adolescents. BJU Int 86:490–493, 2000.
2. Biggers RD, Soderhal DW: The painful varicocele. Mil Med 146:440–441, 1981.
3. Bonduelle M, Camus M, DeVos A, et al: Seven years of intracytoplasmic sperm injection and follow-up of 1987 subsequent children. Hum Reprod 14 (Suppl):243–264, 1999.
4. Braedel HU, Steffens J, Ziegler M, et al: A possible ontogenic etiology for idiopathic left varicocele. J Urol 151:62–66, 1994.
5. Cayan S, Kadioglu TC, Tefekli A, et al: Comparison of results and complications of high ligation surgery and microsurgical high inguinal varicocelectomy in the treatment of varicocele. Urology 55:750–754, 2000.
6. Cayan S, Erdemir F, Ozbey I, et al: Can varicocelectomy significantly change the way couples use assisted reproductive technologies? J Urol 167:1749–1752, 2002.
7. Chehval MJ, Purcell MH: Deterioration of semen parameters over time in men with untreated varicocele: Evidence of progressive testicular damage. Fertil Steril 57:174–177, 1992.
8. Comhaire F, Vermeulen A: Plasma testosterone in patients with varicocele and sexual inadequacy. J Clin Endocrin Metab 40:824–829, 1975.
9. Comhaire F, Vermeulen A: Varicocele sterility: cortisol and catecholamines. Fertil Steril 25:88–95, 1974.
10. Dubin L, Amelar R: Varicocele size and the results of varicocelectomy in selected subfertile men with varicocele. Fertil Steril 21:606–609, 1970.
11. Dubin L, Amelar R: Varicocelectomy: 986 cases in a 12 year study. Urology 10:446–449, 1977.
12. Jarow JP, Coburn M, Sigman M: Incidence of varicoceles in men with primary and secondary infertility. Urology 47:73–76, 1996.
13. Jarow JP, Ogle SR, Eskew LA: Seminal improvement following repair of ultrasound detected subclinical varicoceles. J Urol 155:1287–1290, 1996.
14. Jarow JP: Effects of varicocele on male fertility. Hum Reprod Update 7:59–64, 2001.

15. Jarow JP, Sharlip ID, Belker AM, et al: Best practice policies for male fertility. J Urol 167:2138–2144, 2002.
16. Kamal KM, Jarvi K, Zini A: Microsurgical varicocelectomy in the era of art: Influence of initial semen quality on pregnancy rates. Fertil Steril 75:1013–1016, 2001.
17. Kim ED, Leibman BB, Grinblat DM, Lipshultz LI: Varicocele repair improves semen parameters in azoospermic men with spermatogenic failure. J Urol 162:737–740, 1999.
18. Laven JS, Haans LC, Mali WP, et al: Effects of varicocele treatment in adolescents. Fertil Steril 58:756–762, 1992.
19. Lipshultz LI, Corriere JN: Progressive testicular atrophy in the varicocele patient. J Urol 117:175–176, 1977.
20. Lund L, Larsen SB: A follow-up study of semen quality and fertility in men with varicocele testis and in control subjects. Br J Urol 82:682–686, 1998.
21. Macleod J: Seminal cytology in the presence of varicocele. Fertil Steril 16:735–757, 1965.
22. Madgar I, Weissenberg R, Lunenfeld B, et al: Controlled trial of high spermatic vein ligation for varicocele in infertile men. Fertil Steril 63:120–124, 1995.
23. Marmar JL, Kim Y. Subinguinal microsurgical varicocelectomy: A technical critique and statistical analysis of semen and pregnancy data. J Urol 152:1127–1132, 1994.
24. Matkov TG, Zenni M, Sandlow J, Levine L: Preoperative semen analysis as a predictor of seminal improvement following varicocelectomy. Fertil Steril 75:63–68, 2001.
25. Matthews GJ, Matthews ED, Goldstein M: Induction of spermatogenesis and achievement of pregnancy after microsurgical varicocelectomy in men with azoospermia and severe oligospermia. Fertil Steril 70:71–75, 1998.
26. Mulhall JP, Stokes S, Andrawis R, Buch JP: Simultaneous microsurgical vassal reconstruction and varicocele ligation: Safety profiles and outcomes. Urology 53:239–240, 1997.
27. Nieschlag E, Hertle L, Fischdick A, et al: Treatment of varicocele: counseling as effective as occlusion of the vena spermatica. Hum Reprod 10:347–353, 1995.
28. Nieschlag E, Hertle L, Fischdick A, et al: Update on treatment of varicocele: counseling as effective as occlusion of the vena spermatica. Hum Reprod 13:2147–2150, 1998.
29. Nilsson S, Edvinsson A, Nilsson B: Improvement of semen and pregnancy rate after ligation and division of internal spermatic vein: Fact or fiction? Br J Urol 51:591–596, 1979.
30. Oster J: Varicoceles in children and adolescents. Scand J Urol Nephrol 5:27–32, 1971.
31. Peterson AC, Lance RS, Ruiz HE: Outcomes of varicocele ligation done for pain. J Urol 159:1565–1567, 1998.
32. Rajfer J, Turner TT, Rivera F, et al: Inhibition of testicular testosterone biosynthesis following experimental varicocele in rats. Biol Reprod 36:933–937, 1987.
33. Rodriguez-Rigau LJ, Smith KD, Steinberger E: Varicocele and the morphology of spermatozoa. Fertil Steril 35:54–57, 1981.
34. Scaramuzza A, Tavana R, Marchi A: Varicoceles in young soccer players. Lancet 348:1180–1181, 1996.
35. Scholler R, Nahoul K, Castanier M, et al: Testicular secretion of conjugated and unconjugated steroids in normal adults and in patients with varicocele. Baseline levels and time course response to hCG administration. J Steroid Biochem 20:203–215, 1984.
36. Steckel J, Dicker AP, Goldstein M: Relationship between varicocele size and response to varicocelectomy. J Urol 149:769–771, 1993.
37. Su LM, Goldstein M, Schlegel PN: The effect of varicocelectomy on serum testosterone levels in infertile men with varicoceles. J Urol 154:1752–1755, 1995.
38. World Health Organization (WHO): The influence of varicocele on parameters of fertility in a large group of men presenting to infertility clinics. Fertil Steril 57:1289–1292, 1992.
39. Yaman O, Ozdiler E, Anafarta K Gogus O: Effect of microsurgical subinguinal varicocele ligation to treat pain. Urology 55:107–108, 2000.
40. Zini A, Buckspan M, Berardinucci D, Jarvi K: The influence of clinical and subclinical varicocele on testicular volume. Fertil Steril 68:671–674, 1997.
41. Zorgniotti AW, MacLeod J: Studies in temperature, human semen quality, and varicocele. Fertil Steril 24:854–863, 1973.

16. VASECTOMY

Peter T. K. Chan, M.D., and Marc Goldstein, M.D., FACS

If it ain't broken, break it!
—Peter T. K. Chan, MD

1. When was the first vasectomy performed? What was its purpose?
The first human vasectomy was performed in 1894 by a British surgeon in the mistaken belief that it could cure swelling and hardening of the patient's prostate gland.

2. For what other purposes has vasectomy been mistakenly performed?
In 1916, an Austrian surgeon Eugen Steinach began performing vasectomies for many men (possibly including his neighbor Sigmund Freud) for the purpose of rejuvenation by restricting the production of hormones that cause aging. Steinach ended his operations in the 1940s when his theory was discredited. In 1928, an American surgeon performed a vasectomy for impotence. Other mistaken goals of vasectomy include improvement of muscular firmness and general health and controlling "excessive" masturbation.

3. How effective is vasectomy compared with other methods of contraception?
As seen in the table below, vasectomy is an effective mean of contraception.

Failure Rates of Various Common Methods of Contraception

METHOD	FAILURE RATE
Vasectomy	0.02–0.2%
Tubal ligation	0.2–0.4%
Hormone implant/injection	0.2–0.4%
Oral contraceptive pills	0.2–2%
Intrauterine device (IUD)	0.5–5%
Diaphragm	1–21%
Condom	1–30%
Spermicides	13–28%
Rhythm method	14–47%
Ejaculation "withdrawal"	19%

4. Is vasectomy performed for sterilization more frequently than tubal ligation in women?
Worldwide far fewer vasectomies are performed than female sterilizations by tubal ligation—despite the fact that vasectomy is less expensive and associated with much less morbidity and no mortality compared with tubal ligation for women.

5. Why is male sterilization with vasectomy less popular than female sterilization with tubal ligation?
The reasons are multifactorial. First, the responsibility/burden of family planning in many cultures worldwide is placed on women. Some men fear pain and complications, whereas others falsely equate vasectomy with castration or loss of masculinity. In addition, many men mistakenly believe they will "shoot blanks" after vasectomy when in fact there is no noticeable changes in semen volume after vasectomy.

6. How popular is vasectomy in North America?
Vasectomy is currently the third most commonly used contraceptive method after oral contraceptives and tubal ligation for women. In the North America, nearly 12% of all married couples employ vasectomy as a mean of contraception. This percentage translates into over 0.5 mil-

lion men per year, making vasectomy the most frequently performed urologic surgical procedure in North America.

7. How popular is vasectomy worldwide?

Vasectomy represents 8% of all contraceptive methods used worldwide. Among the countries where vasectomy is most popular are Australia, Canada, The Netherlands, New Zealand, Korea, the United Kingdom, and the United States.

8. What are the two procedural components of vasectomy?

Many techniques have been described in the literature for vasectomy. Regardless of the technique used, the first part of the procedure, after appropriate anesthesia, is to identify and deliver the vas. The second part of the procedure is to occlude the vas. The various techniques currently used and throughout history generally have unique features in either the delivery or the occlusion method.

9. What is no-scalpel vasectomy?

In 1974, no-scalpel vasectomy (NSV) was first described in China by Dr. Shunqiang Li of the Sezchuan Province. In this elegant method of vasectomy, access to the vas is gained though a single tiny puncture hole in the scrotum, eliminating the need for a scalpel or sutures for wound closure. This technique was first introduced to the United States in 1986 by Marc Goldstein, M.D.

10. What is the original name of NSV?

In Chinese the original name of NSV was "Shu Jing Guan Zhi Shi Qin Chuan Fa," or "vasectomy by clamp puncturing under direct vision."

11. What are the major advantages of NSV?

The advantages of NSV include a smaller opening in the scrotal skin, fewer hematomas, and lower infection rates. Generally, no incision is required with NSV. Instead, one small mid-line scrotal opening is used to access both vasa. In addition, no sutures are required to close the puncture wound. Upon delivery of the vas, the vasal vessels are generally spared during vasal occlusion. Since the vasal vessels also supply blood to the testes and epididymides, preservation of the vasal vessels not only reduces the risk of hematoma but also lowers the risk of ischemic injury to the scrotal organs. Finally, the authors believe that the term "no-scalpel" helps reduce the fear of vasectomy for men electing this method of contraception.

12. What special instruments are needed for NSV?

Two instruments have been designed specifically for NSV. A special atraumatic ring-tipped vas fixation clamp (Fig 1) is used to deliver the vas without crushing the scrotal skin. A sharp, curved mosquito hemostat with a sharp tip (Fig. 2) is used to puncture the vasal lumen through the scrotal skin and to push the vasal vessels away from the vas during vasal occlusion.

13. Describe the "three-finger" technique in NSV.

This maneuver securely isolates the vas for anesthesia or vasal access (Fig. 3). The vas is first isolated by rolling the thumb on the anterior scrotal wall and the middle finger on the posterior scrotal wall. Upon securing the vas, the index finger presses down from the anterior scrotal wall to stretch the scrotal skin while the middle finger pushes anteriorly to deliver the vas close to the scrotal wall.

14. In NSV, how is access to the vas gained?

1. After adequate local anesthesia via a "cord-block," the vas is manipulated to the mid-line raphae using the three-finger technique.
2. A special ring-tipped vas clamp (Fig. 4) is used to isolate the vas. Alternatively, a puncture hole can first be made in the median raphe of the scrotum, followed by introduction of the ring-tipped clamp through the hole to grasp the vas.

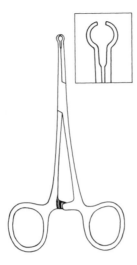

FIGURE 1. Ring-tipped vas fixation clamp.

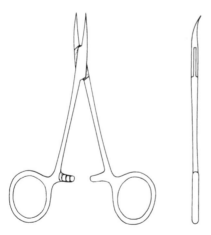

FIGURE 2. Sharp, curved mosquito hemostat.

3. Using one blade of the special sharp mosquito clamp, the vas is punctured through the scrotal skin to the vasal lumen (Fig. 5).

4. Both blades of the mosquito clamp are then introduced through the same puncture hole and are gently opened, spreading all layers until the bare vas can be visualized.

5. Using the right blade of the hemostat, the vas wall is skewered from inside the lumen outward at a 45° angle, and the dissecting clamp is rotated laterally 180° (Fig. 6).

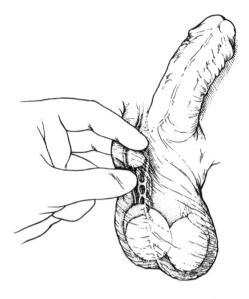

FIGURE 3. The three-finger technique in no-scalpel vasectomy.

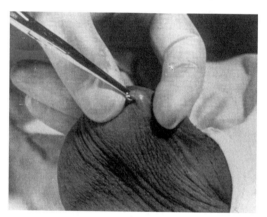

FIGURE 4. The vas is isolated with the ring-tipped clamp.

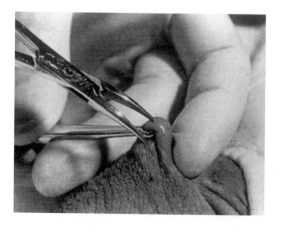

FIGURE 5. The vas is punctured through the scrotal skin to the vassal lumen.

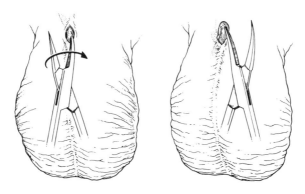

FIGURE 6. The vas is skewered from inside the lumen outward to a 45° angle, and the dissecting clamp is rotated laterally 180°.

6. The vas is delivered through the puncture hole while the ringed clamp is used to secure the delivered vas (Fig. 7).

7. The sharp hemostat is used to push the vasal vessels way from the vas, yielding a clean segment of at least 2 cm in length (Fig. 8).

15. How is the vas occluded during a vasectomy?

Various methods can be used to occlude the vasa.

Suture ligature is still the most common method worldwide. It may result in necrosis and sloughing of the cut end distal to the ligature. If both ends slough, recanalization is more likely to occur.

Titanium hemoclips. The wide diameter of hemoclips distributes pressure on the vasal wall more evenly, resulting in less necrosis than with suture ligature.

Intraluminal occlusion with needle electrocautery or battery-driven thermal cautery further reduces recanalization of the vasal ends.

Removal of a length of vas. Undoubtedly, removal of a very long segment of vas reduces the possibility of recanalization. However, such a destructive procedure is more likely to be as-

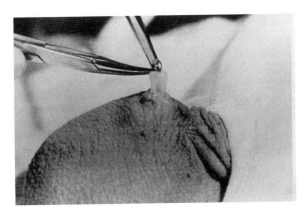

FIGURE 7. The vas is delivered through the puncture hole while the ringed clamp is used to secure the delivered vas.

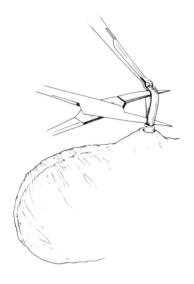

FIGURE 8. The sharp hemostat is used to push the vasal vessels away from the vas, yielding a clean segment of at least 2 cm in length.

sociated with post-perative hematomas and to lessen the possibility of postvasectomy reversal. Generally, removal of 0.5 cm of vas is recommended.

Other techniques include interposition of a fascia between the cut ends, folding back of the vasal ends, and securing one end within the dartos muscle.

16. Does NSV have a higher success rate or lower reanastomosis rate?

Not necessarily. NSV is a technique to deliver the vas during vasectomy. Although NSV has a lower complication rate compared with conventional incisional vasectomy, the success rate or reanastomosis rate depends instead on the occlusion method and the length of vas resected.

17. What is the best way to acquire expertise in NSV?

Although NSV appears deceptively simple, it is more difficult to learn than conventional vasectomy and requires intensive hands-on training. Its use, however, may enhance the popularity of vasectomy and make it a more significant part of the urologist's practice. Various academic institutions, specialists' conferences, and specialty organizations offer workshops for NSV. The many surgical atlases and video materials about NSV can greatly reduce the learning curve of the technique, but there is no substitute for hands-on experience with a qualified and experienced instructor.

18. How is a vasectomy performed if the scrotum is too tight?

Among the most common difficulties faced by surgeons performing vasectomy is a tight scrotum. With the dartos muscle contracted, it can be difficult to isolate the vas. In this setting, the following steps can be taken to relax the scrotum:
1. Use a warm electric blanket to cover the scrotum for a minimum of half an hour.
2. Keep the procedure room warm and humid.
3. Allow the patient to keep on his socks.
4. Use warm antiseptic prep solution.
5. Make the puncture hole in the scrotum first.
6. As a last resort, perform the procedure under anesthesia.

19. Is it necessary to send a piece of vas for pathology confirmation?

Some urologists insist on the removal of a segment of vas for pathologic verification, primarily for medicolegal reasons, whereas others do so because of hospital policy. A report confirming that two pieces of vas were sent does not rule out the possibility of vasectomy failure. The same vas may have to be ligated and resected twice during a vasectomy. Even in a well-performed vasectomy, failure may occur at a rate of 0.6%. Thus, in reality, even from the legal point of view, a pathologist's report confirming the presence of vas in the vasectomy specimen offers little or no protection from litigation. Documented counseling, diligent follow-up to obtain at least one and preferably two azoospermic semen specimens postoperatively, and careful selection of appropriate candidates for vasectomy in the first place provide the best protection from malpractice suits.

20. What are the common complications of vasectomy?

1. Hematoma is a common complication of vasectomy, with an average incidence of 4% with conventional vasectomy but less than 1% with no-scalpel vasectomy.

2. Infection is surprisingly common, with an average rate of 4%.

3. Sperm granulomas are formed when sperm leak from the testicular end of the vas. Approximately 10–30% of men have sperm granulomas at the vasectomy site. They are generally asymptomatic, although rare instances may be associated with pain.

4. Chronic pain after vasectomy can be caused by inflammatory reaction to sperm granuloma, nerve entrapment at the vasectomy site, or congestive epididymitis. About 2% of postvasectomy patients may seek medical help for chronic scrotal pain, but the true incidence may be higher. In some cases when conservative management fails to relieve the pain, a vasectomy reversal may be necessary.

21. What are the signs of vasectomy failure?

1. Presence of motile sperm in the ejaculate after 12 weeks suggests the possibility of vasectomy failure. Most spermatozoa remaining in the excurrent ductal system distal to the vasectomy site should be cleared with regular ejaculation by 12 weeks aftervasectomy.

2. Pregnancy of female partners is another sign of vasectomy failure. Pregnancies due to true vasectomy failure (as opposed to those that are due to intercourse with another fertile male partner) occur rarely (1 in 2000 cases).

22. What causes "vasectomy failure"?

1. In rare cases, the vasectomized vasal ends may recanalize, resulting in the return of sperm to the ejaculate. Recanalization can occur with virtually any techniques of occlusion, although some techniques may have a higher risk than others. Overall, the rate of recanalization is approximately 0.6 %. Recanalization generally occurs within the first 2 years after a vasectomy despite established azoospermia in the initial follow-up period. Although generally it is not practical to check semen analysis for all postvasectomy patients regularly for years, when counseling patients for vasectomy, the possibility of recanalization must be discussed.

2. Although rare, surgical error may occur during a vasectomy. Cutting a structure other than the vas deferens, such as a nerve, blood vessel, or piece of fascia may lead to vasectomy failure. Even a pathology report confirming the presence of two pieces of vas does not rule out the possibility of surgical error, since the same vas may have been resected twice.

23. In men who previously had a varicocelectomy, are any particular precautions needed when a vasectomy is performed?

Although previous varicocelectomy is not a contraindication for vasectomy, one should be careful to preserve the vasal vessels during the vasectomy. Varicocelectomy, especially when it is not performed microsurgically, involves the risk of accidental ligation of the testicular artery. Although collateral vessels to the testes through vasal arteries and the cremasteric artery are possible, damage to the vasal artery during a vasectomy may significantly jeopardize the testicular arterial supply, resulting in testicular atrophy. Similarly, after ligation of the internal spermatic veins, venous drainage of the testes depends on vasal veins and cremasteric veins. Thus, preservation of the vasal vessels during a vasectomy in men with a previous varicocelectomy is important. Doing the vasectomy with optical magnification aids in preservation of the vasal vessels.

24. Where do sperm go after vasectomy?

After vasectomy, sperm are still produced actively by the testes. When sperm pass through the rete testes and the rest of the excurrent ductal system, including the epididymides and the vasa, they are degraded by intraluminal macrophage phagocytosis and absorbed by the epithelial cells.

25. How does the semen change after vasectomy?

Ejaculate or semen is a mixture of secretions from the seminal vesicles (60%), prostate (30%), Cowper's and Littre's glands (5%), and the testis and epididymis ($< 3\%$). Since the testis and epididymis contributes less than 7% of the volume of the ejaculate, there is generally no significant change in semen volume, appearance, texture, odor, or taste after vasectomy.

26. Does vasectomy affect potency or libido?

As mentioned previously, many men who fear vasectomy falsely associate vasectomy with castration. Physiologically, vasectomy should have no negative impact on potency or libido. On the contrary, many men who have had a vasectomy noticed an increase in libido and frequency of intercourse, probably due to freedom from the fear of unwanted pregnancy.

27. What should the patient expect after a vasectomy?

In addition to routine wound care, the authors generally recommend the use of scrotal ice packs for 24 hours to reduce pain and swelling. The patient may resume normal daily activities, including sexual intercourse with temporary contraception, within 2–3 days if he feels comfortable.

28. How many semen analyses are required after a vasectomy?

After a vasectomy, sperm may still be present in the seminal vesicles and vasa distal to the vasectomy sites. The authors generally recommend temporary contraception for 12 weeks or 20 ejaculations, whichever comes first. Every man should have at least one or preferably two semen analyses documenting azoospermia to be reasonably sure that the operation has been a success.

29. A man who had a vasectomy was found to have rare nonmotile sperm in the centrifuged semen specimen. What should be done?

Nothing. In approximately 10% of postvasectomy patients, microrecanalization of the vasal ends—through the formation of microscopic channels—can occur years after vasectomy, resulting in passage of a small quantity of sperm (usually nonmotile) to the distal vas and ejaculate. There is generally not enough viable sperm to be concerned about pregnancy. However, if motile sperm are seen in an uncentrifuged semen specimen, recanalization may be occurring. Additional semen analyses and even a repeat vasectomy may be necessary if recanalization is evident.

30. Is it necessary to vasectomize a cryptorchid testis?

In a cryptorchid testis with hypotrophy or atrophy, often it may be difficult to find the vas for vasectomy. However, since it is not possible to rule out the presence of active spermatogenesis based solely on testicular size, the side with the cryptorchid or atrophic testis should also be vasectomized. If it is difficult to perform vasectomy under local anesthesia in this setting, regional or general anesthesia may be necessary.

31. What forms of counseling should be given to men seeking vasectomy?

In addition to a complete history and physical examination, counseling should be provided to make sure that the man has received appropriate information and has given informed consent. Patients should be counseled about the permanence of vasectomy, potential for reversal, and sperm banking. Risks of complications, early and late failure, need for follow-up semen analyses, and the use of temporary contraception until consistent azoospermia is demonstrated must be discussed.

32. How should a vasectomy be performed to allow an easy reversal in the future?

First, when counseling patients for vasectomy, the surgeon should always emphasize that it is a "permanent" method of sterilization. That being said, the following points can be put into practice to increase the feasibility of vasectomy reversal by minimizing tissue damage without significantly increasing the risk of vasectomy failure:

1. Remove a segment of the vas no longer than 0.5 cm.
2. Use battery-driven thermal cautery to avoid damage of mucosa through electric current injury that extends far beyond the areas of contact with electrocautery.
3. Use the hemoclip instead of suture ligature.
4. Perform vasectomy at the straight portion of the vas, and avoid the convoluted vas.

33. What factors in patients seeking vasectomy are associated with a higher chance of desiring vasectomy reversal in the future?

Approximately 5% of all vasectomized men ultimately seek vasectomy reversal. Most men seek vasectomy reversal because they are involved in a new relationship. This factor makes it impossible to identify the majority of patients who may seek vasectomy reversal in the future. However, factors that may increase the likelihood for men to seek a reversal include:

- Age < 30 years
- Not involved in a relationship at the time of vasectomy
- Involved in a relationship for less than 3 years at the time of vasectomy
- No children prior to vasectomy

Counseling is thus essential before performing a vasectomy in such men.

34. What are the contraindications to vasectomy?

- Congenital bilateral absence of vasa
- High risk of developing complications (infection risk in immunocompromised men, bleeding diathesis).
- Active scrotal disorders, such as infection or hydroceles
- Inability to give an informed consent, such as in cases of mental incompetence.
- Expectancy of reversal in future

35. Does vasectomy increase the risk of prostate cancer?

Several large-scale studies with long-term follow-ups have clearly established that vasectomy does not increase the risk of prostate cancer. Detection bias may be one of the explanations for the increased risks of prostate cancer reported in earlier studies, because vasectomized men are more likely to visit a urologist and therefore are more likely to have the cancer diagnosed earlier.

BIBLIOGRAPHY

1. Cox B, Sneyd, MJ, Paul C, et al: Vasectomy and risk of prostate cancer. JAMA 287:3110–3115, 2002.
2. Goldstein M: Surgical management of male infertility and other scrotal disorders. In Walsh PC, Retik AB, Vaughan ED, Wein AJ (eds): Campbell's Urology, 8th ed. 2002, pp 1532–1587.
3. Goldstein M, Feldberg M: The Vasectomy Book. Tarcher Inc., Los Angeles, 1982.
4. Gonzales B, Marston-Ainley S, Vansintejan G, Li PS: No-scalpel Vasectomy: An Illustrated Guide for Surgeons. AVSC International, 1995.

17. REPRODUCTIVE TRACT RECONSTRUCTION AND VASECTOMY REVERSAL

Peter T.K. Chan, M.D., and Marc Goldstein, M.D., F.A.C.S.

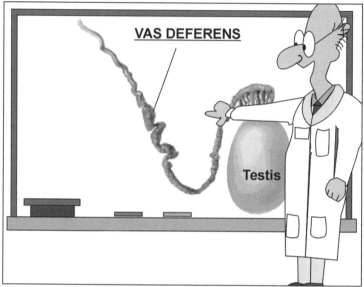

"There is a "Vas Deferens" between fertility and sterility."

A1 Intellectual Media

1. What are the common sites of obstruction in the male reproductive tract?
Theoretically obstruction may occur anywhere along the excurrent ductal system. In reality, the most common sites of obstruction include ejaculatory ducts, epididymides, and vasa.

2. What are the common causes of obstruction in the male reproductive tract?
Vasal obstruction
- Previous vasectomy
- Iatrogenic vasal injury from groin surgery such as hernia repair
- Congenital absence of vas

Epididymal obstruction
- Previous vasectomy (usually > 5 years),
- Inflammation/infection,
- Iatrogenic injury from scrotal surgery (e.g., hydroclelectomy, spermatocelectomy)
- Trauma
- Congenital absence of vas

Ejaculatory ductal obstruction
- Congenital malformation
- Compression by prostatic cysts
- Prostatitis/urethritis
- Rectal injury/surgery

3. What are the contraindications for reproductive tract reconstruction?

Obviously in the absence of an obstruction, reconstruction such as vasovasostomy or vasoepididymostomy should not be performed. Examples include testicular failure or nonobstructive azoospermia, oligospermia due to hypogonadism, or other genetic abnormalities (such as AZFc deletion of the Y-chromosome).

Preoperative clinical investigations for azoospermic or severely oligospermic men may not always allow a diagnosis of obstruction to be made with a 100% certainty. Often a diagnostic testicular biopsy to establish normal spermatogenesis is required to establish a diagnosis of obstruction. At the time of surgical reconstruction, intraoperative vasography may be indicated before proceeding with the appropriate type of reconstructive surgery.

The condition of congenital bilateral absence of vas represents a special situation. Generally such men are not amendable to reconstruction but are excellent candidates for microsurgical epididymal sperm aspiration (MESA) to be used for in vitro fertilization (IVF) or intracytoplasmic sperm injection (ICSI).

4. What surgical procedures are commonly used for male reproductive tract reconstruction?

Sites of Obstruction	Reconstructive Surgery
Vasa	Vasovasostomy
Epididymides	Vasoepididymostomy
Ejaculatory ducts	Transurethral resection or dilatation of ejaculatory ducts

5. With the availability of assisted reproductive technology such as IVF and ICSI, why is vasectomy reversal necessary?

1. Most couples prefer to have children naturally. Vasectomy reversal can allow couples to have multiple children with natural intercourse.

2. Vasectomy reversal or other forms of reconstruction are outpatient procedures. Minimal surgical risks are involved, and the procedures are generally safe with an uncomplicated recovery period.

3. Assisted reproduction with IVF or ICSI is not risk-free. Frequent hormonal injection given to the female partners for ovulation induction may have significant medical complications such as ovarian hyperstimulation syndrome.

4. Even when the couple wants to have only one child, various studies have clearly established that reconstruction with vasovasostomy or vasoepididymostomy remains a more cost-effective option than upfront assisted reproduction. Even in cases when the quality and quantity of sperm returning to the ejaculate are not adequate to achieve natural pregnancy, less invasive options such as intrauterine insemination (IUI) may be used instead of the more advanced, invasive, and expensive forms of assisted reproduction.

5. Even if IVF or ICSI is eventually required, the return of fresh sperm to the ejaculate obviates the need for the men to go through additional surgeries for sperm retrieval for each assisted reproduction trial.

6. What is vasectomy reversal?

The most common cause of excurrent ductal obstruction is previous vasectomy. Although vasectomy should be considered permanent, it can be successfully reversed surgically. Procedures for vasectomy reversal may involve vasovasostomy or vasoepididymostomy.

7. What should patients expect when going through vasectomy reversal?

Vasectomy reversal with vasovasostomy or vasoepididymostomy generally is an outpatient procedure. Depending on the complexity of the case, the surgery may last 2–4 hours or longer, especially if performed using advanced microsurgical techniques. In addition to anesthesia-related complications, there is a very low risk of wound infection, scrotal hematoma, and pain. We generally recommend keeping the incision dry for 24 to 48 hours. Oral analgesic, wound compression with ice-pack, and scrotal support are simple measures to relive postoperative pain. We recommend semen analyses at 1 month, 3 months, and 6 months postoperatively to evaluate patency.

8. What prognostic signs can predict a higher success rate for vasectomy reversal?

1. **Presence of granuloma.** A sperm granuloma is an inflammatory nodule at the testicular end of the vas. It can be palpable on a carefully performed physical examination in certain men who have undergone vasectomy. It is a sign that sperm has been leaking at the vasectomy site, venting the high pressures away from the epididymis, and is associated with a better prognosis for restored fertility regardless of the time interval since vasectomy.

2. **Time since vasectomy.** The longer the time since vasectomy (> 3–5 years), the lower the chance for a successful vasectomy reversal. We have shown that naturally conceived pregnancy rates remain above 80% until greater than 15 years since vasectomy, when pregnancy rates drop to 44%. The reason for this observation is that the longer the time of obstruction, the higher the chance for a "blow-out injury" to the epididymal tubule due to building up of fluid pressure. In the presence of an epididymal obstruction, vasovasostomy has a poor success rate. However, if a vasoepididymostomy is performed as indicated, the overall patency rate even in men with prolonged obstruction remains higher than 80% with experienced surgeons.

3. **Absence of other factors for reduced fertility** (e.g., lifestyle, varicocele, hormonal problem, inflammation). Conditions such as concomitant varicoceles, hypogonadism, recurrent reproductive tract infection or inflammation, and exposure to gonadotoxic agents (e.g., drugs, tobacco consumption, excessive alcohol, heat) can impair postoperative sperm quality and quantity despite a patent surgical anastomosis.

4. **Same female partner.** Recent studies suggest that men who undergo vasectomy reversal while remaining with the same female partners achieved pregnancy at a significantly higher rate than men in a new relationship, despite the older age of the female partner in the former cases. This surprising observation may be in part related to their previously proven fecundity as a couple or a higher dedication in trying to achieve pregnancy.

5. **Age of the man.** In the absence of age-related hypogonadism (andropause), age of the man does not appear to affect the success rate of vasectomy reversal.

9. What investigations are required before vasectomy reversal is performed?

Athorough history and physical examination focusing on the reproductive health and surgical risks for the patients must be performed. Generally, fertility has been previously established in these patients before vasectomy. Otherwise, or when there are reasons to suspect a change in the reproductive health since the vasectomy, a serum level of follicle-stimulating hormone (FSH) or, rarely, a testicular biopsy, may be necessary to confirm active spermatogenesis before a vasectomy reversal is performed.

10. What are the anesthesia choices for vasectomy reversal?

Depending on the complexity of the surgery, it may require 3–4 hours or longer for completion. In addition, slight movements of the patient are greatly magnified by the operating microscope and disturb performance of the anastomosis. For these reasons, light general anesthesia is preferred. In carefully selected and cooperative patients with short interval since vasectomy, regional or even local anesthesia with sedation can be employed.

11. What is a vasogram?

For reconstructive surgery of the male reproductive tract, a vasogram or vasography is used to establish patency of the excurrent ductal outflow. In addition, a vasogram can be used to locate the site of blockade in the excurrent ductal system. Thus, for all reconstructive procedures of the male reproductive tract, whether it is vasovasostomy, vasoepididymostomy, or transurethral resection of the ejaculatory ducts (Fig. 1), a vasogram should be performed in the same setting.

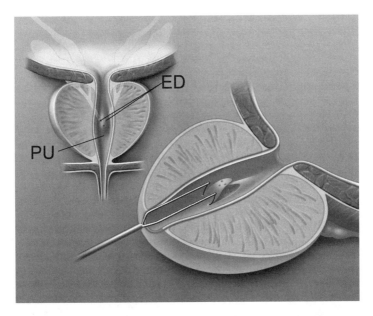

FIGURE 1. Transurethral resection of the ejaculatory ducts. ED ≥ ejaculatory duct, PU ≥ prostatic urethra.

12. Should a vasogram be performed alone as a diagnostic procedure?

No. Unless reconstruction is to be performed immediately in the same setting, a diagnostic vasogram alone should not be performed. The reason is that vasography can lead to stricture at the vasogram site. Furthermore, injection of dye or contrast materials into an obstructive system may lead to postoperative pain, inflammation, and infection, which may further complicate further management of infertility.

13. What are the different types of vasograms?

1. **Saline vasogram.** In this most frequently used and least invasive type of vasogram, a slow injection of saline solution with a 24-gauge angiocatheter cannulating the vas can establish patency of the excurrent ductal outflow provided that there is no resistance during injection. If there is any doubt, a dye vasogram should be performed.

2. **Dye vasogram.** Indigo-carmine (1:1 dilution) can be injected slowly in a similar fashion. The presence of blue/green color in the urine confirms patency of the ipsilateral outflow. If no dye enters the urinary bladder, a radiocontrast vasogram should be performed.

3. **Radiocontrast vasogram.** Since radiation and contrast materials are required for this procedure, it is not routinely performed unless both saline vasogram and dye vasogram fail to establish patency of the excurrent ductal outflow. A blunt-tip, 2–0 Prolene suture can first be passed gently toward the seminal vesicle and a clamp placed on the suture when it passes no further. This technique is particularly useful for delineating the site of inguinal obstruction from prior groin surgery (such as a hernia repair). Radiocontrast vasography is then performed by passing a no.3 whistle-tip ureteral catheter toward the seminal vesicle end of the vas. 16-French Foley catheter is placed in the bladder with the balloon filled with 5 ml of air. Placing the balloon on gentle traction before vasography prevents reflux of contast medium into the bladder, which can obscure details. Vasograms are performed with the injection of 0.5 ml of water-soluble contast media (Fig 2).

14. How is a vasogram performed?

1. Choose the appropriate site. The most common sites of obstruction in the male excurrent ductal system are the vas (from previous vasectomy or groin injury), ejaculatory ducts, and epi-

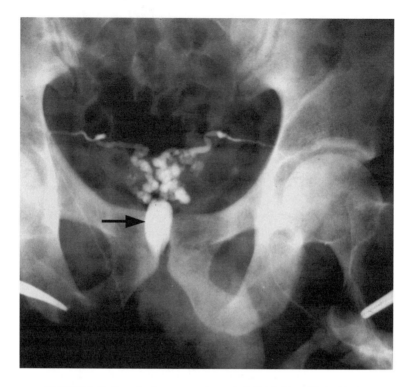

FIGURE 2. Radiocontrast vasogram. Arrow indicates balloon filled with air.

didymis. Unless the site of vasal obstruction is obvious and easily assessed, as in cases of previous vasectomy, a vasogram should be performed at the straight portion of the vas closest to the testis/epididymis. A small segment of the vas is isolated microsurgically with the vasal sheath and vessels dissected off and preserved. Under 25× magnification, the vas is hemitransected to gain access to the vasal lumen.

2. **Evaluation of fluid.** The fluid should then be examined microscopically to look for sperm. The absence of sperm or sperm parts indicates the presence of obstruction in the epididymis (assuming that active spermatogenesis is present) and, after establishing the patency of the ductal outflow, a vasoepididymostomy should be performed (Table 1).

3. **Choose vasogram materials.** Generally one should begin with a saline vasogram. Only when patency cannot be established unequivocally is it necessary to proceed to other types of vasogram.

4. **Closure.** If the obstruction is at the epididymis only, the vas can be completely transected at the vasogram site to proceed to a vasoepididymostomy. Otherwise, after completing the vasogram and when vasal access is no longer needed, it should be closed microsurgically to minimize scarring and obstruction at the vasogram site.

15. What are the complications of vasogram?

1. **Strictures** may occur at the site of hemitransection of the vas. In addition, contrast materials (especially the non-water-soluble types) injected during a vasogram can lead to mucosal inflammation of the vas.

2. **Injury to the vasal blood supply** may occur during a vasogram when the vas is cut. For this reason, hemitransection of the vas should be performed microsurgically to allow sparing of the vasal vessels.

3. **Hematoma** can occur in the preivasal sheath. Bipolar cautery can be used for meticulous hemostasis at the time of vasography to prevent hematomoma formation.

Table 1. Relationship between Gross Appearance of Vasal Fluid and
Microscopic Findings

VASAL FLUID APPEARANCE	MOST COMMON FINDINGS ON MICROSCOPIC EXAMINATION	SURGICAL PROCEDURE INDICATED
Copious, crystal clear, watery	No sperm in fluid	Vasovasostomy
Copious, cloudy thin, water soluble	Usually sperm with tails	Vasovasostomy
Copious, creamy yellow, water soluble	Usually many sperm heads, occasional sperm with short tails	Vasovasostomy
Copious, thick white toothpaste-like, water insoluble	No sperm	Vasoepididymostomy
Scant white thin fluid	No sperm	Vasoepididymostomy
Dry, spermless vas; no granuloma at vasectomy site	No sperm	Vasoepididymostomy
Scant fluid, granuloma present at vasectomy site	Barbitage fluid reveals sperm	Vasovasostomy

4. **Sperm granuloma.** Leaky closure of a vasography site may lead to development of a sperm granuloma, which can result in stricture or obstruction of the vas.

16. What is the success rate of vasovasostomy?
Even among experts who have reported their vasectomy reversal techniques in the literature, the success rates varies widely depending on the surgeon's technique and experience. The overall success rate for vasovasostomy in the literature ranges from 70% to 99.5% for return of sperm to the ejaculate (a.k.a. patency rate). The success rate for vasoepididymostomy in the literature is somewhat lower, ranging from 40% to 90%. Microsurgical longitudinal intussusception vasoepididymostomy (see below) currently has a patency rate of over 90%.

17. What is the definition of success in vasectomy reversal?
One should be careful when evaluating the success of vasectomy reversal. Besides simply being a patent anastomosis, a successful vasectomy reversal should provide good quality and quantity of sperm in the ejaculate. In addition, these parameters should be durable with time, since a poorly performed anastomosis may be patent initially but shut down later due to fibrosis.

Many surgeons consider simply the presence of sperm (even at a very low count) in the ejaculate to indicate successful surgery. Even when evaluating the literature, one should keep in mind that, besides comparing simply the patency rate, quantity (sperm counts) and quality (motility rate, normal morphology rates) should also be taken into consideration.

18. What is the pregnancy rate after vasectomy reversal?
For microdot multilayer vasovasostomy, the cumulative pregnancy rate at 1 year postoperatively is 70%. For microsurgical intussusception vasoepididymostomy, the rate at 18 months postoperatively is 45%.

Although some may consider pregnancy rate to be a better parameter to evaluate vasectomy reversal success, one should keep in mind that the pregnancy rates depend significantly on the age of the female partners and the presence of coexisting female infertility factors. For these reasons, most studies in the literature evaluating the surgical technique of vasectomy reversal report the patency rates for comparative purposes.

19. What are the differences in the techniques of vasosvasostomy?
Nonmicrosurgical vasovasostomy is a crude technique that is generally not recommended by most infertility specialists. The anastomosis is generally performed using 6–0 or larger sutures. Surgeons who use this technique generally do not have the expertise to perform a vasoepididymostomy when necessary.

Microsurgical single-layer vasovasostomy. With the introduction of microsurgical technique using finer suture for the mucosal anastomosis (8–0 or finer), the success rate of this technique is superior to the nonmicrosurgical technique, ranging from 75% to 90% in the literature.

Microsurgical microdot multilayer vasovasostomy. The special features of this advanced technique include mapping of the two ends of the vas with microdot to allow an even distribution of the mucosal anasotmostic suture (generally 10–0 in size). This strategy is necessary because there is generally a large discrepancy between the luminal sizes of the vasal ends in the testicular (proximal) side and the abdominal (distal) side (Fig. 3). Without proper matching of the suture points, a dog-ear may form in the mucosal anastomosis, resulting in leakage of fluid. In addition, the anastomosis with this technique is closed in four layers using a total of 24 microsutures. This technique allows a watertight and secure anastomosis. The patency rate of this technique is 99.5%.

20. What is the significance of the appearance of vasal fluid during a vasectomy reversal?

The vasal fluid from the testicular end should be examined microscopically to determine the presence of sperm. The gross appearance of the vasal fluid can correlate with microscopic findings (see Table 1).

21. When should a vasoepididymostomy be performed instead of a vasovasostomy?

The microscopic findings of the vasal fluid (see Table 1) can help determine whether the vasectomy reversal should be performed with vasovasostomy or, in the presence of epididymal obstruction, with vasoepididymostomy.

22. Can a vasovasostomy be performed in the presence of epididymal obstruction?

Vasovasostomy generally fails in the presence of an epididymal obstruction. The success of vasectomy reversal depends significantly on the technical skills of the surgeon. If the surgeon is not comfortable performing vasoepididymostomy, a vasovasostomy should be performed instead. Attempting a vasoepididymostomy without proper surgical technique can result in significant scarring, making subsequent reconstruction less likely to succeed.

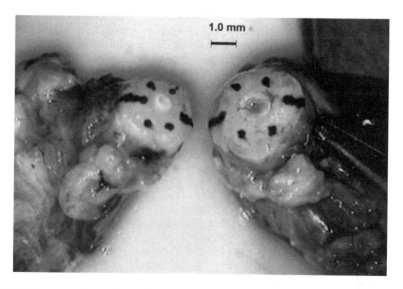

FIGURE 3. Microsurgical microdot multilayer vasovasostomy. This technique is especially useful because of the generally large discrepancy between the luminal sizes of the vasal ends in the testicular (proximal) side and the abdominal (distal) side.

23. How was early vasoepididymostomy performed?

Vasoepididymostomy is considered the most technically challenging reconstructive surgery. Historically, the oldest procedure of vasoepididymostomy was attempted by creation of a fistulous communication between the multiply incised epididymal tubule and the opened lumen of the vas deferens. In 1918 Lespinasse became the first to attempt a precise epdidymal tubule anastomosis to the vasal lumen. The success rate of these nonmicrosurgical vasoepididymostomies was generally poor interms of both patency and subsequent pregnancy.

24. What techniques are currently used for vasoepididymostomy?

All current vasoepididymostomy techniques require advanced microsurgical training and expertise. There are currently three types of microsurgical vasoepididymostomy (Table 2):

1. **End-to-end vasoepididymostomy.** In 1978, with the introduction of optical enhancement in surgery, Silber performed an end-to-end single epididymal tubule anastomosis to the vas. With this method, the epididymis is dissected completely to the vasoepididymal junction and then serially and transversely transected until a gush of fluid is seen exuding from the cut surface, indicating the correct level of the anastomosis. The single tubule from which fluid is effluxing is identified and anastomosed directly to the vas mucosa with three to five interrupted sutures of 10–0 monofilament nylon (Fig. 4).

2. **End-to-side vasoepididymostomy.** In the 1980s, an end-to-side anastomosis was introduced using 6 to 8 microsutures (Fig. 5). The patency rate of vasoepididymostomy ranged from 50% to 85%. Extreme precision and surgical skills, however, are required to anastomose an epididymal tubule to the vasal lumen. Hence, the outcomes of these techniques are highly dependant on the experience of the surgeons.

3. **Intussusception end-to-side vasoepididymostomy.** In the 1990s Berger introduced a triangulation intussusception vasoepididymostomy, which uses only three double-armed microsutures to achieve a 6-point anastomosis. This technique was later modified using only two double-armed sutures placed longitudinally to achieve a 4-point anastomosis (Fig. 6). The unique feature of this technique is that the epididymal tubule intussuscepts into the vasal lumen upon tying of the mucosal sutures. This method allows a more secure anastomosis. The patency rate of the longitudinal intussusception vasoepididymostomy approach is over 90% in current clinical series and is our preferred method of vasoepididymostomy

25. How does one select the level of the epididymis to perform a vasoepididymostomy?

1. **Size of tubules.** Generally, the diameter of the epididymal tubule increases from efferent ductules to caput and from corpus to cauda. Although vasoepididymostomy can be performed at any of these levels, anastomosis to a larger, more dilated, and distal tubule may in theory increase the success rate and allow greater maturation of sperm. The epididymis should also be carefully

Table 2. Comparison of Three Common Techniques for Vasoepididymostomy

TECHNIQUES	ADVANTAGES	DISADVANTAGE
Intussusception	Two to three sutures placed in epididymal tubule provide 4 and 6 points of fixation Virtually bloodless anastomosis	Cannot assess tubular fluid for sperm before anastomosis set-up
End-to-side	Virtual bloodless anastomosis Epididymal fluid can be examined before anastomosis	Difficult suture placement to collapsed tubule
End-to-end	Epididymal fluid can be examined before anastomosis Easy and rapid identification of level of obstruction in the epididymis. Allows upward mobilization of epididymis to bridge a large vasal gap	Difficult hemostasis on transected epididymis Difficult to identify proper tubule for anastomosis Difficult outer layer closure Vasal blood supply from inferior epididymal artery is sacrificed

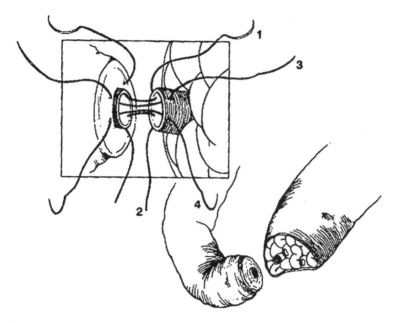

FIGURE 4. End-to-end vasoepididymostomy.. The single tubule from which fluid is effluxing is identified and anastomosed directly to the vas mucosa with three to five interrupted sutures of 10–0 monofilament nylon.

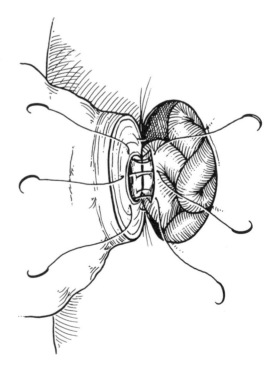

FIGURE 5. End-to-side vasoepididymostomy. An end-to-side anastomosis uses 6 to 8 microsutures.

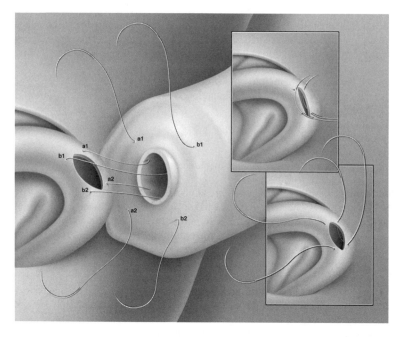

FIGURE 6. Intussusception end-to-side vasoepididymostomy. This technique uses only two double-armed sutures placed longitudinally to achieve a 4-point anastomosis.

examined under the operating microscope to look for signs such as dilatation or discoloration of tubules to help identify an unobstructed segment for the anasotmosis.

2. **Presence of sperm.** The epididymal fluid should be examined microscopically for sperm. Intact sperm, whether motile or not, should be found before proceeding to the anastomosis. Sperm heads or sperm parts, if found in abundant quantity, also indicate that the selected location is proximal to the obstruction, and the anastomosis may be performed. In the absence of sperm, however, a more proximal level should be evaluated for the anastomosis.

26. What is a "cross-over" vasovasostomy or vasoepididymostomy?

In complex cases of obstruction characterized by a solitary functioning testis with an ipsilateral obstructed vas that is not reconstructable (such as multiple vasal obstruction, concomittent vasal and ejaculatory ductal obstruction, unbridgeable gap in the vasal segment), it is better to connect the functioning testis to the patent vas on the contralateral side. This goal may be achieved either by bringing the contralateral vas through the scrotal septum to reach the functioning testis or by bringing the functioning testis to the contralateral hemiscrotum. Either vasovasostomy or vasoepididymostomy can be performed with the cross-over technique with a success rate similar to the corresponding ipsilateral version of the surgery.

27. In which situations can a reconstruction not be performed?

Rarely, an obstruction may be unreconstructable. Examples include epididymal obstruction proximal to the efferent ductules. In this setting, no sperm can be found even at the most proximal epididymal tubule accessible. Hence, a vasoepididmostomy cannot be performed.

Multiple vasal obstructions is another example. After resecting the obstruction segment of the vas, there may be too large of a gap to bridge despite various mobilization maneuvers. Vasovasostomy should not be performed at more than one site in the vas, since the segment of the vas between the two anastomoses will not have any blood supply and will become ischemic.

Finally, the site of obstruction in the ejaculatory ducts may be too proximal to be safely resected transurethrally. In such situations, surgical reconstruction is generally not possible, and sperm retrieval with cryopreservation for future use with assisted reproduction should be performed.

28. What are the surgical principles of a successful vasectomy reversal?

1. Accurate mucosa-to-mucosa approximation
2. Leakproof anastomosis
3. Tension-free anastomosis
4. Good blood supply to tissues
5. Healthy mucosa and muscularis
6. Precise and atraumatic anastomotic technique.

29. What factors can affect the success rate of a vasoepididymostomy?

1. **Skill/experience.** The most important factor for a successful vasoepididymostomy is the surgical skill and experience of the surgeon. This procedure should be attempted only by surgeons who have expertise and experience in microsurgery for male reproductive tract reconstruction.

2. **Technique.** Intussusception techniques appear to be easier to perform and to have a higher success rate than conventional techniques. However, surgeons should choose a technique with which they have the highest and most consistent success rates.

3. **Presence of sperm in the fluid.** In the absence of sperm or sperm parts in the epididymal fluid, vasoepididymostomy always fails. Thus, surgeons should select carefully the epididymal tubule for the anastomosis.

4. **Location.** At least in theory, performing the anastomosis to the distal/caudal epididymis where the tubules are of a larger diameter may have a higher patency rate and leave a greater length of epididymis available for sperm maturation.

30. What should one do if the vasectomy reversal fails?

Studies have shown that in failed vasectomy reversal, whether vasovasostomy or vasoepididymostomy, it is more cost-effective to perform a repeat surgical reconstruction than to attempt assisted reproduction.

Technically, if the failure of a vasovasostomy is due to epididymal obstruction, a vasoepididymostomy, but not a repeated vasovasostomy, should be performed. In cases of vasoepididymostomy failure, a repeat vasoepididymostomy should be performed. Surgeons should not hesitate to refer these difficult cases to more experienced colleagues for management.

31. Is it necessary to cryopreserve sperm during vasectomy reversal?

The answer depends on the likelihood of success in the experience of the surgeon and whether the patient and his female partner are willing to have advanced assisted reproduction in the future. Generally, the success rates of vasovasostomy with most experienced surgeons are above 90%; thus, routine sperm cryopreservation is not necessary for all vasovasostomies. With vasoepididymostomy, since the success rate varies significantly from 60% to 90%, routine cryopreservation should be considered, especially if vasoepididymostomy has to be performed bilaterally.

32. When should sperm return to the ejaculate after vasectomy reversal?

Compared to vasoepididymostomy, vasovasostomy typically yields a higher patency rate, higher quality and quantity of sperm in the ejaculate, and a shorter postoperative time for return of sperm to the ejaculate. Generally, if vasovasostomy is performed on at least one side, sperm should return at the first semen analysis, which is usually performed at 1 month postoperatively. The quantity and quality of sperm may not be optimal initially but will improve in subsequent analyses, provided that the vasovasostomy anastomosis is well performed.

In cases of bilateral vasoepididymostomy, more than 60% of men should have some sperm returned to the ejaculate at the first semen analysis at 1 month postoperatively. By 3–6 months, sperm should return to the ejaculate in most men with a patent anastomosis. As in vasovasostomy cases, in a properly performed vasoepididymostomy, the sperm quality and quantity usually improve further with time.

33. At what point should one deem the surgery a failure?

Generally, if the anastomosis is performed properly, sperm should return to the ejaculate no later than 3 months after vasovasostomy and by 6 months after a vasoepididymostomy is performed. After bilateral vasoepididymostomy, occasionally it may take 1 year for sperm to return.

34. What is delayed failure in vasectomy reversal?

The anastomosis in vasovasostomy and vasoepididymostomy may shut down after an initial period of patency. This shut-down is generally due to fibrosis of the anastomosis. The delayed failure rate is 5–12% for vasovasostomy and 10–21% for vasoepididymostomy at 18 months after surgery.

35. If sperm return to the ejaculate postoperatively, is it necessary to bank them?

This answer also depends on whether a vasovasostomy or vasoepididymostomy (especially if done bilaterally) was performed and whether the patient and his female partner are willing to attempt advanced assisted reproduction (IVF/ICSI) in the future. Since vasoepididymostomy is associated with a significant rate of delayed failure, banking of sperm is advisable. Often the quality and quantity of sperm returning to the ejaculate may be better than the quality and quantity of sperm that are cryopreserved intraoperatively. Hence additional cryopreservation should be considered. When in doubt, it is always more advisable to cryopreserve sperm postoperatively.

36. What is "money-back guarantee" for vasectomy reversal?

Many surgeons advertise a "money-back guarantee" for vasectomy reversal. To a certain extent, this approach may provide assurance to patients undergoing surgery, but often it is viewed as a gimmick to attract business. Surgeons who offer such a guarantee often specify that the surgery is successful as long as sperm (regardless of quality and quantity) are persent in at least one semen analysis postoperatively. Such a guarantee does not necessarily have any relevance to the couple's success in achieving pregnancy. Therefore, one should not falsely assume that surgeons who offer such a guarantee are necessarily providing better surgical results than surgeons who do not.

37. Should vasectomy reversal be performed only at one side?

The patency rate of our microsurgical microdot multilayer vasovasostomy is close to 100%. Nonetheless, we do not advocate performing the surgery on only one side for the following reasons:

1. As seen below, the overall success rate decreases significantly when the procedure is performed only one side (especially if the bilateral patency rate is lower, as with vasoepididymostomy).

2. Having an extra side with sperm production may contribute to higher sperm counts in the ejaculate, allowing a higher chance for achieving pregnancy.

3. Leaving one side obstructed may put patients at a higher risk to continue to produce antisperm antibodies, which may have a negative impact on the quality of the sperm. Therefore, relieving the obstruction may, at least in theory, allows better quality of sperm.

38. What is the "theoretical" success rate of vasectomy reversal if it is performed only on one side?

If the bilateral patency rate for vasovasostomy is 99%, the unilateral patency rate is 90% (see below). If bilateral patency rate for vasoepididymostomy is 84%, the unilateral patency rate decreases to 60%.

For vasovasotomy

Assuming that the bilateral patency rate is 99% and that the probability of patency for the left and right sides is equal and independent of each other:

Probability of patency = P (both side patent) + P (left patent and right blocked) + P (left
                          blocked and right patent)
                        = 99%
Probability of failure   = P (left blocked) x P (right blocked)
                        = 1%
Hence, P (left blocked) = P (right blocked) = 10%
P (one side patent) = 100% − P (one side blocked) = **90%**
For vasoepididymostomy
Assuming that the bilateral patency rate is 84% and that the probability of patency for the left
and right sides is equal and independent of each other:
Probability of patency = P (both side patent) + P (left patent and right blocked) + P (left
                          block and right patent)
                        = 84%
Probability of failure   = P (left blocked) × P (right blocked)
                        = 16%
Hence, P (left blocked) = P (right blocked) = 40%
P (one side patent) = 100% − P (one side blocked) = **60%**

Table 3. Advantages and Disadvantages of Robot-assisted Vasectomy Reversal

ADVANTAGES	DISADVANTAGES
Reduction of fine tremor	Extra time required to set up the bulky robot for the anastomosis
Potential to perform "tele-surgery"	High cost to acquire a robotic unit
	Inferior vision at high magnification through camera and television monitor (compared to direct observation through the operating microscope)

39. Discuss the role of robot-assisted vasectomy reversal.

Robot-assisted microsurgical vasovasostomy and vasoepididymostomy have been used as experimental procedures in several infertility centers. The advantages and disadvantages are summarized in Table 3. Despite the technical advantages of using robot assistance for fine maneuvers, robot assistance does not obviate the need for prudent surgical judgment. The majority of the time during a vasectomy reversal is generally spent on selecting healthy tissue with good blood supply, choosing the appropriate level of anastomosis during a vasoepididymostomy, or properly setting up a tension-free anastomosis. Hence, one should be aware that robot assistance is unlikely to reduce the surgical time significantly, since it is most useful only during the placement of micro-needles in the anastomosis (in reality, about 20% of surgical time).

BIBLIOGRAPHY

1. Belker AM, Thomas AJ Jr, Fuchs EF, et al: Results of 1,469 microsurgical vasectomy reversals by the Vasovasostomy Study Group. J Urol 152:505–511, 1991.
2. Berger RE: Triangulation end-to-side vasoepididymostomy. J Urol 159:1951, 1998.
3. Boorjian S, Lipkin M, Goldstein M: The impact of obstructive interval and sperm granuloma on outcome of vasectomy reversal. J Urol 171:304–306, 2004.
4. Chan PT, Li PS, Goldstein M: Microsurgical vasoepididymostomy: A prospective randomized study of 3 intussusception techniques in rats. J Urol 169:1924, 2003.
5. Chan PTK, Brandell RA, Goldstein M: Prospective analysis of the post-operative outcomes of microsurgical intussusception vasoepididymostomy. J Urol 167:310, 2002.
6. Chan PTK, Goldstein M: Superior outcomes of microsurgical vasectomy reversal in men with the same female partner. Fertil Steril 2004 [in press].

7. Chan PT, Libman J: Feasibility of microsurgical reconstruction of the male reproductive tract after percutaneous epididymal sperm aspiration (PESA). Can J Urol 10(6):2070–2073, 2003.

8. Donovan JF Jr, DiBaise M, Sparks AE, et al: Comparison of microscopic epididymal sperm aspiration and intracytoplasmic sperm injection/in-vitro fertilization with repeat microscopic reconstruction following vasectomy: Is second attempt vas reversal worth the effort? Hum Reprod 13:387, 1998.

9. Goldstein M, Li PS, Matthews GJ: Microsurgical vasovasostomy: The microdot technique of precision suture placement. J Urol 159:188–190, 1998.

10. Goldstein. M: Surgical management of male infertility and other scrotal disorders. In Walsh PC, Retik AB, Vaughan ED, Wein AJ (eds): Campbell's Urology, vol. 2, 8th ed. Philadelphia, W.B. Saunders, 2002, pp 1532–1587.

11. Goldstein M, Chan PTK, Li PS: Ultra-precise multi-layer microsurgical vasovasostomy: Tricks of the trade. Ortho-McNeil AUA Video HV2266.

12. Goldstein M, Chan PT, Li PS: Microsurgical intussusception vasoepididymostomy: Tricks of the trade. J Urol 169:387, 2003.

13. Kolettis PN, Thomas AJ: Vasoepididymostomy for vasectomy reversal: A critical assessment in the era of intracytoplasmic sperm injection. J Urol 158:467, 1997.

14. Matthews GJ, Schlegel PN, Goldstein M: Patency following microsurgical vasoepididymostomy and vasovasostomy: Temporal considerations. J Urol 154:2070, 1995.

15. Pavlovich CP, Schlegel PN: Fertility options after vasectomy: A cost-effectiveness analysis. Fertil Steril 67:133, 1997

16. Schlegel PN, Goldstein M: Microsurgical vasoepididymostomy: Refinements and results. J Urol 150: 1165, 1993

18. TESTICULAR BIOPSY

Yefim Sheynkin, M.D.

1. What is the main indication for a diagnostic testicular biopsy?

Testis biopsy is indicated in azoospermic men with testes of normal size and consistency, palpable vasa deferentia, and normal serum levels of follicle-stimulating hormone (FSH).

The main purpose for diagnostic testis biopsy remains to distinguish between obstructive and nonobstructive causes of azoospermia (e.g. to differentiate between normal spermatogenesis and hypospermatogenesis, maturation arrest, Sertoli-cell-only syndrome, and other histologic changes associated with testicular failure). Sperm (if found) may also be harvested at the time of testicular biopsy.

2. In addition to histologic evaluation of the testes, what are the other uses for testicular biopsy?

Testicular tissues can be sampled, not for diagnostic purposes, but for retrieval of sperm.

Advances in assisted reproduction and development of the intracytoplasmic sperm injection (ICSI) procedure have expanded the indications for a testis biopsy to virtually all azoospermic patients. The procedure can provide successful sperm harvesting for ICSI. In addition, retrieved sperm can be cryopreserved. Azoospermic men with small, soft testes and FSH levels elevated more than twice normal (nonobstructive azoospermia) generally have primary testicular failure. In such patients biopsy may be helpful to rule out intratubular germ-cell neoplasm (carcinoma in situ).

3. What is the goal of a diagnostic testis biopsy?

The goal of testis biopsy is to obtain sufficient sampling of testicular tissue for histologic diagnosis while avoiding trauma to the specimen (which may lead to artifacts) and injury to the epididymis and testicular blood supply. Additionally, sperm harvesting may be performed if a sperm cryopreservation facility is available.

4. What are the methods of performing testicular biopsy?

Testicular biopsy may be performed with (1) conventional open surgical technique, (2) atraumatic microsurgical technique, and (3) percutaneous techniques.

5. Explain the percutaneous testis biopsy techniques.

Percutaneous testis biopsy can be performed with a 14-G biopsy gun, similar to what is used for prostate biopsy, to obtain a core of tissue. It can also be done with testicular needle aspiration.

6. What type of testicular biopsy is considered the gold standard?

Open testicular biopsy remains the gold standard to obtain an optimal amount of tissue for diagnosis and sperm retrieval for IVF.

7. What are the advantages of microsurgical testicular biopsy?

The use of optical magnification (loupes or operating microscope) allows a clear identification of blood vessels on the testicular tunica, thus minimizing bleeding. Bleeding during a testicular biopsy may contaminate the biopsy specimen and lead to devascularization of testicular tissue, resulting in a higher risk of testicular atrophy.

8. What are the disadvantages of the percutaneous testicular biopsy?

Percutaneous testicular biopsy is a blind procedure and may result in unintentional injury to the epididymis or the testicular artery. If bleeding occurs, it cannot be easily controlled. Particularly with needle aspiration, the amount of specimen obtained is often small, making proper interpretation of histology difficult.

9. What are the complications of testicular biopsy?

Testicular biopsy is associated with few complications when carefully performed. The most serious complication is inadvertent biopsy of the epididymis. Such iatrogenic injury results in epididymal obstruction and significantly complicates subsequent reconstructive surgery in patients with obstructive azoospermia by creating additional areas of obstruction. Significant hematoma may result from unrecognized hemorrhage if the testicular artery on the surface of the tunica albuginea has been injured. Thanks to the rich blood supply to the testicles, infection is rare in the absence of hematoma. Blind percutaneous biopsy or biopsy performed under local anesthesia with cord block may result in inadvertent vascular injury and testicular atrophy.

10. How should the testicular biopsy specimen be handled?

To protect the biopsy specimen, tissue traumatization by forceps or excessive handling in any way must be avoided. For most practical purposes, testicular biopsy specimens are usually fixed with Bouin's solution (picric acid, formaldehyde, and acetic acid) to preserve nuclear morphology. Improper handling of the biopsy specimen with the use of the wrong fixative is a nuisance and may necessitate repeat biopsy. Other common fixatives, such as formalin, result in distortion of histology and tissue shrinkage.

11. What are the possible histologic findings in the testicular biopsy of an infertile man?

Normal spermatogenesis, hyposeprmatogenesis, maturation arrest, germ cell sloughing, and Sertoli-cell-only syndrome (germ cell aplasia).

12. What are the most common histologic findings in infertile men?

Hypospermatogenesis and maturation arrest.

13. Describe hypospermatogenesis.

Hypospermatogenesis means reduced spermatogenesis. In pure hypospermatogenesis, all stages of the spermatogenic cycle are present, but the germinal epithelium is thin and the number of germ cells at each level is proportionally reduced. Most fertility specialists agree that less than 20 spermatids per cross-section of a seminiferous tubule is consistent with hypospermatogenesis.

14. Describe Sertoli-cell-only syndrome (SCO).

SCO syndrome or germ-cell aplasia is characterized by reduced diameter of seminifereous tubules lined only by Sertoli cells, with complete absence of all germ cells. It is found in 13% of patients with azoospermia. Clinically patients may present with azoospermia with normal external genitalia, well-developed male sex characteristics, elevated serum FSH, normal or slightly elevated luteinizing hormone (LH), and normal or slightly decreased testosterone

15. Describe maturation arrest.

Spermatogenesis proceeds normally through a specific stage, at which point no further maturation of germ cells is identified. Hence, by definition, histologically no spermatozoa are seen in the seminiferous tubule. The "arrest" usually occurs at the stage of primary spermatocytes (early arrest) or at the stage of spermatids (late arrest).

16. Describe germ-cell elements in the normal adult seminiferous tubule.

The germ-cell elements compose the bulk of the cells in the seminiferous tubule. Maturation of germ cells proceeds in an orderly and nonrandomized fashion along the length of the seminiferous tubule. Groups of germ cells at one level of development tend to be found in association with specific germ cells at another level of development. Six cellular associations of germ-cell elements in the human have been described. Germ cells recognized in the cross-sectional view of a seminiferous tubule include spermatogonia, different stages of primary spermatocytes, secondary spermatocytes, early and late spermarids, and spermatozoa. However, not all stages of differentiation may be seen in any one cross-sectional view of seminiferous tubule.

17. Describe histologic appearance of germ cell elements of normal adult seminiferous tubule.

Spermatogonia are located in the basal compartment close to basement membrane, Their nuclei are dense with homogenous chromatin pattern. The nucleolus can be easily identified. **Primary spermatocytes** include preleptotene, leptotene, zygoten, pachyten, and diploten. In the leptotene spermatocytes, chromatin becomes filamentous with fine beading arrangement. Zygotene spermatocytes are characterized with coarse granularity and eccentrical chromatin location. Pachytene and diplotene spermatocytes are easily recognized by their very large nucleus and thick, short chromatin filaments. **Secondary spermatocytes** present in much smaller number than primary spermatocytes and can be recognized by their smaller size and fine granular chromatin pattern **Early spermatids** may have identifiable slight depression on the surface, the beginning of acrosome. The nucleus of **late spermatids** changes to an oval and then an elongated form, eventually assuming the configuration of a mature spermatozoon.

18. What are the compartments of seminiferous tubule?

The seminiferous tubule can be divided into the basal and adluminal compartments.

19. Which germ cells are located in the basal compartment?

Spermatogonia and preleptotene primary spermatocytes.

20. Testicular biopsy reveals normal spermatogenesis. Describe the appearance of germ cells in the adult seminiferous tubule.

Spermatogonia at the basement membrane, primary spermatocytes in different stages, secondary spermatocytes, and spermatids/spermatozoa. Not all stages of differentiation may be seen in any one cross-sectional view of the seminiferous tubule.

21. What is the prognostic significance of testicular biopsy for subsequent sperm retrieval?

Studies reveal an association between distinctive histologic pattern and possibility of local sperm findings/harvesting:

- Sertoli cell-only   24%
- Maturation arrest   42%
- Hypospermatogenesis   81%

22. Should testicular biopsy be performed unilaterally or bilaterally?

Most clinicians usually perform bilateral testicular biopsy, regardless of the size discrepancy between the two testes. Histologic findings cannot be reliably predicted by testicular size. Good spermatogenesis is sometimes present in a small, firm testis, and maturation arrest may be seen in a large, healthy testis. Intraindividual variation is reported in the literature in up to 47% of cases after bilateral biopsies.

23. Bilateral testicular biopsy in an azoospermic man revealed normal spermatogenesis. What does this finding mean?

This finding is pathognomonic for bilateral obstruction of the excurrent ductal system.

24. What is a "touch-prep"?

When the tunica albugenia is open during a testicular biopsy, a sample of the seminiferous tubules is first removed for histologic diagnosis. The opened seminiferous tubules are then blotted several times with a glass slide. A drop of normal saline is added to the blotted areas of the slide and covered with a cover slip. The "touch-prep" slide is examined using a light microscope.

The presence of mature sperm on the slide invariably indicates the presence of normal spermatogenesis. A "touch-prep" should always be performed in a testicular biopsy. On paraffin histologic section, it is difficult to distinguish normal spermatogenesis (in which mature spermatozoa are present) from late maturation arrests (in which only elongated/late spermatids and no mature spermatozoa are present). Evaluation of "touch prep" is necessary to differentiate between the two entities.

25. Describe testicular blood supply.
- Testicular (internal spermatic) artery from the aorta (main blood supply)
- Deferential artery from the internal iliac (hypogastric) artery
- Cremasteric (external spermatic) artery from the inferior epigastric artery

26. Which areas of the testes are most likely to contain a major superficial artery?
The areas of the testis most likely to contain a major superficial arterial branch are the medial, anterior, and lateral surfaces of the lower pole.

27. Incision of which areas of the tunica albuginea is least likely to cause arterial injury?
The areas of the human testis that are least likely to contain a major superficial artery are the medial and lateral surfaces of the upper pole. Incisions on the tunica albugenia should be made in these areas during a biopsy.

BIBLIOGRAPHY

1. Buch JP, Johansson SL: Testis biopsy in male infertility: Current status. Adv Urol 5:209–237, 1992.
2. Kevin HS: Testicular biopsy in the study of male infertility. Hum Pathol 10:584, 1979.
3. Kim ED, Lipschultz LI: Testis biopsy: Indications and interpretation in male infertility. AUA Update Series 17:314–319, 1998.
4. Nistal M, Paniagua R: Testicular biopsy. Urol Clin North Am 26:555–595, 1999.
5. Su LM, Palermo GD, Goldstein M, et al: Testicular sperm extraction with intracytoplasmic sperm injection for nonobstructive azoospermic: Testicular histology can predict success of sperm retrieval. J Urol 161:112–116, 1999.
6. Trainer TD: Histology of normal testis. Am J Surg Pathol 11:797–809, 1987.

19. MANAGEMENT OF
EJACULATORY DISORDERS

*Dana A. Ohl, M.D., Susanne A. Quallich, CNP, CUNP,
and Jens Sonksen, M.D., Ph.D., D.M.Sc*

1. List the components of the genitourinary system involved with ejaculation.

The organs involved in the ejaculatory process include the epididymis, vas deferens, seminal vesicles, prostate, bladder neck, and periurethral skeletal muscle.

2. What neurologic and anatomic events are involved in ejaculation?

Ejaculation is a complex process that involves the coordination of three distinct processes: emission, bladder neck contraction, and projectile ejaculation. During sexual stimulation and before ejaculation, the cauda epididymis contracts, slowly pushing sperm into the vas deferens to prepare for its rapid expulsion. In addition, the bulbourethral (Cowper's) gland secretes a mucoid fluid, commonly called "pre-ejaculate."

3. Describe the process of emission.

Emission is initiated by the throracolumbar sympathetic nerves, which arise from T10–L2 and cause contraction of the smooth muscle in the vas deferens, seminal vesicles, and prostate. The result is rapid distal flow of sperm, which merges with fluid from the seminal vesicles at the ejaculatory ducts. Seminal vesicle fluid is expelled by smooth muscle contraction, and, along with the vas contribution, these components constitute the seminal fluid, which is deposited into the posterior urethra. During this time, the local genital pleasure sensation (orgasm) is perceived.

4. Describe the function of bladder neck contraction.

At the time of seminal emission, the bladder neck forcefully contracts to prevent the seminal fluid from flowing into the bladder (retrograde ejaculation). Bladder neck closure is also under sympathetic control.

5. How is projectile ejaculation achieved?

Shortly after emission, rhythmic contractions of the periurethral muscles expel the seminal fluid from the urethra (projectile ejaculation). The periurethral muscles are under the control of the pudendal nerve, which originates from S2–S4.

6. Can a man ejaculate without having an erection?

The neurologic control of erection has some overlap with that of ejaculation, since both involve spinal levels S2–S4. Therefore, if a man is unable to have an erection due to a neurologic condition, it is likely that projectile ejaculation may also be impaired. However, in this setting, it is possible that seminal emission may occur without projectile expulsion of the semen.

Most erectile dysfunction, however, is due to vascular disease. Therefore, erection may be impaired by a process that has nothing to do with the nervous system. In such men, erection may be absent, but the ejaculatory reflex may be entirely intact. In fact, when a patient describes this situation, it is highly likely that his erectile dysfunction is due to vascular disease.

7. List the disorders of ejaculation.

- Premature ejaculation
- Retarded ejaculation
- Retrograde ejaculation
- Anejaculation

8. Describe premature ejaculation. How is it treated?

Premature ejaculation, the most common form of ejaculatory dysfunction, is characterized by inability to delay orgasm. Sometimes ejaculation may occur immediately after or even before intromission. Since semen is commonly deposited into the vagina, premature ejaculation is not usually associated with infertility, but it is considered a sexual dysfunction. Premature ejaculation is treated with behavioral therapy and/or drugs known to delay ejaculation, such as selective serotonin-reuptake inhibitors (SSRIs).

9. Define retarded ejaculation. How is it treated?

Retarded ejaculation (delayed ejaculation, idiopathic anejaculation, psychogenic anejaculation) is a condition in which the patient is seemingly neurologically intact but unable to reach climax. The lack of orgasm in an otherwise intact man differentiates this condition from other types of anejaculation noted below. This condition is treated with psychotherapy, although results have been mixed. In refractory cases, electroejaculation has been used to retrieve sperm for the purposes of causing a pregnancy.

10. What is retrograde ejaculation? How is it treated?

Retrograde ejaculation into the bladder is due to inability of the bladder neck to close during seminal emission. This condition can be neurogenic, medication-induced, or anatomic (see question 15). In refractory cases, sperm can be retrieved from the bladder and used for artificial insemination.

11. Define anejaculation. How is it treated?

Anejaculation is total absence of release of seminal fluid, whether in antegrade or retrograde direction. This condition is due to disruption of the neural pathways (described above) that control seminal emission. These disruptions can occur at many levels of this neurologic control. Depending on the dysfunction responsible for anejaculation, orgasm may be present or absent.

12. In which medical conditions are ejaculatory problems common?

Spinal cord injury (SCI) is the most common cause of anejaculation, accounting for about 80% of men who seek medical treatment for anejaculatory infertility. Any condition that impairs spinal cord function, such as transverse myelitis, multiple sclerosis, congenital spinal bifida, or spinal cord ischemia can also result in dysfunctions that are similar to hose with traumatic SCI.

Because peripheral autonomic nerves are necessary to preserve ejaculatory function, any disease leading to peripheral neuropathy can also lead to dysfunction. The most common cause is diabetes mellitus, but problems can also be seen with any disease that leads to autonomic neuropathy. The disease may be manifest by problems with bladder neck closure, leading to retrograde ejaculation, or complete absence of seminal emission.

13. What are the sexual and fertility capabilities of a man with SCI?

Approximately 80% of all men with SCI have some preservation of erectile function. Most men with an injury above T9 level have reflex erections. However, they are usually ill-timed and do not persist long enough for satisfactory sexual activity. Erectile dysfunction treatment is usually necessary. Men with lower motor neuron injuries typically do not have erections.

Men with SCI do not fare as well with ejaculatory function. Only 5–15% of men have any evidence of ejaculation after SCI, and this ejaculatory dysfunction is the major factor contributing to the infertility problem in this population. Even when ejaculation is preserved, semen quality is also quite poor. Only about 5% of men with SCI are able to initiate a pregnancy without medical intervention.

14. Describe the typical presentation of ejaculatory dysfunction in diabetic men.

Diabetic neuropathy tends to be a slowly progressive condition. Men with neuropathy of the autonomic nerves leading to the ejaculatory organs typically have manifestations of neuropathy at other sites. The first symptom is a decrease in the amount of ejaculate rather than complete absence of ejaculation. The amount decreases further, until orgasm occurs without visible ejaculate. If medical attention is sought at this early stage, evaluation of the postorgasm urine usually demonstrates evidence of retrograde ejaculation. Although no change in symptoms is usually noted with time, presentation at a later stage typically demonstrates total absence of seminal emission, verifying progression of the neuropathy to a more complete stage.

15. Which surgical procedures can cause or contribute to ejaculatory dysfunction?

Y-V plasty of the bladder neck, which was a relatively common procedure in the 1950s and 1960s used to treat everything from bedwetting to recurrent urinary infections, commonly results in retrograde ejaculation due to anatomic factors. Transurethral resection of the prostate for benign prostatic hyperplasia (BPH) usually results in retrograde ejaculation, although the age group at risk for BPH is less likely to desire preservation of fertility.

Any surgery to the pelvic region can damage peripheral nerves, resulting in either an incompetent bladder neck with retrograde ejaculation or total anejaculation. Examples may include colon resection, rectal prolapse surgery, and major bladder surgery. Men who have retroperitoneal surgery, such as retroperitoneal lymph node dissection for testis cancer, or aortic surgery are at risk for injury to the retroperitoneal sympathetic nerve and anejaculation. Because testis cancer is most commonly seen in men aged 20–40 years, fertility may be an important issue.

16. Which is more common after retroperitoneal surgery—retrograde ejaculation or anejaculation?

After retroperitoneal surgery patients are usually referred to the urologist for "retrograde ejaculation." Orgasm is preserved, and patients and doctors alike believe that if orgasm is present, fluid must have been produced and ejaculated into the bladder. However, despite the sensation of fluid expulsion, most men with ejaculatory dysfunction after retroperitoneal surgery actually suffer total absence of seminal emission.

17. Can medications contribute to ejaculatory dysfunction?

Many medications and pharmacologic substances have been implicated as affecting ejaculatory function. The antidepressants typically cause anorgasmia, whereas agents with alpha-blocking properties may cause either retrograde ejaculation or anejaculation.

Drugs That May Contribute to Ejaculatory Dysfunction

CLASS	EXAMPLES
Monoamine oxidase inhibitors	Furazolidone, isocarboxazid, pargyline, phenelzine sulfate, tranylcypromine
Selective serotonin inhibitors	Fluoxetine, paroxetine, sertraline
Tricyclic antidepressants	Amitriptyline, clomipramine, doxepin, imipramine hydrochloride
Antipsychotics	Chlorpromazine, chlorprothixene, haloperidol, perphenazine, thioridazine, trifluorperazine hydrochloride
Benzodiazopines	Alprazolam, chlordiazepoxide, lorazepam
Antihypertensives/antiarrhythmics	Bethanidine, bretylium, guanethidine sulfate, hexamethonium, phenoxybenzamine hydrochloride, phentolamine, prazosin hydrochloride, reserpine, thiazides

18. Discuss the congenital disorders of ejaculation.

Neurogenic congenital causes of anejaculation, including spina bifida and other spinal cord malformations, are generally obvious to the treating physicians. Structural problems with the posterior urethra, such as urethral valves, and corrective surgery can lead to retrograde ejaculation. Obstructive causes include malformation of the prostate in exstrophy of the bladder, congenital absence of the vas deferens when the seminal vesicles are also atretic, and congenital ejaculatory duct obstruction.

19. Describe the common presentation of a man with ejaculatory dysfunction.

The presentation depends on the type of dysfunction. Men with retarded ejaculation typically have either a lifelong history of anorgasmia (primary retarded ejaculation) or a new-onset problem after previously normal function (secondary retarded ejaculation). The key feature in this patient population is the absence of orgasm. In men with primary retarded ejaculation, this history may be difficult to obtain, because patients may have no concept of what an orgasm is. Some may believe that the scant mucoid discharge from the bulbourethral glands represents an ejaculate. A highly detailed (and personal) history may be necessary to define this condition. Intermittent nocturnal emissions are common in this type of patient.

Otherwise neurologically intact patients with retrograde ejaculation or anejaculation usually are able to describe all of the events of the ejaculatory reflex, including the sensation of orgasm, release, and rhythmic contractions of the periurethral muscles. It is a fallacy that such contractions are absent in the absence of seminal emission. Patients with retrograde ejaculation may notice cloudy urine or debris in the urine after climax, whereas those with anejaculation will not.

20. What are the components of the initial history and physical examination in the evaluation of suspected ejaculatory dysfunction?

A **detailed sexual history** is essential to define the dysfunction. In most cases of neurogenic dysfunction, the cause is obvious, as in men with SCI or severe diabetic neuropathy. Patients with new-onset dysfunction, however, may have no knowledge of their pre-existing condition. Occasionally, ejaculatory dysfunction is the first sign of diabetes mellitus. Any surgical procedures that may cause dysfunction must be noted.

The **physical examination** should assess secondary sex characteristics as a measure of hormonal deficiency. Genital examination includes assessment of testicle size and consistency and palpation to confirm the presence of the vas deferens bilaterally.

21. What type of testing should be done in men with suspected ejaculatory dysfunction?

Hormonal assessment (follicle-stimulating hormone and testosterone) may assist in determining the adequacy of sperm production. In men with low-volume ejaculate, the antegrade specimen should be submitted for semen analysis. In these patients and in patients with orgasm with no antegrade ejaculate production, examination of the postorgasm urine for the presence or absence or sperm should be performed. In men with no sperm present on either antegrade or retrograde specimen, it may be necessary to perform testis biopsy to assess whether spermatogenesis is present. When it is difficult to differentiate an obstructive problem from a neurogenic etiology, transrectal ultrasound may be needed. In men with SCI or other obvious risk factors for ejaculatory dysfunction, the history may take precedence, with additional tests deferred in many of these patients.

22. How is anejaculation differentiated from ejaculatory duct obstruction?

This distinction can be difficult at times because of significant overlap in the presenting symptoms, signs, and test results. Prostate ultrasound usually shows dilation of the seminal vesicles in obstruction, but dilation also may be seen in men with a functional problem. The most distinctive feature of ejaculatory dysfunction is the presence of a medical condition that places the patient at risk.

23. Can medications be used to promote ejaculation?

Results of medications used to treat retrograde ejaculation depend on the underlying etiology. Drug therapy works only on men with a preserved sensation of orgasm. In other words, men with retarded ejaculation or SCI typically do not respond. Pharmaoctherapy is most promising in men with a peripheral neurologic problem of recent onset, such as patients who have had a recent retroperitoneal surgery or a diabetic with new onset of changes in ejaculation. Alpha-adrenergic agonists, such as pseudoephedrine, are used. A man with retrograde ejaculation may be converted to an antegrade ejaculator, or a man with anejaculation may respond with either retrograde or antegrade ejaculation. In diabetes, even if the man responds initially to medical therapy, it typically fails after a certain period due to worsening of the neuropathy over time.

24. Is it possible to induce ejaculation in anejaculatory males?
Yes. The two procedures currently in use to induce ejaculation are penile vibratory stimulation and electroejaculation.

PENILE VIBRATORY STIMULATION

25. Describe the process of penile vibratory stimulation (PVS).
A vibrator is placed on the penile frenulum and held in place until ejaculation occurs or for a total of 3 minutes. After a rest of 1 minute, another attempt can be performed. An assistant holds a collection cup ready to retrieve the ejaculate. Multiple ejaculations may be obtained during a single session from an optimal subject.

26. How does PVS work?
PVS depends on a vibratory stimulus placed on the penis to supply a strong afferent input into the central nervous system. Through reflex activity, the response is initiation of the ejaculatory reflex. All components of the central and peripheral nervous system must be intact for PSV to work, including:
- Dorsal nerves of the penis, which carry the afferent signals to their entry into the sacral spinal cord (S2–S4)
- Ascending tracts within the spinal cord, which allow the information to reach the ejaculatory center in regions T10–L2
- Sympathetic outflow from the thoracolumbar cord
- Descending pathways back to S2–S4
- Pudendal nerves to carry efferent signals to the periurethral muscles to contract

27. Which patients are candidates for PVS?
Since PVS requires the neurologic components mentioned above, the best candidates for PVS are men with SCI above the level of T10. These SCIs generally involve upper motor neuron lesions with an intact reflex arc in the ejaculatory neuro-pathway.

28. Why does PVS not work in all patients with anejaculation?
SCI below T10 typically involves lower motor neuron lesions and a generalized lack of reflex activity. Since components of the reflex are missing, it cannot succeed. Of interest, men with *incomplete* lesions above T10 have a lower chance of success with PVS, because input from the brain may "overrule" the basic reflex that PVS is trying to achieve.

For the same reason, men who are neurologically intact, such as those with retarded ejaculation, do not always respond to PVS, although there have been reports of small numbers of successes. To compound the problem, patients with peripheral neuropathic problems, such as diabetic neuropathy, or retroperitoneal surgery also do not respond due to interruption of the peripheral efferents.

29. Do any signs indicate that ejaculation is imminent during the PVS procedure?
When the vibrator is applied to the penis in a suitable subject, signs of leg muscle or abdominal contraction are typical. There may be jerking motions and changes in the contractions during the stimulation period. Immediately before ejaculation, there is usually a very strong, tonic, generalized muscle contraction that lasts a few seconds, followed by an abrupt release of contraction. Ejaculation usually occurs within seconds of this release.

30. Is a PVS-induced ejaculation physiologically normal?
Since PVS induces a normal ejaculatory reflex mechanism, it is physiologically normal. There is coordination between seminal emission, bladder neck closure, and contraction of the

periurethral muscles, resulting in a normal, antegrade, projectile ejaculation. It is prudent during the first session to examine the postejaculate urine, but significant retrograde ejaculate from PVS is uncommon.

31. What are the potential complications of PVS?

The vibrator can cause local skin bruising, but it is usually minor, and requires no treatment. Spasticity may be generally decreased for several hours after the procedure, which is usually a good effect. However, if the patient depends on reflex bladder activity for urination, retention of urine may occur. Autonomic dysreflexia may also occur in susceptible men.

32. What is autonomic dysreflexia?

Men with a complete SCI lesion located above T6 may have an effective disconnection of the peripheral sympathetic nervous system from the brainstem. This disconnection allows changes in blood pressure in response to peripheral events without modulation by the medulla. Therefore, with application of noxious stimuli, such as PVS or electroejaculation, the blood pressure may elevate to dangerously high levels. This pressure elevation can be partially abrogated by the administration of 10–30 mg of nifedipine sublingually before the procedure. It is essential that the first PVS in any man be performed in a clinic setting with blood pressure monitoring to ensure that the procedure is safe.

33. What prognostic factors predict success with PVS in men with SCI?

Higher success rates are seen in men with complete lesions, lesion level > T10, and intact hip flexion and bulbocavernosus reflexes. Patients who are obviously spastic tend to do better. Anecdotally, we believe that patients who would normally be considered optimal for PVS may fail the procedure due to medications given to reduce spasticity, either oral agents or agents given through intrathecal pumps.

34. What equipment should be used for PVS?

Sønksen and colleagues demonstrated that high ejaculation rates depend on the amplitude of vibration. Optimal parameters of vibration are 2.5-mm amplitude at 100 Hz. In difficult cases, one may need to go to higher levels of amplitude to exceed the ejaculatory threshold. Most commercially available vibrators have unreliable vibration parameters. We favor the FertiCare vibrator (Multicept APS, Copenhagen, DK), which has undergone FDA scrutiny and has an excellent record of providing accurate vibration delivery.

35. Must all PVS procedures be done in the clinic setting?

No. Once safety has been demonstrated in the clinic, a vibrator may be prescribed for home use. Men with SCI may use the device for sexual activity or to obtain semen specimens for home self-insemination to achieve pregnancy.

ELECTROEJACULATION

36. Describe the steps in the process of electroejaculation (EEJ).

1. The bladder is catheterized with a plastic catheter using a minimal amount of nonspermicidal lubricant.

2. After the urine is drained, 10 ml of buffered insemination media is instilled into the bladder to protect any sperm that may be ejaculated in a retrograde direction.

3. The patient is turned on his side, and rectoscopy is done to ensure that no rectal lesions are present.

4. A transrectal probe is placed in the rectum with electrodes facing anteriorly.

5. Electricity is delivered in a wave-like fashion, increasing progressively, until ejaculation is complete.

6. An assistant collects the antegrade ejaculate in a specimen container.

7. Rectoscopy is repeated to look for rectal lesions.

8. The bladder is again catheterized and rinsed with media to extract any retrograde sperm.

37. What is the appropriate way to deliver voltage during electroejaculation?

To limit the amount of heat generated at the probe electrodes, careful control of voltage delivery is crucial. Typically, initial stimulation may begin at 5 volts and then be increase by 5 volts for every two additional stimulations until ejaculation is seen. There may be a small amount of output of semen either during or just after each stimulation is given. The peak voltage for the session should usually be 5–10 volts above the voltage that produced the initial amount of ejaculate. Thus, the procedure should be stopped when two or more consecutive stimulations are given that produce no more ejaculate or when probe temperature exceeds 38.5° C.

Based on animal experience, early methods described for EEJ in humans suggested that a continuous electrical baseline should be maintained between stimulations. However, physiologic studies of sphincteric contractions during the procedure, which were later confirmed in clinical studies, suggested that this practice would cause continuous contraction of the external sphincter, which would lead to increased retrograde ejaculation. Therefore, we currently recommend that the maximum voltage for the stimulation be reached rather quickly, held at that level for 5 seconds, and then abruptly discontinued. Ejaculation may actually occur during the rest period, when the electricity is off. The ejaculation usually lasts 10–20 seconds; when it stops, the next stimulation can then be delivered.

38. How does the ejaculation from an EEJ procedure differ from a PVS procedure?

There are some similarities as well as important differences. First, rather than depending on the reflex response, there is some degree of direct stimulation of the ejaculatory organs. When the electrical delivery is discontinued, some men clearly exhibit a persistent and possibly coordinated reflex, but it tends to be short-lived. In a study that measured sphincteric activity during the two procedures, the internal sphincter of the urinary bladder contraction was less sustained during EEJ. For this reason, EEJ induces a significant portion of retrograde ejaculate in nearly all patients. Finally, because of the more direct route of stimulation, EEJ is successful in obtaining sperm from nearly all patients in whom it is attempted.

39. Which patients with anejaculation should be considered candidates for EEJ?

All patients with anejaculation, including cases believed to be psychogenic, can be considered candidates for EEJ. However, cost-effectiveness needs to be considered in comparing EEJ coupled with artificial insemination vs. other options for procreation. This analysis is discussed below.

40. Can EEJ be performed in the clinic setting?

In men who have complete SCI lesions, EEJ can usually be performed in the clinic setting without incident. In men with incomplete lesions, men with preserved sensation, and all men without a spinal cord problem who are relatively neurologically intact, the procedure is too painful to undergo without anesthesia. General and spinal anesthesia have been successfully used for EEJ procedures in this subgroup.

41. What are the risks of electroejaculation?

In men with SCI lesions above T6, autonomic dysreflexia may occur, and it tends to be more severe with EEJ than with PVS. Sublingual nifedipine may be used prophylactically as with PVS.

Because of the rectal probe insertion and electrical delivery, rectal injury is a possibility. However, with modern equipment that has continuous probe temperature monitoring, the risk of rectal burn or perforation is less than 1 in 1000 procedures.

42. Can the retrograde ejaculate be used for artificial insemination?

Yes, but the sperm quality tends to be poorer after exposure to urine. This effect can be minimized by urine alkalinization with oral administration of bicarbonate (1.5 gm 12 hours and 2 hours before the procedure), and immediate catheterization following stimulation with laboratory processing.

43. Since EEJ is uniformly successful in inducing ejaculation, should it be the preferred procedure for all patients rather than PVS?

Although success rates are higher for EEJ, there are a number of reasons why PVS should be attempted first in men with SCI and favorable prognostic factors:

1. The ejaculate is uniformly antegrade; thus, problems associated with urine contamination are not seen.

2. Evidence suggests that the sperm in the antegrade ejaculate from PVS may be of better quality and have better function that that seen with EEJ.

3. There is no chance of rectal injury with PVS.

4. A crossover study of the two procedures showed that PVS was much better tolerated and accepted by patients.

5. PVS has the ability to be applied in the home setting in acceptable subjects.

Therefore, we attempt PVS first in men with upper motor neuron lesions and move to EEJ in PVS nonresponders.

EJACULATORY DYSFUNCTION AND ASSISTED REPRODUCTION

44. Is the sperm from EEJ and PVS procedures normal?

Sperm obtained from anejaculatory men exhibit multiple abnormalities, including poor motility and viability, decreased ability to penetrate cervical mucus, and decreased fertilizing capability, as measured by the hamster oocyte sperm penetration assay. These semen abnormalities are doubtless responsible for poor results with assisted reproductive techniques.

45. How can sperm from EEJ or PVS be used to initiate pregnancy?

Home insemination can be performed by patients who have adequate sperm quality and in whom PVS can be safely performed in the home setting. A specimen can be obtained, drawn into a syringe, and then placed vaginally on the day of ovulation. This approach is patient-driven and inexpensive. However, the success rate is lower with home insemination than with other methods. Approximately 25% of couples deemed good candidates for home insemination will be successful within 1 year of attempts.

Intrauterine insemination (IUI) is used to improve the chance of pregnancy without extreme cost. Semen that has been processed is placed into the uterine cavity, which allows improved delivery to the site of fertilization. Cycle fecundity for IUI is approximately 10–12%, with 35–40% of couples succeeding after multiple cycles. A minimum of 5 million total motile sperm after processing is necessary for IUI.

In vitro fertilization (IVF) is performed for patients who have failed IUI and patients in whom the total motile sperm count after processing is < 5 million. The IVF experience in anejaculatory men is that success rates typically mimic the general rates of the IVF program.

IVF with intracytoplasmic sperm injection (IVF/ICSI) is used to ensure that fertilization will take place. In subjects with < 1 million total motile sperm, strict morphology values less than 5%, and/or very poor sperm motility and viability, ICSI can ensure that fertilization is achieved. Some argue that ICSI should be used for all PVS and/or EEJ specimens.

46. Are home insemination and IUI cost-effective? Should all patients consider IVF as an initial method of achieving pregnancy?

If the total motile sperm count is > 20 million, home insemination has a low but measurable success rate. Since the cost is negligible, it is reasonable for suitable couples to attempt this method. They should be informed that the success rate is somewhat low.

Because of the relatively low cost of performing PVS or EEJ in the clinic setting in men with

SCI, IUI has been shown to be cost-effective if the inseminated total motile sperm count exceeds 5 million.

However, in subjects who require anesthesia to perform EEJ, we have found that IUI is not cost-effective. Such couples should be counseled to go directly to IVF. We typically then perform a sperm extraction procedure rather than EEJ to supply sperm for IVF/ICSI.

47. What is the role of surgical extraction of sperm in anejaculatory men?

Studies have shown that the sperm from the vas deferens in men with SCI is of better quality than ejaculated sperm. This finding has led some specialists to abandon PVS and EEJ altogether in favor of surgical extraction. However, extracted sperm numbers are low enough that IVF with ICSI is used for these specimens. Therefore, the advantage of better quality sperm is really moot. Patients with SCI are better served by undergoing ejaculation induction in the clinic, with IUI used first. IVF is then performed in couples who do not become pregnant with IUI, but the sperm used for IVF is still obtained with either PVS or EEJ.

BIBLIOGRAPHY

1. Biering-Sørensen F, Sønksen J: Sexual function in spinal cord lesioned men. Spinal Cord 39:455–470, 2001.
2. Brackett NL, Padron OF, Lynne CM: Semen quality of spinal cord injured men is better when obtained by vibratory stimulation versus electroejaculation. J Urol 157:151–157, 1997.
3. Buch JP, Zorn BH: Evaluation and treatment of infertility in spinal cord injured men through rectal probe electroejaculation. J Urol 149:1350–1354, 1993.
4. Denil J, Ohl DA, Menge AC, et al: Functional characteristics of sperm obtained by electroejaculation. J Urol 147:69–72, 1992.
5. Master VA, Turek PJ: Ejaculatory physiology and dysfunction. Urol Clin North Am 28:363–375, 2001.
6. Ohl DA, Bennett CJ, McCabe M, et al: Predictors of success in electroejaculation of spinal cord injured men. J Urol 142:1483–1486, 1989.
7. Ohl DA, Sønksen J, Menge AC, et al: Electroejaculation versus vibratory stimulation in spinal cord injured men: sperm quality and patient preference. J Urol 157:2147–2149, 1997.
8. Ohl DA, Wolf LJ, Menge AC, et al: Electroejaculation and assisted reproductive technologies in the treatment of anejaculatory infertility. Fertil Steril 76:1249–1255, 2001.
9. Schuster TG, Ohl DA: Diagnosis and treatment of ejaculatory dysfunction. Urol Clin North Am 29:939–948, 2002.
10. Sønksen J, Biering-Sørensen F, Kristensen JK: Ejaculation induced by penile vibratory stimulation in men with spinal cord lesion. The importance of the vibratory amplitude. Paraplegia 32:6–60, 1994.
11. Sønksen J, Ohl DA: Penile vibratory stimulation and electroejaculation in the treatment of ejaculatory dysfunction. Int J Androl 25:324–332, 2002.
12. Sønksen J, Ohl DA, Giwercman A, et al: Quality of semen obtained by penile vibratory stimulation in men with spinal cord injuries: observations and predictors. Urology 48:453–457, 1996.
13. Sønksen J, Ohl DA, Wedemeyer G: Sphincteric events during penile vibratory ejaculation and electroejaculation in men with spinal cord injuries. J Urol 165:426–429, 2001.
14. Szasz G, Carpenter C: Clinical observations in vibratory stimulation of the penis of men with spinal cord injury. Arch Sex Behav 18:461–474, 1989.

III. Female Reproductive Disorders

20. FEMALE REPRODUCTIVE PHYSIOLOGY
Ina Cholst, M.D.

1. What are the main hormones of the female menstrual cycle?
- **Gonadotropin-releasing hormone** (GnRH) is a decapeptide secreted by the hypothalamus.
- **Follicle-stimulating hormone** (FSH) and **luteinizing hormone** (LH) are complex glycoproteins secreted by the anterior lobe of the pituitary
- **Estradiol** and **progesterone** are the main steroids produced in the ovary.
- **Inhibins are** glycoproteins composed of two subunits: alpha and beta. Two different alpha subunits exist, defining the two different inhibin molecules (inhibin A and B).

In addition, **other endocrine and paracrine factors,** including insulin-like growth factor (IGF), interleukins, epidermal growth factor, transforming growth factor, and vascular endothelial growth factor, are known to play a role in the regulation of the menstrual cycle.

2. Explain the law of negative feedback.
Several laws govern the behavior of the reproductive hormones. The most basic—and intuitive—of these laws is negative feedback. Negative feedback can be considered to work in the same way as a thermostat in a house. When the house is cold, the thermostat sends a signal to the furnace to make heat. As the house warms, the thermostat senses the warmth and decreases its signal to the furnace. Similarly, at the beginning of the menstrual cycle, estrogen levels are low. In response to the low levels of estrogen, the pituitary secretes FSH. The FSH stimulates the ovary to make estrogen (and eggs). In turn, the rising levels of estrogen suppress pituitary FSH.

3. How does pharmacology make use of negative feedback?
Several commonly used drugs make use of negative feedback. Oral contraceptive pills contain estrogen and progesterone. These steroids suppress pituitary FSH; therefore, the ovaries remain relatively quiet. By contrast, the fertility drug clomiphene citrate acts on the pituitary as an anti-estrogen, blocking its ability to detect circulating levels of ovarian estrogen. Thus, high levels of FSH are secreted, driving the ovary.

4. What is positive feedback?
Positive feedback means that when the pituitary senses a high enough level of estrogen for a long enough period, it responds paradoxically, not with suppression of gonadotropin, but with a gonadotropin surge. Positive feedback is responsible for the LH surge that triggers ovulation. Thus, positive feedback is ultimately responsible for the monthly cyclicity of the menstrual cycle.

5. Do any other endocrine systems make use of positive feedback?
No. Although most endocrine systems make use of negative feedback for regulation (thyroid-stimulating hormone and thyroid hormone, adrenocorticotropic hormone and cortisol), the female reproductive system is the only endocrine system in the body to make use of positive feedback.

6. Explain the role of GnRH.

Pulsatile GnRH is considered necessary to the secretion of gonadotropins from the pituitary. Without GnRH, there is no FSH or LH secretion. When the pituitary stalk has been severed and GnRH does not reach the pituitary, the pituitary does not respond to either negative or positive feedback.

7. Is pulsatile secretion necessary to the action of GnRH?

Yes. Similar concentrations of GnRH infused continuously rather than in a pulsatile manner result in a paradoxical suppression of LH and FSH secretion. Pharmacologically, this means that potent, long-acting GnRH analogs act like continuous infusions and *suppress* rather than stimulate gonadotropins. Clinically, such long-acting analogs are used in situations in which suppression is considered desirable, such as precocious puberty or endometriosis.

GnRH pulses correlate strictly with LH pulses. The frequency of the pulses in the follicular phase is about one pulse every 90 minutes. At midcycle, the frequency is briefly increased. Finally, probably due to the feedback of progesterone on the hypothalamus, the pulses gradually slow to every 4 to 6 hours during the luteal phase.

8. The ovary of the female fetus contains about 7 million germ cells. Obviously, they are not all ovulated. What happens to them?

Apoptosis, genetically programmed cell death, is the ultimate fate of all but about 300 of these 7 million oocytes. Therefore, ovulation can be considered the exception rather than the rule.

9. What determines ovulation?

In effect, ovulation is determined by the presence of "anti-apoptotic" factors that interfere with the natural tendency of the oocyte toward atresia. The most potent of these anti-apoptotic factors is FSH, but local concentrations of estradiol and ovarian peptides play a lesser—and still incompletely understood—role.

The majority of the ovarian growth factors (IGF, transforming growth factor beta, fibroblast growth factor, and activin) appear to enhance the action of FSH and can therefore be considered anti-apoptotic. By contrast, a number of ovarian peptides including inhibin, epidermal growth factor/transforming growth factor alpha (EGF/TGFα), and insulin-like growth factor binding proteins (IGF-BPs) decrease FSH activity and are considered to enhance atresia.

10. Give a clinical example of the anti-apoptotic role of FSH.

Controlled ovarian hyperstimulation—for ovulation induction or in vitro fertilization—is a clinical example of the anti-apoptotic role of FSH. Pharmacologic doses of FSH are used to overcome the tendency toward atresia and to "rescue" some of the developing follicles, otherwise destined for cell death.

11. How many stages are involved in follicular development?

Follicular development can be considered to take place in three stages.

12. What happens in the first stage?

The first stage is the initiation of growth of the primordial follicle, up to a size of about 0.2 mm in diameter. This phase is independent of gonadotropin stimulation and is very slow, with a (highly variable) duration of about 6 months.

13. Describe the second stage of follicular development.

The second stage is the development of the antral cavity. This phase takes the follicle from a size of about 0.5 mm to 2 mm in diameter and is also slow—lasting about 70 days—and also relatively independent of FSH. The independence from FSH stimulation is demonstrated by the presence of this stage of follicular development in females with absent or undetectable FSH concentrations (for example, prepubertal girls, women using oral contraceptives, patients with anorexia nervosa, patients with other forms of hypogonadotrophic hypogonadism, and patients with mutations of either the FSH receptor or the FSH beta subunit).

14. Describe the third stage of follicular development.

The third and final stage of follicular growth—from 2 mm to 16 mm—takes place over about 15 days and involves the recruitment of a cohort of antral follicles and the selection of one of them to become the dominant follicle. FSH is absolutely indispensable for this stage of development (it does not take place in patients with inactivating mutations of FSH hormone or receptor). Essentially, the demise of the previous cycle's corpus luteum (and the subsequent decrease in progesterone, estradiol, and inhibin A concentrations) allows plasma FSH to rise. The rise in FSH, in turn, allows recruitment of a cohort of about 30 follicles. About day 7, under the influence of FSH and estradiol, one of the cohort moves slightly ahead of the rest, granulosa cells proliferate, and the selected follicle is able to "press its advantage" by making more efficient use of the decreasing concentrations of FSH. At this stage, the remainder of the cohort of recruited follicles undergo atresia, leaving (in most cases) a single preovulatory follicle.

15. What is the corpus luteum?

After the egg leaves the follicle, a follicular scar containing large numbers of active granulosa cells is left behind. The scar is called the corpus luteum (Latin for "yellow body"), and the granulosa cells are now called granulosa luteal cells. They secrete estrogen, progesterone, and inhibin A, under the control of LH. If a pregnancy results, the corpus luteum continues to support the early pregnancy until the developing placenta is able to take over steroidogenesis. If there is no pregnancy, the corpus luteum regresses, and levels of estrogen, progesterone, and inhibin A fall. The fall of these hormones allows pituitary FSH levels to rise and a new ovarian cycle to begin.

16. How does the endometrium respond to these rising and falling hormone levels? What causes menstruation?

A series of morphologic changes occurs over the course of the menstrual cycle. Three distinct phases are identified: proliferative, secretory and menstrual. The preovulatory endometrium contains relatively hypertrophied glands and stroma. The endometrial surface and glandular surfaces are covered with cilia and microvilli. After ovulation, under the influence of luteal phase progesterone, the endometrium undergoes a rapid secretory differentiation. Glands, stroma, and vessels become compacted and tightly coiled, mucus vacuoles rise to the surface, and mucus is secreted into the lumens of the glands. If implantation does not occur, a process of vasoconstriction and ischemia lead to bleeding and shedding of the endometrial layer.

17. Patients say that they eat more and crave sweets premenstrually. Is this a myth?

Numerous studies, using various methodologies, document that cyclic fluctuations in food intake do indeed occur across the menstrual cycle. Lowest food intake is associated with ovulation, and highest caloric intake occurs in the late luteal phase of the cycle. The mechanisms of these changes remain to be elucidated but may have implications for understanding the biologic determinates of appetite. If estrogen, as seems possible, is an appetite suppressant, understanding the mechanism of that suppression may shed light on other aspects of the control of appetite.

BIBLIOGRAPHY

1. Buffenstein R, Poppitt SD, McDevitt RM, Prentice AM: Food intake and the menstrual cycle: A retrospective analysis, with implications for appetite research.
   Physiol Behav 58:1067–1077, 1995.
2. Chabbert Buffet N, Djakoure C, Christin Maitre S, Bouchard P: Regulation of the human menstrual cycle.
   Front Neuroendocrinol 19:151–186, 1998.

21. EVALUATION OF FEMALE REPRODUCTIVE DISORDERS

Ina Cholst, MD

1. When should evaluation of the infertile woman take place?

Infertility is defined as 12 months of unprotected intercourse without a resulting pregnancy. Therefore, it is always appropriate to evaluate at 1 year. However, it is reasonable to begin the evaluation of the woman who is over 35 years old at 6 months of infertility. Likewise, it is not sensible to delay evaluation when an obvious cause of infertility, such as amenorrhea or severe endometriosis, is known to exist.

2. What is the first step in an infertility evaluation?

As in most areas of medicine, the first step in an infertility evaluation should be a careful history and physical exam. A previous history of sexually transmitted disease, pelvic inflammatory disease (PID), ruptured appendix , or use of an intrauterine device (IUD) may suggest tubal disease. Menstrual irregularity, galactorrhea, or hot flashes may suggest ovarian dysfunction. Severe dysmenorrhea or dyspareunia may suggest endometriosis.

3. What percent of infertility is related to a male factor?

Approximately 30–40% of infertility is due to a male factor. A semen analysis, therefore, should be obtained early in the course of infertility evaluation.

4. How is ovulation assessed?

Assessment of ovulation may begin with a basal body temperature chart. The patient is asked to take her temperature every morning, at about the same time, before getting out of bed. The temperature chart usually shows some "bounce" but tends to rise about 0.5°F after ovulation. The rise in basal body temperature is a response to progesterone, which is secreted by the corpus luteum after ovulation. Alternatively, or in addition, home kits allow the patient to detect the preovulatory surge of luteinizing hormone (LH). Finally, a blood test showing an elevation in luteal phase progesterone is diagnostic of ovulation.

5. How is hyperprolactinemia diagnosed and evaluated?

Even in the absence of menstrual irregularity, amenorrhea, or galactorrhea, serum prolactin levels should be assessed in all female patients presenting with infertility. In most cases, if discovered, hyperprolactinemia should be further evaluated with an MRI scan of the pituitary before treatment or conception.

6. How is polycystic ovarian syndrome (PCO) diagnosed?

PCO can be suspected in patients with menstrual irregularity, hirsutism, a body mass index (BMI) > 25, a ratio of LH to follicle-stimulating hormone (FSH) > 2, or a typical ovarian ultrasound showing peripheral follicles ("necklace sign"). If PCO is suspected, androgens (testosterone, free testosterone, androstenedione, and dehydroepiandrosterone sulfate [DHEAS]) as well as baseline 17-OH progesterone should be measured. According to the results, if late-onset congenital adrenal hyperplasia is suspected, an adrenocorticotropic hormone (ACTH) test should be done. In the absence of signs or symptoms of PCO, it is not necessary to check androgens in regularly cycling infertile women.

7. Define inadequate luteal phase.

The term *inadequate luteal phase* refers to a situation in which ovulation occurs, but the corpus luteum does not produces adequate progesterone to properly prepare the endometrium to receive the fertilized embryo.

8. How is inadequate luteal phase evaluated?

The syndrome is diagnosed by late luteal phase endometrial biopsy. The biopsy is dated by pathology, and then the histologic dating is compared with the actual date of the biopsy, as determined by counting backward from the date of the next menstrual period. A biopsy that is three or more days out of phase suggests an inadequate luteal phase.

9. How is premature ovarian failure detected?

Premature ovarian failure, or incipient premature failure, is suspected in patients with oligomenorrhea or amenorrhea or shortened cycle length, especially when hot flashes are present. Levels of FSH, LH, and estrogen on day 3 allow the diagnosis to be made.

10. What is the effect of maternal age on infertility and how can it be assessed?

Age has a significant effect on fertility. Both infertility and early pregnancy loss increase rapidly after age 35 years. About one-third of women who delay childbearing until their mid-to-late 30s and half of women who delay childbearing until after age 40 will be unable to conceive. At present, women in their mid-to-late 30s and early 40s constitute the largest portion of the population with total infertility.

11. What population studies have been done to assess the effects of maternal age on infertility?

Studies to assess age-related infertility have been done in Hutterite populations, communities who use no contraception and value large families. These studies have found that 11% of Hutterite women bear no children after 34 years of age, 33% bear no children after 40 years of age, and 87% are infertile after 45.

12. How is the individual woman assessed for age-related infertility?

Provocative tests, such as the clomiphene citrate (Clomid) challenge, may have some value, but the most information can be obtained from a basal assessment of the concentrations of FSH, LH, and estradiol on day 2 or day 3 of the cycle. Norms must be established for the particular assay being used, because of considerable interassay variability. FSH alone is insufficient for diagnosis: a low FSH level in combination with an elevated estradiol level denotes a poor prognosis.

13. When should the age-related assessment be done?

Identifying women with a poor prognosis due to advanced maternal age should be an early part of the infertility evaluation. Although many patients will wish to pursue evaluation and treatment despite a low likelihood of success, it is important to inform such patients honestly and empathetically of their poor prognosis before embarking on invasive and expensive evaluation and treatment.

14. What is a hysterosalpingogram?

Ahysterosalpingogram (HSG) is a radiologic test in which dye is passed into the fundus of the uterus under fluoroscopic guidance. The test can be used to diagnose the patency of the tubes and also to assess the normalcy of the uterine cavity. If present, an intrauterine septum, bicornuate uterus, submucus myoma, or polyp can usually be identified.

Extratubal adhesions and endometriosis are not evaluated by the hysterosalpingogram. When indicated, a laparoscopy can be considered complementary to the hysterogram.

15. When in the cycle should an HSG be performed?

An HSG should be performed after the menstrual flow has ceased but before ovulation. The test should be done after bleeding has stopped so that endometrial cells are not pushed retrograde through the tubes and into the peritoneal cavity, which may increase the risk of seeding endometriosis. The test is done after ovulation so that an early pregnancy would not be inadvertently exposed to radiation.

Anecdotal evidence suggests that, perhaps by cleaning the tubes of debris, conception rates may rise after the HSG. Patients should be encouraged to have well-timed intercourse in the cycle of HSG.

16. How can I assess the uterine cavity of a patient who is allergic to iodine dye?

In most cases, the uterine cavity can be adequately assessed on midcycle ultrasound. When a submucus myoma or polyp is suspected, saline can be introduced into the cavity (sonohysterogram) to delineate the lesion.

17. Does magnetic resonance imaging (MRI) have a role in the evaluation of female infertility?

MRI can be useful to differentiate a septate uterus from a bicornuate uterus. The images must be obtained in a plane coronal and perpendicular to the long axis of the uterus. In some cases the ability of MRI to localize myomas and differentiate them from adenomyosis may be useful preoperatively.

18. I have done the entire work-up but have not discovered the cause of my patient's infertility. What did I miss?

Nothing. Approximately 15% of infertility is idiopathic. Although frustrating for doctor and patient, this diagnosis carries a good prognosis. Pregnancy rates are reasonable even with expectant management (if the woman is young and patient) and very good with in vitro fertilization (IVF).

19. How have the success and availability of assisted reproductive technology (ART) affected the infertility evaluation?

In an era of highly successful and available ART, the infertility evaluation should be tailored to the age, preferences, and even financial capability of each infertile couple. Costly or invasive diagnostic tests that will not alter the course of treatment should not be performed.

For example, in cases of known extensive adhesions and tubal occlusion or oligo-azoospermia, it may be advisable to proceed to IVF directly, with essentially no other evaluation than assessment of the uterine cavity, day 3 test, and semen analysis. In such cases, postcoital testing, endometrial biopsy, and laparoscopy are unnecessary.

Multiple attempts at tubal surgery are rarely indicated at any age. In the older patient or the patient with a borderline day 3 test, even a diagnostic laparoscopy or initial lysis of adhesions may be superfluous. Likewise, the patient with severe endometriosis, even with tubal patency, should not undergo multiple cycles of controlled ovarian hyperstimulation (which may exacerbate the endometriosis) but should usually go directly to IVF.

BIBLIOGRAPHY

1. Balasch J: Investigation of the infertile couple in the era of assisted reproductive technology: A time for reappraisal. Hum Reprod 15:2251–2257, 2000.
2. Forti G, Krausz C: Clinical review 100: Evaluation and treatment of the infertile couple. J Clin Endocrinol Metab 83:4177–4188, 1998.
3. Rosene-Montella K, Keely E, Laifer SA, Lee RV: Evaluation and management of infertility in women: The internists' role. Ann Intern Med 132:973–981, 2000.

22. THYROID AND ADRENAL DISORDERS

Owen K. Davis, M.D.

1. What are the nonreproductive symptoms and signs of thyroid diseases?

Symptoms of hypothyroidism may include cold intolerance, dry skin, coarse hair, lethargy, paresthesias, and weight gain. On physical examination, goiter, edema, bradycardia, and prolongation of the relaxation phase in deep tendon reflexes may be noted. Severe cases may have myxedema (deposition of mucoprotein ground substance in soft tissues) and cardiac abnormalities, including pericardial effusion and cardiomyopathy. Myxedema coma, which is rare in reproductive-age women, is characterized by an inability to maintain body temperature, hypercapnia, respiratory acidosis, and coma.

Symptoms of hyperthyroidism may include heat intolerance, nervousness, emotional lability, weight loss, perspiration, palpitations, and diarrhea. On physical examination, the skin may be warm and moist. Tachycardia may also be observed. With Graves' disease, diffuse goiter, lid lag, proptosis, and, less commonly, pretibial myxedema may be noted. Thyroid storm, an uncommon but life-threatening manifestation of thyrotoxicosis, may be precipitated by stresses, including labor and infection.

2. What are the causes of thyroid diseases?

The most common cause of **hypothyroidism** in industrialized society is Hashimoto's autoimmune thyroiditis, which is characterized in part by high titers of antithyroid antibodies and, in some cases, antithyroid peroxidase. The second leading cause of hypothyroidism is iatrogenic hypothyroidism following ablative surgery or treatment with radioactive iodine. Hypoothyroidism secondary to iodine deficiency is virtually nonexistent in North America.

The most common cause of **hyperthyroidism** is Graves' disease, which is associated with production of a thyroid-stimulating autoantibody (IgG). Less common causes of hyperthyroidism include iatrogenic or factitious hyperthyroidism, functioning thyroid adenoma, and subacute thyroiditis. Rare gynecologic causes include gestational trophoblastic disease and struma ovarii.

3. Describe the basic laboratory evaluation of thyroid function.

The standard serologic evaluation of thyroid function is a serum thyroid profile, including the thyroid-stimulating hormone (TSH) level and direct or indirect assessment of free (unbound, active) thyroxine (T_4). Primary hypothyroidism (most commonly Hashimoto's disease) is characterized by an elevated TSH level and a reduced free thyroxine level. Secondary or central hypothyroidism is marked by low circulating levels of both free thyroxine and TSH. Primary hyperthyroidism (e.g., Graves' disease) manifests a suppressed TSH in the setting of an elevated free thyroxine. This profile also is seen with factitious and iatrogenic hyperthyroidism. Less commonly, a suppressed TSH level and normal free thyroxine level are observed in instances of T_3-toxicosis. Assay of triiodothyronine (T_3) is useful in these cases.

Hyperestrogenic states (e.g., pregnancy, treatment with oral contraceptives) result in increased hepatic production of thyroxine-binding globulin (TBG) and consequently increased levels of total thyroxine. Free thyroxine and TSH levels remain within the normal range in a euthyroid person, despite the effect of estrogens on TBG and total thyroxine.

4. What are the reproductive effects of hypothyroidism?

Primary hypothyroidism in childhood may be associated with precocious puberty and should be sought in such cases. In women of reproductive age, hypothyroidism has been associated with menstrual disturbances, particularly menorrhagia or hypermenorrhea. Primary hypothyroidism may result in secondary hyperprolactinemia via the stimulatory effects of thyrotropin-releasing hormone (TRH) at the level of the lactotrope. Evaluation of thyroid status, including measurement of TSH, is therefore warranted in cases of hyperprolactinemia.

Hypothyroidism may be associated with recurrent spontaneous abortions. Thus, thyroid functions are often assessed in the evaluation of the infertile couple. The impact of subclinical hypothyroidism (elevated TSH in the setting of compensated, normal free thyroxine) on fertility, however, is unclear.

5. What are the reproductive effects of hyperthyroidism?

Excessive production of thyroid hormone may result in shortening or lengthening of the menstrual cycle. Characteristically, hyperthyroidism is associated with decreased menstrual flow (hypomenorrhea) and may cause anovulation and amenorrhea.

6. What are the effects of abnormal thyroid function on sex steroid metabolism?

Hypothyroidism results in decreased production of sex hormone-binding globulin (SHBG) and thus a reduction in total estradiol. The two major metabolic pathways for estrogens are 2-hydroxylation and 16-hydroxylation. In hypothyroidism 16-hydroxylation is favored, with preferential conversion to estriol.

Hyperthyroidism increases the hepatic production of SHBG, which may contribute to the overall increase in plasma estrogen levels. Thyroid hormone excess leads to increased 2-hydroxylation of estrogens to catechol estrogens (2-hydroxyestradiol and 2-hydroxyestrone), which are weak estrogen agonists.

7. How is hypothyroidism treated?

The goal of treatment is clinical euthyroidism. Hypothyroidism can be treated with thyroid hormone replacement with the oral administration of thyroxine, triiodothyronine (T_3), or combined regimens. It is not clear whether T_3 confers any distinct benefit over thyroxine therapy alone. Thyroxine is generally initiated at doses of 0.1–0.15 mg/day, and replacement is usually life-long. The effects of a given treatment dose will be observed in 4–8 weeks. The best index of biochemical euthyroid status is a normal TSH level. Adequate thyroid replacement results in normalization of the TSH level with normal to mildly elevated levels of T_4 and T_3. A low or undetectable level of TSH may indicate excessive replacement with attendant risks, including osteoporosis.

8. How is hyperthyroidism treated?

Graves' disease is a chronic disorder with no specific, definitive therapy. Management is directed toward decreasing thyroid hormone secretion. Medical maintenance may be achieved with a thionamide such as propylthiouracil (PTU), which is usually the drug of choice for women in their reproductive years. PTU decreases both thyroxine secretion and the peripheral deiodination of thyroxine to triiodothyronine. An infrequent but serious potential risk of PTU therapy is the development of agranulocytosis, a decline in the number of circulating neutrophils. Administration of PTU is generally long term; permanent remission after 6 months of treatment is seen in fewer than 20% of patients.

Control of Graves' disease may also be accomplished through ablative surgery or radiation. Surgical thyroidectomy entails risks, including hypoparathyroidism (due to simultaneous removal of parathyroid glands in the thyroid gland) and accidental recurrent laryngeal nerve damage. Radioablation with administration of ^{131}I , predicated on the fact that the thyroid is the only organ that concentrates iodine (with the exception of renal excretion) is safe and effective. Although gonadal exposure to ionizing radiation results from the transit of the radioisotope through the bladder, no evidence indicates that it has a significant impact on ovarian function or reserve. Thyroid ablation generally renders the patient hypothyroid, at which point thyroid replacement is instituted.

9. How is treatment of thyroid disease modified by pregnancy?

The treatment of **maternal hypothyroidism** is essentially unchanged by pregnancy. Thyroid replacement is continued with routine monitoring. The increase in maternal TBG results in an overall increase in total thyroid hormone levels, but free T_4 and T_3 are unchanged. The administered thyroxine and/or triiodothyronine do not cross the placenta to an appreciable degree. *Recent evidence suggests that fetal neurologic development may be impaired if maternal hypothyroidism is undetected or not adequately treated.*

The treatment of **maternal hyperthyroidism** is more complex. Radioiodine is not an option, because transplacental transfer occurs readily and leads to ablation of the fetal thyroid gland. The treatment of choice for maternal hyperthyroidism is PTU at the lowest dose that can satisfactorily maintain the patient in a normal to slightly hyperthyroid state. PTU does cross the placenta and may potentially cause fetal goiter and hypothyroidism. Moderate doses of PTU (100–200 mg/day) have been observed to suppress T_4 and increase TSH levels in the newborn, with normalization occurring within the first week of extrauterine life. Clinical follow-up of these infants has not revealed any developmental impairment. Finally, as previously noted, hyperthyroid women are at increased risk for thyroid storm during labor or cesarean delivery.

10. What is postpartum thyroiditis?

Postpartum thyroiditis may occur in approximately 5% of pregnancies and is characterized by transient hyperthyroidism followed by transient hypothyroidism. This disorder usually develops 3–6 months postpartum. The hyper- and hypothyroid phases each last approximately 1–3 months. Spontaneous recovery is seen in 90% of cases. The cause of postpartum thyroiditis is most likely autoimmune, suggested in part by the frequent presence of antithyroid microsomal autoantibodies in this disorder. Postpartum thyroiditis commonly recurs with subsequent pregnancies and may herald the development of future hypothyroidism. This disorder should be considered in cases of postpartum depression or anxiety.

11. What is the potential role of thyroid disease in disordered puberty in girls?

Primary hypothyroidism (e.g., Hashimoto's disease) can give rise to precocious puberty in affected girls. This particular type of sexual precocity is uniquely characterized by short stature with *delayed* bone age. The resultant hyperprolactinemia may cause galactorrhea. Thyroid replacement therapy permits regression of the precocious sexual development and resolution of the galactorrhea.

Childhood Graves' disease can provoke early onset of puberty accompanied by *advanced* bone age due to hypermetabolism. Primary hypothyroidism is an infrequent cause of pubertal delay. Thyroid function evaluation should be obtained if the clinical picture warrants.

12. How does adrenal gland anatomy differ in the fetus and the adult?

The fetal adrenal gland, which is differentiated by 7 weeks of gestation, is characterized by an inner fetal zone, comprising approximately 80% of the gland, and a thin outer zone, which is the precursor to the adult adrenal cortex. The fetal adrenal glands are prominent structures, often exceeding the size of the kidneys by the end of the first trimester.

13. How does the fetal adrenal gland contribute to maternal estrogen levels?

Maternal estrone and estradiol are predominantly derived from a complementary interplay of the maternal, placental, and fetal adrenal compartments. The importance of the fetal adrenal gland's contribution to maternal estrogens is underscored by the extremely low levels of maternal circulating estrogens in cases of fetal anencephaly, a condition marked by the absence of normal fetal adrenal glands.

The fetal adrenal gland is unique in that it utilizes sulfated steroids in its biosynthetic pathways. Additionally, the fetal adrenal is deficient in 3B-hydroxysteroid dehydrogenase and consequently produces steroids (pregnenolone sulfate and dehydroepiandrosterone sulfate [DHEAS]) by the delta 5 pathway.

Maternal cholesterol is first converted to pregnenolone by the placenta, which is in turn conjugated to pregnenolone sulfate by the fetal adrenal. This, in turn, is converted by the fetal adrenal gland to DHEAS, which is then cleaved to DHEA by placental sulfatase. The placenta then produces androstenedione and testosterone by the delta 4 pathway; both are in turn aromatized to estrone and estradiol. Circulating maternal levels of these estrogens at term are approximately 100-fold those in the nongravid state. Maternal estriol levels are increased 1000-fold due to placental aromatization of 16-OH-DHEA, which derives from 16-hydroxylation of DHEAS by the fetal liver.

14. What are the signs and symptoms of hypercortisolism?

Patients with endogenous or exogenous cortisol excess may manifest centripetal obesity with relatively thin extremities, facial plethora, purple abdominal striae, weakness due to muscle catabolism, and hypertension. In reproductive-aged females, hypercortisolism frequently results in varying degrees of hyperandrogenemia with hirsutism and oligo- or amenorrhea. Hyperandrogenism results primarily from adrenal overproduction of DHEAS and androstenedione, particularly when the syndrome is adrenocorticotropic hormone (ACTH)-dependent (Cushing's disease) or in cases of adrenal carcinoma. Osteoporosis is also seen frequently and can lead to fractures and back pain. Less common clinical features include emotional changes (depression, psychosis), peptic ulcer disease, and easy bruisability.

15. Describe the evaluation of suspected hypercortisolism.

Confirmation of hypercortisolism may be obtained by measuring 24-hour excretion of urinary free cortisol, which typically exceeds 100 μg/24 hours in cases of Cushing's syndrome. Alternatively, an overnight dexamethasone suppression test may be performed with administration of 1 mg of dexamethasone orally at 11 PM and with assay of the plasma cortisol concentration at approximately 8 AM the following morning. Cushing's syndrome is excluded if the cortisol level suppresses to below 5 μg/dl. A false-positive result may be seen in cases of obesity, depression, pregnancy or oral contraceptive use, anorexia nervosa, and chronic alcoholism.

If cortisol excess is documented, the differential diagnosis of Cushing's syndrome can be facilitated by performing a high-dose dexamethasone suppression test. Dexamethasone is administered at a dose of 2 mg orally every 6 hours for 8 doses (two days). A 50% reduction in urinary 17-OHCS or plasma cortisol suggests a diagnosis of Cushing's disease, which is ACTH-dependent (pituitary microadenoma or, less frequently, macroadenoma). Suppression does not occur in cases of primary hypercortisolism due to adrenal tumors (adenoma or carcinoma) or ectopic ACTH production (e.g., from lung, thymus, or pancreatic tumors). Measurement of the plasma ACTH level may also be useful, with low-to-undetectable levels (< 20 pg/ml) seen with adrenal tumors, normal-to-slightly elevated levels with Cushing's disease, and markedly elevated levels in cases of ectopic ACTH (> 200 pg/ml). Further localization of the pathology may be undertaken with imaging procedures (e.g., CT/MRI of the pituitary, CT of the adrenals, CT of the lungs) in cases of ectopic ACTH and/or selective venous sampling.

16. Describe the treatment of Cushing's syndrome.

Therapy is determined by the underlying cause. Primary hypercortisolism is generally treated by unilateral adrenalectomy. Cushing's disease is primarily treated via transsphenoidal resection of the pituitary adenoma, although irradiation is an alternative. Ectopic ACTH syndrome can be successfully treated by surgical resection of a benign adenoma. In cases of a metastatic malignancy, however, resection is seldom possible, and treatment of the cortisol excess is undertaken with enzyme inhibitors (e.g., aminoglutethimide) or, less commonly, bilateral adrenalectomy.

17. Can adrenocortical insufficiency have reproductive effects?

Primary adrenocortical failure (Addison's disease) can result in amenorrhea, diminished libido, and scant pubic/axillary hair in addition to nonreproductive signs and symptoms such as fatigue, weakness, hypotension, weight loss, nausea/vomiting, and hyperpigmentation. In the U.S., adrenal insufficiency is most commonly due to autoimmunity and may be associated with other autoimmune endocrinopathies, including thyroid dysfunction, hypoparathyroidism, diabetes, and occasionally premature ovarian failure. The diagnosis is confirmed by the finding of "normal" or diminished basal cortisol levels that are hyporesponsive to standard ACTH stimulation testing (e.g., no increase 60 minutes after administration of intravenous Cortrosyn, 250 μg). Treatment consists of glucocorticoid and, when necessary, mineralocorticoid replacement for life.

18. What is adrenarche?

The phase of pubertal development associated with maturation of the adrenal glands and increased production of adrenal androgens is termed *adrenarche*. Specifically, increasing size and function of the inner zone (reticularis) of the adrenal cortex results in a rise in peripheral levels of DHEA, DHEAS, and androstenedione, which progress from approximately age 6–7 years throughout pubertal maturation.

19. What is the role of the normal adrenal gland in sex steroid production in the female?

In the reproductive years, the adrenal cortex directly gives rise to approximately 90% of circulating DHEA, virtually 100% of DHEAS, 50% of androstenedione, and 25% of testosterone. Roughly 50% of circulating testosterone derives from peripheral conversion of androstenedione, which in turn is secreted by the adrenal glands and ovaries.

20. Which adrenal disorders can cause hyperandrogenism/hirsutism?

Although a relatively uncommon cause of hirsutism, Cushing's syndrome can present with androgen excess (see discussion above). Hyperandrogenism can also result from adrenal enzyme defects, including 21-hydroxylase deficiency, 3B-hydroxysteroid dehydrogenase deficiency, and 11 B-hydroxylase deficiency. Finally, androgen-producing tumors (adenomas or carcinomas) can arise in the adrenal gland.

21. How do androgen-secreting adrenal tumors present?

A tumor should be suspected in a woman presenting with rapidly progressing masculinization, typically over a course of months. Masculinization represents more profound androgenic effects than hirsutism alone, including clitoromegaly, deepening of the voice, increased muscle mass, and male pattern hair loss. An adrenal tumor should be suspected in the presence of markedly increased circulating androgen levels (e.g., testosterone > 200 ng/dl, DHEAS > 700 μg/dl).

The diagnosis of an adrenal tumor is facilitated by the use of imaging techniques, including abdominal CT, MRI, or nuclear scan. Functioning adrenal carcinomas generally secrete both excess glucocorticoids and androgens. They also tend to be larger than benign lesions; most adrenal lesions < 2 cm in diameter are benign. In the absence of identifiable adrenal or ovarian lesions, selective retrograde catheterization with venous sampling may be undertaken for tumor localization. Treatment is surgical resection. The prognosis for adrenal carcinomas tends to be poor.

22. How do late-onset and classic 21-hydroxylase deficiency differ?

Classic 21-hydroxylase (P450c21) deficiency is an autosomal recessive disorder with clinical manifestations in homozygous individuals. The severe forms present with either simple virilization at birth (female pseudohermaphroditism with ambiguous genitalia, e.g., clitoromegaly and labial fusion) or virilization with salt-wasting, which is life-threatening if not diagnosed and treated promptly. Hyperandrogenism results from shunting of cortisol precursors toward androgens (e.g., androstenedione), whereas salt-wasting is a manifestation of mineralocorticoid deficiency.

Late-onset or nonclassic 21-hydroxylase deficiency is due to homozygous expression of alleles with milder forms of clinical manifestation. Symptoms and signs generally do not appear until puberty or adulthood. This milder form of 21-hydroxylase deficiency typically presents with hirsutism and is in the differential diagnosis of polycystic ovary syndrome (PCOS).

Classic forms present at birth and can be confirmed by the presence of markedly elevated 17-hydroxyprogesterone (17-OHP) levels. In adult females suspected of harboring the late-onset form, early morning (8 AM) follicular phase 17-OHP levels are elevated (> 200 ng/dl) and will rise dramatically with ACTH testing. After an intravenous dose of Cortrosyn, 250 μg, the stimulated level of 17-OHP at 1 hour typically exceeds 1200 ng/dl in affected individuals. Effective treatment of this disorder entails glucocorticoid replacement, which suppresses the elevated ACTH levels that fuel the clinical manifestations.

23. How is suspected congenital adrenal hyperplasia managed prenatally?

The male partners of pregnant women with 21-hydroxylase deficiency should undergo genetic testing for carrier status. If both partners carry one or more abnormal genes, a female fetus is at risk for congenital virilization with ambiguous genitalia. Prenatal diagnosis can be accomplished either through amniocentesis with measurement of 17-OHP, androstenedione, and 21-deoxycortisol or via chorionic villus sampling (CVS) with sex determination and molecular diagnosis. Given that normal differentiation of the female external genitalia begins in the latter half of the first trimester, preventive treatment must be instituted before a definitive prenatal diagnosis can be made. Typically, maternal dexamethasone therapy is initiated at 5–6 weeks of gestation (up to 1.5 mg/day) to suppress fetal androgen secretion. If CVS or amniocentesis demonstrates the presence of either a male fetus or an unaffected female fetus, the dexamethasone can be discontinued.

24. What other forms of congenital adrenal hyperplasia can cause virilization?

11 B-hydroxylase (P450c11) deficiency is a less common form of congenital adrenal hyperplasia. In this disorder the final step in cortisol synthesis is blocked, resulting in increased levels of precursors, including 11-deoxycorticosterone (DOC) and 11-deoxycortisol, proximal to the defective metabolic step. This disorder is generally associated with hypertension and hypokalemia. Virilization can occur due to shunting of steroidogenic precursors to androgens (DHEA, DHEAS, androstenedione). A milder, nonclassic form of this deficiency causes milder virilization and, rarely, hypertension. Diagnosis is confirmed through documentation of elevated levels of DOC and 11-deoxycortisol. Treatment again consists of glucocorticoid replacement to suppress ACTH.

3B-hydroxysteroid dehydrogenase deficiency, in contrast to the foregoing, affects *both* the adrenal gland and the ovary. Complete deficieny is incompatible with life. Incomplete forms with milder clinical manifestation also exist and may be diagnosed only later in adulthood. In this disorder, mild virilization is seen due to increased levels of DHEA and DHEAS, which can be converted to more potent androgens in peripheral tissues. Effective therapy entails glucocorticoid and mineralocorticoid replacement.

25. What form of congenital adrenal hyperplasia causes primary amenorrhea with sexual immaturity?

17α-Hydroxylase (P450c17) deficiency affects both the adrenal gland and the gonads and results in the absence of sex steroid synthesis. Shunting of precursors toward DOC and corticosterone results in hypertension and hypokalemia. Affected males present with pseudohermaphroditism. Affected females manifest an immature female external genital phenotype with failure of sexual maturation at puberty. Primary amenorrhea results, with elevated levels of FSH and LH. Treatment includes replacement of both glucocorticoids and sex hormones to allow secondary sexual development and maintenance.

26. Do the adrenal glands play a role in PCOS and its management?

DHEAS, a steroid almost exclusively of adrenal origin, is elevated in approximately 50% of women with PCOS. Suppression of DHEAS by GnRH-agonist therapy suggests that such increases are secondary to the ovarian hormonal perturbations. It has been proposed that adrenal suppression may be useful as an adjunct to ovulation induction in women with PCOS resistant to clomiphene citrate. Patients with elevated DHEAS levels may benefit from the addition of a low dose of glucocorticoid (e.g., dexamethasone, 0.5 mg at bedtime) in conjunction with clomiphene therapy.

Various pharmacologic agents used in the treatment of hirsutism (PCOS-associated or idiopathic) have some adrenal effects. Spironolactone exhibits multiple actions, including primary, direct effects at the hair follicle, but also has inhibitory effects on adrenal (and ovarian) androgen secretion through suppression of the cytochrome P450 system. Ketoconazole also inhibits androgen biosynthesis through a similar mechanism but is usd infrequently due to adverse effects, including hepatic toxicity.

27. Should adrenal status be evaluated in cases of premature ovarian failure?

Premature ovarian failure (POF) has many etiologies, including iatrogenic causes (surgery, antineoplastic therapy), karyotypic abnormalities (Turner's mosaicism), and galactosemia. One prominent cause of POF is autoimmune disease. POF may be one manifestation of the polyglandular autoimmune syndromes, which can also include autoimmune thyroiditis, hypoparathyroidism, and adrenal insufficiency. Generally, POF precedes adrenal failure in such cases, suggesting the advisability of adrenal function screening at the time of diagnosis of POF with periodic surveillance thereafter. In the absence of other clinical evidence for adrenal insufficiency, an 8 am cortisol level is a reasonable screening test. ACTH stimulation testing may also be undertaken.

BIBLIOGRAPHY

1. Azziz R, Zacur H: 21-Hydroxylase deficiency in female hyperandrogenism: screening and diagnosis. J Clin Endocrinol Metab 69:577, 1989.
2. Glinoer D, DeNayer P, Bourdoux P, et al: Regulation of maternal thyroid during pregnancy. J Clin Endocrinol Metab 71:276, 1990.
3. Haddow JE, Palomaki GE, Allan WC, et al: Antenatal thyroid deficiency during pregnancy and subsequent neuropsychological development of the child. N Engl J Med 341:549, 1999.
4. Karaviti L, Mercado AB, Mercado MB, et al: Prenatal diagnosis/treatment in families at risk for infants with steroid 21-hydroxylase deficiency. J Steroid Biochem Mol Biol 41:445, 1992.
5. Walfish PG, Chan YYC: Postpartum hyperthyroidism. Clin Endocrinol Metab 14:417, 1985.

23. HYPOGONADOTROPIC HYPOGONADISM

Owen K. Davis, M.D.

1. What is hypogonadotropic hypogonadism?

Hypogonadotropic hypogonadism (HH), also commonly called *hypothalamic amenorrhea,* refers to a state of gonadal hypofunction (hypoestrogenemia and anovulation/amenorrhea) due to anatomic and/or functional disorders of the hypothalamic/pituitary compartments. The endocrine basis for HH is disordered and deficient secretion of hypothalamic gonadotropin-releasing hormone (GnRH) and/or pituitary gonadotropins (follicle-stimulating hormone [FSH] and luteinizing hormone [LH]).

2. How does HH present?

In childhood, HH can present as pubertal delay or arrest, with primary amenorrhea. In sexually mature women, HH generally presents as secondary amenorrhea.

3. How is HH diagnosed in childhood?

In evaluating females with delayed puberty and/or primary amenorrhea, other more frequently encountered disorders must first be excluded. Physical examination may point to a diagnosis of mullerian agenesis, transverse vaginal septum, or complete androgen insensitivity in a genotypic male (testicular feminization). Levels of thyroid-stimulating hormone (TSH) and prolactin should be measured to rule out hypothyroidism and hyperprolactinemia, respectively. Gonadotropin levels are markedly elevated in girls with primary ovarian failure due to gonadal dysgenesis or 17α-hydroxylase deficiency.

In cases of HH (including physiologic delay of puberty, a diagnosis of exclusion), circulating gonadotropin levels are low. Prepubertal estradiol and androgen levels can be inferred in girls lacking secondary sexual development (i.e., delayed thelarche and pubarche).

If HH occurs after the initiation or completion of puberty, low estradiol levels can be documented by serum assay. Assessment of the maturation index on vaginal cytology can be helpful. In addition, failure to exhibit withdrawal bleeding following a progestin challenge (after documenting the absence of pregnancy) may provide further evidence of the diagnosis. Neither serum estradiol determinations nor the progestin challenge are definitive, however, and the diagnosis should be made in accordance with the clinical picture.

4. How is HH diagnosed in adults?

Once pregnancy is excluded, secondary amenorrhea due to HH can be established by documentation of low (or "normal") gonadotropin levels in the presence of hypoestrogenemia. Hypoestrogenemia can be established through the finding of low peripheral estradiol levels, failure to elicit uterine bleeding after a progestin challenge (e.g., oral medroxyprogesterone acetate, 10 mg for 5 days), vaginal cytology exhibiting a hypoestrogenic maturation index, and/or scant cervical mucus. Hyperprolactinemia can present with an HH-like clinical picture (with or without galactorrhea); thus, serum prolactin testing should be included in the investigaton.

5. What are the possible causes of HH?

Common hypothalamic causes of HH include postradiation hypothalamic dysfunction, tumor, Kallmann's syndrome, isolated GnRH deficiency, physiologic delay of puberty, eating disorders and weight loss, stress, and exercise. Common pituitary causes of HH include prolactinomas, other central nervous system (CNS) tumors, inflammatory or infiltrative processes, and pituitary infarction.

6. How can the cause of HH be determined?

A thorough history and physical examination may suggest iatrogenic causes, stress, eating disorders/weight loss, or strenuous exercise and may reveal galactorrhea or anosmia (one manifestation of GnRH deficiency due to Kallmann's syndrome). Hyperprolactinemia can be identified with measurement of the prolactin level. Imaging of the hypothalamus and pituitary (MRI or CT) is generally indicated to diagnose or exclude a mass lesion, particularly in the setting of an elevated prolactin level, which may be due to a prolactinoma or mass lesion compressing the pituitary stalk.

7. How does Kallmann's syndrome present?

Although more frequently seen in males, Kallmann's syndrome does occur in females and is characterized by lack of spontaneous secondary sexual maturation and primary amenorrhea in the setting of a normal female karyotype and low gonadotropin levels. Affected people also exhibit anosmia, an inability to perceive odors. This syndrome can occur sporadically but is often inherited by X-linked, autosomal dominant or autosomal recessive transmission.

The cause of Kallmann's syndrome is failure during embryologic development of migration of GnRH-secreting neurons from the olfactory placode to the arcuate nucleus. Isolated congenital GnRH deficiency may also be seen, with preservation of olfactory perception. People with Kallmann's syndrome may be unaware of their anosmia; olfactory perception can be tested with aromatic substances such as coffee and perfume.

8. What is the relationship between eating disorders and HH?

Anorexia nervosa and bulimia are potentially life-threatening causes of HH and thus mandate appropriate diagnosis and intervention. The typical age of onset of anorexia is between 10 and 30 years. This syndrome is characterized by distorted body image, dieting with typical loss of 25% of body weight, and amenorrhea. Other manifestations include hyperactivity, increased lanugo hair, bradycardia, hypotension, and constipation. Hypercarotenemia is a frequent finding and may manifest as yellow discoloration of the palms. Eating disorders are associated with a number of endocrinologic phenomena, including (in addition to HH) increased levels of cortisol, increased levels of reverse T_3 with decreased triiodothyronine, and diabetes insipidus. This diagnosis requires appropriate psychiatric referral.

9. What is the association between exercise and HH?

Intense exercise, as in competitive female athletes and dancers, can result in amenorrhea. In adolescents, it can also result in delay of menarche. Weight loss and a low level of body fat significantly contribute to the HH associated with exercise, but the stress of intense physical activity appears to play an independent role. Menstrual function can return after the cessation of intense physical training even prior to significant weight gain or increase in percent body fat. The mechanism of exercise-induced amenorrhea is suppression of pulsatile GnRH secretion, possibly through an increase in central endorphin activity.

10. What are the causes of nonphysiologic hyperprolactinemia?

Categorized by size as microadenomas (< 1 cm) or macroadenomas (> 1 cm), prolactin-secreting adenomas of the pituitary are a relatively common cause of hyperprolactinemia. Given that pituitary secretion of prolactin is modulated via tonic inhibition by hypothalamic dopamine, any mass lesion that compresses the pituitary stalk can also result in elevated levels of prolactin, although usually to a lesser degree than with prolactin-secreting adenomas. Primary hypothyroidism can lead to secondary hyperprolactinemia due to the stimulatory effects of thyrotropin-releasing hormone (TRH). Thus, in addition to pituitary/hypothalamic imaging (MRI/CT), the evaluation of hyperprolactinemia should include determination of thyroid function through measurement of the TSH level.

Iatrogenic causes of hyperprolactinemia include medications that inhibit central dopaminergic activity through a direct effect on secretion or on receptor blockade. Common examples include receptor antagonists (e.g., metoclopramide), opioids, and phenothiazines. Less common causes of hyperprolactinemia include chronic renal failure and, rarely, ectopic prolactin secretion by an extrapituitary tumor.

11. How is hyperprolactinemia treated?

Non–prolactin-secreting CNS tumors (e.g., craniopharyngiomas) are treated with surgical resection and/or irradiation. Primary hypothyroidism is successfully treated with thyroid replacement therapy.

Pituitary prolactinomas can be treated surgically (e.g., via transsphenoidal resection), but a high recurrence rate of 50% has been reported. Furthermore, surgery has attendant risks, including cerebrospinal fluid leaks and panhypopituitarism. Currently the mainstay of therapy for prolactinomas is pharmacologic. Dopamine agonists (e.g., bromocriptine, cabergoline) are highly effective in the management of hyperprolactinemia and induce the regression of prolactinomas in most cases.

Bromocriptine, a lysergic acid derivative, is most commonly administered at a dosage of 2.5 mg orally (or vaginally) twice daily. Serum prolactin levels should be monitored to confirm normalization and for adjustment of dosage. Side effects, which include postural hypotension and nausea, can be minimized by initiating therapy at a low, bedtime dose (e.g., 1.25 mg) with gradual escalation to the targeted dosage. Longer-acting dopamine agonists, such as cabergoline, are administered less frequently, typically at a dosage of 0.25–1.0 mg twice weekly. Menstrual function is generally restored within 1–6 months of therapy. Pregnancy rates of up to 70% have been reported in large-scale outcome trials. In the U.S., dopamine agonist therapy is typically discontinued on establishment of pregnancy.

12. Describe the natural history of prolactinomas in pregnancy.

Fewer than 2% of microadenomas and approximately 15% of macroadenomas grow significantly during gestation. Thus, despite the normal stimulatory effects of pregnancy on the pituitary lactotropes, which include hypertrophy and hyperplasia, progression of symptoms of hyperprolactinemia during pregnancy is relatively uncommon. Likewise, breast feeding after pregnancy can be pursued without significant tumor growth. Tumor growth is best monitored through symptoms, such as the development of headaches or visual changes. In the absence of these symptoms visual field testing and imaging are generally not warranted. Clinically significant tumor expansion in pregnancy can be managed with dopamine agonist therapy. Serious acute events, including pituitary hemorrhage, occur rarely.

13. What is Sheehan's syndrome?

The increased size and vascularity of the pituitary gland in pregnancy render it susceptible to ischemic injury. Sheehan's syndrome is pituitary necrosis due to massive obstetric hemorrhage with hypovolemic shock. Pituitary injury of variable degrees may be seen. One of the first indications of Sheehan's syndrome is the failure of postpartum lactation/breast engorgement due to deficient prolactin secretion. The syndrome can result in panhypopituitarism, which can be diagnosed with appropriate hormonal testing and may require subsequent maintenance therapy with thyroxine, glucocorticoid, and sex hormone replacement.

14. What are the general health consequences of HH?

In childhood, HH results in the absence or arrest of pubertal secondary sexual development and/or primary amenorrhea. In adulthood, HH can result in secondary amenorrhea and partial regression of secondary sexual characteristics. Hypoestrogenemia typically causes vaginal dryness and variable degrees of vulvar atrophy. In addition, HH-associated estrogen deficiency causes loss of bone mass and can result in osteopenia or osteoporosis and thus an increased risk of fractures. Finally, as in all anovulatory states, infertility will result.

15. Describe the role of hormone replacement therapy in HH.

If the underlying cause of HH cannot be corrected, hormone replacement therapy is warranted, particularly for the purpose of maintenance of bone density. Adequate estrogen replacement can be achieved with either oral estrogens (e.g., conjugated equine estrogens: CEE, 0.625 mg daily, micronized estradiol, 1.0 mg daily) or transdermal systems (estradiol skin patches delivering 0.025–0.05 mg daily). Progestins (e.g., medroxyprogesterone acetate [MPA]) should be administered either cyclically (10 mg daily for 10–13 days) or continuously (2.5 mg daily) to protect the endometrium from the neoplastic risks associated with unopposed estrogens. Some patients, particularly those desiring contraception, achieve effective replacement with a low-dose oral contraceptive pill. Calcium supplementation should also be encouraged (1,000–1,500 mg daily).

16. What are the options for treatment of HH-associated infertility?

Anovulation due to HH is unresponsive to treatment with antiestrogens (clomiphene citrate, tamoxifen). Effective treatment of HH-associated infertility entails ovulation induction with exogenous gonadotropin injection therapy. If pituitary function is intact, pulsatile GnRH therapy may be considered. The goal of ovulation induction in cases of HH is a monofollicular response in contrast to the superovulation (multifollicular recruitment) used in the assisted reproductive technologies (ART) or in conjunction with intrauterine inseminations (IUI) for the treatment of unexplained or mild male factor infertility. In cases of anovulation secondary to hyperprolactinemia, normalization of the prolactin level with a dopamine agonist (see above) is generally successful.

17. Which gonadotropin preparations are effective for HH?

Available gonadotropin preparations include urinary-derived products (human menopausal gonadotropins [hMG] and purified FSH) and recombinant gonadotropins (rFSH). Gonadotropins are formulated in single-dose ampules/vials (generally 75 IU/ampule) and multidose vials. HMG can be administered intramuscularly or subcutaneously. Purified urinary or recombinant FSH is generally administered by subcutaneous injection, although intramuscular administration is effective.

LH secretion is highly variable in women with HH. In some, there is an absence or near absence of endogenous LH. Given that at least a minimum level of LH is required for biosynthesis of thecal androgens, which serve as estrogen precursors, many clinicians prefer hMG (which has LH-like action in addition to FSH-like action) for ovulation induction in cases of HH. However, many women with HH who produce adequate levels of LH may respond adequately to treatment with FSH alone.

18. How are gonadotropins administered in cases of HH?

Gonadotropins are typically self-administered at a starting dosage of 75–150 IU daily, and the initial dose is adjusted based on a combination of sonographic and hormonal (estradiol) monitoring. When maturation of the oocyte(s) is evident (when a mean diameter of 16–18 mm is achieved), ovulation is effected by the administration of human chorionic gonadotropin (hCG) at a dose of 5,000–10,000 IU intramuscularly or subcutaneously. Although a monofollicular response is sought, the incidence of multiple gestations is approximately 20%. The aggregate pregnancy rate among patients with HH treated with gonadotropins is approximately 25% per cycle. Risks, in addition to multiple gestation, include ovarian hyperstimulation syndrome (OHSS), although this risk can be minimized with less aggressive stimulation using the lowest effective doses of gonadotropins and diligent monitoring.

19. How is GnRH administered in cases of HH?

As mentioned previously, GnRH therapy is effective only in cases of HH with intact pituitary function (i.e., when the primary defect is inadequate secretion of endogenous GnRH by the hypothalamus). Pulsatile GnRH is generally administered at a dose of 5 μg intravenously every 60–90 minutes or 10 μg subcutaneously every 90 minutes via a portable infusion pump. Once ovulation has been documented, the GnRH can be discontinued with subsequent administration of 1,000–2,000 IU of hCG every third day (for 3 doses) for luteal support. In cases of HH, pulsatile GnRH therapy results in an approximately 80% rate of ovulation and a per-cycle conception rate of roughly 25%. Advantages over gonadotropin treatment include a negligible risk of OHSS and fewer multiple pregnancies (on the order of 5%). The principal disadvantage of pulsatile GnRH therapy is the requirement for a portable infusion pump and indwelling catheter for intervals ranging from approximately 10 to 22 days.

20. How is sexual development induced in girls with delayed puberty due to HH?

In contrast with physiologic pubertal delay, which is generally managed expectantly and with reassurance, sexual infantilism due to HH requires identification and treatment of the underlying pathology. When this is not possible (e.g., Kallman's syndrome), administration of exogenous sex steroids should be considered. Once the diagnosis has been established, estrogen therapy is initiated between the ages of 12 and 13 years, starting with a low daily dosage (CEE, 0.3 mg; micronized estradiol, 0.5 mg; or ethinyl estradiol, 5 μg) for 6 months to 1 year. The estrogen dosage is then doubled and cycled, with subsequent addition of a progestin (e.g., MPA, 10 mg on days 1–12 of each month) for breakthrough bleeding. Pulsatile GnRH, although effective in the initiation and sustenance of pubertal development, is both expensive and technically impractical.

BIBLIOGRAPHY

1. Al-Suleiman SA, Najashi S, Rahman MS: Outcome of treatment with bromocriptine in patients with hyperprolactinaemia. Aust NZ J Obstet Gynaecol 29:176, 1989.
2. Filicori M, Flamigni C, Meriggiola MC, et al: Ovulation induction with pulsatile gonadotropin-releasing hormone: technical modalities and clinical perspectives. Fertil Steril 56:1, 1991.
3. Fluker MR, Urman B, Mackinnon M, et al: Exogenous gonadotrophin therapy in World Health Organization Groups I and II ovulatory disorders. Obstet Gynecol 83:189, 1994.
4. Garner DM: Pathogenesis of anorexia nervosa. Lancet 341:1631, 1993.
5. Knorr JR, Ragland RL, Brown RS, et al: Kallmann's syndrome: MR findings. Am J Neuroradiol 14:845, 1993.

24. AGE-RELATED INFERTILITY

Isaac Kligman, M.D., and Zev Rosenwaks, M.D.

1. Summarize the demographic impact of maternal age on reproduction.
Due to the availability of contemporary birth control methods as well as educational and career aspirations, women in developed nations are delaying childbearing. As a result of this trend, increasing numbers of older women are presenting for assisted reproductive technology (ART) treatments after failing to conceive. The decreased fertility observed with advancing age may also contribute to the dramatic drop in birth rates in the United States in recent years.

2. What physiologic principle underlies the decline in fertility associated with advancing maternal age?
The physiologic principle behind age-dependent decline in female fertility is multifactorial, involving both quantitative and qualitative decline in oocyte production.
Quantitative decline. Although many factors are responsible for the age-dependent decline in female fertility, the most compelling is the well-known decline in oocyte numbers. Women are endowed with a finite and nonreplenishable number of germ cells. At mid-gestation the fetal ovaries contain a peak number (6–7 million) of oogonia. At birth, a female has a total of one million oogonia, and by onset of puberty this complement declines to 300,000. Such attrition is further accelerated by ages 37 to 38, at which time the number of available follicles reaches 25,000.
Chromosomal anomalies. Chromosomal aneuploidy is known to be increasingly common with advanced maternal age.
DNA fragmentation. Rates of DNA fragmentation have been noted to be significantly higher in aged mice compared with younger mice.
Chromosomal degeneration. Chromosomal investigations on unfertilized oocytes following IVF revealed a significantly increased rate of chromosomal degeneration associated with advanced age.
DNA deletion in organelles. It has also been reported that oocytes from older women are more likely to contain mitochondrial DNA deletions than oocytes from younger women.

3. What is ovarian reserve?
The number and functional competence of primordial follicles and germ cells in a woman's ovary constitutes her ovarian reserve—a concept that appears to have a significant impact on a woman's fertility potential. Functional ovarian reserve may or may not correlate with chronological age. For example, in certain pathologic conditions, an accelerated rate of follicular loss may result in diminished ovarian reserve (or ovarian failure) at any age.

4. How is ovarian reserve assessed?
Basal and dynamic tests are available to estimate ovarian reserve. **Basal tests** include evaluation of serum levels of follicle-stimulating hormone (FSH), estradiol and inhibin B levels in the early follicular phase, generally at day 2–3 of the menstrual cycle. **Dynamic tests** include the clomiphene (Clomid, Serophene) challenge test and the leuprolide (Lupron) screening test.

5. What physiologic principles support the basal FSH test?
With advancing age, basal levels of FSH increase before and to a greater extent than basal levels of luteinizing hormone (LH) and are highest in the early-to-mid follicular phase of the menstrual cycle; therefore, FSH levels obtained at this time can serve as sensitive indicators of endocrinologic changes associated with declining ovarian reserve. Presumably, the observed FSH elevation is a consequence of the reduced negative inhibition by steroids and peptides elaborated

by the smaller follicular cohort. Some authors have demonstrated that serum FSH levels in the early follicular phase begin to rise at least 5 to 6 years before menopause.

6. How is basal FSH measured?
Serum FSH levels are generally measured on the second or third day of the menstrual cycle. Different assays are available to determine these levels. There is a wide variation in what constitutes "normal" FSH values, depending on the particular hormonal assay used. Levels below 20 mIU/ml are considered normal with the radioimmunoassay (RIA); with the chemoluminescence assay (DPC) levels below 12 mIU/ml are considered normal. Each laboratory should optimally establish its own normative data.

7. Discuss the relationship between elevated FSH levels and infertility.
Several authors have suggested that subtle elevations of basal FSH may signal declining ovarian reserve despite the presence of regular menstrual cycles; similarly, others have suggested that an increase of FSH early in the menstrual cycle is associated with "unexplained" infertility.

8. What is the impact of elevated FSH levels on ART outcome?
A distinct relationship between basal FSH levels and ART success rates has been described: pregnancy rates decline significantly as day 3 FSH levels rise above 15 mIU/ml, and very few pregnancies have been described when FSH levels exceed 25 mIU/ml (by RIA). With increasing basal FSH levels, there is a decrease in the number of follicles available for aspiration, the number of eggs retrieved, and the number of embryos available for transfer. There is also a direct relationship between increasing FSH levels and cycle cancellation for inadequate response. Furthermore, day-3 FSH concentrations, at any age, predict ART outcome and represent a sensitive indicator of ovarian reserve. Even a single elevated FSH level in a woman who exhibits cycle-to-cycle FSH fluctuations denotes a poorer prognosis.

9. What physiologic principle supports the basal estradiol (E_2) test?
Elevated basal E_2 levels may also serve as markers of diminished ovarian reserve in older (> 35 years) patients. The observed elevated E_2 concentrations, in the presence of seemingly "normal" FSH levels, are the result of **early follicular recruitment,** which may occur as the result of a premature luteal elevation of FSH. The resulting higher estrogen, in turn, feeds back centrally to suppress FSH secretion, thus potentially masking the patient's overall FSH status. Such **early luteal recruitment** may occur when relatively less inhibin is produced by a diminished follicular cohort.

10. Summarize the impact of elevated E_2 levels on ART outcome.
Elevated basal E_2 concentrations have been associated with poor IVF outcome in older patients. A study conducted at our center noted that the ongoing pregnancy rates per retrieval for patients with day 3 (basal) E_2 levels lower than 30 pg/ml was significantly higher than for patients with E_2 levels at 31 to 75 pg/ml. No pregnancies occurred when the day 3 E_2 in the treatment cycle exceeded 75 pg/ml (in nonagonist cycles). Furthermore, the simultaneous evaluation of FSH and E_2 levels appeared to be superior in predicting pregnancy outcome than either of these hormone levels alone. The pregnancy rate was highest when both basal FSH and E_2 levels were low. No pregnancies were seen when the FSH level was greater than 17mIU/ml and the E_2 level was greater than 45pg/ml by RIA.

11. What physiologic principle support the basal inhibin B determination?
Inhibin is a potent inhibitor of FSH secretion. Granulosa cells obtained from women with low basal FSH levels ($\leq$ 6IU/l) have been shown to secrete significantly more dimeric inhibin than cells isolated from women with high day 3 serum FSH levels ($\geq$ 10 IU/l). This finding can be explained either by lower follicular (or granulosa cell) numbers or by impaired inhibin-B production. Other studies have shown that granulosa-luteal cells from older women obtained at the time

of follicular aspiration for IVF have a significantly reduced ability to secrete immunoreactive inhibin in vitro.

12. What is the role of inhibin B determination as an indicator of ovarian reserve?

Assessment of day 3-serum dimeric inhibin-B concentrations may also serve as a predictor of ART outcome. Women with day 3 serum inhibin-B concentrations < 45 pg/ml have been shown to exhibit lower E_2 responses, retrieval of fewer oocytes, higher cycle cancellation rates, and lower clinical pregnancy rates than women with day 3 inhibin-B levels ≥ 45pg/ml. However, the additional utility of the inhibin-B assay beyond the routine assessment of basal FSH and estradiol is not yet established.

13. What is the clomiphene citrate challenge test (CCCT)?

The CCCT is an indirect method of evaluating ovarian reserve. The test assesses the ability of clomiphene-induced FSH secretion to stimulate ovarian steroid and peptide production through the measurement of the degree of subsequent suppression of endogenous FSH. Normal ovarian reserve is manifested by normal or low FSH concentrations after the administration of clomiphene. Women with diminished ovarian reserve are unable to mount adequate ovarian feedback, resulting in elevated FSH concentrations.

14. How is the CCCT conducted?

Baseline (day 2–3) and response levels (day 10) of FSH are measured before and after the administration of 100 mg of clomiphene on days 5–9 of the menstrual cycle. An abnormal test is characterized by an elevated FSH concentration (> 2 SD from basal levels) after clomiphene ingestion. The original study was conducted on 51 women aged 35 years or older, diagnosed with idiopathic infertility. In the group of patients with an abnormal test, one of 18 patients conceived over the ensuing year, whereas in the group with normal results 14 of 33 (42%) patients achieved pregnancy.

15. What is the leuprolide screening test?

The early E_2 response to leuprolide acetate administered in the early follicular phase has also been postulated as a prognosticator of diminished ovarian reserve. Patients with early E_2 elevations followed by a fall exhibited better implantation and pregnancy rates than patients with persistent E_2 elevations or those exhibiting no response through cycle day 5. This test is rarely used to assess ovarian reserve.

16. Summarize the impact of diminished ovarian reserve and advanced maternal age on ART outcome.

Both diminished ovarian reserve and advanced maternal age have a direct and profound impact on the success of ART; advanced maternal age is the most important factor determining outcome. Advancing maternal age is associated with decreased responses to ovarian stimulation as reflected by lower peak estradiol levels, decreased mean numbers of total oocytes retrieved, and lower rates of oocyte fertilization and embryo cleavage. Increased rates of spontaneous abortions and, ultimately, sharply decreased delivery rates are also a consequence of advancing maternal age.

17. Explain what is meant by embryo implantation rate.

The implantation rate can be defined by the number of intrauterine sacs or the number of fetal hearts detected per embryos transferred. Thus, a twin pregnancy (two gestational sacs) following the transfer of four embryos connotes a 50% implantation rate.

18. How does maternal age affect implantation rates and pregnancy outcome?

Implantation rates are inversely related to advancing maternal age. A recent study conducted at our center demonstrated that implantation rates remained relatively constant until age 34. At age 35, implantation rates fall significantly at a linear rate of approximately 2.7% per year. The implantation rate for day 3 embryos is approximately 33–34% for women who are 34 years or younger and declines to about 3–4% per embryo in women who are older than 44 years.

Similarly, success rates with IVF diminish significantly with advancing maternal age. The delivery rate per embryo transfer in couples undergoing intracytoplasmic sperm injection (ICSI) by age groups in our center is represented in Figure 2 of the chapter about in vitro fertilization.

19. What is the impact of advancing maternal age on the spontaneous abortion rate?

Maternal age plays a significant role in determining the spontaneous abortion rate after implantation is established. We have demonstrated that the major cause for these spontaneous losses appears to be chromosomal abnormalities. An analysis of 2014 consecutive clinical IVF pregnancies—defined by positive heart beats on 7 week gestational age ultrasound—revealed an overall pregnancy loss rate of 11.6%. A significant increase in fetal loss was demonstrated with advancing maternal age (Fig. 1). Cytogenetic analysis of fetal tissue in a representative subgroup of women older than 40 years demonstrated that 91.3% of the losses were due to chromosomal abnormalities.

20. What strategies can be used to improve pregnancy success rates in older patients?

Although it is generally believed that the overwhelming determinant of poor success in older women undergoing IVF is related to the genetic make-up of their oocytes and embryos, several strategies aimed at increasing oocyte yield and improving embryo quality have been used in efforts to optimize outcome. Examples include:
- Novel ovarian stimulation strategies
- Embryo co-culture techniques
- Assisted hatching
- Preimplantation genetic analysis (PGD). Genetic testing of preimplantation embryos allows the selection of normal (euploid) embryos.
- Donor oocyte. When success cannot be achieved with a woman's own oocytes, oocyte donation using eggs from younger women has been the most successful strategy.

21. How can the response to ovarian stimulation be improved?

In a significant proportion of cases, a poor ovarian response in the older woman is directly related to diminished ovarian reserve. Poor responders have lower peak E_2 levels, fewer eggs re-

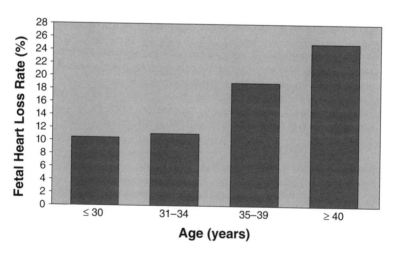

FIGURE 1. Total fetal heart loss as a function of age.

trieved, and fewer embryos available for transfer with a resulting decrease in clinical pregnancy rates. Efforts to enhance the response to ovarian stimulation in this difficult patient group include the following:

- Decreasing the dose of gonatropin-releasing hormone analog (GnRHa).
- Increasing the dose of gonadotropins.
- Avoiding GnRH agonists.
- Using antagonists in the mid-follicular phase to ablate premature ovulation
- Using GnRHa "flare" protocols in the early follicular phase (cycle day 2).
- Using "microdoses" of GnRHa in the early follicular phase (cycle day 2), with or without prior suppression with oral contraceptive pills
- Combining clomiphene citrate with high doses of gonadotropins
- Using growth hormone as an adjuvant for ovarian stimulation (evidence for growth hormone use is controversial)

22. Explain endometrial cell co-culture.

It has been proposed that growing embryos in the presence of somatic cells may enhance embryo viability. Although various cell lines have been used for co-culture, including bovine endometrial cells, kidney cells, and granulosa cells, the authors have adapted a method that uses the patient's own secretory endometrial cells for this purpose. Briefly, an endometrial biopsy is performed in the mid-to-late luteal phase of a cycle preceding the IVF treatment cycle. The endometrial tissue is enzymatically digested with collagenase, and the stromal and glandular cells are separated by differential sedimentation, then cultured to confluence and cryopreserved for later use. These cells are thawed in a subsequent IVF cycle, at which time the one-day old zygotes (2pn) are placed in the co-culture system until day 3 after retrieval.

Several studies support the use of this method in patients with multiple implantation failures and/or poor embryo quality. It has been demonstrated that co-culture is associated with an increase in embryo cell number and a decrease in fragmentation rates compared with embryos that are simultaneously cultured in conventional media. Moreover, pregnancy rates appear to be enhanced when co-culture is used in this challenging group of IVF candidates. It is postulated that somatic cells may improve embryo development by elaborating growth factors or possibly by acting as detoxifiers of metabolic wastes in the microenvironment. An impact of co-culture specifically on age-associated infertility has yet to be established.

23. What is assisted hatching?

The human embryo must hatch (or free itself) from the zona pellucida before implantation. It has been proposed that the in vitro environment may cause zona hardening and thus could impede the hatching process. Assisted hatching is a procedure whereby a small opening is made in the zona pellucida, either by a chemical method (acidic Tyrode's solution) or by a mechanical method (e.g., laser) to facilitate the hatching process and implantation. At our institution, assisted hatching with acidified Tyrode's solution has been selectively implemented in older patients, especially those with highly fragmented embryos or thick zonae and those who have had multiple IVF failures. The impact of assisted hatching on age-associated infertility is still being investigated.

24. What is preimplantation genetic diagnosis (PGD)?

PGD consists of removing one or two blastomeres from a day-3 developing embryo using micromanipulation techniques. Embryo biopsy is used in conjunction with polymerase chain reaction (PCR) techniques, applied clinically to detect single gene defects (e.g., cystic fibrosis, Tay-Sachs disease, sickle cell disease) or with fluorescent in situ hybridization (FISH) to detect numerical chromosomal abnormalities. FISH involves the use of fluorochrome-labeled, chromosome-specific probes that are allowed to hybridize in situ with single interphase nuclei.

Initial studies with FISH demonstrated that the technique can be successfully applied in a high percentage of blastomeres in a time frame that allows embryo transfers to take place within

1–2 days of biopsy. It should be emphasized that removing a single cell (blastomere) from the 3-day-old, 6- to 8-cell embryo does not appear to harm the embryo. Initial reports described the analysis of five chromosomes most commonly observed in human aneuploidy (X,Y,18,13,21), although the use of FISH has expanded to other chromosomes. However, due to the limitation of the techniques only 7–9 chromosomes can be examined in a time frame compatible with embryo transfer.

Comparative genomic hybridization (CGH) following whole genome amplification, an emerging analytic technique, may allow testing of all 23 chromosomes simultaneously. To date, the complexity of CGH does not ensure consistent and dependable results within the required few days necessary to permit IVF transfer.

25. Discuss the role of PGD in older patients.

The authors and others have demonstrated that embryonic chromosomal abnormalities increase with advancing maternal age. This increase in aneuploidy appears to be independent of embryo morphology. Theoretically, the use of FISH to evaluate for aneuploidy should permit the selection and transfer of normal (euploid) embryos, resulting in higher implantation rates and diminished miscarriage rates. However, it should be emphasized that there are limitations to this procedure. For example, analysis of a single blastomere may not be reflective of all the remaining cells, as may be observed in instances of mosaicism. Moreover, there may be limitations in the ability to pick up the chromosome signal, thus resulting in either false-positive or false-negative diagnoses. It should also be realized that in older patients, who often exhibit poor ovarian response and who have few embryos, embryo biopsy may not be a practical approach.

26. What is oocyte donation?

Oocyte donation is the IVF procedure that uses eggs from younger donors for women with ovarian failure or diminished ovarian reserve as well as for women of advanced age who cannot achieve pregnancies with their own oocytes.

Simply described, the donor undergoes ovarian stimulation to achieve multiple follicle development. The recipient's endometrium is prepared with estrogen and progesterone. Careful synchronization of donor and recipient ensures that egg retrieval and insemination of the donor eggs is precisely timed with endometrial development in the recipient. Donor stimulation is controlled with the use of GnRH agonist downregulation. The recipient begins estrogen supplementation 5–7 days before gonadotropin stimulation starts in the donor. The recipient continues estradiol supplementation in increasing doses. Synchronization of the embryo transfer is critically dependent on the initiation of progesterone treatment; as such, the recipient begins progesterone supplementation one day before the donor's retrieval (or one day after HCG administration of human chorionic gonadotropin [HCG]). This synchronization scheme is driven by the timing of HCG administration of the donor, ensuring that day-3 embryos are transferred on day 19 of the recipient cycle (day 15 is arbitrarily designated as the first day of progesterone administration).

Because, with a few exceptions, oocyte donors are young women, this form of ART treatment results in pregnancy success rates that can exceed 50% per embryo transfer. Recently, extended embryo in vitro culture (resulting in day-5 or blastocyst transfer) techniques have yielded pregnancy rates that can exceed 70% per transfer, with implantation rates that exceed 50% per embryo.

BIBLIOGRAPHY

1. Damario M A, Davis O K, Rosenwaks Z: The role of maternal age in assisted reproductive technologies. Reprod Med Rev 7:41–60, 1999.
2. Kligman I, Rosenwaks Z: Differentiating clinical profiles: Predicting good responders, poor responders and hyperresponders. Fertil Steril 76:1185–1190, 2001.
3. Licciardi FL, Liu H-C, Rosenwaks Z: Day 3 estradiol serum concentrations as prognosticators of stimulation response and pregnancy outcome in patients undergoing in vitro fertilization. Fertil Steril 64:991–994, 1995.

4. Lim AST, Tsakok MFH: Age-related decline in fertility: A link to degenerative oocytes? Fertil Steril 68:265–271, 1997.
5. Muasher SJ, Oehninger S, Simonetti S, et al: The value of basal and/or stimulated serum gonadotropin levels in prediction of stimulation response and in vitro fertilization outcome. Fertil Steril 50:298–307, 1988.
6. Navot D, Rosenwaks Z, Margalioth EJ: Prognostic assessment of female fecundity. Lancet i:645–647, 1987.
7. Scott RT, Toner JP, Muasher SJ, et al: Follicle-stimulating hormone levels on cycle day 3, are predictive of in vitro fertilization outcome. Fertil Steril 51:651–654, 1989.
8. Soderstrom-Antilla V, Foudila T, Hovatta O: Oocyte donation in infertility treatment. Acta Obstet Gynecol Scand 80:191–199, 2001.
9. Spandorfer S, Chung P, Kligman, I, et al: An analysis of the effect of age on implantation rates. J Assist Reprod Genet 17(6):303–306, 2000.
10. Spandorfer S, Davis OK, Barmat LI, et al: IVF pregnancy loss: Relationship between maternal age and aneuploidy. Fertil Steril 2004 [in press].
11. Spandorfer SD, Rosenwaks Z: The impact of maternal age and ovarian age in infertility. Postgrad Obstet Gynecol 20(11):1–5, 2000.
12. Spandorfer SD, Rosenwaks Z: The impact of maternal age and ovarian age on implantation efficiency. In Embryo Implantation: Molecular, Cellular and Clinical Aspects. Serono Symposia USA. Norwell, MA, 1999, pp 12–19.
13. Thornhill AR, Snow K: Molecular diagnostics in pre-implantation genetic diagnosis. J Mol Diag 4(1):11–29, 2002.

25. IDIOPATHIC/UNEXPLAINED INFERTILITY

Owen K. Davis, M.D.

1. What is idiopathic infertility?

By definition, idiopathic (unexplained) infertility has no identified pathophysiologic basis and, as such, is a diagnosis of exclusion. Idiopathic infertility may be categorized as primary (no prior pregnancies) or secondary (history of prior pregnancy). Infertility is generally defined as a failure to conceive after an interval of approximately 1 year of regular, unprotected intercourse. Given the profound impact of maternal age on fertility, a clinical evaluation is warranted after 6 months when the female partner is 35 years or older.

2. What constitutes an adequate evaluation for idiopathic infertility?

The infertility evaluation should include, at minimum, a semen analysis of the male partner. For the female partner, it includes documentation of ovulation either by history (regular menses accompanied by molimina), biphasic basal body temperature charting, serum progesterone levels, endometrial biopsy and/or documentation of the luteinizing hormone (LH) surge, and documentation of tubal patency and a normal endometrial cavity, generally by hysterosalpingography or endoscopic evaluation (laparoscopy/hysteroscopy).

Given that advanced female age alone can result in infertility, the contemporary evaluation should also include ovarian reserve testing, such as determination of basal, early follicular phase (typically day 2 or 3) FSH and estradiol, clomiphene challenge testing, and/or sonographic determination of ovarian volume and basal antral follicle counts.

3. What additional fertility testing is warranted?

In the presence of normal ovulatory function and ovarian reserve, patent fallopian tubes, normal uterine anatomy, and a normal semen analysis, other ancillary tests are frequently performed, but a consensus regarding their *routine* utility is lacking. Examples of these tests include postcoital testing, diagnostic laparoscopy, cervical cultures for bacteria such as *Mycoplasma* and/or *Ureaplasma* species, evaluation of thyroid function and prolactin levels in the absence of clinical signs or symptoms, assessment of histologic luteal phase adequacy, antisperm antibody testing, and sperm function tests (e.g., hamster egg penetration assay). Some or all of these ancillary tests may be useful when selectively applied, but their routine use cannot be deemed essential to the fertility investigation.

4. What proportion of infertility is idiopathic?

Approximately 10–15% of infertile couples receive a diagnosis of unexplained infertility. The prevalence may be somewhat lower if laparoscopy is routinely performed, but the role of minimal-to-mild endometriosis as a cause of infertility is debatable. It should be noted that "unexplained" infertility in the setting of advanced age of the female partner (nearing or exceeding 40 years) is often attributable to diminished ovarian reserve, despite the finding of "normal" tests results.

5. Describe the natural history of idiopathic infertility.

The per-cycle fecundity rate in normal, young, fertile couples is approximately 20–25%. With expectant management, monthly pregnancy rates in couples with idiopathic infertility have been determined to range between 1.3% and 4.1%. It has been estimated that roughly 60% of couples with unexplained infertility of less than 3 years' duration will *spontaneously* conceive within 3 years. Baseline fecundity rates, therefore, must be taken into account in any critical appraisal of empirical therapy. The option of expectant management should be discussed with these couples but may be inadvisable, particularly when the female partner is 35 years or older. In some instances, it is likely that treatment of idiopathic infertility serves simply to hasten conception that would ultimately have occurred without intervention.

6. What are the possible mechanisms of idiopathic infertility?

In the setting of a normal fertility evaluation, possible causes of idiopathic infertility include abnormalities of oocyte release or pick-up by the fallopian tubes, perturbations of sperm/oocyte/embryo transport, fertilization failure, disorders of implantation of the blastocyst, and/or intrinsic functional abnormalities of the gametes or embryos. Repetitive preclinical pregnancy loss is another theoretical mechanism; it should be noted, however, that approximately 40% of early conceptions are lost in studied fertile women.

7. What are the therapeutic options for treatment of idiopathic infertility?

A number of therapeutic strategies may be considered in the management of idiopathic infertility. Apart from expectant management, specific interventions may include natural cycle (nonmedicated) intrauterine inseminations (IUI), IUI following ovulation induction/superovulation with clomiphene citrate (CC), and/or exogenous gonadotropins, superovulation alone (i.e., with timed intercourse), and assisted reproductive technologies (ARTs), such as in vitro fertilization (IVF). Given the apparent short-term enhancement of fecundity following hysterosalpingography (HSG), it is often reasonable to defer further therapy for a few (e.g., three) months after the procedure.

8. Discuss the utility of natural cycle IUI for idiopathic infertility.

IUI entails the periovulatory introduction of washed, processed sperm into the uterine cavity via a transcervical catheter. Semen is washed via centrifugation and resuspended in culture medium. Further sperm "selection" can be achieved through techniques such as "swim-up" procedures and density centrifugation in an effort to enhance sperm concentration and/or motility. IUI has been compared with timed intercourse and appears to confer a modest enhancement in fecundity, but per-cycle pregnancy rates appear to be just under 5%. This treatment strategy has been estimated to result in one additional pregnancy per 37 treatment cycles compared with control cycles. The principal, albeit infrequent, risk of IUI is pelvic infection.

9. Is clomiphene citrate combined with intercourse an effective treatment for idiopathic infertility?

The "empirical" use of CC with intercourse is widespread. In theory, CC may enhance fecundity through the ovulation of more than one oocyte or through the correction of a subtle luteal phase defect. On the other hand, the antiestrogenic effects of CC at the end-organ level may have an adverse impact on fecundity (e.g., through a decrease in cervical mucus secretion or via deleterious endometrial effects). An examination of published trials of CC with intercourse vs. control cycles suggests, at best, a minimal positive effect and possibly no significant benefit at all in the treatment of idiopathic infertility.

10. Discuss the efficacy of CC/IUI for idiopathic infertility.

In aggregate, the published data suggest that the empiric administration of CC combined with timed IUI is more effective than either timed intercourse, IUI or CC alone. One randomized study of CC/IUI vs. timed intercourse suggested an approximately 50% enhancement in treatment cycles, yielding an estimated benefit of one additional pregnancy in 16 CC/IUI cycles compared with no treatment. The most common adverse effects of CC include an 8–10% incidence of multiple gestations (predominately twins) and an approximately 5–10% incidence of functional ovarian cysts.

11. What are the success rates and risks of gonadotropin/IUI?

The injection of exogenous gonadotropins for the treatment of infertility is commonly termed superovulation (SO). A number of gonadotropin preparations are available, including recombinant FSH, purified urinary FSH and human menopausal gonadotropins (hMG). By and large, success rates and safety profiles are comparable among the various formulations. SO/IUI is significantly costlier than CC/IUI due both to the cost of the injectable gonadotropin preparations and the requisite monitoring, most often consisting of a combination of sonographic follicular studies and peripheral estradiol measurements. As with ovulation induction, ovulation is triggered with the injection of hCG once follicular maturation (optimally between 2 and 4 follicles) has been attained.

One large, randomized, controlled multicenter study indicated that combined SO/IUI resulted in pregnancy rates double those achieved with either SO or IUI alone. A review of 27 clinical studies suggested per-cycle pregnancy rates of approximately 18% following SO/IUI. SO is associated with an increased risk of multiple gestation (approximately 20% twins and 5% higher-order multiple pregnancies) and severe ovarian hyperstimulation syndrome (OHSS) compared with CC/IUI.

12. Discuss the role of IVF in the treatment of idiopathic infertility.

Although few well-designed studies have directly compared conception rates following IVF with control treatments, there is a practical consensus that IVF is effective, particularly when simpler and less costly treatments have failed. Some European trials have suggested that SO/IUI may be a more cost-effective primary approach than IVF, but relative fecundity rates and cost-effectiveness are expected to differ among clinics given the variability in IVF pregnancy rates. At highly successful IVF centers, per-transfer live birth rates following IVF can exceed those with SO/IUI by 2- to 3-fold.

The relative risks of IVF vs. SO/IUI also vary from center to center. The overall rate of multiple gestations following IVF in the U.S. exceeds 35%. Given the inherent control over the number of embryos replaced, however, IVF is less likely to result in the highest-order multiple pregnancies (quadruplets and greater) than SO/IUI. With meticulous cycle management the risk of clinically significant OHSS should not exceed 5% with either treatment, and at many centers the incidence is in fact considerably lower.

Finally, IVF may also be of diagnostic utility in instances of idiopathic infertility. Fertilization failure or persistently poor oocyte/embryo quality may indicate an intrinsic abnormality of the gametes. Thus failure of IVF may direct affected couples to more effective therapies or adoption.

BIBLIOGRAPHY

1. Collins JA, Burrows EA, Willan AR: The prognosis for live birth among untreated infertile couples. Fertil Steril 64:22, 1995.
2. Crosignani PG, Walters DE, Soliani A: The ESHRE multicentre trial on the treatment of unexplained infertility: a preliminary report. Hum Reprod 6:953, 1991.
3. Deaton JL, Gibson M, Blackmer KM, et al: A randomized, controlled trial of clomiphene citrate and intrauterine insemination in couples with unexplained infertility or surgically corrected endometriosis. Fertil Steril 54:1083, 1990.
4. Guzick DS, Carson SA, Coutifaris C, et al: Efficacy of superovulation and intrauterine insemination in the treatment of infertility. N Engl J Med 340:177, 1999.
5. Guzick DS, Sullivan MW, Adamson GD, et al: Efficacy of treatment for unexplained infertility. Fertil Steril 70:207, 1998.

26. EARLY MENOPAUSE AND AMENORRHEA

Ina Cholst, MD

1. How is premature menopause defined?

Premature menopause is defined as the cessation of ovarian function before the age of 40. Normal menopause occurs in the United States at the average age of 51. Because there is a bell-shaped curve of incidence around this mean, ovarian failure occurring after age 40 should be considered a natural variant, with the term "premature" reserved for ovarian failure occurring before age 40.

2. What is the clinical hallmark of premature menopause?

A clinical history of true hot flashes can be considered pathognomonic. A true hot flash is characterized by its brevity. An intense sensation of warmth may or may not be followed by flushing and sweating. This sensation may be followed by a brief chill. The true hot flash may be mild or severe, but it is always brief,

3. What causes the hot flash?

Hot flashes are centrally mediated. There is a resetting downward of a thermoregulatory set point in the hypothalamus. The discrepancy between core temperature and this set point results in the sensation of warmth. Physiologic mechanisms—such as sweating and peripheral vasodilatation—are set in motion to correct the discrepancy. However, as quickly as it came, the hot flash disappears. The hypothalamic set point returns to baseline, and the hot flash is over.

4. What laboratory tests are used to confirm the diagnosis?

Elevations in gonadotropins (follicle-stimulating hormone and luteinizing hormone) are diagnostic of premature ovarian failure. However, since the ovarian failure may be sporadic or "sputtering," gonadotropins at any particular time may be normal. *Normal gonadotropins do not exclude the diagnosis of premature ovarian failure.* It may be helpful to measure gonadotropins on day 2 or 3 of the cycle in order to diagnose cases of more subtle or incipient ovarian failure.

5. Describe the mechanism behind intermittent or "sputtering" ovarian function.

Primordial follicles appear to migrate slowly from deep within the ovarian cortex toward the more vascular surface of the ovary. Periods of seemingly normal ovarian function may be associated with follicles that have migrated to the surface of the ovary. Here they have access to a more abundant blood supply and to high levels of intravascular follicle-stmiulating hormone. In response, they begin estrogen production and even normal ovulatory function. By contrast, at periods when there are no follicles near the surface of the ovary, little estrogen production leads to amenorrhea and symptoms of menopause.

6. What is the differential diagnosis for premature ovarian failure?

Amenorrhea in young women is more commonly due to anovulatory states, such as polycystic ovary syndrome, or to hypothalamic suppression of various etiologies. A simple work-up includes a pregnancy test and prolactin level, followed by a progesterone challenge test. A withdrawal bleed occurring after the administration of progesterone suggests anovulation. By contrast, failure of withdrawal bleeding is more often associated with ovarian failure or hypothalamic suppression. Gonadotropin levels differentiate between the two. When the gonadotropins are elevated, chromosomal evaluation and adrenal and thyroid function tests are indicated.

7. Is premature ovarian failure an autoimmune disease?

Most cases of premature ovarian failure are idiopathic. However, the following autoimmune endocrinopathies have been associated with ovarian failure:

- Hypoadrenalism, hypoparathyroidism, and mucocutaneous candidiasis
- Schmidt's syndrome (Addison's disease and chronic lymphocytic thyroiditis with or without diabetes mellitus)
- Idiopathic Addison's disease (plus hyperthyroidism and diabetes mellitus)
- Idiopathic hypoparathyroidism
- Pernicious anemia (thyrogastric antibodies)
- Diabetes mellitus and vitiligo
- Myasthenia gravis

8. Explain the significance of premature ovarian failure for fertility.
Documented premature ovarian failure with elevated gonadotropins carries a poor prognosis for pregnancy. Pregnancies do occur, with an incidence of about 1–5%. There is little evidence that high-dose estrogen or high-dose steroids improve this low baseline rate. If the patient responds to high-dose gonadotropins, one or two cycles of in vitro fertilization can be attempted. If the patient is amenable, donor egg remains the best option for achieving pregnancy.

BIBLIOGRAPHY

1. Edwards RG: Genetics of human premature ovarian failure. Reprod Biomed Online 2:139–140, 2001.
2. Larsen EC, Muller J, Schmiegelow K, et al: Reduced ovarian function in long-term survivors of radiation- and chemotherapy-treated childhood cancer. J Clin Endocrinol Metab 88:5307–5314, 2003.
3. Luborsky JL, Meyer P, Sowers MF, et al: Premature menopause in a multi-ethnic population study of the menopause transition. Hum Reprod 18:199–206, 2003.
4. McDonough PG: Selected enquiries into the causation of premature ovarian failure. Hum Fertil (Camb) 6:130–136, 2003.
5. Ross JL, Stefanatos GA, Kushner H, et al: The effect of genetic differences and ovarian failure: Intact cognitive function in adult women with premature ovarian failure versus turner syndrome. J Clin Endocrinol Metab 89:1817–1822, 2004.

27. POLYCYSTIC OVARIAN SYNDROME

Dan Goldschlag, M.D.

1. What is polycystic ovarian syndrome (PCOS)?

It is a term used to describe a group of conditions causing the ovaries to produce excessive androgens. In many cases of PCOS, the ovaries become enlarged with many small cysts; hence the name "polycystic." Symptoms of PCOS include hirsutism, acne, obesity, irregular menstrual periods, lack of ovulation, and infertility.

2. What is Stein-Leventhal syndrome?

Described originally by two Chicago gynecologists, Irving Freiler Stein and Michael Leo Leventhal in 1935, Stein-Leventhal syndrome is another term for PCOS.

3. What are the minimal diagnostic criteria for PCOS?

1. Menstrual irregularity due to oligo- or anovulation
2. Evidence of hyperandrogenism, whether clinical (e.g., hirsutism, acne, male pattern baldness) or biochemical (elevation of androgen levels)
3. Exclusion of other causes of excess androgen production
4. Evidence of hyperandrogenism

4. What should the differential diagnosis of PCOS include?

- Hyperprolactinemia
- Nonclassic congenital adrenal hyperplasia
- Ovarian and adrenal androgen production
- Exogenous medication usage

5. What percent of reproductive age women are affected by PCOS?

PCOS may be one of the most common endocrinopathies in women. Approximately 5% of women in the United States are affected by PCOS.

6. What types of menstrual irregularity are seen in PCOS?

Menstrual irregularities often begin in the peripubertal period. Menarche may be delayed. Women with PCOS may have oligomenorrhea, amenorrhea, or other menstrual irregularities.

7. Does the diagnosis of PCOS require the presence of polycystic ovaries on ultrasound examination?

No. Only 80% of women with PCOS have polycystic ovaries on ultrasound examination. Likewise, many women without endocrinopathies may have polycystic-appearing ovaries.

8. Why does PCOS affect fertility?

Oligo-ovulation or anovulation is the cause of PCOS-related infertility. This type of infertility is usually readily corrected through ovulation induction.

9. How can the infertility associated with PCOS be treated?

After a comprehensive fertility evaluation of both partners, ovulation induction can be initiated. If appropriate, weight loss can be attempted before medication is used to induce ovulation. For many women, ovulation can be restored with weight loss. Approximately 80% of women with PCOS ovulate in response to clomiphene citrate. Metformin has also been shown to induce ovulation. Other medications include gonadotropins.

10. What risks do women with PCOS face when undergoing ovulation induction?
- Multiple pregnancies
- Ovarian hyperstimulation syndrome

11. How is ovulation induction with gonadotropins different for women with PCOS?
Very low doses of gonadotropins are used with careful monitoring to avoid ovarian hyperstimulation and multiple pregnancies.

12. What biochemical findings may be present in women with PCOS?
- Elevation in free testosterone concentrations
- Elevation in serum luteinizing hormone (LH) concentrations
- Normal early follicular serum estradiol
- Increased serum estrone concentrations
- Impaired glucose tolerance

13. What risks are associated with chronic anovulation, as seen in women with PCOS?
Chronic anovulation is associated with an increased risk of the development of endometrial hyperplasia or carcinoma.

14. Explain the pathogenesis of endometrial hyperplasia in obesity and PCOS.
Obese women can have high levels of endogenous estrogen due to the peripheral conversion of androstenedione to estrone and the aromatization of androgens to estradiol. In addition, the lower levels of sex hormone-binding proteins in women with PCOS can lead to an increase in the available estrogen. Furthermore, a chronic anovulatory state lacks the physiologic progesterone secretion normally present in the luteal phase. These factors act synergistically to enhance the effect of estrogens on the endometrium.

15. How can the endometrium be protected?
Oral contraceptives (OCPs) provide a daily exposure to progestins. Progesterones antagonize the proliferative effect of estrogens on the endometrium. Oral contraceptives also raise sex hormone-binding globulin production, thereby decreasing the availability of testosterone. Other progesterone-containing agents are also effective in protecting the endometrium in women with PCOS.

16. How do oral contraceptives affect women with PCOS?
Depending on the type of progesterone, OCPs may decrease glucose intolerance and lower serum insulin levels. OCPs decrease free testosterone concentrations.

17. How is obesity related to PCOS?
Obesity is present in about half of patients with PCOS. The obesity is android in type, with a waist-to-hip ratio exceeding 0.85.

18. Why types of weight loss diets may be effective in PCOS?
Caloric monitoring and low-carbohydrate diets. Most diets resulting in weight loss seem to have the same affect on restoring ovulation and improving insulin sensitivity.

19. What is hirsutism?
Hirsutism is excessive male-type pattern of growth in women. It is important to differentiate hirsutism from generalized hair growth. Hirsutism can be caused by excessive androgens.

20. Adrenal androgen excess can be demonstrated by elevation of what biochemical markers?
- 17-hydroxyprogesterone
- Plasma and total testosterone
- DHEA sulfate

21. How is hirsutism treated?

Hirsutism can be treated through mechanical removal of hair. New hair growth can be slowed through the use of oral contraceptives and/or antiandrogens.

22. How are PCOS and insulin resistance related?

Many women with insulin resistance have marked hyperandrogenism. Insulin and IGF-1 receptors are present within ovarian tissue. Stimulation of these receptors increases androgen production. Reducing insulin resistance by the administration of *metformin* lowers serum free testosterone concentrations.

23. What is the role of insulin in androgen production?

Theca cells respond to LH stimulation with an increase in androgen production. Insulin has a synergistic effect to further increase androgen levels.

BIBLIOGRAPHY

1. Azziz R, Ehrmann D, Legro RS, et al: Troglitazone improves ovulation and hirsutism in the polycystic ovary syndrome: A multicenter, double blind, placebo-controlled trial. J Clin Endocrinol Metab 86:1626–1632, 2001.
2. Barbieri RL: Metformin for the treatment of polycystic ovary syndrome. Obstet Gynecol 101:785–793, 2003.
3. Barbieri RL, Smith S, Ryan KJ: The role of hyperinsulinemia in the pathogenesis of ovarian hyperandrogenism. Fertil Steril 50:197–212, 1988.
4. Knochenhauer ES, Key TJ, Kahsar-Miller M, et al: Prevalence of the polycystic ovary syndrome in unselected black and white women of the southeastern United States: A prospective study. J Clin Endocrinol Metab 83:3078–3082, 1998.
5. Moll GW Jr, Rosenfield RL: Testosterone binding and free plasma androgen concentrations under physiological conditons: chararacterization by flow dialysis technique. J Clin Endocrinol Metab 49:730, 1979.
6. Nestler JE, Jakubowicz DJ, Evans WS, Pasquali R: Effects of metformin on spontaneous and clomiphene-induced ovulation in the polycystic ovary syndrome. N Engl J Med 338:1876, 1998.
7. Nestler JE, Powers LP, Matt DW, et al: A direct effect of hyperinsulinemia on serum sex hormone-binding globulin levels in obese women with the polycystic ovary syndrome. J Clin Endocrinol Metab 72:83, 1991.
8. Rosenfield RL: Plasma testosterone binding globulin and indexes of the concentration of unbound androgens in normal and hirsute subjects. J Clin Endocrinol Metab 32:717, 1971.

28. PELVIC INFLAMMATORY DISEASE AND TUBAL INFERTILITY

Dania Al-Jaroudi, M.D., and Togas Tulandi, M.D.

1. What is pelvic inflammatory disease (PID)?

PID is a spectrum of infections of the female genital tract, including endometritis, salpingitis, oophoritis, myometritis, parametritis, tuboovarian abscess, and peritonitis. In practice, it refers mainly to infection involving the fallopian tubes.

2. How common is PID?

It is estimated that 10–15% of women of reproductive age have had an episode of PID. In the United States, nearly 1 million women develop PID each year.

3. Who is likely to develop PID?

PID can occur at any age, but sexually active women under the age of 25 years are at the greatest risk (almost 70%); 33% of cases develop before the age of 19.

4. Who is less likely to develop PID?

- Rates of PID are low in women over the age of 35.
- Due to lack of menses, PID is rare in pregnant, premenarchal, amenorrheic, or post-menopausal women.
- Women who use oral contraceptive pills (OCPs) have 40–60% reduction in risk of PID because of thicker cervical mucus throughout the menstrual cycle. However, due the large area of cervical ectopy, the risk of endocervical chlamydial infection is increased.
- Women who have undergone tubal sterilization.

5. What are the risk factors of PID?

- Young age
- Low socioeconomic status (low levels of education, unemployment, low income)
- Single, divorced, or separated
- Urban residence
- Multiple sexual partners (4.6 times more likely to develop PID)
- High frequency of sexual intercourse
- Young age at first intercourse
- Previous PID or current PID (2.3 times more likely to develop another episode of PID), including gonorrhea, chlamydial infection, and bacterial vaginosis
- Intrauterine device (2- to 4-fold higher risk of developing PID, which is limited to the first 1–3 months after insertion, possibly due to transient bacterial contamination of the endometrial cavity)
- Menstruation (up to 75% of women with gonorrheal or chlamydial PID develop symptoms in the first 7 days of menses. The cervical mucus plug usually helps in preventing ascension of microorganisms to the upper genital tract; however, it is lost during menses.)
- Cigarette smoking (2-fold increase in risk)
- Substance abuse
- Vaginal douching (douching once a week or more has 3.9-fold higher risk)

6. Why are adolescents at greatest risk?

- Early age at first intercourse
- Multiple lifetime and new partners (more than 2 partners within 30 days)

- More likely to have unprotected intercourse
- Low prevalence of protective chlamydial antibodies
- Anovulatory cycles with cervical mucus that is easier to penetrate.
- Binding and ascend of infectious agents is more likely because of larger zone of cervical ectopy and more columnar cells.

7. How do women get PID?
- Spontaneous infections (85%)
- After certain procedures (15%), such as intrauterine device insertion, dilation and curettage, endometrial biopsy, hysterosalpingography, and hysteroscopy

8. How does PID develop?
- PID is caused by organisms ascending to the upper female genital tract from the vagina and cervix in more than 99% of the cases. The organisms colonize and infect the endometrium and the fallopian tubes. Infection can spread to the surface of ovaries, nearby peritoneum, and, in rare cases, the broad ligament and pelvic blood vessels.
- Transperitoneal spread from a perforated appendix or intrabdominal abscess can cause PID.
- Spread to the tubes and ovaries can occur via hematogenous and lymphatic routes.

9. What organisms are most commonly involved in PID?
Multiple organisms have been isolated. However, *Chlamydia trachomatis* and *Neisseria gonorrhoeae* are among the most common. In untreated cases, about 10–17% of women with gonorrhea and 10% of women with chlamydial infection develop PID. Anaerobic bacteria such as peptococci, peptostreptococci, and bacteroids have also been isolated. The genital *Mycoplasma* and *Ureaplasma* species and the gut coliforms have been isolated from the upper genital tract of women with PID. Other facultative (aerobic) bacteria such as *Gardnerella vaginalis, Streptococcus* species, *Escherichia coli,* and *Haemophilus influenzae* have also been linked to the etiology of PID; in 50% of cases they coexist with gonorrhea and chlamydial infection.

10. What patient complaints are associated with PID?
- Bilateral lower abdominal pain (90% of cases begin a few days after the onset of the last menstrual period)
- Pelvic pain
- Vaginal discharge
- Low back pain
- Irregular vaginal bleeding (35%)
- Dysuria (20%)
- None (silent or asymptomatic PID)

11. What are the common symptoms of PID?
Patients may present with toxic symptoms of fever (30%), nausea, vomiting, and severe lower abdominal pain.

12. What is Fitz-Hugh–Curtis syndrome?
Characterized by intense pain in the right upper quadrant of the abdomen, Fitz-Hugh–Curtis syndrome is a severe presentation of PID occurring in 15–30% of women with PID. It is caused by spreading of infection to the liver capsule. It is associated with gonoccocal PID in around 1–10% of the patients. It can also occur following chlamydial PID. The syndrome is synonymous with perihepatitis (inflammation of the liver capsule along with adhesions between the liver capsule and the diaphragm or the anterior peritoneum, classically known as "violin strings"). Diagnosis is usually made by direct visualization during laparoscopy.

13. What are the findings on pelvic examination?
- Mucopurulent cervical discharge
- Cervical motion tenderness
- Uterine tenderness
- Adnexal tenderness (usually bilateral)
- An adnexal mass may be found (suggestive of tuboovarian abscess)

The sensitivity of pelvic exam is 60%.

14. What are the minimal clinical criteria for initiating therapy?
According to the Centers for Disease Control and Prevention (CDC) guidelines for diagnosis of acute PID, empirical treatment of PID should be instituted based on the presence of all of the following three minimal clinical criteria for pelvic inflammation in the absence of an established cause other than PID:
1. Lower abdominal tenderness
2. Adnexal tenderness
3. Cervical motion tenderness

15. What other criteria can be used for diagnosis?
In addition to the minimal criteria, additional criteria to increase the specificity of diagnosing PID are based on clinical information.
Routine criteria for diagnosing PID
- Oral temperature > 38.3°C
- Abnormal cervical or vaginal discharge
- Elevated erythrocyte sedimentation rate > 15 mm/hr
- Elevated C-reactive protein
- Laboratory documentation of cervical infection with *N. gonorrhoeae* or *C. trachomatis*

Elaborate criteria for diagnosing PID
- Endometrial biopsy with histopathologic evidence of endometritis (presence of leucocytes and plasma cells)
- Transvaginal sonography or other imaging techniques showing thickened fluid-filled tubes with or without free pelvic fluid or tuboovarian complex
- Laparoscopic abnormalities consistent with PID. Examples may include hyperemia, ischemia, edema, or necrosis of the fallopian tubes plus at least one of the following signs: pus inside the tube or coming out of the tube (pyosalpinx), fresh periadnexal adhesions, or sticky exudate on the tubal surface. In diagnosing PID, laparoscopy has up to 95% sensitivity.

16. What other diseases can mimic the presentation of PID?
- Appendicitis
- Meckel's diverticulum
- Ectopic pregnancy
- Adnexal torsion
- Hemorrhagic ovarian cyst
- Rupture of adnexal mass
- Endometriosis
- Urinary tract infection
- Renal calculus
- Acute peritonitis
- Mesenteric adenitis
- Crohn's disease

17. What are the management options of PID?
In 2001, the CDC published recommendations for both outpatient and inpatient management of PID.
CDC ambulatory management of PID
Regimen A
Cefoxitin, 2 gm IM, *plus* probenecid, 1 gm orally in a single dose concurrently, *or* ceftriaxone, 250 mg IM, *or* other parenteral third-generation cephalosporin (e.g., ceftizoxime or cefotaxine) *plus* doxycycline, 100 mg orally 2 times/day for 14 days.

Regimen B
Ofloxacin, 400 mg orally 2 times/day for 14 days, *plus* clindamycin, 450 mg orally 4 times/day, *or* metronidazole, 500 mg orally 2 times/day for 14 days.

CDC inpatient management of PID
Regimen A
Cefoxitin, 2 gm IV every 6 hr, *or* cefotetan, 2 gm IV every 12 hr, *plus* doxycycline, 100 mg every 12 hr orally or IV. (This regimen is given for at least 48 hours after the patient clinically improves.) After discharge from the hospital, continue doxycycline, 100 mg orally twice daily for a total of 14 days.

Regimen B
Clindamycin, 900 mg IV every 8 hr, *plus* gentamycin, loading dose of 2 mg/kg IV or IM followed by maintenance dose (1.5 mg/kg) every 8 hr. (This regimen is given for at least 48 hours after the patient improves.) After discharge from the hospital, continue doxycycline, 100 mg orally twice daily for a total of 14 days, *or* clindamycin, 450 mg orally 5 times/day for 10–14 days.

18. What are the indications for surgery in PID?
Operative treatment of acute PID is restricted to life-threatening cases, such as ruptured tubo-ovarian abscesses; persistent masses in some women who have completed their families; and removal of a persistent symptomatic mass. However, some evidence suggests that the recovery time of patients with tubo-ovarian abscess is shorter after laparoscopic drainage of the abscess.

19. What operative procedures are used in PID?
- Unilateral removal of tubo-ovarian complex or abscess either by laparotomy or laparoscopy
- Laparoscopic drainage of the abscess
- Drainage of a cul-de-sac abscess via a colpotomy incision
- Percutaneous aspiration or drainage of pelvic abscesses under ultrasonic or computed tomographic guidance

20. Who should be hospitalized?
In practice, most women with PID are treated as outpatients. However, according to CDC recommendations, hospitalization should be considered for the following:
- All nulliparous women
- Presence of tubo-ovarian complex or abscess
- Pregnancy
- All adolescents
- Concurrent infection with HIV
- Uncertain diagnosis
- Gastrointestinal symptoms
- Peritonitis in upper quadrants
- Presence of an intrauterine device
- History of operative or diagnostic procedures
- Inadequate response to outpatient therapy

21. What are the short-term sequelae after PID?
- Tubo-ovarian abscess (TOA) occurs in 15–30% of women with acute PID. In 60–100% of cases, anaerobic organisms are isolated from the abscess. *N. gonorrhoeae* and *C. trachomatis* are uncommonly isolated. Diagnosis can be made by ultrasound, computed tomography (CT), or magnetic resonance imaging (MRI) scans. Treatment with antimicrobials is usually successful with clindamycin plus metronidazole or clindamycin and an aminoglycoside. Approximately 75% of women with TOA respond to antimicrobial therapy alone. Traditionally, surgical drainage is performed only if rupture occurs (which can happen in 3–15% of TOAs) or if medical therapy fails. Recent reports, however, suggest that laparoscopic drainage facilitates the recovery.

- Peritonitis, sepsis, shock, and death (5–10%), usually due to rupture of TOA
- Fitz-Hugh–Curtis syndrome

22. What are the long-term sequelae of PID?

- Chronic pelvic pain due to pelvic adhesions occurs in 17–24% of cases after acute PID.
- Ectopic pregnancy (up to 10% of women who conceive will have an ectopic pregnancy).
- Infertility occurs in approximately 20% of women who have had PID. The infertility rate is proportional to the number and severity of episodes of acute PID. The risk is 8% after the first episode, 20% after the second episode, and 40% after the third episode.
- Repeated attacks of PID. Around 25–30% of women who have had PID will have another attack.
- Salpingitis isthmica nodosa (SIN) follows PID in 70% of cases. It is characterized by diverticular eversion of the endosalpinx protruding into the tubal muscularis and is often associated with tubal occlusion. Diagnosis is made during hysterosalpingography. SIN has been associated with ectopic pregnancy.

23. How can we prevent PID?

- Behavioral changes such as delaying age at first intercourse, decreasing the number of sex partners, and partner selection
- Use of barrier contraception, such as condoms and diaphragms, combined with spermicides and use of oral contraceptive pills
- Avoiding unsafe sex practice
- Identifying and treating infections
- Periodic screening for sexually transmissible diseases (STDs), especially in women at high risk
- Ensure partner's compliance with treatment
- Public awareness and education about STDs

24. What causes infertility following PID?

Infertility after PID is usually due to tubal blockage or adhesions surrounding the ovaries or fallopian tubes (found in 30–40% of infertile women). Tubal blockage can occur distally or proximally. Tubal damage can also occur after ectopic pregnancy, endometriosis, and adhesions as a result of previous abdominal or pelvic surgery.

25. What is the contribution of adhesions to tubal infertility?

The surface of the ovary holds onto the ovulated oocytes. The fimbria of the tube picks up the ovum, and the muscular movements and cilia in the fallopian tube facilitate ovum transfer within the tube so that it eventually meets with the sperm. Peritubal adhesions may impede this mechanism, thus leading to infertility.

26. What is the risk of infertility after PID?

In a classic Swedish study of women with laparoscopically confirmed PID, Westrom reported 10–15% incidence of infertility after 1 episode, 20–25% incidence after 2 episodes, and 50–55% incidence after 3 episodes. After an episode of PID, the risk of infertility was correlated to the woman's age (presumably younger women may delay medical intervention), number of infections, and severity of infection. He also reported a 6- to 10-fold increase in the ectopic pregnancy rate after an episode of PID.

27. Is distal obstruction more common than proximal obstruction?

Yes. Among women with tubal disease, 85% have distal obstruction; 15% have proximal obstruction.

28. How do we assess for tubal damage?

- Usually, the hysterosalpingogram (HSG) can determine whether the tubes are obstructed. This method is widely used.
- Sonohysterography is a procedure whereby saline is injected into the uterine cavity. Simultaneously ultrasonography is performed, demonstrating migration of the saline along the tubes. The image is clearer with a special contrast medium (hystero-contrast sonography, or hycosy), but the procedure is costly. In contrast to HSG, this method does not provide a good image.
- Salpingoscopy is an endoscopic visualization of the ampullary portion of the tube during laparotomy or laparoscopy.
- Falloposcopy aided by hysteroscope is another method to visualize the lumen of the tubes. Salpingoscopy and faloposcopy are not widely used.
- Laparoscopy is used for diagnostic purposes in infertility investigation, usually in association with hydrotubation to determine tubal patency. During laparoscopy, reconstruction of the tube can be performed. Laparoscopy also allows identification and treatment of other condition such as endometriosis.

29. Is there a discrepancy between the results of HSG and laparoscopy?

Yes. The agreement between the two techniques varies between 55% and 76%. It was also reported that a good percentage of patients with normal HSG have an abnormal finding during laparoscopy.

30. When can we perform HSG?

HSG usually is performed after cessation of menses by 2–5 days. HSG should be avoided in women with a history of previous PID because the risk of reinfection is as high as 15%. Alternatively, prophylactic antibiotics are given.

31. When is laparoscopy needed?

Laparoscopy is a mandatory examination in infertile women who have had PID. It provides a clear picture of the tubal status and the pelvic organs in general. Surgical treatment can also be performed at the same time. However, for the purpose of in vitro fertilization, laparoscopy is not needed.

32. How can distal tubal occlusion be repaired?

In most cases, adhesions surrounding the tubes and ovaries have to be first liberated (salpingo-ovariolysis). Sometimes, the adhesions surround the fimbrial opening of the tube, blocking the tube partially (fimbrial phimosis). In such cases, a fimbrioplasty (removal of band of adhesions surrounding the tube) can be done. If the distal end of the tube is completely occluded (hydrosalpinx), a salpingostomy is performed. The procedure can be done using laser, electrocautery, or sutures. The clinical outcome is similar.

33. What is the outcome after salpingo-ovariolysis?

At 24 months follow-up, the cumulative pregnancy rate was 45% in women who had salpingo-ovariolysis for periadnexal adhesions vs. only 16% in women who had not received treatment. The incidence of ectopic pregnancy was similar in both groups.

34. What factors favor the success of salpingostomy?

The success rate of salpingostomy is related to the tubal findings, such as the diameter of hydrosalpinx and tubal wall thickness, and the percentage of ciliated cells in the fimbria.

35. What is the pregnancy rate after salpingostomy?

The pregnancy rate after terminal salpingostomy can be as high as 80% if the tubal damage is not extensive. If the tube is rigid and has thick-walled hydrosalpinx without rugae, the pregnancy rate is almost nil. In general, the pregnancy rate after repair of distal tubal blockage (hydrosalpinx) is poor (about 25–30%).

36. What do we do if the tubes are occluded proximally?

The diagnosis of proximal tubal blockage is usually made when no dye reaches the tube during HSG; however, spasm may give false-positive results. Accordingly, if the tubes are not visualized on a hysterosalpingogram, a selective tubal catheterization under fluoroscopy or hysteroscopic control is performed. Using a guide-wire, the "occluded" portion of the tubes is cannulated. Most proximal tubal occlusion is due to mucus plug or amorphous material that can be easily unblocked.

Tubal catheterization is usually successful in about 60–80% of cases, and pregnancy rates range between 20% and 50% in several reports. In one report, the intrauterine pregnancy rates after hysteroscopic tubal cannulation was 57%.

37. Are the results after tubocornual anastomosis as good?

Tubocornual anastomosis is surgical correction of the blocked proximal portion of the tube. The pregnancy rates depend on the extent of tubal damage. After tubocornual anastomosis, pregnancy rates range between 16% and 55%; the rate of ectopic pregnancy is between 7% and 30%.

38. When should IVF be considered in managing infertility due to PID?

In vitro fertilization is often preferable to surgery when tubal damage is more advanced, large hydrosalpinges is seen on hysterosalpingogram, or a previous surgical approach has been unsuccessful.

39. Should laparoscopic salpingectomy be performed for women with hydrosalpinx?

Hydrosalpinx fluid can escape into the uterine cavity to impair embryo implantation. Women with hydrosalpinx undergoing IVF should be given the option of laparoscopic salpingectomy since the pregnancy rates and live births are higher after removal of the blocked tubes. Alternatively, antibiotics can be administered to counteract the toxic effects of the fluid.

BIBLIOGRAPHY

1. Adelusi B, Khashoggi T, Al-Nuaim L, et al: Accuracy of hysterosalpingography and laparoscopic hydrotubation in diagnosis of tubal patency. Fertil Steril 63:1016–1020, 1995.
2. Benaim J, Pulaski M, Coupey S: Adolescent girls and pelvic inflammatory disease: Experience and practice of emergency department pediatricians. Arch Pediatr Adolesc Med 152:449–454, 1998.
3. Canis M, Manhes H, Mage G, et al: Laparoscopic distal tuboplasty: report of 87 cases and a 4-year experience. Fertil Steril 56:616–621, 1991.
4. Centers for Disease Control and Prevention: Recommendations for the prevention and management of Chlamydia trachomatis infections. MMWR 42(RR-12), 1993.
5. Centers for Disease Control and Prevention. Pelvic inflammatory disease: Guidelines for prevention and management. MMWR 2001.
6. Corfman R, Badran O: Effect of pelvic adhesions on pelvic pain and fertility. Infertil Reprod Med Clin North Am 5:405–411, 1994.
7. Das K, Nagel TC, Malo JW: Hysteroscopic cannulation for proximal tubal obstruction: A change for the better? Fertil Steril 63:1009–1014, 1995.
8. Donnez J, Casanas-Roux F: Prognostic factors influencing the pregnancy rate after microsurgical corneal anastomosis. Fertil Steril 46:089–1094, 1986.
9. Donnez J, Casanas-Roux F: Prognostic factors of fimbrial microsurgery. Feril Steril 46:200–204, 1986.
10. Droegemueller W: Infections of the upper genital tract. In Mishell D, Stenchever M, Droegemueller W, Herbest A (eds): Comprehensive Gynecology, 3rd ed. St. Louis, Mosby, 1997.
11. Guerreiro D, Gigante M, Teles LC: Sexually transmitted diseases and reproductive tract infections among contraceptive users. Int J Gynecol Obstet 63(1):S167–S173, 1998.
12. Johnson NP, Mak W, Sowter MC: Surgical treatment for tubal disease in women due to undergo in vitro fertilization (Cochrane Review). The Cochrane Library, Issue 4, 2002. Oxford: Update Software.
13. Mishell D: Tubal causes of infertility. In Mishell D, Stenchever M, et al (eds): Comprehensive Gynecology, 3rd ed. St. Louis, Mosby, 1997.

14. National Institute of Allergy and Infectious Diseases: Pelvic Inflammatory Disease; Washington, DC, National Institutes of Health, 1998
15. Pastorek J: Sexually transmitted diseases. Obstet Gynecol Clin North Am 16(3), 1989.
16. Rock JA, Katayama P, Martin EJ, et al: Factors influencing the success of salpingostomy techniques for distal fimbrial obstruction. Obstet Gynecol 52:591–596, 1978.
17. Tulandi T: Infertility: Surgical management. In Copeland LJ (ed): Textbook of Gynecology. Philadelphia, W.B Saunders, 1993.
18. Yudin M, Landers D: Pelvic inflammatory disease. Curr Probl Obstet Gynecol Fertil 25:1–24, 2002.

29. ENDOMETRIOSIS

Durga Rao, M.D., and Togas Tulandi, M.D.

1. What is endometriosis?

Endometriosis is the presence of endometrial glands and stroma outside the uterine cavity in association with evidence of cellular activity and progression such as adhesion formation.[1]

2. Where are the most common sites of endometriosis?

The ovary and posterior cul de sac are the most common sites of involvement (Fig. 1). Other areas are the uterosacral ligaments, posterior uterus, and posterior broad ligament.[2] There is a predisposition of endometriosis and endometrioma for the left side, possibly due to reduced fluid movement secondary to the presence of sigmoid colon in the left hemipelvis.[3]

Extrapelvic sites of endometriosis are bowel, ureter, bladder, lungs, umbilicus, rectus abdominis muscle, omentum, liver, pancreas, gallbladder, and surgical scars, including episiotomy scars, laparoscopic trocar sites, and amniocentesis tracts. A few cases of endometriosis of the sciatic nerve and the central nervous system have been reported.[4]

3. What causes endometriosis?

The exact mechanism is still unknown, but several hypotheses have been proposed to explain the development of endometriosis:

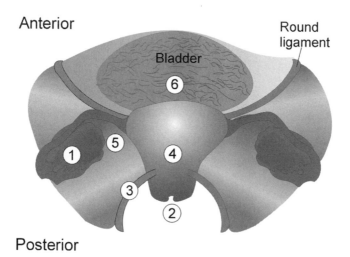

FIGURE 1. Posterior view of the uterus and associated structure. Common sites of endometriosis are (1) ovary, (2) posterior cul de sac, (3) uterosacral ligaments, (4) posterior uterus, (5) posterior broad ligament, and (6) urinary bladder.

1. In 1927 Sampson suggested retrograde flow of menstrual blood through the fallopian tubes into the abdominal cavity as the probable cause .[5] The fact that most women have retrograde menstruation, although not all of them have endometriosis, suggests that other factors play a role.

2. Endometriosis at distant sites may be due to vascular or lymphatic transport of endometrial tissue.[6]

3. Metaplastic transformation of other tissue or activation of cells of mullerian origin (embryonic cell rest theory) to endometrial tissue.

4. Coelomic metaplasia theory[7]: transformation of coelomic epithelium to endometrial tissue. This theory may explain the occurrence of endometriosis in prepubertal girls and in unusual sites such as thumb, thigh, and knee.

5. Immunologic theory.

4. Does endometriosis have a genetic predisposition?

Simpson reported that 6.9% of first-degree relatives of patients with endometriosis had the disease compared with 1.0% in a control group.[8,9] This incidence is comparable to that found in United Kingdom and Montreal (unpublished data). In addition, monozygotic twins have a strong tendency to be concordant for endometriosis.[10] No association with any particular HLA type has been found. However, one research team has demonstrated particular genetic polymorphisms and allelic imbalances in women with endometriosis and suggests that a gene at 9p21 may be involved in the disease.[11,12]

5. What is the role of immune system in the mechanism of endometriosis?

Endometriotic lesions in women with endometriosis have an elevated cytokine concentrations, T- and B-cell abnormalities, and reduced apoptosis similar to lesions found in autoimmune diseases such as rheumatoid arthritis. An autoimmune origin may be difficult to accept due the lack of association between endometriosis and any particular HLA type. But some reports show that women with endometriosis tend to suffer from autoimmune disorders such as thyroid disease, lupus, allergies, and candidal infections.

Endometriotic lesions have significantly higher concentrations of both interleukin-1 and interleukin-6 and a lower concentration of tumor necrosis factor-α than normal endometrium.[13] The ability of numerous cytokines to stimulate or inhibit the growth of endometrial cells[14,15] suggests a role of an inappropriate balance of these proteins in the pathophysiology of endometriosis.

6. What environmental factors may be associated with endometriosis?

Recent reports suggest that exposure to dioxins is associated with endometriosis.[16] Dioxins are toxins found in plastic and chemical industries. Investigators have also found associations between endometriosis and heavy use of alcohol, high doses of caffeine, use of tamoxifen, and cigarette smoking.[17]

7. How common is endometriosis?

Approximately 10–15% of women in the reproductive age group and 25–35% of infertile women have endometriosis

8. What are the common misconceptions about endometriosis?

- Endometriosis occurs only in goal-oriented women over the age of 30 years.
- It does not occur in black women.
- It does not occur in teenage girls.
- It is seen only in nulliparous women.
- Pregnancy cures endometriosis.

9. What are the symptoms of endometriosis?

Many women with endometriosis are asymptomatic, and the diagnosis is made only during laparoscopy for other indications.[18] Little evidence suggests that these women may later become

symptomatic. Some women with extensive endometriosis have little or no pain, but deeply infil-
trating endometriosis is usually associated with pain.

Typical symptoms are pelvic pain, painful bowel movements, back pain, abdominal bloat-
ing, and dyspareunia, often accentuated around the time of menstruation. Rarely women with endometriosis suffer from premenstrual spotting or menorrhagia.

Involvement of various segments of the bowel occurs in up to 15% of patients and may cause
painful defecation. Intussusception of the terminal ileum, acute obstruction, and pseudo-obstruction
with malnutrition are rarely found.[4]

Approximately 4% of patients with endometriosis have urinary signs and symptoms, including dysuria, suprapubic pain, and hematuria. They are due to involvement of the bladder or, less
often, the ureter.[4]

Pleural and pulmonary involvement, causing hemoptysis, bilateral pneumothorax, and
bronchial obstruction, has been reported.

Involvement of the central nervous system can cause subarachnoid hemorrhage and catame-
nial epilepsy.

Common Symptoms of Endometriosis

Dysmenorrhea	Suprapubic pain
Dyspareunia	Hematuria
Low back pain	Painful defecation
Dysuria	Infertility

10. What are the clinical signs of endometriosis?

Adnexal mass with tenderness on palpation, fixed retroverted uterus, and nodularity of the
uterosacral ligaments and cul-de-sac are some signs of endometriosis. However, in most cases
physical examination is negative and not helpful in suspecting endometriosis.

11. What are the differential diagnoses of endometriosis?

Gynecologic

Adenomyosis	Ovarian cyst
Pelvic inflammatory disease	Leiomyoma
Ectopic pregnancy	Vascular congestion

Urologic

Chronic cystitis	Detrusor hypertrophy
Interstitial cystitis	Urethral syndrome
Calculi	

Gastrointestinal

Irritable bowel syndrome	Diverticulitis
Inflammatory bowel disease	Constipation
Chronic appendicitis	

Psychological

Depression	Physical or sexual abuse

Other

Multiple sclerosis	Acute intermittent porphyria
Sickle cell anemia	

12. Are there serum markers for endometriosis?

The two markers that have been studied are the CA125 and CA19–9. Recent study has shown
that CA19–9 is higher in the serum of women with severe endometriosis than in those with mild
endometriosis or in normal women without the disease. However, its sensitivity is not high.[19]
CA125 is a cell surface antigen that is often elevated in the serum of women with endometriosis.
The low sensitivity limits its use, and CA125 can also be elevated by pregnancy, pelvic inflammatory disease, fibroids, ovarian cancer, and menstruation

13. How is endometriosis diagnosed?
- History and pelvic examination may help the diagnosis.
- Imaging studies such as ultrasound and magnetic resonance imaging can detect ovarian endometrioma, but not endometriotic implants or adhesions
- Diagnosis is established by laparoscopy, laparotomy, or histopathology.

14. Describe the appearance of endometriosis on laparoscopy.
The classic lesions look like blue or black powder burns. The lesions can also be red, bluish, nonpigmented, pink, or clear; they may look like red vesicles. Red lesions have been shown to be the most active. Peritoneal defects and adhesions are often observed.

15. What is a chocolate cyst?
Endometrioma or endometriotic cyst is often called a chocolate cyst because of the brownish chocolate-colored fluid content. Formation of typical chocolate cysts can be due to (1) inversion and progressive invagination of the ovarian cortex containing endometriotic implants, (2) secondary involvement of functional ovarian cysts by endometriosis, or (3) metaplasia of the invaginated celomic epithelium.

16. What is rectovaginal endometriosis? How is it treated?
Two hypotheses have been proposed for rectovaginal endometriosis: metaplasia of the mullerian rest cells into endometriotic glands and infiltration of endometriosis of the pouch of Douglas into the rectovaginal septum. Surgical treatment of endometriosis in this location is challenging and should be performed only by skilled surgeons. Most patients need postoperative medical therapy to relieve symptoms.

17. How does endometriosis impair fecundity?
Anatomic damage to the pelvis by tubo-ovarian adhesions or impairment of tubal anatomy impairs gamete transfer. In women with normal anatomy, the cause may be related to impairment of ovulation, reduced response to ovarian stimulation, low embryo quality, and impaired implantation.

18. How is endometriosis classified?
The American Fertility Society Revised Classification of Endometriosis is the standard format for staging of endometriosis. Using a point system, the classification is based on the amount of endometriosis and the number of adhesions.
- Stage I (minimal): 1–5 points
- Stage II (mild): 6–15 points
- Stage III (moderate): 16–40 points
- Stage IV (severe): > 40 points

19. What are the goals of treatment?
1. Alleviation of symptoms
2. Prevention of progression
3. Promotion of fertility[20]

20. What are the different treatment modalities for endometriosis?
Expectant management, medical management, and surgical management (laparoscopy or laparotomy) .

21. What are the medical treatments of endometriosis?
Medical treatments of endometriosis include estrogen-progestin combinations, progestogens, gonadotropin-releasing hormone (GnRH) analogs, and danazol. In general, these agents inhibit growth of endometriotic implants by suppression of ovarian steroids and induction of a hypoestrogenic state. The treatments are associated with a symptomatic improvement in 45–65% of

patients, but the problem often recurs in 6–12 months after treatment.[21] The recurrence rate after medical therapy is 5–15% in the first year, increasing to 40–50% in the fifth year. Potential drugs for treating endometriosis are SERMS and aromatase inhibitors.

22. What is the role of medical management in endometriosis?

The main use of medical treatment is for symptom control and managing recurrence.[22] All current medical therapies are equally effective in controlling dysmenorrhea, dyspareunia, and pelvic pain. Medical therapy improves the AFS scores and the rate of recurrence compared with placebo. Due to their low side effects, progestins alone or in combination with estrogens are commonly used. The best supression is with the use of GnRH analogs. All of these regimens are of limited value in patients who wish to conceive, because they prevent spontaneous ovulation. Moreover, pain recurs in about half of women once therapy is discontinued. No data have demonstrated the protective effect of the drugs against recurrence. Medical treatment has no effect on adhesions or on endometrioma larger than 1cm.[23]

Usual Drug Doses for the Treatment of Endometriosis

DRUGS	DOSE	ADMINISTRATION
Danazol	200–800 mg daily	Oral
Progestins		
Medroxyprogesterone acetate	30 mg daily	Oral
Depot medroxyprogesterone acetate	150 mg every 3 months	Intramuscular
Megestrol	40 mg daily	Oral
GnRH analogs		
Leuprolide acetate	3.75 mg monthly	Intramuscular
Goserelin	3.6 mg monthly	Subcutaneous
Nafarelin	200 μgm twice/day	Intranasal

23. What is the most effective medical treatment?

All of the described medical treatments have been shown to be equally effective in controlling dysmenorrhea, dyspareunia, and pelvic pain and in decreasing the bulk of endometriotic tissue.[24] However, the follow-up period in most of the trials was short (only 3–6 months). The reported recurrence rate of endometriosis is 10% at 1-year follow-up.[25] The following points should be kept in mind:

1. The combined oral contraceptive pill can be prescribed continuously without a withdrawal bleed.

2. Danazol is a derivative of a synthetic steroid of testosterone. It produces high serum androgen and hypoestrogenic environment. The common side effects are weight gain, fluid retention, fatigue, decreased breast size, acne, oily skin, growth of facial hair, atrophic vaginitis, hot flushes, and muscle cramps. It can also irreversibly deepen the voice. It should not be given if there is a possibility of pregnancy. Today danazol is not commonly used.

3. Progestational agents such as medroxyprogesterone acetate are cost-effective and have fewer side effects. Side effects include weight gain, fluid retention, breakthrough bleeding, and depression. The use of the depot preparation is limited by the prolonged time required for resumption of ovulation after treatment discontinuation. Its effectiveness in reducing the amount of endometriosis, however, is low.

4. GnRH analogs produce a hypogonadotrophic state. They have a better side-effect profile than danazol in terms of weight gain and acne, whereas danazol is associated with fewer hot flushes and better bone mineral density. In general, GnRH analogs are more effective and better tolerated than danazol. However, long-term therapy carries a risk of osteoporosis. Addback therapy with a progestational agent (e.g., norlutate) reduces the loss of bone mineral density and does not interfere with effectiveness.

5. That medical therapy is not effective for endometriosis-related infertility has been well established in large-scale, randomized controlled trial.[26]

24. What is the role of surgery in endometriosis?
Surgery helps to restore normal anatomy and is better performed by laparoscopy. The following points should be kept in mind:
- During surgery, endometriosis can be excised.
- Surgery can treat adhesive disease.
- Endometriomas of more than 1 cm is best treated by excision.
- Diagnosis and treatment can be done at the same setting.
- Surgery requires no delay for starting infertility management.

25. Describe surgical options for endometriosis.
The definitive treatment of endometriosis-related pain is hysterectomy and bilateral salpingo-oophorectomy. It should be reserved for women in whom medical therapy and conservative surgery have failed.[27] However, some women who have completed childbearing may elect it as the primary surgical option.

The objectives of conservative surgical treatment of endometriosis are to remove foci of endometriosis and to restore anatomy. Surgical treatment includes excision of endometriosis, vaporization by laser or electrocautery, removal of the endometrioma, and lysis of adhesions.[28]

The surgery may be performed laparoscopically or as an open procedure. Laparoscopic surgery is preferable when performed by experienced laparoscopic surgeons because it provides the same results as laparotomy but with less morbidity and lower cost.

Surgery directed at the pelvic nerves has had variable success in relieving pain. Presacral neurectomy probably is indicated only for women with midline dysmenorrhea that does not respond to conservative treatment.[29] Laparoscopic uterosacral nerve ablation (LUNA) has been done for women with chronic and unresponsive midline pain. However, the recurrence rate at 1 year after LUNA has been high (50%).[29] Most surgeons have abandoned this procedure.

26. What are the different laparoscopic methods for treating ovarian endometrioma?
Excision of endometrioma is superior to aspiration, fenestration, and ablation of the cyst wall either with laser or electrocautery. It provides tissue for histopathologic examination and is associated with a more complete removal of the endometriotic tissue. The concerns of increased adhesion formation are not well substantiated in various human and animal studies.[30] Recurrence of symptoms is significantly lower, and the interval between operation and pain is longer in the excision group than in the vaporization group.[31]

27. Describe the treatment of stage I and stage II endometriosis.
Surgical treatment has been shown to be more effective in pain relief than expectant management. Compared with medical treatment, surgical treatment is also associated with increased fecundity with minimal complications.[32]

28. Describe the treatment of stage III and stage IV endometriosis.
In advanced endometriosis (AFS stage III or IV), surgery to remove endometrial implants or endometrioma, to remove adhesions (scar tissue), or to interrupt neural pathways is the treatment of choice because an endometrioma > 1 cm responds poorly to medical therapy. Furthermore, hormonal suppression has no effect on adhesions, which are often associated with endometriosis.[27]

29. Should women with endometriosis undergoing assisted reproductive technology (ART) be treated medically after surgery?
Postoperative treatment with GnRH analogs after surgery increases the in vitro fertilization (IVF) pregnancy rate in patients with endometriosis. Similar results in patients with stage III or IV endometriosis undergoing intrauterine insemination (IUI) or IVF have been reported.[33,34]

30. Is endometriosis associated with malignancy?

The malignant transformation rate of endometriosis is estimated to be 0.7% to 1.0%. Data suggest that endometriosis may be the precursor of some, and possibly all endometrioid and clear-cell ovarian cancers.[35] More studies are needed to clarify this matter.

BIBLIOGRAPHY

1. Milingos S, Mavromnatis C: Fecundity of infertile women with minimal or mild endometriosis: A clinical study. Arch Gynecol Obstet 267:37–40, 2002.
2. Jenkins S, Olive DL, Haney AF: Endometriosis: Pathogenic implications of the anatomic distributions. Obstet Gynecol 67:335–338, 1986.
3. Al-Fozan H, Tulandi T: Left lateral predisposition of endometriosis and endometrioma. Obstet Gynecol 101:164–166, 2003.
4. Honore GM: Extrapelvic endometriosis. Clin Obstet Gynecol 42:699–671, 1999.
5. Sampson JA: Peritoneal endometriosis due to the menstrual dissemination of endometrial tissue into the peritoneal cavity. Am J Obstet Gynecol 14:422–426, 1927.
6. Ueki M: Histologic study of endometriosis and examination of lymphatic drainage in and from the uterus. Am J Obstet Gynecol 165:201–209, 1991.
7. Suginami H: A reappraisal of the coelomic metaplasia theory by reviewing endometriosis occurring in unusual sites and instances. Am J Obstet Gynecol 165:214–218, 1991.
8. Simpson JL, Elias J, Malinak LR, Buttram VC: Heritable aspects of endometriosis. I: Genetic studies. Am J Obstet Gynecol 137:327–331, 1980.
9. Kennedy S, Mardon H, Barlow D: Familial endometriosis. J Assist Reprod Genet 42:32–34, 1995.
10. Hadfield RM, Mardon HJ, Barlow DH, Kennedy SH: Endometriosis in monozygotic twins. Fertil Steril 68:941–942, 1997.
11. Arvanitis DA, Goumenou AG, Matalliotakis IM, et al: Low-penetrance genes are associated with increased susceptibility to endometriosis. Fertil Steril 76:1202–1206, 2001.
12. Goumenou AG, Arvanitis DA, Matalliotakis IM, et al: Microsatellite DNA assays reveal an allelic imbalance in p16 (Ink4), GALT, p53, and APOA2 loci in patients with endometriosis. Fertil Steril 75:160–165, 2001.
13. Bergqvist C, Bruse M, Carlberg L, Carlstrom K: Interleukin-1 beta, interleukin-6, and tumor necrosis factor-alpha in endometriotic tissue and in endometrium. Fertil Steril 75:489–495, 2001.
14. Harada T, Iwabe T, Terakawa N: Role of cytokines in endometriosis. Fertil Steril 76:1–10, 2001.
15. Gazvani R, Smith L, Fowler PA: Effect of interleukin-8 (IL-8), anti-IL-8, and IL-12 on endometrial cell survival in combined endometrial gland and stromal cell cultures derived from women with and without endometriosis. Fertil Steril 77:62–67, 2002.
16. Rier S : Environmental dioxin and endometriosis. Toxicol. Sci 70:161–170, 2002.
17. Zeyneloglu B, Arici A, Olive DL: Environmental toxins and endometriosis. Obstet Gynecol Clin North Am 24:307–329, 1997
18. Moen MH, Stokstad T: A long-term follow-up study of women with asymptomatic endometriosis diagnosed incidentally at sterilization. Fertil Steril 78:773–776, 2002.
19. Harada T, Kubota T, Aso T: Usefulness of CA19–9 versus Ca 125 for the diagnosis of endometriosis. Fertil Steril 78:733–739, 2002.
20. Paulson JD, Asmar P: Mild and moderate endometriosis. Comparison of treatment modalities for infertile couples. J Reprod Med 36:151–155, 1991.
21. The evidence for the management of endometriosis. Database of abstracts of reviews of effectiveness. EBM Reviews. Issue 4, December 2002.
22. Miller JD, Shaw RW: Historical prospective cohort study of the recurrence of pain after discontinuation of treatment with danazol or a gonadotrophin-releasing hormone agonist. Fertil Steril 70:293–296, 1998.
23. Saleh A, Tulandi T: Surgical management of ovarian endometrioma. Controversies in reproductive surgery. Infertil Clin North Am 11:61–76, 2000.
24. Prentice A, Deary AJ, Goldbeck-Wood S, et al: Gonadotrophin- releasing hormone analogues for pain associated with endometriosis (Cochrane Review). The Cochrane Library, Issue 1, 2002. Oxford, Update Software.
25. Schenken RS, Malinak LR: Reoperation after initial treatment of endometriosis with conservative surgery. Am J Obstet Gynecol 131:416–424, 1978.
26. Hughes E, Fedorkow D, Collins J, Vandekerckhove P: Ovulation suppression for endometriosis (Cochrane Review). Cochrane Library, Issue 1, 2002. Oxford, Update Software.
27. Shaw RT: Treatment of endometriosis. Lancet 340:1267–1271, 1992.

28. Sutton CJG, Ewen SP, Whitelaw N, Haines P: Prospective, randomized, double blind, controlled trial of laser laparoscopy in the treatment of pelvic pain associated with minimal, mild, and moderate endometriosis. Fertil Steril 62: 696–700, 1994.

29. Kim AH, Adamson GD. Surgical treatment options for endometriosis. Clin Obstet Gynecol 42:633–644, 1999.

30. Tulandi T: Reproductive outcome after treatment of mild endometriosis with laparoscopic excision and electrocoagulation. Fertil Steril 69:229–231, 1998.

31. Beretta P, Franchi M,Ghezzi F, Busacca M, et al: Randomised clinical trial of two laparoscopic treatments of endometriomas, cystectomy versus drainage and coagulation. Fertil Steril 70:1176–1180, 1998.

32. Marcoux R, Maheux R, Bérubé S , and the Canadian Collaborative Group on Endometriosis : Laparoscopic surgery in infertile women with minimal or mild endometriosis. N Engl J Med 337:217–222, 1997.

33. Rickes D, Nickel I, Kropf S, Kleinstein J: Increased pregnancy rates after ultralong postoperative therapy with gonadotrophin-releasing hormone analogs in patients with endometriosis. Fertil Steril 78:757–762, 2002.

34. Surrey ES, Silverberg KM, Surrey MW, Schoolcraft WB: Effect of prolonged gonadotropin-releasing hormone agonist therapy on the outcome of in vitro fertilization-embryo transfer in patients with endometriosis. Fertil Steril 78:699–704, 2002.

35. Vignali M, Infantino M, Matrone R, et al: Endometriosis: Novel etiopathogenetic concepts and clinical perspectives. Fertil Steril 78:665–678, 2002.

30. CONTRACEPTION

Steven Spandorfer, M.D.

1. What are the most common methods of contraception?
Common methods of contraception include sterilization, oral contraceptive pills, condoms, diaphragm, cervical cap, sponge, intrauterine devices, long-term hormonal implantation, and natural "rhythm" methods.

Most Common Methods Used to Prevent Conception in the U.S.

CONTRACEPTIVE METHOD	PERCENT WOMEN WHO USE
Oral contraceptives	26
Surgical sterilization	25
Withdrawal	19
Condom	10
None	19

2. Compare family planning for teenagers in the United States and the rest of the world.
More young women become pregnant in the United States than in any other country. For women under the age of 25 years, western European rates are approximately half of the rate in the U.S. Unfortunately, three-quarters of U.S. teenage pregnancies are unintended, and many are aborted.

3. List the typical failure rates during the first year of use for the most commonly used contraceptive methods.
- Oral contraceptive pill: 3.0%
- Intrauterine device: 0.1–2.0%
- Long-term hormonal implantation: 0.05%
- Tubal sterilization: 0.05%
- Condoms: 14%
- Diaphragm: 18%

4. List the most common methods of surgical female tubal sterilization and their 10-year failure rates.
- Unipolar coagulation: 0.75%
- Postpartum tubal ligation: 0.75%
- Silastic ring: 1.77%
- Interval tubal excision: 2.01%
- Bipolar coagulation: 2.48%
- Hulka clip: 3.65%

5. What type of risk factors should be discussed with the patient before proceeding with surgical female tubal sterilization?
The patient should be counseled that tubal sterilization is a "permanent" procedure. Not a small number of patients later may regret undergoing the procedure, particularly younger patients (< 30 years). Surgical reversal of tubal sterilization and in vitro fertilization are possible options for patients who desire pregnancy after a tubal sterilization is performed. Patients should also understand the low but significant long-term failure rates of tubal sterilization procedures. If a pregnancy is diagnosed after tubal sterilization is performed, the suspicion for an ectopic pregnancy is high.

6. How does vasectomy for men compare with female surgical tubal sterilization?
Male vasectomies are safer, easier, and less expensive. Few long-term sequelae have been reported after vasectomy.

7. What is the most commonly used estrogen in the combined oral contraceptive pill (OCP)?
Ethinyl estradiol. The addition of an ethinyl group to estradiol makes this substance a highly potent oral estrogen.

8. What is the progestin component of the OCP?
Various progestins are used. Biochemically, they are mostly derivatives of testosterone with removal of the 19th carbon, which changes the predominant activity from androgenic to a progestin-like activity.

9. What are the major actions of the OCP in preventing pregnancy?
The combined OCP works via many actions at once. Ovulation is inhibited at both the pituitary and hypothalamic levels. The progestational dominance in the OCP leads to an increase in cervical mucus, making it less hospitable to sperm transport. The endometrium also becomes unfavorable for implantation. Tubal peristalsis is also thought to be diminished.

10. During the daily usage of combined OCP, missing which days of the pills is more likely to result in "accidental" pregnancy or contraception failure?
Missing the first pill or two is most commonly associated with OCP failure and pregnancy. This is thought to be due to "early escape" of follicles from hormonal ovarian suppression, which results in the production of a dominant follicle.

11. Are rates of idiopathic venous thromboembolism (VTE) increased in OCP users?
The risk of VTE appears to be higher in patients taking OCPs. This risk is increased by a magnitude of 3- to 4-fold. Note that this rate remains lower than the risk of VTE in pregnant patients. Most cases of VTE are found in the patients with factor V Leiden mutation, a hereditary disorder that produces a defective coagulation factor V, which cannot be destroyed in the bloodstream.

12. What effect does the combined OCP have on anemia?
Women taking the combined OCP are less likely to have iron deficient anemia. The bleeding with the menses is usually lighter and of shorter duration.

13. How do progestin-only contraceptive pills differ from the combined OCPs in respect to mechanism of action?
The combined pill is more consistent than progestin-only pills in preventing ovulation. Both types effectively thicken cervical mucus, decrease fallopian tube motility, and alter the receptiveness of the endometrium for implanatation.

14. Which patients are generally not thought to be good candidates for combination OCPs?
Patients older than 35 years and patients who are heavy users of tobacco are generally not good candidates for the combined OCP. In addition, patients with a history of thromboembolism, coronary artery disease, congestive heart failure, cerebrovascular disease, severe diabetes, or lupus are not good candidates.

15. How does the use of combined OCPs affect the risk of gynecologic cancers?
Use of the OCP for at least 12 months is associated with a decrease in endometrial cancer by 50%. Ovarian cancer is decreased by 40% after the use of OCPs. Studies have found an increase in cervical cancer after the use of OCPs for at least 1 year. The association of breast cancer and OCPs

is controversial. There may be a small increase in premenopausal breast cancer. Overall, post-menopausal breast cancer does not appear to be increased in women with a history of using OCPs.

16. Describe the components of the long-term hormonal implant for contraception.
The implant consists of a subdermal system designed for long-term release of hormone for contraception. Six capsules, each measuring 34 mm in length with a 2.4 mm outer diameter, are included. Each capsule contains 36 mg of crystalline levonorgestrel.

17. What are the major adverse effects of Depot-Provera (injectable long-term progesterone)?
Abnormal uterine bleeding is most predictably seen, particularly after the first 3-month dose. Only one-third of patients achieve amenorrhea after the first injection. After discontinuing the medication, on average, it takes 6 months before regular ovulation resumes. Several studies have demonstrated a 3- to 10-pound weight gain within the first year of use. Mood changes have been described as well, but the incidence of depression is generally below 5%. Many women also develop headaches, usually of mild severity, while on the medication. A slight deterioration in glucose metabolism is also noted. HDL levels also appear to fall. Studies have found no increase in reproductive cancers associated with the use of Depo-Provera.

18. What are the mechanisms of action of the intrauterine device (IUD)?
The major action of the IUD in preventing pregnancy is thought to be a spermicidal effect against a foreign body placed in the endometrium. A sterile inflammatory response appears to promote spermicidal action. In addition, copper IUDs can also promote a decrease in sperm transport in the cervical mucus, but the major contraceptive activity of the copper IUDs is via the spermicidal effect. Progesterone IUDs can also decrease the receptivity of the endometrium for implantation.

19. List the contraindications to placement of an IUD.
• Pregnancy
• Undiagnosed vaginal bleeding
• History of pelvic inflammatory disease
• Recent endometritis
• Acute cervicitis

20. How common are uterine perforations after placement of an IUD?
Perforation of the uterus after placement of an IUD is very rare. It almost always occurs at the time of placement. In large studies, it occurred in < 0.1% of placements. If a perforation is suspected, a sonogram or abdominal x-ray should be performed to locate the IUD. It is best to remove the IUD if indeed perforation has occurred.

21. Who is a candidate for emergency contraception?
Any woman of reproductive age who has had unprotected intercourse during the previous 72 hours. It appears that the earlier the first dose of the emergency contraception is given, the more effective it will be.

22. What forms of emergency contraception are available?
Emergency contraception is most commonly offered as a high dose of hormonal contraception. Many formulations have been used and appear to be equally effective with reductions in unintended pregnancies by at least 75%. IUDs with hormonal manipulations also appear to be effective as emergency contraception.

23. Describe the techniques of natural family planning with the rhythm method.
These techniques rely on the woman's awareness of several physical clues to when she may be ovulating so that she may avoid intercourse at the appropriate time. Patients often use a com-

bination of calendar charting, cervical mucus tests, and temperature methods to determine when intercourse is least likely to result in pregnancy. These methods are more successful for women with a regular, predictable cycle.

24. Other than the rhythm method, what other common natural family planning method is available?

Withdrawal of the penis from the vagina before orgasm and ejaculation, commonly known as the "withdrawal" method, has been practiced commonly as a method of contraception.

25. What is the failure rate of the withdrawal method?

The withdrawal method is highly unreliable compared with other commonly used method of contraception; it is associated with a 19% accidental pregnancy rate during the first year of use.

26. How does the female condom compare with the male condom?

Both are excellent barrier contraception methods that can prevent transmission of sexually transmitted diseases in addition to pregnancy. The female condom can be placed before sexual activity and can remain in place for a longer time after intercourse. They are important alternatives because most failures of male condom usage as a means of contraception are thought to be due to the placement of male condom shortly before orgasm/ejaculation. Keep in mind that preejaculation discharge from the male accessory glands may contain sperm that can result in unwanted pregnancy. Finally, the female condom is less likely to rupture during intercourse.

BIBLIOGRAPHY

1. Collaborative Group on Hormonal Factors in Breast Cancer: Breast cancer and hormonal contraceptives: Collaborative reanalysis of individual data from 54 epidemiological studies. Lancet 347:1713, 1996.
2. Hellgren M, Svensson PJ, Dahlbach B: Resistance to activated protein C as a basis for VTE associated with pregnancy and OCP. Am J Obstet Gynecol 173:210, 1995.
3. Henshaw SK: Unintended pregnancies in the U.S. Fam Plann Perspect 30:24, 1998.
4. Peterson HB, Xia Z, Hughes JM, et al for the U.S. Collaborative Review of Sterilization Working Group: The Risk of pregnancy after tubal sterilization. Am J Obstet Gynecol 174:16, 1996.
5. Schwallie PC, Assenzo JR: Contraceptive use: Efficacy study utilizing medroxyprogesterone acetate administered as an intramuscular injection. Fertil Steril 24:331, 1973.
6. Task Force on Postovulatory Methods of Fertility Regulation: Randomised controlled trial of levonorgestrel versus the Yuzpe method for emergency contraception. Lancet 352:428–433, 1998.
7. Trussell J: Contraceptive efficacy. In Hatcher RA, Trussell J, Stewart P, et al (eds): Contraceptive Technology, 17th ed. New York, Irvington Publishers.
8. World Health Organization: The Tcu220C, multiload 250 and Nova T IUDs at 3.5 and 7 years of use. Contraception 42:141, 1990.

31. RECURRENT PREGNANCY LOSS

Robert Straub, M.D., and Pak H. Chung, M.D.

1. What is the definition of recurrent pregnancy loss (RPL)?

RPL, or habitual abortion is classically defined as 3 or more consecutive spontaneous miscarriages before 20 weeks of gestation.

2. What is the incidence of RPL?

Approximately 1% of pregnant women have had at least two prior spontaneous abortions.

3. What is the likelihood of a live birth after three or more spontaneous miscarriages have occurred?

In 1938, Malpas used theoretical calculations and estimated that there was a 73% chance of a subsequent pregnancy loss after three miscarriages. However, more recent clinical studies have indicated that the risk should be 30–45%. The chance of a live birth after RPL is diagnosed with or without a previous live birth is 70% and 55% respectively. These statistics, however, apply only to young women. It is not unusual that RPL in older women is complicated by secondary infertility with aging.

4. What are the common causes for RPL?

The causes of RPL can be many. It is useful to consider the following categories in evaluating RPL:

Idiopathic loss	Anatomic causes
Genetic factors	Infectious causes
Environmental factors	Immunologic causes
Endocrine factors	

5. What is the likelihood of a parental chromosomal problem in RPL?

For a couple experiencing RPL, there is an increased chance of a chromosomal defect in either of the partners. Various studies suggest that when both partners undergo karyotyping, there is a 3–8% chance of detecting any chromosomal defect; the most common is a balanced translocation. Other abnormalities that are often detected are sex chromosome mosaicism, chromosome inversions, and ring chromosomes.

6. Can all genetic defects be detected by karyotyping?

Karyotyping detects only structural or numeric chromosomal aberrations related to RPL. Other defects, such as single gene defects, are not detected by karyotyping. It is possible that undetected genetic defects play a role in RPL that is otherwise unexplained.

7. In the era of advanced reproductive technology, is there any way to minimize the risk of RPL in couples with balanced translocation?

If karyotype testing reveals parental balanced translocations, preimplantation genetic diagnosis (PGD) can be used to increase the chance of a healthy pregnancy. PGD used in conjunction with in vitro fertilization (IVF) allows screening of embryos for genetic abnormalities. In PGD, a single blastomere is removed from a 6- to 8-cell embryo and subjected to fluorescent in situ hybridization (FISH) to determine chromosome number and a variety of other chromosomal defects. This technique reveals whether an embryo is normal (balanced vs. unbalanced). Only the normal or balanced embryo is considered for transfer.

8. What is the contribution of fetal chromosomal abnormalities to RPL?
Despite normal parental karyotypes, about 70% of early spontaneous miscarriages are associated with fetal chromosomal abnormalities. These abnormalities are often a result of an error in maternal or paternal gametogenesis. If products of conception are available, as in the setting of dilatation and curretage or tissue collection by the patient, they should be sent for cytogenetic analysis. If fetal karyotype is normal, other etiologies of RPL deserve much more attention.

9. What are the most common fetal chromosomal abnormalities in first-trimester miscarriages?
Autosomal trisomy (16, 22, 21, 15, 14, and 18 in that order) is the most common anomaly as a group (50%) and usually results from nondisjunction. The single most common anomaly is 45,X, or classic Turner syndrome (25%).

10. Have any specific environmental factors been linked to RPL?
Tetrachloroethylene (chemical used in dry cleaning) has been implicated as a causative agent in spontaneous miscarriage. Reports also suggest that alcohol and tobacco abuse increase the risk for RPL. Caffeine and anesthetic gases were once thought to be causative agents in RPL, but recent studies have not supported these associations.

11. Which endocrinopathies are associated with RPL?
Uncontrolled diabetes mellitus or significant thyroid disease may be associated with an increased risk for spontaneous miscarriage. Routine screening for these conditions is not productive in apparently asymptomatic and healthy women. However, thyrotropin-stimulating hormone (TSH) level is often used to rule out mild or subclinical hypothyroidism. Polycystic ovarian syndrome has also been associated with RPL.

12. Explain the concept of luteal phase defect (LPD).
LPD has long been debated as a causative factor in RPL. The concept is that inadequate secretion of progesterone from the corpus luteum during the secretory phase retards the development of the endometrial lining. The underdeveloped endometrium is unable to support the developing pregnancy, and spontaneous miscarriage results.

13. How is LPD diagnosed?
To determine whether LPD is present, an endometrial biopsy is scheduled close to an upcoming menses (e.g., day 26 or 27 in a 28-day cycle). Sometimes the biopsy can be timed according to urine surge of luteinizing hormone (around day 9 or 10 after the surge). To date the endometrium by histology, the patient has to be reminded to notify her physician once menses starts after the biopsy. The day of the menses is arbitrarily designated as day 28, and the day of biopsy can then be determined retrospectively. The biopsy is then evaluated histologically. If there is a lag of more than 2 days between the endometrium and the biopsy day, LPD may exist. The diagnosis of LPD should be based on two biopsies from two different cycles.
Alternatively, a quick and less invasive evaluation of the luteal phase can be performed by measuring serial mid-luteal progesterone levels. Any level less than 10 ng/ml may indicate a luteal insufficiency.

14. How do we treat LPD?
LPD is believed to be due to poor folliculogenesis. Any drug that can improve follicular development, such as clomiphene citrate or gonadotropin, can potentially correct LPD. Progesterone can also be given in the luteal phase via oral, vaginal, or intramuscular administration. Mid-luteal progesterone levels should be checked.

15. How is RPL related to the anatomy?
Anatomic causes for RPL can be congenital or acquired. Depending on the type of uterine anomaly or pathologic condition, there may be impaired vascularization or a mechanical distor-

tion of the uterus that prevents implantation or inhibits the pregnancy from developing properly. Anatomic conditions that can increase the chance of RPL include the following:

- Type V anomalies (septate)
- Congenital mullerian anomalies related to diethylstilbestrol (DES) exposure
- Asherman's syndrome
- Other intrauterine filling defects (e.g,, submucous myoma)

16. Can bicornuate uterus cause RPL?

Congenital anomalies involving incomplete mullerian fusion resulting in type II (unicornuate), type III (didelphys), and type IV (bicornuate) anomalies are not associated with RPL.

17. How can an anatomic cause be detected?

Multiple methods are available to evaluate the reproductive tract for anatomic defects. Ultrasonography is readily available in the office setting and allows initial evaluation of the uterus. Saline infusion sonography (SIS) allows more accuracy in diagnosing any intracavitary lesions. Hysterosalpingography (HSG) is still the gold standard to evaluate the uterine cavity and also offers information about tubal patency. Magnetic resonance imaging (MRI) is necessary to discriminate between possible suspected anomalies such as uterine septum or bicornuate uterus. Hysteroscopy is another direct way to evaluate the uterus, although it is more invasive. It can be used to treat uterine anomalies such as fibroids, polyps, septums, and Asherman's syndrome. Laparoscopy and hysteroscopy are sometimes required in combination to distinguish between a bicornuate uterus and a septate uterus.

18. What is a typical history of an anatomic cause of pregnancy losses?

Depending on the type of anatomic defect, one may see a variety of pregnancy histories. With a large filling defect such as a fibroid, a patient may experience infertility, first- and/or second-trimester losses, and even preterm labor. A patient with a congenital defect such as a uterine septum may experience earlier pregnancy losses; each subsequent loss typically occurs later in the gestation. At times, a subsequent pregnancy may last till a viable gestational age is achieved. DES exposure is associated with increased risk for spontaneous miscarriage as well as ectopic pregnancies and preterm deliveries.

19. What is the appropriate course of action to distinguish between a uterine septum and a bicornuate uterus?

If there is suspicion of a congenital uterine anomaly such as a uterine septum or a bicornuate uterus, an MRI should be performed for definitive diagnosis before surgical correction is attempted. If the MRI is not conclusive, laparoscopy should be performed in conjunction with operative hysteroscopy to properly diagnose and treat the defect. Never should a patient be scheduled for a hysteroscopic septum removal based only on HSG findings. One may risk uterine perforation if the diagnosis turns out to be a bicornuate uterus.

20. Describe the surgical procedure for correction of a septate uterus.

Hysteroscopic resection is the procedure of choice, with 1.5% glycine solution as the distention medium. Continuous flow pump has to be used during surgery to keep track of fluid balance. Scissors can be used to cut the septum in the middle, which usually will retract. Therefore, no tissue is removed. Some surgeons prefer to remove the septum from the base using cautery, but this approach may risk scarring the underlying myometrium if resection is overly aggressive.

21. Summarize the postoperative management of uterine septum removal.

Removal of a small septum does not require postoperative hormone treatment. Otherwise, postoperative estrogen (e.g., conjugated estrogen, 1.25 mg /day) for 30 days, followed by 10 days of overlap with medroxyprogesterone at the end of the regimen, can be considered. Postoperative intrauterine Foley placement is rarely indicated in septum removal.

22. Why do we have to be very cautious when glycine is used as distention fluid in operative hysteroscopy?

Glycine, a low-viscosity fluid at 1.5% concentration, is a common distention medium used during operative hysteroscopic procedures and offers great resolution. During operative hysteroscopy, glycine solution may gain access to the uterine vasculature when these vessels are opened during the procedure (e.g., submucosal resection of myoma). Because the distention medium is under pressure, it readily passes into the vasculature. The influx of hypotonic glycine can lead to hyponatremia, hypo-osmolality, and hypervolemia, which in turn can cause pulmonary edema, water intoxification, and cerebral edema. To minimize the risks associated with the use of glycine, one should maintain a low intrauterine pressure and carefully monitor the fluid deficit (total fluid = fluid in + fluid out) by a continuous flow pump. Any deficit of glycine during surgery of greater than 500 ml should alert the surgeon to consider termination of the procedure. In any patient whose fluid deficit exceeds 500 ml, electrolytes should be monitored postoperatively. Treatment for the complications of glycine overload consists of diuresis with furosemide and careful monitoring of vital signs and electrolytes.

23. What microorganisms have been implicated in RPL?

Despite a fair number of anecdotal reports and occasional studies suggesting a link between various bacterial or viral agents and RPL, no studies conclusively support an infectious etiology for RPL. However, *Ureaplasma urealyticum* and *Listeria monocytogenes* have received considerable attention and are thought by some to play a role in RPL or sporadic pregnancy loss. *Toxoplasma gondii* and several viruses (i.e., rubella, herpes simplex, and measles virus, cytomegalovirus, coxsackievirus) have been implicated in sporadic pregnancy losses.

24. Do antibiotics have any place in the treatment of RPL?

Routine prophylaxis is not recommended. If a culture grows *Ureaplasma urealyticum*, both partners should be treated with doxycycline (100 mg orally for 14 days).

25. What is the current status of an immunologic etiology for RPL?

Immunologic causes for RPL have been the most controversial in terms of diagnosis and treatment. So far only antiphospholipid antibodies have fulfilled the criteria for causality. Examples include anticardiolipin antibodies and lupus anticoagulant. Otherwise, HLA sharing in couples, phosphatidylserine antibodies, antinuclear antibodies, antithyroid antibodies, other less common thrombophilic conditions, and some alloimmune conditions have been implicated in RPL.

26. Do thrombophilias affect the risk for RPL?

The association between thrombophilias and RPL, with the exception of antiphospholipid antibodies, remains controversial. Certain conditions predispose a patient to a thrombotic event. Examples include sporadic mutations and familial patterns. The debate continues as to whether conditions that increase the risk for a thrombotic event have an effect on early pregnancy loss and RPL or on second- and third-trimester pregnancy losses and complications. No studies have conclusively linked thrombophilias with RPL. However, several small studies and case series suggest that thrombophilias may be associated with RPL when no other cause can be identified.

27. What laboratory blood tests can be used to rule out a thrombophilic etiology for RPL?

The list of laboratory tests to evaluate for a possible thrombophilia is long, and the battery of tests can be quite expensive. The parameters in italics should be ordered first for screening. It is often best to consult a hematologist with a special interest in this topic.

- *Activated partial thromboplastin time (aPTT)*
- *Anticardiolipin antibodies*
- *Antinuclear antibodies (ANA)*
- *Lupus anticoagulant*

- Antithrombin III
- Protein C
- Protein S
- Activated protein C resistance ratio
- Fibrinogen
- Prothrombin G mutation
- Thrombin time
- Factor V Leiden mutation
- Homocysteine level
- Complete blood count

28. How do you treat thrombophilic problems associated with RPL?
If a diagnosis of thrombophilia is made, the patient should be treated with baby aspirin and prophylactic doses of heparin. Despite some disagreement about the exact dose to be recommended, 5,000 units twice daily, given subcutaneously, should suffice. The patient usually commits to this treatment throughout the entire pregnancy, but it is best managed by a perinatologist. In the event that IVF is indicated for RPL, aspirin and heparin must be stopped before oocyte retrieval. Monitoring the bleeding profile in patients treated with prophylactic doses of heparin is not necessary.

29. What is the current status of the use of immunotherapy for RPL?
Some early studies have suggested that activation of the immune system leads to RPL. Although this theory has not yet been clearly delineated, some have proposed various treatment protocols. Immunotherapy with intravenous immunoglobulin (IVIG) is a popular though unproven treatment for a suspected immunologic cause of RPL. Others have proposed immunizing the woman with paternal lymphocytes. Neither therapy has proved effective, nor has either been evaluated by randomized controlled studies. In addition, immunotherapies are generally quite expensive, and risks are associated with any blood product usage. They should remain as experimental therapies and be used under research protocols.

30. What should you recommend if patients with RPL cannot naturally achieve pregnancy again?
When a couple with a history of RPL is unable to conceive naturally, several treatment modalities are available. Options for improving the odds of conception per month, such as the use of superovulation agents coupled with IUI or even IVF, can be considered. In difficult cases, the use of donor egg or donor sperm, surrogate gestational carrier, and adoption may be indicated.

31. In summary, what tests should be first considered in the evaluation of RPL?
- Parental and fetal (if available) karyotypes
- Cervical cultures for *Mycoplasma*, and *Ureaplasma* species
- HSG or saline sonogram
- TSH, prolactin
- Mid-luteal progesterone levels
- Endometrial biopsy
- Autoimmune evaluations: antiphospholipid antibodies, ANA, aPTT

BIBLIOGRAPHY

1. ACOG Practice Bulletin Number 24: Management of recurrent early pregnancy loss, 2001 In 2003 Compendium of Selected Publications. Washington, DC, American College of Obstetricians and Gynecologists, 2003, pp 425–436.
2. Adashi EY, Rock JA, Rosenwaks Z (eds): Reproductive Endocrinology, Surgery, and Technology. New York, Lippincott-Raven, 1996.

3. Cunningham FG, Clark SL, Leveno KJ (eds): Williams Obstetrics, 21st ed. New York, McGraw-Hill, 2001.
4. Hill JA: Recurrent pregnancy loss. In Creasy RK, Resnick R, Bralow L (eds): Maternal Fetal Medicine, 4th ed. Philadelphia, W.B. Saunders, 1999.
5. Lobo RA, Branch DW Jr, Reindollar RH, Carson SA: Current management of recurrent pregnancy loss. Cont Obstet Gynecol 1–23, 2000.
6. Speroff L, Glass RH, Kase NG: Recurrent early pregnancy losses. In Clinical Gynecologic Endocrinology and Infertility, 6th ed. Philadelphia, Lippincott Williams & Wilkins, 1999.
7. Witz CA, Silverberg KM, Burns WN, et al: Complications associated with the absorption of hysteroscopic fluid media. Fertil Steril 60:745–756, 1993.

32. IMAGING IN REPRODUCTIVE MEDICINE

William M. Buckett, M.D., and Seang Lin Tan, M.D.

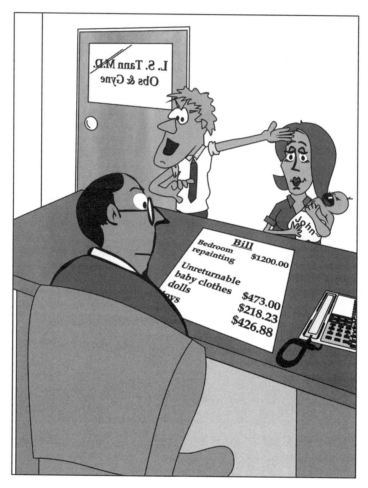

"C'mon doc, fair is fair. You were sure it would be a girl".

IMAGING TECHNIQUES

1. What imaging modalities are commonly used in reproductive medicine?

The imaging techniques most commonly used in reproductive medicine are x-rays (most notably during hysterosalpingogram to delineate the uterine cavity and to determine tubal patency) and ultrasound (both for the evaluation of uterine and ovarian morphology and for the monitoring of ovarian response during treatment).

X-ray particles (or photons) are high-energy electromagnetic radiation that can pass through tissue and are detected by x-ray sensitive film. Structures that are dense (such as bone) block most of the photons and appear white on the developed films. Structures containing air are black on the films, and muscle, fat, and fluid appear as shades of gray. Metal and contrast media (intravenous or oral contrast) block almost all of the photons and appear bright white. The energy of the absorbed photons can break apart, or ionize, compounds that may cause cell damage. This process is known as ionizing radiation. Most cell damage is soon repaired, although some is permanent. For the exposures encountered in conventional radiography, the risk of cancer or heritable defects (via damaged ovarian cells or sperm cells) is extremely low.

Ultrasound is high-frequency sound energy. Transducers in the ultrasound probe emit short pulses of ultrasound and then receive echoes returning from the interface between the tissues in the area under examination. Processing at high speed produces a real-time two-dimensional gray scale image. Conventionally, ultrasound examination of the abdomen and pelvis may be performed transabdominally with a full bladder to allow better visualization of the structures of the pelvis. The development and widespread availability of the transvaginal ultrasound probe during the 1980s has led to enhanced image resolution. Transvaginal ultrasound is now the approach of choice in reproductive medicine (Fig. 1).There is no ionizing radiation exposure with ultrasound.

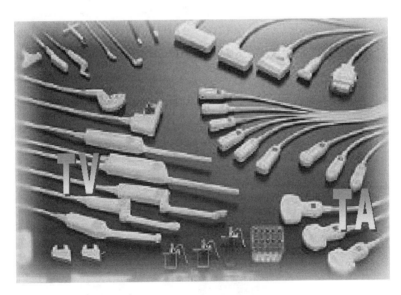

FIGURE 1. An array of ultrasound probes, showing both transvaginal (TV) and transabdominal (TA) approaches.

2. Discuss the roles of computed tomography (CT) and magnetic resonance imaging (MRI).

In **CT,** a thin x-ray beam rotates around the area under examination and its absorption is measured. The differences in absorption are used to generate a cross-sectional image. The role of CT scanning in the abdomen or pelvis is limited. In reproductive medicine, however, CT scans are still used to diagnose and monitor treatment of pituitary tumours—particularly prolactinomas—in both men and women who present with infertility (Fig. 2).

MRI, or nuclear magnetic resonance (NMR), uses the establishment of a strong magnetic field to align the magnetic nuclei in the tissues under examination. Then focused radiowave pulses are emitted and received from the MRI transducers. The subtle differences in the signal from various body tissues and tomographic analysis allow the generation of cross-sectional images that are able to differentiate many tissues. These features make MRI scanning particularly effective in the assessment of many tumours or congenital anatomic anomalies. MRI, where available, is now the investigation of choice for the diagnosis and monitoring of treatment of prolactinomas. Because of its ability to detect subtle differences in tissue , MRI also has a role the evaluation of uterine anomalies such as bicornuate or septate uteri (Fig. 3). Further possible indications currently under research include the assessment and monitoring of percutaneous laser treatment of fibroids and the evaluation of uterine peristaltic activity. Finally, MRI has also been used to detect testicular, prostatic, ejaculatory ductal, and other anatomic abnormalities in men, although its use in the evaluation of male factor infertility is not widespread at the moment.

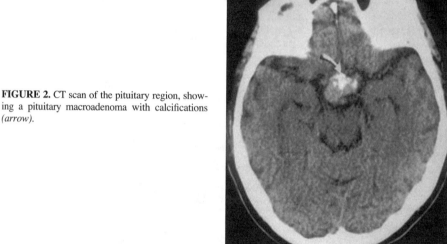

FIGURE 2. CT scan of the pituitary region, showing a pituitary macroadenoma with calcifications *(arrow)*.

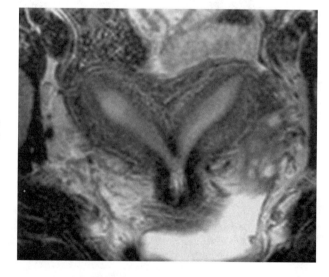

FIGURE 3. MRI scan of the pelvis showing a bicornuate uterus.

PELVIC ULTRASOUND

3. Is ultrasound completely safe?

It is generally acknowledged that transabdominal and transvaginal gray-scale imaging is unlikely to cause any significant biologic effect. Acoustic output intensity is measured by the spatial peak-temporal average intensity I_{SPTA} (the intensity and power of the ultrasonic beam over time), the spatial peak pulse average I_{SPPA} (the average intensity during the ultrasound pulse), and the maximum or peak intensity I_M. Values of maximum acoustic output for ultrasound in different tissues have been produced by the Center for Devices and Radiological Health (CDRH) of the United States Food and Drug Administration (FDA) in the document entitled *The 510 (k) Guide for Measuring and Reporting Acoustic Output of Diagnostic Medical Devices*. The maximum acoustic outputs used in transabdominal and transvaginal gray-scale imaging are significantly below the FDA maximum values for ultrasound exposure in fetal tissue.

Maximum Acoustic Output of Transabdominal and Transvaginal Gray-scale Imaging

ACOUSTIC OUTPUT	TRANSABDOMINAL	TRANSVAGINAL	FDA FETAL VALUE
I_{SPTA} (mW/cm^2)	10	5	180
I_{SPPA} (mW/cm^2)	250	150	350
I_M (mW/cm^2)	400	200	550

4. Who should have ultrasound assessment of the pelvis?

An ultrasound assessment of the pelvis should be performed in all women undergoing infertility investigation prior to treatment. It is a noninvasive investigation allowing assessment of the uterine and ovarian function and morphology as well as a screening test for other pelvic pathology.

Baseline ultrasound scan allows the diagnosis of polycystic ovary syndrome (PCOS), which is important because affected women are at increased risk of ovarian over-response or ovarian hyperstimulation syndrome (OHSS), functional ovarian cysts (which may delay or reduce the efficacy of treatment), endometrial polyps, or, occasionally, undiagnosed early pregnancy. The presence of endometriomata, submucosal or large fibroids, and hydrosalpinges can also be made at the baseline ultrasound scan.

5. What features should be routinely assessed during pelvic ultrasound?

A methodologic ultrasound assessment of the pelvis is recommended. Initially the uterus and uterine cavity should be examined for any anomalies and/or tumours (e.g., fibroids), the dimensions should be measured, and the uterine volume should be calculated. The endometrial thickness should also be measured and its appearance assessed, along with the presence or absence of any intraendometrial abnormalities (e.g., polyps). Then ovarian morphology (normal, polycystic, or multicystic) should be assessed, followed by the position, mobility, total volume, and antral follicle count for both ovaries. During treatment or monitoring, follicular size should also be measured. Finally, the presence or absence of any free fluid, masses, or tubal abnormalities within pelvis should be noted.

Role of the Initial Baseline Ultrasound Examination

- Assess total ovarian volume, stromal volume, and morphology (PCOS criteria)
- Exclude functional ovarian cysts or endometriomata
- Assess the uterus for any fibroids or endometrial polyps and the presence of other pelvic pathology (e.g., hydrosalpinx)
- Extended role may include assessment of tubal patency or intrauterine pathology

6. When should an initial baseline ultrasound be performed?

Initial baseline ultrasound should ideally be performed in the early follicular phase of the menstrual cycle (day 2–5 following the onset of bleeding). This timing allows full assessment of ovarian morphology while the ovaries are at their most quiescent as well as assessment of ovarian reserve. It also allows the diagnosis of polycystic ovaries and other ovarian pathology such as a functional ovarian cyst or endometrioma. Because of rhythmic changes in uterine and ovarian blood flow during the day, when the use of Doppler ultrasound (see question 26) is planned, ultrasound assessment should be performed in the morning.

When a patient undergoes treatment, such as ovulation induction or intrauterine insemination, further ultrasound examinations in the late follicular and early ovulatory phase need to be performed to confirm the development of a dominant follicle and subsequent ovulation. Occasionally, ultrasound in the luteal phase is also indicated to confirm appropriate endometrial response.

More recently, the concept of a single "pivotal" ultrasound in the late follicular phase has been proposed. Although this approach can reduce the number of ultrasound scans needed and may also allow the possibility of saline sonohysteroscopy and assessments of tubal patency at the same time (see question 21), the presence of any functional cyst or endometrioma may confuse the findings.

7. What is ovarian reserve? How is it determined by ultrasound?

The ability of an ovary to respond to stimulation during ovulation induction or in vitro fertilization (IVF) is known as the ovarian response or ovarian reserve. It is thought to be a reflection of the decreasing pool of primordial follicles in the ovary as a woman ages. Because of the wide variation among women, age itself is not a reliable predictor. Several endocrine and dynamic tests have been used, such as assessment of follicle-stimulating hormone (FSH) levels in the early follicular phase and the clomiphene citrate challenge test.

Ultrasound has been used as an adjunct to endocrine assessment of ovarian reserve. Decreased ovarian volume and low number of antral follicles of 2–10 mm (the antral follicle count), measured during the early follicular phase, are signs of ovarian aging that may be observed earlier than a rise in FSH levels. Small ovaries (less than 4 cm^3) and a low antral follicle count (AFC < 5) are associated with poor response to superovulation and a high cancellation rate in IVF. More recently, the measurement of ovarian stromal blood flow with color Doppler may also have a role in the assessment of ovarian reserve.

8. What are the diagnostic criteria for polycystic ovaries?

In repeated studies, three main ultrasound features are used in the diagnosis of polycystic ovaries: (1) increased ovarian size or volume, (2) a "polycystic" or polyfollicular pattern, and (3) hypertophic, echogenic stroma (an increased, bright ovarian stroma). The ovarian volume should be > 10 cm^3, and the polycystic pattern is typically peripheral with the follicles encircling the ovarian cortex like a string of pearls, although this pattern is sometimes incomplete (Fig. 4).

The absolute number of follicles needed to diagnose polycystic ovaries remains controversial. The diagnostic criteria range from > 8 follilces to > 10 follicles or even > 15 follicles within any given ultrasound plane. Other experts suggest that an effort should be made to determine the total number of follicles.

9. Does detection of polycystic ovaries by ultrasound mean that a particular women has PCOS?

Not necessarily. The diagnosis of PCOS requires the presence of clinical manifestations, such as anovulatory cycles or oligomenorrhea, and evidence of mild hyperandrogenism, such as acne or hirsuitism, as well as the ultrasound findings of typically polycystic ovaries and the disordered endocrine indices of PCOS. The presence of polycystic ovaries in otherwise asymptomatic women with regular ovulatory cycles are better termed "ultrasound-only'" polycystic ovaries. Such women are still at greater risk of ovarian over-response or developing OHSS when they undergo ovarian stimulation.

10. What if I cannot determine the position and nature of the ovaries?

The easiest way to view the ovaries by transvaginal ultrasound scan is first to identify the uterus longitudinally at the fundus and in the midline and then to move the ultrasound probe laterally. In most cases the ovary will come into view. Occasionally, it is difficult to visualize the

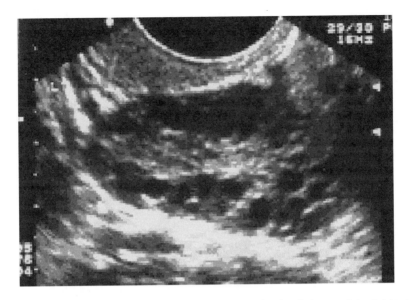

FIGURE 4. Transvaginal ultrasound image of a polycystic ovary, showing the increased size, bright stroma, and typical polycystic pattern.

ovary, particularly in women who have a large uterus distorted by multiple fibroids, who have had previous ovarian or tubal surgery, or who have severe endometriosis or severe tubal disease. In such cases, the ultrasound probe should be moved more laterally until the internal iliac vessels are seen. These vessels should then be followed until the ovary is found. Using a deeper field of vision may be necessary, but in most cases the ovary will be identified.

11. How is the ovarian response to ovulation induction or superovulation monitored?
    After initiation of ovulation induction treatment, the ovaries undergo an enhanced follicular response, often resulting in multiple follicular development. Ultrasound allows the number and sizes of the developing follicles to be observed easily. Although the technique is not standardized, most workers measure the internal diameter of the follicle in two diameters in each of two different ultrasound planes and then calculate the mean diameter. Following the initial ultrasound scan performed during menstruation, most programs monitor follicular development with ultrasound on day 8–10 of the cycle and then as appropriate, until the development of a mature follicle. Follicles grow approximately 2 mm per day; 18–23 mm is regarded as the optimal size for mature follicles. Therefore, once the largest follicle reaches a mean diameter of at least 18mm, ovulation or final oocyte maturation may be triggered with an injection of human chorionic gonadotropin (hCG), if necessary.

12. How accurate is ultrasound monitoring?
    With the technique outlined above, the intraobserver standard deviation has been reported at 0.6 mm and the interobserver standard deviation at 1.2 mm. For any single measurement, therefore, the 95% confidence limits would be ± 2.4 mm. Therefore, after appropriate training, usually there is no need for the same ultrasonographer to perform the serial ultrasound scans for any particular woman.

13. How is the endometrial response to ovulation induction or superovulation monitored? Is it important?
    The value of measuring the endometrial thickness and studying the endometrial reflectivity remains contentious. Initial work suggested that, immediately prior to ovulation, endometrial

thickness and a multilayered pattern were significantly greater in pregnant than nonpregnant women, possibly predicting implantation. However, a number of subsequent studies have suggested that endometrial thickness has no predictive value for pregnancy. There appears to be a minimal threshold of endometrial response that is nearly always achieved in a normal cycle. However, where the endometrium remains thin throughout the cycle despite good ovarian response, the possibility of additional endometrial pathology (e.g., uterine synechiae) must be excluded before continuing further treatment.

Features of Ultrasound Monitoring of Treatment

- All patients undergoing ovulation induction should be monitored by ultrasound.
- Ultrasound scans should be performed at day 8–10 of the cycle and then until development of the dominant follicle.
- Follicles should be measured in two diameters in two different planes.
- Endometrial thickness remains contentious, but additional endometrial pathology should be excluded if the endometrium remains thin despite a good ovarian response.

14. How are the nature and significance of fibroids assessed?

The ultrasound assessment of any fibroid should include the dimensions of the fibroid (in at least two planes of vision), echogenicity and appearance (e.g., presence of any calcifications), and position of the fibroid. The localization of the fibroid (fundal, anterior, posterior, or cervical) needs to be accompanied by an assessment of whether the fibroid is submucosal, myometrial, or serosal. Ultrasound photographs are a useful adjunct (Fig. 5). Further assessment of the fibroid and any effect on the uterine cavity can also be assessed by saline hysterosonography (see below). When fibroids are small and do not distort the uterine cavity, they are unlikely to have a major impact on fertility.

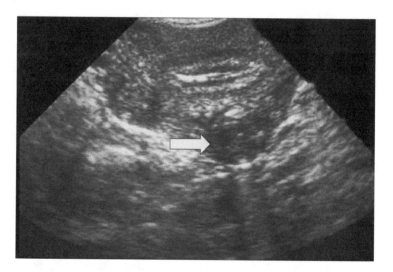

FIGURE 5. Transvaginal ultrasound image demonstrating a subserosal fibroid (*arrow*).

15. Can adenomyosis be diagnosed at ultrasound scan?

The diagnosis of adenomyosis is histologic. However, certain features during ultrasound assessment of the uterus may be suggestive of adenomyosis, such as a diffuse heterogenous pattern and myometrial cysts. Although sensitivity and positive predictive values are high in symptomatic women, the efficacy of ultrasound to screen asymptomatic women for adenomyosis is poor.

16. What are the tell-tale features of hydrosalpinx?

A normal fallopian tube is rarely visible by ultrasound, even with high-resolution transvaginal ultrasound. However, the development of a hydrosalpinx and the subsequent tubal distention allow visualization at ultrasound. The ultrasound features of hydrosalpinx are the presence of an elongated, thin-walled, fluid-filled structure, with incomplete septae , which result from the folding of the tube once it has become distended with fluid. (Fig. 6). Additional evidence is the presence of hyperechoic tubal-wall nodules, often known as the "'beads-on-a string" sign.

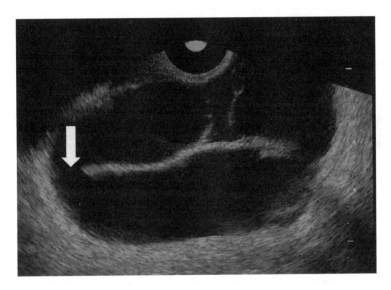

FIGURE 6. Transvaginal ultrasound image of a hydrosalpinx, demonstrating the typical elongated shaped and the incomplete septae (*arrow*).

17. What is the difference between a follicle, a functional cyst, and a complicated cyst?

Both **follicles** and **functional cysts** are unilocular cystic structures within the ovary. In many cases a functional cyst may be large (e.g., mean diameter over 4 cm). The easiest way to differentiate between a growing follicle and a functional cyst, however, is to perform serial ultrasound examinations. A follicle demonstrates follicular growth (about 2 mm per day). This distinction highlights the importance of an initial baseline ultrasound.

A **complicated cyst** is, therefore, any other cystic structure. It may be multiloculated, with septae and have internal echoes or solid material within it. Any complicated cystic structure needs further evaluation. Often a persistent corpus luteal cyst gives a complicated appearance, and a repeat ultrasound examination at the following menses is an appropriate first step. When a complicated cyst is large and has multiple abnormalities, MRI and surgical evaluation are appropriate.

18. What does an endometrioma look like?

The typical appearance of an endometriosis "chocolate" cyst or endometrioma is a thick-walled, round-shaped cystic structure with regular margins, containing homogenous low-level echoes. The appearance of the cystic fluid is often described as having "ground-glass" consistency (Fig. 7). Bilateral or multiple endometriomas may be present. Although ultrasound is a useful and effective tool in the diagnosis of ovarian endometriomas (positive likelihood ratios reach 25), the noninvasive diagnosis of endometriosis without endometriomas remains difficult.

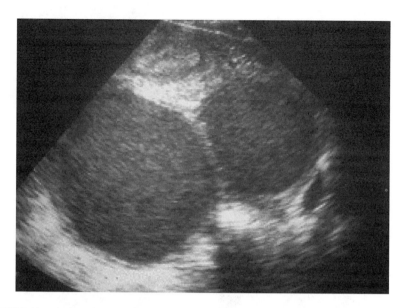

FIGURE 7. Transvaginal ultrasound image of bilateral ovarian endometriomas.

19. Can ovarian cancer be diagnosed at ultrasound?

The diagnosis of ovarian cancer is histologic. In most cases, because of the importance of staging the disease and the risks of metastases associated with percutaneous or transvaginal biopsy, the diagnosis of ovarian cancer is surgical. However, certain ultrasound features of any ovarian neoplasm are associated with an increased risk of malignancy, including the presence of papillary protrusions, solid parts, thick septae, highly echogenic refection patterns, low vascular resistance (measured by color Doppler; see below) associated with vascular neogenesis, and peritoneal fluid (Fig. 8).

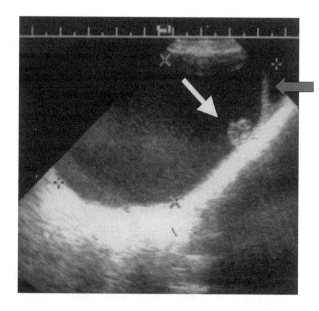

FIGURE 8. Abdominal ultrasound image of early papillary ovarian cancer, showing the papillary protrusion (*white arrow*) and the thickened septa (*dark arrow*).

20. Does abdominal ultrasound have a role in reproductive medicine?
Since the advent of transvaginal ultrasound in the 1980s and its subsequent widespread use, transvaginal assessment of the female pelvis has become the ultrasound approach of choice in reproductive medicine. However, in the cases of large pelvic masses or when previous surgery or disease has distorted the pelvic anatomy, full ultrasound evaluation is impossible without recourse to the transabdominal approach. The increasing use of ultrasound-guided embryo transfer also requires the transabdominal approach. Therefore, any person performing ultrasound in the field of reproductive medicine must be appropriately trained in both transvaginal and transabdominal ultrasound.

SALINE HYSTEROSONOGRAPHY

21. What is saline hysterosonography and for whom should it be considered?
Saline hysterosonography is the infusion of saline, as a negative contrast agent, into the uterine cavity through the cervix with continuous gray-scale, real-time ultrasound. It was first described in the early 1990s and is superior to conventional ultrasound in the evaluation of submucous and myometrial fibroids as well as the demonstration of any structural abnormality of the endometrium (Fig. 9).

Any woman in whom the endometrial cavity appears to be distorted at the initial baseline ultrasound examination should be considered for saline hysterosonography. This test further evaluates any endometrial abnormality. Similarly, any woman with evidence of uterine cavity abnormality at hysterosalpingography (HSG) should be considered for saline hysterosonography before considering operative hysteroscopy.

The role of saline hysterosonography as a routine test for all women undergoing infertility evaluation or for women with recurrent miscarriage or recurrent implantation failure after embryo transfer is unclear.

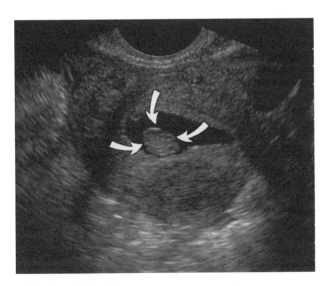

FIGURE 9. Saline hysterosonography demonstrating an endometrial polyp (*white arrows*) within the uterine cavity and an intramural myometrial fibroid (*dark arrow*), which is not distorting the cavity.

22. Are any risks associated with saline hysterosonography?
Saline hysterosonography is well tolerated and acceptable to many women. Pain scores are consistently lower than those for HSG and outpatient hysteroscopy. No significant complications with saline hysterosonography have been reported, although, as with all intrauterine interventions,

there remains the possibility of cervical trauma and introduction of infection. Any high vaginal or intracervical infection should be excluded prior to saline hysterosonography.

23. How does saline hysterosonography compare with HSG and hysteroscopy for evaluation of the uterine cavity?

Many studies have compared saline hysterosonography, HSG, and outpatient hysteroscopy. No significant difference among the different investigative modalities has been shown, either singly or when used in combination, although hysteroscopy may be better at discriminating between small pedunculated submucous fibroids and large endometrial polyps. Saline hysterosonography has the advantage of decreased procedure time and less pain compared with the other modalities.

24. Can tubal patency be tested at ultrasound?

The development of an echo-enhancement contrast material led to the possibility of hysterosalpingo contrast sonography (HyCoSy) and the subsequent assessment of tubal patency. However, the technique in most hands is associated with a high number of false-negative results (namely, apparently blocked normal tubes). It appears, therefore, that its main role is as a possible screening test before considering HSG or laparoscopy and chromotubation for assessment of tubal patency.

The use of color flow Doppler examination and three-dimensional ultrasound (see below) may lead to an increased ability to detect and assess tubal disease.

25. How can I reduce patient discomfort following instrumentation of the uterus?

Before any uterine instrumentation is undertaken, particularly saline hysterosonography, HyCoSy, or HSG, vaginal or cervical infection should be excluded. At least 1 hour before any such procedure, an effective nonsteroidal anti-inflammatory analgesic (e.g., mefenamic acid, ibuprofen, or naproxen) should be given to decrease discomfort during the procedure and the need for analgesics afterward.

DOPPLER ULTRASOUND

26. What is Doppler or color-flow Doppler ultrasound?

As ultrasound passes through a body, it is either absorbed or reflected. If the reflecting interface is stationary, the frequency of the reflected wave remains unchanged. However, if the interface is moving, the reflected frequency will be shifted to a higher or lower frequency; this phenomenon is called the Doppler shift.

Pulsed Doppler is the addition of a pulsed ultrasound source and receiver with a range gate that allows a sample region to be selected for Doppler analysis. Color-flow Doppler is essentially a multigate pulse Doppler system with simultaneous real-time, gray-scale imaging.

Doppler ultrasound, therefore, is used to measure flow. Clinically, it is most often used in the evaluation of blood flow. Besides a subjective interpretation of vascularity, certain objective measurements or assessments of the Doppler waveform can be made (Fig. 10): maximum velocity (V_{max}), pulsatility index (PI), and resistive index (RI). Most ultrasound machines now calculate these parameters automatically.

27. Is Doppler ultrasound safe?

As discussed in question 3, ultrasound energy has the potential to cause thermal bio-effects, although the FDA values have a significant safety margin. The increased ultrasound pulse repetition rate in Doppler ultrasound leads to significantly higher spatial peak-temporal average intensities (I_{SPTA}) that can approach FDA limits (see table below). Care must be taken not to exceed these values during ultrasound Doppler examination; in most ultrasound machines a maximum power can be set. *Note:* Figure 10 shows the maximum power at 50 mW/cm^2.

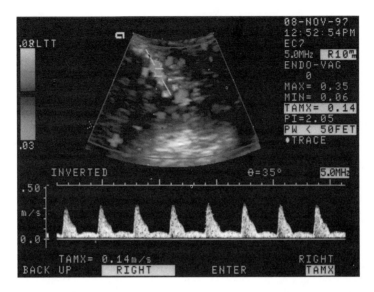

FIGURE 10. Ultrasound image showing the Doppler waveform of the right uterine artery.

Maximum and Minimum Acoustic Output of Pulsed Doppler in Transabdominal and Transvaginal Ultrasound Examination

ACOUSTIC OUTPUT	TRANSABDOMINAL	TRANSVAGINAL	FDA FETAL VALUE
I_{SPTA} (mW/cm^2)			
Minimum	150	50	180
Maximum	850	150	
I_{SPPA} (mW/cm^2)			
Minimum	50	10	350
Maximum	150	40	
I_M (mW/cm^2)			
Minimum	50	10	550
Maximum	200	50	

28. Are there ultrasound markers for implantation failure?

Doppler ultrasound may allow indirect assessment of implantation failure. Waveform analysis of the uterine artery throughout the menstrual cycle has shown that the pulsatility index (PI) falls to a nadir 9 days after the preovulatory LH peak. This finding is consistent with maximum uterine perfusion at the time of peak luteal function. It has also been shown that uterine artery PI, measured on the day of embryo transfer, is significantly lower in women who become pregnant. Recent evidence shows that a uterine artery PI of greater than 3.0, when measured immediately before hCG administration following ovarian stimulation, is associated with a significantly reduced chance of pregnancy. These findings suggest that the measurement of uterine artery PI, during the ultrasound monitoring of ovulation induction or assisted reproduction, may allow the option of delaying hCG administration for 1 or 2 days until the PI falls and therefore increases the chance of pregnancy.

The role of Doppler analysis of subendometrial blood flow has been elucidated recently and suggests that the absence of pulsatile subendometrial blood flow is associated with a very low pregnancy rate.

29. Is ovarian vascular assessment necessary?

Although it is possible to assess the uterine arteries and endometrial flow at the initial baseline ultrasound scan, the value of this technique is limited. However, Doppler assessment of the ovarian stromal blood vessels is of value. A raised peak blood flow velocity (V_{max}), generally > 10 cm/sec, or a raised time-averaged maximum velocity (TAMX), generally > 8 cm/sec, in these small vessels is consistent with a diagnosis of PCOS and also associated with an excellent response to gonadotropins. Therefore, these values should be taken into account in tailoring any ovarian stimulation regimen. Finally, some investigators suggest that peak blood flow velocity (V_{max}) may also have a role in the assessment of ovarian reserve.

30. Discuss the other roles of Doppler ultrasound.

Doppler ultrasound can help in the elucidation of complicated ovarian and uterine structures during the initial baseline ultrasound scan. Another advantage of Doppler assessment of blood flow at the baseline ultrasound scan may be to help diagnose intramural and submucous fibroids (often in conjunction with the saline hysterosonography; see above). Typically, blood flow is increased around the leiomyoma compared with the surrounding myometrium and endometrium.

In the context of IVF after ovarian stimulation, the presence of perifollicular blood flow increases the likelihood of obtaining an oocyte at retrieval and developing an embryo for transfer. Spontaneous ovulation is also associated with characteristic changes in the perifollicular blood flow. These findings suggest that there may be a potential value in the measurement of perifollicular flow as a guide to subsequent management.

Key Points of Doppler Ultrasound in Reproductive Medicine

1. Initial analysis
   - Raised V_{max} and TAMX in PCOS
   - Can help assessment of complicated uterine and ovarian structures
2. Doppler monitoring
   - Uterine artery PI > 3.0 on the day of hCG administration is associated with reduced chance of pregnancy
   - Absent subendometrial blood flow is associated with a very poor chance of pregnancy and further assessment is indicated
   - Possible role for perifollicular blood flow assessment

THREE-DIMENSIONAL ULTRASOUND

31. What is three-dimensional (3D) ultrasound? What are its indications?

Standard two-dimensional (2D) ultrasound allows images of the longitudinal and transverse sections of the field of interest. However, standard 2D ultrasound does not allow visualization of the transverse plane of the pelvis (i.e., the plane parallel to the transducer face or perpendicular to the ultrasound beam). If the third plane (often described as the C-plane) could be seen, complete ultrasound examination would be possible. Stored volume data can lead to computer-generated planar reformatted sections of the three orthogonal planes. These views allow excellent spatial evaluation of the organ or structure of interest, visualization of the C-plane, volume calculation, and 3D reconstruction and retrospective evaluation of the volume.

Initial reports using 3D ultrasound have shown reduced intra- and interobserver error in measuring endometrial and ovarian volumes (Fig. 11). More accurate spatial visualization is of particular interest in the assessment of uterine abnormalities and also follicular volume. Three-dimensional ultrasound has been shown to accurately differentiate bicornuate and subseptate uteri without the need for a hysterosalpingogram (Fig. 12), and has a role in the evaluation of submucus fibroids and endometrial polyps—particularly in association with saline hysterosonography.

Three-dimensional ultrasound has also been shown to be more accurate in the measurement of follicular volume than conventional 2D ultrasound.

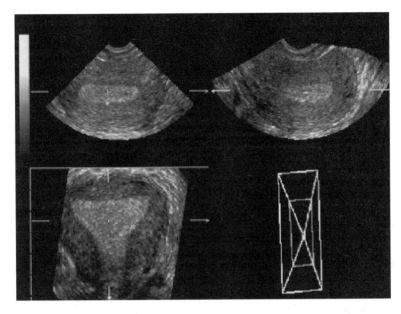

FIGURE 11. Three-dimensional ultrasound photograph of the endometrium, showing the three planes and allowing more accurate volume measurement.

32. What is four-dimensional ultrasound?

Four-dimensional (4D) ultrasound uses advanced signal processing to allow real-time 3D imaging without waiting for the ultrasound machine computer software to produce the third plane image as is the case with conventional 3D ultrasound. Although there appear to be many advantages for obstetric ultrasound, during which movement of the fetus may make conventional 3D imaging difficult, in reproductive medicine at present 4D ultrasound appears to offer little advantage over conventional 3D ultrasound.

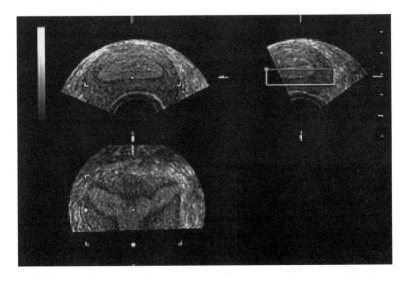

FIGURE 12. Three-dimensional ultrasound photograph of a septate uterus, showing the three planes.

SCROTAL AND TESTICULAR ULTRASOUND

33. Which men should have scrotal or testicular ultrasound?

Evaluation of all couples presenting with infertility should include a history and examination of the male partner. Any testicular mass, cyst, or irregularity should be further investigated by ultrasound. The presence of subclinical varicoceles can also be confirmed by ultrasound, usually with Doppler confirmation of blood flow.

34. What features should be routinely assessed at scrotal or testicular ultrasound?

Testicular volume and parenchymal consistency should be evaluated in all patients undergoing scrotal or testicular ultrasound. The integrity of the epididymis also should be evaluated (e.g., partial or complete agenesis or the presence of epididymal obstruction). The presence of subclinical varicocele should be excluded.

35. How significant is an ultrasound-diagnosed varicocoele?

There is much debate about the role of subclinical varicocle in the etiology of infertility. However, at present there is insufficient evidence that treatment of varicocele in men from couples with otherwise unexplained subfertility will improve the couple's chances of spontaneous pregnancy.

36. Should the prostate be imaged by ultrasound in infertile men?

There is no role for the routine use of transrectal ultrasonography of the prostate in the evaluation of the infertile couple. However, it has been used to detect and evaluate the treatment of ejaculatory duct obstruction and seminal vesicle hypoplasia. Its role in the diagnosis of inflammation of the prostate and seminal vesicles remains controversial.

ULTRASOUND-GUIDED PROCEDURES

37. For oocyte retrieval in women undergoing IVF and embryo transfer (ET), is ultrasound guidance always used?

When IVF-ET was initially developed, oocyte retrieval was performed under laparoscopic control. However, with advent of routine transvaginal ultrasound oocyte retrieval by ultrasound guidance has become the norm. The advantages of the route include higher retrieval rates and avoidance of the anesthetic and surgical morbidity associated with laparoscopy. In exceptional circumstances, laparoscopic oocyte retreival may be indicated.

38. Can ovarian cysts be drained under ultrasound control?

Ultrasound-guided ovarian aspiration for simple cysts has not shown any advantage over expectant management, because many cysts reaccumulate fluid and cytologic assessment of the aspirated fluid cannot reliably confirm a benign diagnosis in women at risk of ovarian cancers. However, in the context of assisted reproductive treatments, when the formation of a functional cyst may impair ovarian response to stimulation, cyst aspiration is as effective as expectant management and expedites treatment.

39. Is it safe to aspirate endometriomas under ultrasound control?

Aspiration of the "chocolate" endometriotic fluid from ovarian endometriomas, whether performed at laparoscopy or under transvaginal ultrasound control, is an ineffective treatment associated with a high recurrence rate. Furthermore, the transvaginal ultrasound guidance approach is associated with significantly higher risks of ovarian and pelvic infection and abscess formation.

Occasionally, during ultrasound-guided oocyte retrieval for IVF-ET, an endometrioma is encountered. Puncture should be avoided if at all possible. If avoidance is impossible, appropriate antibiotic prophylaxis will reduce the incidence of infection.

40. What is the most appropriate way to manage ascites secondary to OHSS?
Paracentesis, or drainage, of the ascitic fluid that has collected as a result of ovarian hyper-stimulation syndrome (OHSS) is the single strategy that predictably produces clinical and bio-chemical improvement and hastens resolution. Traditional management involved hospitalization and percutaneous paracentesis (under ultrasound control). However, early outpatient transvaginal paracentesis (under ultrasound control), judicious colloid replacement, and careful fluid and biochemical monitoring have led to successful outpatient management in many cases.

HYSTEROSALPINGOGRAPHY

41. Should all woman undergoing infertility evaluation have HSG?
HSG remains the most commonly used test to evaluate the endometrial cavity, tubal patency, and tubal disease. It is the first-line investigation of tubal status for over 96% of reproductive endocrinologists. Nevertheless, the sensitivity and specificity in demonstrating tubal patency, compared with laparoscopy, are 65% and 85%, respectively. HSG is unreliable in the diagnosis of peritubular adhesions. Therefore, in women with a history suggestive of tubal disease or women with risk factors for tubal disease, laparoscopy and chromotubation are the appropriate first choice in the absence of operative contraindications.

42. Are any risks associated with HSG?
Like any procedure that involves instrumentation of the cervix or uterine cavity, HSG is associated with certain risks, however small. Occasionally, damage (trauma) to the cervix during insertion of the dye may cause significant pain and bleeding. In rare patients, severe anaphylaxis to the x-ray contrast dye may occur. The principal risk, however, which affects about 1/1000 low-risk patients, is ascending infection within the cavity or fallopian tubes. To reduce this risk, careful patient selection and preprocedure screening or prophylactic antibiotics should be used.

No reported risks of x-ray irradiation of the pelvis have been associated with the low levels used for hysterosalpingogram. Obviously, however, there are real risks of miscarriage or fetal abnormality if the procedure is performed during pregnancy. Therefore HSG should be performed only in the follicular phase of the menstrual cycle.

43. What is the gold standard for the assessment of tubal patency and disease?
As mentioned above, laparoscopy and chromotubation are the gold standards for the assessment of tubal patency and disease, although they are associated with increased patient morbidity.

44. Explain selective salpingography and tubal canalization.
Selective salpingography is the opacification of the fallopian tube under x-ray control at HSG via a catheter placed in the uterine cornua or the first 1 cm of the tube. **Tubal recanalization** is the interventional radiologic procedure whereby a catheter is pushed through the tubal ostium and dilated to recanalize a tube that has been blocked at the cornua. In all cases, selective salpingography is performed prior to tubal recanalization.

45. What is SIN?
Salpingitis isthmica nodosa (SIN) is a pathologic and radiologic finding characterized by a diverticulum or diverticula of the fallopian tubal epithelium in the isthmic region of otherwise patent tubes. The finding is often bilateral and usually accompanied by nodular hyperplasia of the surrounding muscularis. Typically 2-mm accumulations of contrast medium are observed within the diverticula, with associated irregularities in the tubal lumen (Fig. 13).

46. How important is SIN?
Traditional teaching suggested that tubes affected by SIN are not amenable to recanalization or tubal microsurgery because of an increased risk of tubal perforation or technical failure. How-

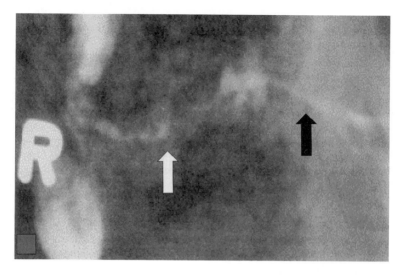

FIGURE 13. HSG showing severe nodular SIN in the isthmic portion of the right tube and normal distal tubal appearance.

ever, several recent studies have demonstrated successful outcomes following excision and tubal reimplantation as well as tubal recanalization. Nevertheless, there remain concerns that the association of SIN and ectopic pregnancy will result in increased tubal pregnancy rates.

IV. Management of Female Reproductive Disorders

33. OVULATION INDUCTION DRUGS

Isaac Kligman, M.D., and Zev Rosenwaks, M.D.

1. What are the physiologic principles underlying spontaneous follicular development and ovulation?

Ovarian follicular development and ovulation involve a complex interaction between anterior pituitary production of follicle-stimulating hormone (FSH) and luteinizing hormone (LH); hormonal feedback from the ovary in the form of estrogen, inhibin, and activin; and other ovarian paracrine and autocrine factors. Human folliculogenesis normally yields a single mature egg each cycle through the selection of a single dominant follicle and regression of smaller follicles within its cohort.

2. What are ovulatory disorders?

Most ovulatory disorders fit into one of three categories:

1. Hypogonadotropic hypogonadism (WHO class I). Gonadotropin secretion is lower in women with this disorder than in women who ovulate regularly.

2. Euestrogenic ovulatory dysfunction (WHO class II). Affected women have serum gonadotropin concentrations in the normal range or occasionally present with elevated serum LH levels.

3. Hypergonadotropic hypogonadism (WHO class III). Affected women have severely compromised or absent ovarian function.

3. Is there a difference between induction of ovulation (OI) and controlled ovarian hyperstimulation (COH)?

Traditionally, OI is indicated for patients with ovulatory disturbances with the purpose of establishing monofollicular ovulation and thus conception. In contrast, COH targets patients with regular menstrual cycles and infertility not necessarily due to ovulatory disorders. The objective is to achieve the development of competent oocytes to be used for assisted reproductive technologies (e.g., IVF), or intrauterine insemination (IUI).

4. What drugs are available for OI and COH?

Agents used alone or in combination for OI or COH include clomiphene citrate (CC), human menopausal gonadotropins (hMG), and, more recently, purified urinary and recombinant FSH, recombinant LH, and pulsatile gonadotropin-releasing hormone (GnRH). Adjuvants to these therapies include dexamethasone and insulin-sensitizing agents such as metformin. Other adjuvant drugs include GnRH analogs and antagonists that help prevent premature LH surges, especially in the context of COH for IVF.

5. What is CC?

Clomiphene citrate is an oral nonsteroidal estrogen antagonist that disrupts estrogen's inhibitory effects within the hypothalamus and pituitary by binding estrogen receptors and blocking normal negative feedback. The result is an increase in pulse frequency of GnRH, which increases FSH and LH release from the anterior pituitary, resulting in stimulation of follicular recruitment and growth. Since CC typically results in the production of one or two follicles each cycle, it has been traditionally used as an ovulation induction agent but can be used in combination with gonadotropins for superovulation.

6. How is CC administered?

CC is dispensed in 50-mg tablets. Treatment is administered orally, generally with a starting dose of 50 mg/day, beginning on cycle days 2 to 5 after a spontaneous or progesterone-induced withdrawal bleed. Therapy is typically continued for 5 days. Spontaneous ovulation usually occurs 5–10 days after the last day of medication. If ovulation has been achieved, the patient should remain on this dose for up to 3 or 4 cycles. If the initial dose is ineffective in achieving an ovulatory response, it should be increased in 50-mg increments each cycle until ovulation is documented. The maximum dose of CC is 250 mg daily. Twenty to 25% of oligo-ovulatory or anovulatory women will not ovulate with this dose of medication. Most pregnancies occur at doses of 50 mg (50%) or 100 mg (20%) for 5 days. Some evidence suggests that prolonged (7–8 days) administration may benefit some patients. Ultrasound monitoring of follicular development may be used for timing of intercourse or IUI and reduction in multiple pregnancies in the case of multiple follicular development. In this modality, an ovulatory dose of 10,000 IU of human chorionic gonadotropin (hCG) is given when the diameter of the lead follicle exceeds 18 mm.

7. What are the success rates with CC?

Overall, ovulation rates range from 60% to 90%, and conception rates range from 25% to 50%. Pregnancy rates per treatment cycle range from 12% to 25% in women who ovulate with this regimen.

8. What are the side effects of CC?

The secondary effects are mostly related to the antiestrogenic effects of the drug. Examples include hot flashes (10%); mood swings, depression, and headaches (1%); pelvic pain (5.5%); nausea (2%); and breast tenderness (5%). Visual symptoms such as blurring, halos, streaks of light at night, or scotomas (1.5%) are the most serious secondary effects and are an indication for discontinuation of the treatment. Although the mechanisms responsible for this phenomenon are not fully understood, this side effect is considered self-limited. The symptoms generally disappear within days to weeks after discontinuation of the treatment. The antiestrogenic effects of the drug also affect the quality of the cervical mucus. As many as 15% of women may present with abnormal cervical mucus. Some practitioners have recommended adjuvant estrogen therapy to increase the cervical mucus, but a significant increase in pregnancy rates has not been reported with this approach.

9. What are the potential adjuvants to CC therapy?

Adjuvants to CC therapy include insulin sensitizers (metformin) and dexamethasone.

10. What is metformin?

Metformin hydrochloride (Glucophage) is an oral insulin sensitizer used in the management of patients with type 2 diabetes mellitus, either alone or in combination with sulfonylureas or other agents.

11. What is the relationship between insulin resistance and anovulation?

Polycystic ovarian syndrome (PCOS) is the most common endocrine disorder in euestrogenic anovulation. Most women with PCOS have a variety of signs and symptoms, including hirsutism and obesity. Insulin resistance with compensatory hyperinsulinemia is an important feature and may be in part responsible for the hyperandrogenic state and chronic anovulation. The degree of hyperinsulinemia and glucose intolerance varies greatly.

12. How is insulin resistance diagnosed?

Several tests have been implemented to detect insulin sensitivity. The glucose clamp technique has been accepted as the gold standard for estimating insulin sensitivity. This laboratory test involves

IV administration of glucose, insulin, and other substances in a research setting that makes the test cumbersome and costly. More recently, the fasting glucose/insulin ratio has been used as a marker of insulin resistance in women with PCOS. A ratio of 4.5 or less is lower than the ratio found in 90% of weight-matched control women (without PCOS). This cut-off value of $\leq$ 4.5 can be used as a screening test for detecting insulin resistance. It is a clinically useful parameter for selecting which patients with PCO will have a better response to the administration of insulin-sensitizing agents.

13. How is metformin administered?

It is advisable to start with a low dose (500 mg) with dinner and gradually increase the dose over a period of 3–4 weeks to a maximum dose of 2500 mg. The medication is available in 500-mg, 850-mg, or 1,000-mg tablets; the starting dose is 500 mg twice daily. Dosage is adjusted over the period of 2–3 weeks to the usual dose of 500 mg 3 times daily or 850 mg twice daily with meals. Once the maintenance dose has been achieved, the patient's ovulatory status is reassessed over a 6- to 8-week period. If metformin alone has led to ovulatory cycles, no further intervention is necessary. Otherwise, the drug is administered together with the CC regimen. Several studies have shown that this regimen increases the rate of ovulation in CC-resistant women. Although metformin treatment appears safe during pregnancy, most clinicians discontinue the medication once pregnancy is documented.

14. What is the role of glucocorticoids as adjuvants of CC therapy?

Fifty percent of women with PCOS have a significant adrenal component to their hyperandrogenism, as reflected by elevated serum concentrations of dehydroepiandrosterone sulfate (DHEAS). Such women may benefit from treatment with a glucocorticoid such as dexamethasone as an adjunct to CC therapy.

15. How is dexamethasone administered?

The medication is started with the onset of menses at a dose of 0.25 mg at night. It is continued until ovulation is documented, largely to prevent the possibility of iatrogenic Cushing's syndrome and longstanding adrenal suppression. This regimen has been shown to be effective as an adjuvant to CC therapy mainly in women with DHEAS levels > 200 µg/dl (range: 52–400 µg/dl). Other treatment doses as high as 5 mg at night have been reported with good therapeutic results.

16. What are gonadotropins?

Gonadotropins are preparations that contain FSH and/or LH; they are used to treat ovulatory disorders related to hypogonadotropic or eugonadotropic anovulation, as well as for patients with PCO who are refractory to CC therapy. They are also used to induce multiple follicular development for IVF protocols. They may also be used empirically in combination with intrauterine insemination for women with unexplained infertility.

17. What gonadotropin preparations are available?

Human menopausal gonadotropin (hMG) (Pergonal, Repronex) is extracted from the urine of menopausal women. It contains 75 IU of FSH and 75 IU of LH per ampule. Because the half-life of LH is shorter than the half-life of FSH, the patient receives a greater ratio of FSH to LH.

Highly purified FSH (Fertinex and Bravelle) is presented as 75 IU of FSH and less than 0.1 IU of LH. It is extracted from hMG by immunochromatography, using a monoclonal antibody to FSH. Because of its purity it can be administered subcutaneously.

Recombinant FSH (Gonal-F, Follistim) has become available more recently. It is produced from a genetically engineered Chinese hamster ovarian cell line. It can be administered subcutaneously. Recombinant LH is available in some countries and is produced with the same technology.

18. Discuss the protocols used for COH with gonadotropins.

Protocols used for COH vary greatly depending on the specific application. Protocols applied to COH for IUI aim at developing 1–3 mature follicles in order to maximize the chance for success without exposing the patient to an excessive risk of multiple pregnancy and/or ovarian hyperstimulation syndrome. Protocols of COH for IVF, although following the same safety principles, are tailored to produce a large number of mature eggs for retrieval.

19. What are the most common protocols used for COH with IUI?

With the most commonly used protocol, gonadotropins are typically started at a dose of 150 IU on menstrual cycle day 3; the dose is adjusted according to the ovarian response. The administration of these preparations requires careful monitoring with daily estradiol determinations and ultrasound evaluations for follicle number and growth.

20. What is the principle behind the "low-dose protocol" of ovulation induction for patients with PCOS?

The low-dose protocol, used primarily for patients with PCOS, is based on the concept of the FSH threshold, a critical point at which the ovaries respond with monofollicular development and beyond which multiple follicles develop and the risk of OHSS rises.

21. How is the low-dose protocol administered?

This regimen starts with a very low dose of gonadotropin on cycle day 3 (75 IU or less). The patient is carefully monitored, and the doses of gonadotropins are carefully adjusted throughout the cycle. Typically, the patient remains at each succeeding dose increment for 1 week, until follicular development is observed, at which point that dose is maintained until the dominant follicle reaches the customary size requiring ovulatory triggering with hCG or LH. This regimen has been shown to achieve an ovulation rate of 75%, of which 70–75% is monofollicular. Multiple pregnancy rates are on the order of 6% with this regimen.

22. What are the success rates with COH?

In women with PCOS and hypogonadotropic or eugonadotropic hypogonadism, the rate of ovulation has been documented at greater than 90%. The cycle fecundity rate approaches that observed in the normal fertile population (21%). Couples with idiopathic infertility perform less successfully with this treatment, achieving an overall success rate of 15%.

23. Describe the most common protocol used for COH for IVF.

Such protocols are tailored specifically to each patient, according to her age, ovarian reserve, and response to previous stimulations. They typically include a GnRH analog, started in the midluteal phase of the previous cycle (see below). The most commonly used ("step-down") protocol involves the administration of the highest dose of gonadotopin (300–450 IU) at the beginning of the stimulated cycle, with progressive reduction of the dose according to the ovarian response. The principle behind this protocol is to mimic yet amplify what occurs during the normal menstrual cycle, trying to maximize the number of follicles recruited while limiting the risk of OHSS.

24. What is the role of GnRH in OI?

GnRH has been used successfully in the treatment of hypogonadotropic hypogonadism due to hypothalamic insufficiency. It cannot be used in women with pituitary failure. The aim of this treatment is monofollicular development; hence the risk of multiple pregnancies is greatly reduced.

25. How is GnRH administered?

Pulsatile GnRH can be administered subcutaneously (20 μg every 90 minutes) or intravenously (5 μg every 90 minutes). Intravenous administration is more effective and reliable but requires professional care of the IV line. There is a higher risk of infections such as endocarditis or septicemia. With the advent of other pharmacologic agents to induce ovulation, pulsatile GnRH administration is no longer a common form of treatment for this type of patients.

26. What are GnRH agonists?

GnRH agonists are decapeptides designed to interact with the pituitary GnRH receptors, whereby amino acid substitutions in positions 6 and 10 of the original GnRH decapeptide produce a compound that results in a noncompetitive downregulation of the pituitary hormones, leading to an iatrogenic hypogonadotropic state. They are used in COH for IVF to avoid spontaneous LH surges associated with early follicular luteinization or premature ovulation.

27. What are GnRH antagonists?

GnRH antagonists result from amino acid substitutions in different positions in the native GnRH decapeptide. These preparations produce immediate competitive inhibition of the gonadotropin release and are used as adjuvants for COH protocols for IVF. They are administered in the mid-follicular phase of the treatment cycle to effect immediate blockage of the LH surge.

28. What are the potential complications of OI and COH?

The most common potential complications are OHSS and multiple pregnancies. Spontaneous abortion rates appear to be higher with superovulation; however, common causes of infertility, such as polycystic ovary disease, are independent risk factors for early pregnancy loss. Superovulation increases the risk of tubal pregnancy several-fold, and also increases the risk of heterotopic pregnancy, with simultaneous implantation inside and outside the uterine cavity. Infertile patients, in general, are at increased risk for ectopic pregnancy because of the incidence of tubal disease, although increased embryo numbers and negative effects of gonadotropins on tubal motility have been implicated. A link between ovarian cancer and controlled ovarian stimulation is controversial; however, evidence to date seems to indicate that the increased risk of epithelial carcinomas can be attributed to independent risk factors common to this population of women— namely, lower parity and reduced exposure to oral contraception.

29. What is OHSS?

This syndrome is characterized by ovarian enlargement and increased capillary permeability with accumulation of fluid in third spaces and resulting peritoneal, pleural, and pericardial effusions. Young, thin patients are at risk of developing the syndrome as well as those who exhibit a high ovarian response to gonadotropin treatment, such as women with PCOS. The severity of the syndrome increases in cycles in which pregnancy occurs. The syndrome can range from mild discomfort to severe illness with multiple organ failure and death. The three degrees of OHSS—mild, moderate, and severe—depend on clinical parameters such as severity of discomfort, size of the ovaries, changes in weight, changes in hematocrit, white blood cell count, and renal function tests. The most severe cases can result in renal failure, electrolyte imbalance, and a hypercoagulable state, leading to arterial and/or venous thrombotic events, including pulmonary embolus.

30. How is OHSS prevented?

The syndrome is prevented by withholding hCG administration when a significant risk exists and advising the couple to avoid intercourse to prevent pregnancy in the case of spontaneous ovulation.

31. How is OHSS treated?

For mild and moderate OHSS, rest, fluid management, and avoidance of intercourse to prevent the rupture of the ovarian cysts are adequate methods of treatment. Moderate and severe cases require admission to the hospital for management of fluid imbalance and hypoalbuminemia, prophylaxis of the hypercoagulable state, and pain management. Paracentesis is frequently useful to alleviate severe ascitis.

32. What is the incidence of multiple pregnancies after OI or COH?

Multiple pregnancy occurs in approximately 20% cases; 80% of these are twin pregnancies.

BIBLIOGRAPHY

1. Adashi EY: Ovulation induction: Clomiphene citrate. In Adashi EY, Rock JA, Rosenwaks Z (eds): Reproductive Endocrinology, Surgery, and Technology, vol. 1. Philadelphia, Lippincott-Raven, 1996.
2. Amerian Society for Reproductive Medicine: Guideline for Practice: Induction of Ovulation with Human Menopausal Gonadotropins. Birmingham, AL, YEAR?
3. Balen A: Endocrine methods of ovulation induction. Bailliere's Clin Obstet Gynecol 12:521–539, 1998.
4. Erickson GF: Physiologic basis of ovulation induction. Semin Reprod Endocrinol 14:287–297, 1996.
5. Hillier SG: The Parkes Lecture. Controlled ovarian stimulation in women. J Reprod Fertil 120:201–210, 2000.
6. Phipps WR: Polycystic ovary syndrome and ovulation induction. Obstet Gynecol Clin North Am 28:165–182, 2001.
7. Shushan A, Laufer N: Fertility drugs and ovarian cancer: What are the practical implications of the ongoing debate? Fertil Steril 74:8–9, 2000.
8. Vollenhoven BJ, Healy DL: Short and long term effects of ovulation induction. Endocrinol Metab Clin North Am 27:903–914, 1998.
9. Wolf LJ: Ovulation induction. Clin Obstet Gynecol 43:902–915, 2000.

34. UTERINE FIBROIDS

Steven D. Spandorfer, M.D.

1. What are uterine fibroids?
Histologically, uterine fibroids are benign neoplasms arising from the smooth muscle cells of the uterus. Hence, uterine fibroids are also known as leiomyomata.

2. What are the most common symptoms related to fibroids?
Approximately two-thirds of patients with fibroids are asymptomatic. Symptoms associated with uterine fibroids generally are related to their location and may include a feeling of pressure from an enlarging fibroid that presents with abdominal discomfort and urinary symptoms. Patients also complain of dysmenorrhea and often have dysfunctional uterine bleeding.

3. What are the different types of leiomymata?
Uterine fibroids can be divided into three types (Fig. 1): (1) subserous fibroids (55%, located in the outer wall of the uterus; (2) intramural fibroids (40%), located within the muscular layers of the uterine wall; and (3) submucous fibroids (5%), which are located on the inner wall of the uterus and may protrude into the uterine cavity.

4. What types of genetic mutations are involved in leiomyomata?
Leiomyomata develop as genetically abnormal clones of a single cell. Hence, multiple leiomyomata develop from different clones.

5. How often is cancer associated with leiomyomata?
The development of leiomyosarcoma from leiomyomata is uncommon, occurring in less than 1% of all leiomyomata. It is more commonly suspected when a leiomyoma demonstrates rapid growth.

6. What epidemiologic factors are associated with leiomyomata?
Leiomyomata are more common in African Americans than in Caucasians, Asians, or other racial groups. Leiomyomata are also more commonly found in nonsmokers. Fortunately, the use of oral contraceptives is not linked to an increasd risk of leiomyomata.

7. At what age are leiomyomata most prevalent?
Leiomyomata are most prevalent during the fifth decade of a woman's life. Myomas are rare before puberty and usually shrink after menopause.

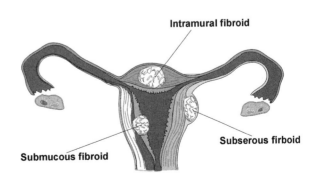

FIGURE 1. Three types of uterine fibroids.

8. Discuss the hormonal environment of leiomyomata.

Leiomyomata exist in a hyperestrogenic environment. Within a leiomyoma the concentration of estrogen and progesterone receptors is increased. Because of the hormonal environment (hyperestrogenemia), it is not surprising that one may find endometrial hyperplasia. Benign endometrial hyperplasia is often found at the periphery of a submucosal fibroid.

9. How do leiomyomata affect infertility?

Leiomyomata rarely are the sole cause of infertility.They are more commonly associated with difficult implantation of fertilized eggs and recurrent spontaneous miscarriage. Leiomyomata can also cause infertility by obstructing the patency of the fallopian tubes.

10. What types of fibroids are more commonly associated with recurrent miscarriages?

Leiomyomata located in a submucous location are more commonly associated with recurrent miscarriages. It is generally thought that the distortion of these fibroids can affect implantation and development of the early pregnancy.

11. What methods are used to determine whether a patient has a submucous fibroid?

- Atransvaginal sonogram is useful in detecting uterine fibroids. Particularly when the patient is in mid cycle, the ultrasound can help elucidate the relationship between the fibroid and the endometrial cavity.
- Hysterosalpingograms are considered an excellent method for detecting intrauterine abnormalities, particularly in infertility patients, because this test allows assessment of tubal patency as well.
- Saline-infusion sonogram is a technique in which saline is infused into the endometrial cavity, allowing the physician to detect intracavitary abnormalities.
- MRI allows detailed assessment of the uterus and its fibroids.
- Finally, hysteroscopy allows the physician to visualize the cavity to detect submucous fibroids and also allows resection of a submucosal fibroid.

12. What are the recurrence risks after myomectomy?

Leiomyomata are commonly treated by myomectomy. Recurrence risks are higher in the younger patient with removal of multiple leiomyomata . Risks of recurrence have been reported to range from 15% to 35%.

13. What are the criteria for consideration of performing a hysteroscopic resection of a leiomyoma?

Submucosal leiomyomata are generally thought to be more closely associated with infertility and recurrent miscarriage. Since they are more accessible from within the uterine cavity, submucosal leiomyomata are good candidates for less invasive surgical removal via hysteroscopy. Leiomyomata that are good candidates for hysteroscopic removal are smaller and protrude at least 50% into the endometrial cavity.

14. Does any preoperative treatment facilitate the hysteroscopic removal of leiomyomata?

Preoperative treatment with a gonadotropin-releasing hormone (GnRH) agonist can be helpful. Preoperative treatment for 3 months with a GnRH agonist is especially indicated for patients with anemia or a larger submucosal leiomyomata. This treatment provides a few months of amenorrhea to allow the patient to increase her hematocrit. Because leiomyomata are hormonally responsive, the induced hypoestrogenism of the GnRH agonist leads to shrinkage of leiomyomata.

15. What role do leiomyomata play in pregnancy?

Leiomyomata affect pregnancies in less than 1% of cases. Leiomyomata are not common causes of premature labor. Most Leiomyomata do not change in size during pregnancy.

16. What is leiomyoma degeneration? What types of degeneration can a leiomyoma undergo?

Leiomyoma degeneration is a condition of breakdown or decay of the fibroid, as when it outgrows its blood supply. Leiomyomata can undergo multiple types of degeneration: fatty, red, hemorrhagic, calcific, and cancerous degeneration. Red degeneration can be problematic, especially when it occurs during late gestation. Patients generally present with acute pain and occasionally with premature labor.

17. When is medical treatment of leiomyomata with GnRH agonists indicated?

Medical treatment of leiomyomata with GnRH agonists is common. The major indication for the use of preoperative medical treatment is to produce amenorrhea and allow the patient to increase her hematocrit. This technique produces a hypoestrogenic environment that reduces the size of the leiomyomata and decreases the bleeding preoperatively. When necessary, this approach can allow the patient to donate autologous blood before a myomectomy is performed.

18. What are the clinical advantages of GnRH agonist treatment before myomectomy?

Many advantages have been ascribed to medical treatment with GnRH agonists for leiomyomata, including reduced need for hysterectomy, less blood loss, reduced need for blood transfusions, and shorter operative time.

19. What are the common side effects of medical treatment with GnRH agonists for leiomyomata?

Because GnRH agonists produce a hypoestrogenic environment, there are many side effects that are similar to menopausal symptoms, including hot flushes, vaginal dryness, headaches, depression, and forgetfulness.

20. Can GnRH agonists be used indefinitely as an alternative to surgical treatment of leiomyomata?

Some have proposed the use of GnRH agonists for long periods as an alternative to surgery. The major problems with long-term, uninterrupted use of GnRH agonists are the development of osteoporosis and unfavorable lipid changes. Once treatment extends beyond 6 months, add-back treatment is mandatory to diminish the risks of long-term GnRH agonist usage. Add-back treatment consists of either pure progestin (norethindrone, 5mg) or a combination of low-dose estrogen (conjugated equine estrogen, 0.625 mg) with a progestin. Add-back treatment significantly decreases the side effects of the GnRH agonist suppression and thus enhances compliance.

21. Define leimyomatosis peritonealis disseminata.

Leimyomatosis peritonealis disseminata is defined by multiple and diffuse implants of fibroid. Usually the implants are contained within the abdominal cavity, but they have been found in the lungs as well. They are hormonally responsive and can best be treated with GnRH agonist therapy.

22. What are the common indications for a myomectomy?

Common indications for myomectomy include symptomatic fibroids. Symptoms may be physical as a result of the size and location of the fibroids. For example, a patient may have constant urinary symptoms from a large fibroid compressing her bladder. Symptoms mayalso include chronic blood loss as well as ureteral obstruction.

23. What role does uterine artery embolization (UAE) have in the management of uterine fibroids?

UAE is a newly developed procedure for the treatment of fibroids. It involves partially blocking the vessels that support the uterus and its fibroids, resulting in a decrease in size of the fibroids. Further investigations are needed to establish the safety of this procedure in the reproductive health of young women, but it appears best to avoid UAE in women who may later wish to conceive. Most patients have noted a significant reduction in the size of fibroids after this procedure. Complications, including infection, severe pain, bleeding, and uterine necrosis requiring emergent surgery, have been reported.

24. Can any intraoperative adjuncts reduce blood loss at the time of myomectomy?

Several small studies have attempted to address this issue. The injection of vasopressin into the serosal surface of the uterine incision site has been shown to reduce blood loss compared with saline sham injection. Other studies have focused on physical attempts to control bleeding by use of a tourniquet, either a Penrose drain with vascular clamps or Foley catheters.

25. How should a physician advise a postmyomectomy patient about delivery of a subsequent pregnancy?

It is generally believed that if the endometrial cavity is entered during the performance of a myomectomy, a cesarean delivery is recommended because of the concern of uterine rupture during vaginal labor. However, the risk of uterine rupture is actually below 1.0%.

BIBLIOGRAPHY

1. Barbieri RL, Andersen J: Uterine leiomyomas: The somatic mutation theory. Semin Reprod Endocrin 10:301, 1992.
2. Buttram VC, Reiter RC: Uterine leiomyomata: Etiology, symptamatology and management. Fertil Steril 36:433, 1981.
3. Cramer DW: Epidemiology of myomas. Semin Reprod Endocrin 10:320, 1992.
4. Deligdish L, Loewenthal M: Endometrial changes associated with myomata of the uterus. J Clin Pathol 23:676, 1970.
5. Frederick J, Fletcher H, Simeon D, Mullings A, Hardie M: Intramyometrial vasopressin as a hemostatic agent during myomectomy. Br J Obstet Gynecol 101:435–437, 1994.
6. Marshall LM, Spiegelman D, Barbieiri RL, et al: Variation in the incidence of uterine leiomyomata among premenopausal women by race and age. Obstet Gynecol 90:967, 1997.
7. Marshall LM, Spiegelman D, Goldman MB, et al: A prospective study of reproductive factors and oral contraceptives use in relation to the risk of uterine leiomyoma. Fertil Steril 70:432, 1998.
8. Parker WH, Fu YS, Berek JS: Uterine sarcoma in a patient operated on for a presumed leiomyoma. Obstet Gynecol 83:414, 1994.
9. Rein M, Freidman AJ, Stuart JM, MacLaughlin JT: Fibroid and myometrial steroid receptors in women treated with GnRH agonist. Fertil Steril 53:1018, 1990.
10. Verkauf BS: Myomectomy for fertility enhancement and management. Fertil Steril 58:1, 1992.

35. LAPAROSCOPY

Kate Dragesic, M.D., and Steven Spandorfer, M.D.

1. What common procedures can be safely performed laparoscopically?
Permanent sterilization, diagnosis and management of ectopic pregnancies, adnexal surgery (salpingo-oophorectomy, ovarian cystectomy, paratubal cystectomy), lysis of adhesions, treatment for endometriosis, and diagnostic laparoscopies are common indications. More advanced surgeries include laparoscopic hysterectomies, myomectomies, lymph node sampling, and urogynecologic procedures.

2. Discuss contraindications to laparoscopy.
A patient who cannot tolerate an intraabdominal pressure of 20 mmHg is not a candidate for laparoscopy. A patient with a large hiatal hernia may not tolerate intra-abdominal insufflation. Suspicion of significant pelvic or abdominal adhesions may lead the surgeon to consider open laparoscopy or an alternative approach to insufflation (see question 5) or to proceed with laparotomy. An unstable patient (e.g., a patient with a bleeding ectopic pregnancy in hemorrhagic shock) may be a better candidate for laparotomy because of the impaired visualization due to bleeding and the physiologic effects of pneumoperitoneum (see question 3).

3. Discuss physiologic considerations during anesthesia for laparoscopy.
The basic problems for laparoscopic patients are associated with carbon dioxide gas insufflation and subsequent hypercarbia and abdominal discomfort. To prevent these problems, laparoscopic patients should be intubated and hyperventilated. Airway pressures may rise with a decrease in lung compliance due to an increase in abdominal pressure and Trendelenburg position. Regurgitation and pulmonary aspiration of stomach contents may occur due to increases in gastric pressure and Trendelenburg position. Because of pneumoperitoneum, venous return is reduced, leading to decreased cardiac output. Bradycardias can result from peritoneal stretching and arrythmias from hypercapnea induced by peritoneal absorption of carbon dioxide. Additionally the pulse pressure narrows due to cardiac compression by the pneumoperitoneum.

4. What are the complications of laparoscopy?
As with any surgery, there are risks of anesthesia as well as bleeding, infection, and injury to internal organs. Injury to both the gastrointestinal tract and the genitourinary system can result from either mechanical dissection or thermal injury. Gas emboli can result when carbon dioxide gas used for insufflation is introduced into the vasculature. Neurologic injury can result from damage to nerves intraoperatively or patient positioning. Phlebitis or venous thromboses can result from prolonged immobilization and pelvic surgery. Patients may have soft tissue emphysema from gas leaking around the trocar or from preperitoneal insufflation. Incisional hernias may occur (see below). Rarely, in gynecologic laparoscopy, procedures such as extensive ovarian cystectomies may lead to ovarian failure.
Preoperative patients should be counseled that the planned procedure may not be able to be safely performed laparoscopically and may need to be converted to a laparotomy.

5. What are the indications for laparoscopic management of an adnexal mass?
Recent trends toward the laparoscopic management of adnexal masses have introduced concern about inadvertently operating on a woman with undiagnosed ovarian cancer as well as the potential morbidity associated with spillage of tumor contents during the operation. It is critical that an adnexal mass be accurately evaluated before laparoscopic management. Clinical history, physical exam, ultrasonographic findings, and CA-125 levels are noninvasive methods of evaluation.

The sonographic criteria include tumor size, number of loculi (unilocular vs. mutilocular), and the presence of internal papillary excrescences, echodensity, solid components, ascites, or adherent bowel. Studies also have examined Doppler flow characteristics of ovarian masses, which may correlate with likelihood of malignancy.

ACA-125 level less than 35 U/ml is considered within the normal range. In premenopausal patients, this level can be elevated for other reasons, such as pelvic inflammatory disease, endometriosis, and fibroids. It is a more useful adjunct in postmenopausal patients.

6. Describe proper positioning of the patient for laparoscopy.

The patient's position should be adjusted once she is intubated, the endotracheal tube is taped in place, and the anesthesiologist confirms that she may be moved. The patient's legs should be placed simultaneously into stirrups, which provide leg and foot support. Care should be taken that the weight of the patient's legs is placed flatly on the heels of the stirrups and that undue pressure is not placed on the posterior calves. For the purposes of operative laparoscopy, the level of the knees should be at the level of the iliac crests. The femoral heads should not be externally rotated. The foot of the bed can be lowered only once attention to the location of the patient's hands is noted.

To avoid extensive abduction of the arms during operative laparoscopy, the arms can be tucked using a draw sheet placed under the patient. The arms should be tucked in the adducted and pronated position, with care to ensure that there is no contact between the hands and metal objects. The use of egg crate foam cushions is quite helpful for arm positioning.

7. How should a patient be positioned while attaining abdominal access?

Access should be attained with the patient flat. Placing a patient in Trendelenburg position decreases the distance between the point of entry and major retroperitoneal vasculature, such as the bifurcation of the aorta. Once a laparoscope is introduced, the patient should not be placed in Trendelenburg position until a thorough inspection of the underlying organs and retroperitoneal vessels has been performed.

8. Describe the anatomic sites most commonly used to obtain abdominal access in laparoscopy.

One of the most common sites of entry is the base of the umbilicus. The umbilicus is the thinnest point of the abdominal wall. At the umbilicus there is no subcutaneous adipose tissue, and the lower border is composed of peritoneum and deep fascia. To enter at the umbilicus, the abdomen must be relaxed and lifted, with hands or other instruments away from the underlying viscera and vessels. Authors recommend inserting a Veress needle or trocar at an approximately 45° angle for thinner patients and almost directly vertical for obese patients.

The infraumbilical space can be used, directing needle insertion into the hollow of the pelvis. Care should be taken to lift the abdominal wall and insert the needle at a 45° angle toward the uterine fundus. Occasionally the peritoneum sags from the overlying fascia, and the needle tip may not puncture the peritoneum, leading to insufflation of the preperitoneal space.

The left upper quadrant site provides a deep space available for safe needle insertion. The stomach and transverse colon lie immediately below but are mobile. A nasogastric or orogastric tube should be placed to drain the stomach contents. The spleen lies high above the lower level of the rib cage and is safe from accidental puncture, but patients should be examined for hepatosplenomegaly before attempting this technique. The exact location for entry is approximately 3 cm from the midline and 3 cm below the left rib cage. The abdominal skin is again lifted or stretched taut by pulling the skin caudally. This method can be used for obese patients, patients who have had prior surgeries, and patients in whom there is concern for pelvic or lower abdominal adhesions; it also can be used in cases in which the preperitoneal space is accidentally insufflated.

A transvaginal cul-de-sac site can be used as a site of insufflation in patients who have a cul-de-sac free of adhesions. This technique can be useful in obese patients.

9. What instruments are most commonly used to obtain abdominal access in laparoscopy?
The Veress needle is the most popular instrument for intra-abdominal insufflation. Following insufflation, the fascia is elevated by the intra-abdominal pressure, allowing the path of insertion in the desired location.

An alternative technique is to bypass the use of the Veress needle and directly insert a trocar into a nondistended abdomen, thus minimizing the number of punctures of the abdominal wall. Direct insertion can be performed also with a relaxed abdominal wall, which can be further elevated and thus allows less force for trocar insertion and greater proprioception of each abdominal wall layer traversed.

A final option is open laparoscopy, which was designed to eliminate the blind entry of the insufflation needle and laparoscope trocar. In this technique developed by Hasson, an incision is made in the base of the umbilicus, and the fat is pulled laterally, exposing the fascia. After securing the fascia with clamps, the fascia is incised. The peritoneum is bluntly punctured and this opening is spread. The fascial edges are sutured to the Hasson open laparoscopy cannula, which contains a blunt trocar to aid in the insertion of the sleeve through the open wound. The insufflation of gas is accomplished through the trocar sleeve via the insufflation port.

10. Describe the mechanics of the Veress needle.
Its design is that of a blunt cannula within the shaft of a sharp, 14- to 16-gauge needle. In the hub of the needle is a spring that allows the blunt inner cannula to retract inside the needle shaft when pressure is placed against the tip of the blunt cannula. When the needle is thrust into the abdominal wall, the blunt inner tip retracts and the outer shaft's cutting edge penetrates the layers of the abdomen. The surgeon may hear "clicks" as the instrument traverses the abdominal wall, and the spring forces the blunt tip ahead of the sharp shaft to protect against laceration of intra-abdominal viscus.

11. Explain the utility of the "hanging droplet test."
Once the Veress needle is introduced into the abdominal cavity, a 10-cc syringe filled with approximately 5 cc of saline can be applied to the Veress needle. First the syringe should be withdrawn to see if blood, air, or bowel contents are drawn back. Saline should not be able to be aspirated. The syringe is removed, and then droplets of water should be dropped into the Veress cannula, which should fall easily with elevation of the abdominal wall. The drawback to this test is the false-positive rate; saline can fall easily into the preperitoneal space as well.

12. Before you start to insufflate the abdominal cavity, what should the carbon dioxide insufflator pressure readings be?
Prior to insufflation, the connection between the insufflation tubing and the insufflator should be checked. When turned to high flow, the insufflation pressure should be close to 0 mmHg.

13. What should the abdominal pressure be during insufflation?
The pressure should be low upon initial entry (less than 6–7 mmHg) and should remain less than 10 mmHg during insufflation.

14. What constitutes "high flow"?
High flow is 6 L/min without the Veress needle through the insufflator tubing. With the Veress needle attached, high flow is 2–2.5 L/min, which is the maximum allowed through the 14-gauge needle of the Veress.

15. What constitutes "low flow"?
Low flow is 1 L/min. This setting is used for initial insufflation of the abdomen.

16. Does body mass index (BMI) correlate with abdominal wall thickness at the umbilicus and left upper quadrant?
Using the spinal needle test, researchers have shown a significant correlation between BMI and abdominal wall thickness at the umbilicus and left upper quadrant. The mean thickness at the um-

bilicus differed significantly between obese (3.0 ± 1.2 cm) and nonobese women (1.7 ± 0.7 cm, p < 0.001), as did mean thickness at the left upper quadrant (4.4 ± 1.0 vs. 2.0 ± 0.7, p < 0.001).

17. Describe the anatomic landmarks pertinent to placing ancillary pelvic trocars in gynecologic laparoscopy.

All secondary trocars should be inserted under endoscopic visualization. The suprapubic midline or lower quadrants are ideal locations. Adnexal disease is best reached through lateral lower quadrant ports. The suprapubic location does not offer the ease of a lateral approach to the adnexa, and a well-drained bladder is a necessity to protect against accidental bladder perforation.

Transillumination of the anterior abdominal wall may help identify the epigastric vessels. The superficial epigastric artery is a branch of the femoral artery that runs within the anterior abdominal wall fascia. The inferior epigastric artery, which is a branch of the external iliac artery, courses under the abdominal wall fascia and may not be seen with transillumination. It can be identified where it courses along the parietal peritoneum lateral to the obliterate umbilical artery (median umbilical ligament).

18. Describe the techniques for placing ancillary pelvic trocars in gynecologic laparoscopy.

In a review of the abdominal computed tomographic images of 21 women of women, Hurd et al. found that immediately above the symphysis pubis both the superficial epigastric and inferior epigastric arteries are at their most lateral locations. To avoid the superficial and inferior epigastric arteries as well as the superficial circumflex iliac artery, the authors recommended placing trocars at 8 cm from the midline and approximately 5 cm above the symphysis. Hurd et al. also recommend placing trocars at a 45° angle, rather than directly vertical, to avoid the external iliac artery below this site. To minimize tracking medially into the peritoneal cavity, other authors recommend coursing perpendicular to the fascia and transversing the fascia prior to directing the trocar medially into the pelvis.

19. What is the incidence of vascular injuries during laparoscopy? Which vessels are most likely to be injured during laparoscopy?

Because of the proximity of the abdominal wall to the retroperitoneal great vessels, life-threatening hemorrhage may result from injury by a Veress needle or trocar. Munro estimated that the incidence of major vascular injuries during laparoscopy ranges from 0.04 to 0.5%, depending on the study.

Bhoyrul et al. reviewed the list of 408 trocar-related major vascular injuries reported to the Food and Drug Administration by the medical device industry between 1993 and 1996. This study found that the aorta was the most common site of injury (23%), followed by the vena cava (15%). Soderstrom conducted a medicolegal review and reported that of 47 injuries reported to major blood vessels during laparoscopy, the most common sites were the iliac vessels (28), followed by the right common iliac (16), aorta (6), left common iliac (5), and vena cava (5).

20. Describe the different settings of electrosurgical current.

The two main waveforms used in laparoscopy are the cutting waveform (high-current, low-voltage, continuous) and coagulation waveform (high-voltage, low-current, noncontinuous). Tissue effects are attained using different waveforms in contact and noncontact settings.

21. Describe the uses of and common indications for *noncontact* modalities of electrosurgical current.

Electrosurgical cutting is performed using a needle or knifelike electrode, not in contact with the target tissue, with cutting current. Current travels through a steam bubble between the active electrode and the tissue. As a result of the constant current flow and the use of low voltage, the width and depth of necrosis of the walls of the incision are minimal.

Fulguration (superficial coagulation) is performed with coagulation current spraying long electrical sparks to the surface of the tissue. The most common indication is when coagulation is needed in a large area that is oozing blood and a discrete bleeder cannot be identified. With fulguration superficial eschar is produced and the depth of necrosis is minimal. A great deal of the energy is dissipated in the air through which the current passes.

22. Describe the uses of and common indications for *contact* modalities of electrosurgical current.

Dessication (deep coagulation) occurs from slow, delicate contact with coagulation current, although cutting current can also be used. The most common indication is a discrete bleeding source. Because electrical energy is not wasted in heating the air between the electrode and the target tissue, increased energy is delivered into the tissue. Deeper necrosis results—as deep as it is wide. Typically for dessication, the power density is lower because the physical size of the active electrode is larger. The larger electrode requires longer activation times to attain the desired tissue effect.

23. Describe the difference between bipolar and monopolar electrosurgery.

In **monopolar** surgery, electrons pass from the active electrode (electrosurgical instrument) through the patient to the ground plate or return electrode. The electrons spread out after leaving a high density of energy at the point of tissue contact by the active electrode and are then dispersed over the broad surface of the return electrode.

The **bipolar** system incorporates an active electrode and a return electrode into a two-poled instrument such as forceps. This technique eliminates the need for a ground plate. It also allows the instrument to produce a high power density at each pole of the forceps, with a discrete amount of tissue effect confined to the shape and size of the forceps in contact with the tissue.

24. What is direct coupling?

In this technique an activated electrode makes direct contact with a metal instrument on the surgical field. If this approach were used with a metal instrument that has an insulator preventing it from being in direct contact with the abdominal wall, the current may take an alternative route through a point of contact with the adjacent tissue.

25. Explain capacitive coupling.

Capacitive coupling involves the introduction of stray current to a surrounding conductor through the intact insulation of an active electrode. The amount of stray current can be significant. For example, between 5% and 40% of the power level can be coupled or transferred from the insulated shaft of the active electrode to the metal trocar cannula. Normally this stray current is returned to the dispersive electrode by conduction through the large area of contact between the metal trocar sheath and the abdominal wall. However, if a metal sheath is in contact with the abdominal wall with an insulating plastic device (such as a grip), the current in the sheath can travel to any organ with which the sheath is in contact. To a lesser degree this phenomenon can also occur when one laparoscopic instrument is crossed with the electrosurgical electrode. To avoid this problem, it is recommended to use all-metal or all-plastic trocar cannulas.

26. Describe the mechanism of the harmonic scalpel.

The harmonic scalpel is an ultrasonically activated laparoscopic device that uses mechanical energy to cut and coagulate tissue. A piezoelectric crystal within the handpiece vibrates the tip of the titanium blade, and energy is transmitted through the tissue in a linear fashion, parallel to the lines of force. Hydrogen bonds that maintain the integrity of proteins are ruptured, leading to a denatured protein coagulum up to 2 mm with minimal dessication or charring.

27. What is the incidence of laparoscopic port site hernias?

A retrospective study by Kadar et al. reported an incidence of 6 hernias in 5560 operative laparoscopies. A self-report questionnaire study by Montz et al. estimated the incidence of incisional hernias after laparoscopic surgery at 21 per 100,000 cases. Of the 840 reported hernias in which port size was noted, 86.3% occurred in sites where the diameter was at least 10 mm in diameter. Of these, 47.6% occurred at sites 12 mm or greater and 52.4% occurred with ports 10–12 mm in diameter. Only 92 hernias (10.9%) occurred at the site of insertion of ports at least 8 mm in diameter but less than 10 mm. The umbilical incision was the most common site of hernia (75.7%), and lateral hernias were found in 23.7% of cases.

28. When should the fascia be closed for laparoscopic port incisions?
Based on the above findings, the authors recommended closing the fascia for any incision 10 mm or greater. However, if a 5-mm incision is extensively stretched due to specimen removal, the surgeon may consider closing the fascia of that incision as well.

29. Give examples of hernia-associated morbidity in post-laparoscopy hernias.
A self-report questionnaire study found that hernia-related morbidity occurred in 69.5% of reported hernias (648 patients). The most common complication was a palpable hernia or fascial defect in 204 patients (31.5%). In at least 157 women (16.8% of all reported hernias), the presenting symptom was related to involvement of the large or small intestine or bowel incarceration, strangulation, or obstruction. Other reported symptoms were protruding or incarcerated omentum or peritoneum, pain, and nausea.

30. What are the common patient complaints after laparoscopy?
Patients typically note shoulder, chest, and upper abdominal pain from insufflated gas left in the abdominal cavity. They may feel bloated or distended. They have some incisional tenderness, which should improve after a few days. If irrigation was performed, patients may note drainage of serous fluid from the incisions.

BIBLIOGRAPHY

1. American College of Obstetricians and Gynecologists: Vascular injury at laparoscopy. In Reproductive Endocrinology and Infertility, 4th ed. Washingto, DC, American College of Obstetricians and Gynecologists, 2000.
2. American College of Obstetricians and Gynecologists: Contraindications to laparoscopy for adnexal mass. In Reproductive Endocrinology and Infertility, 4th ed. Washington, DC, American College of Obstetricians and Gynecologists, 2000.
3. Bhoyrul S, Vierra MA, Nezhat CR, et al: Trocar injuries in laparoscopic surgery. J Am Coll Surg 192:677–683, 2001.
4. Brill AI: Laparoscopic access and instrument ergonomics. In A Primer in Gynecologic Endoscopy. American Association of Gynecologic Laparoscopists, 2002.
5. Hurd WW, et al: The location of abdominal wall blood vessels in relationship to abdominal landmarks apparent at laparoscopy. Am J Obstet Gynecol 171 (3):642–646, 1994.
6. Kadar et al: Incisional hernias after major laparoscopic gynecologic procedures. Am J Obstet Gynecol 168:1493–1495, 1993.
7. Milad MP,Terkildsen MF: The spinal needle test effectively measures abdominal wall thickness before cannula placement at laparoscopy. J Ame Assoc Gynecol Laparosc 9:514–518, 2004.
8. Montz et al: Incisional hernia following laparoscopy: A survey of the American Association of Gynecologic Laparoscopists. Obset Gynecol 1994.
9. Parker WH: Adnexal surgery by operative laparoscopy. In A Primer in Gynecologic Endoscopy. American Association of Gynecologic Laparoscopists, 2002.
10. Soderstrom RM: Injuries to major blood vessels during endoscopy. J Am Assoc Gynecol Laparosc 4:395–398, 1997.
11. Soderstrom RM: Principles of electrosurgery as applied to gynecology. In Rock JA, Thompson JD (eds): Telinde's Operative Gynecology, 8th ed. Philadelphia, Lippincott-Raven, 1997.
12. Soderstrom RM: Physiologic considerations during anesthesia for laparoscopy. In Soderstrom RM (ed): Operative Laparoscopy. Philadelphia, Lippincott-Raven, 1998.
13. Soderstrom RM: Basic operative technique. In Soderstrom RM (ed): Operative Laparoscopy. Philadelphia, Lippincott-Raven, 1998.
14. Soderstrom RM: Biophysics of electrical energy. In Soderstrom RM (ed): Operative Laparoscopy. Philadelphia, Lippincott-Raven, 1998.

36. TUBAL DISEASE, LIGATION, AND RECONSTRUCTION

Glenn L. Schattman, M.D., FACOG

1. What is the major cause of tubal disease?

Most cases of tubal disease are caused by an infection of the upper genital tract. Pelvic inflammatory disease is unquestionably the largest contributor to tubal infertility as well as to ectopic gestations. When salpingitis occurs, luminal endothelial damage destroys the ciliated cells lining the ampullary and infundibular portions of the fallopian tube. These ciliated cells, responsible for transport of the gametes and embryo to their proper location, often do not recover after resolution of the infection. Loss or compromise of ciliated cells leads to fibrosis both within the tube and distally, causing occlusion and possibly pelvic adhesions.

Prior abdominal surgeries, septic abortions, appendicitis associated with rupture, endometriosis, or other inflammatory pelvic and abdominal processes have also been implicated in causing tubal disease. Approximately 50% of patients with tubal infertility or pelvic adhesions, however, have no antecedent history of a pelvic infection or other risk factors.

2. Which bacterial infection is most likely to cause tubal infertility?

Chlamydia trachomatis is the most prevalent sexually transmitted bacterial infection in the United States. Twenty to 40% of sexually active women have positive chlamydial antibody titers indicating prior exposure. *C. trachomatis* is more likely than *Neisseria gonorrhoeae* to cause tubal damage for a variety of reasons. Chlamydial salpingitis has a long incubation period (mean = 10 days) and is more likely to cause minimal-to-no symptoms. Therefore, it is likely to lead to a prolonged, untreated infection causing permanent endothelial damage. Care must be taken in evaluating patients with pelvic infections since 25–40% of women with *N. gonorrhoeae* are also infected with *C. trachomatis*.

3. What is the risk of infertility after pelvic inflammatory disease (PID)?

After successful antibiotic treatment of laparoscopically confirmed PID, the risk of persistent tubal damage leading to infertility is approximately 8–12%. This risk doubles with each subsequent episode of PID so that infertility affects approximately 23–24% of patients after 2 documented episodes of PID, and approximately 40–54% of patients after 3 episodes.

4. After successful treatment of PID, what is the risk of ectopic pregnancy?

After PID, denuded areas within the fallopian tube are a nidus for embryo implantation within the tube due to delayed transport of the conceptus into the uterine cavity. In 1987, the risk of ectopic pregnancy in the general population was 16.8/1000 pregnancies. The risk of ectopic pregnancy after an episode of treated salpingitis increases by 4- to 7-fold.

5. What mechanisms can help reduce the rate of ectopic pregnancy in patients with tubal disease secondary to infections?

1. **Cilia motion of endothelial cells.** The oocyte is initially retrieved by the ciliated cells of the fimbrae at ovulation and transported to the ampullary region of the fallopian tube, where fertilization takes place. The cilia of the fallopian tube always beat in an abovarian direction and are largely responsible for the transport of the ovum and early pre-embryo to the uterine cavity by the third day after ovulation.

2. **Tubal contractions.** Tubal contractions are able to mobilize the embryo, although these contractions are not directional, sometimes pushing the pre-embryo in a forward direction and at other times pushing the pre-embryo away from the uterine cavity. Muscular contractions that are

able to push the pre-embryo beyond the denuded segment or other obstruction allow the conceptus to continue its journey.

6. What methods are available to diagnose tubal disease and occlusion?

Since approximately 50% of women with tubal disease causing infertility have no historical risk factors, an evaluation of tubal patency is warranted in all women unable to achieve pregnancy.

- **Hysterosalpingography** (HSG) is currently the procedure of choice for the initial evaluation of tubal patency. Besides documenting patency, additional information gleamed from the radiographic appearance of the diseased tube(s) can help determine prognosis for surgical repair.
- **Transvaginal ultrasound** can visualize only the tube if there is obvious pathology (e.g., hydrosalpinx formation).
- **Saline infusion sonography** (SIS) involves injection of saline via a transcervical catheter into the uterine cavity while performing a transvaginal ultrasound. SIS can demonstrate patency of at least one tube if free fluid accumulates in the pelvis.
- **Laparoscopy combined with chromopertubation** requires general anesthesia and should be limited to patients with documented, repairable tubal pathology or patients in whom the cause of the infertility remains unexplained despite a careful evaluation.
- **Falloposcopy** can provide information about the health of the endothelial cells and the presence of intratubal adhesions, but the requirements for considerable expertise and general anesthesia limit its usefulness as a screening test.

7. What are the success rates after repair of distal tubal occlusion?

Success rates depend on many factors. First and foremost is age of the female partner. Next, the condition of the tube visualized on HSG can predict in which patients repair is more likely to be successful in terms of achieving patency as well as pregnancy. The degree of tubal damage can be assessed both pre- and intraoperatively. Tubal disease is generally categorized as mild, moderate, or severe based on the following criteria:

	PREOPERATIVE		INTRAOPERATIVE	
	Hydrosalpinx	Rugae	Fimbrae	Adhesions
Mild	< 15 mm	Present	Normal	None
Moderate	15–30 mm	Absent	Patchy	Mild-moderate
Severe	> 30 mm	Absent	Absent	Severe

Intrauterine pregnancy rates following surgery for mild disease are quite high. Approximately 50–70% of patients conceive a spontaneous pregnancy. Tubal surgery for patients with moderate-to-severe disease tends to have a much worse prognosis; fewer than 30% of patients conceive after surgical repair. The presence of visible rugae alone on HSG is associated with pregnancy rates > 60% after repair compared with < 10% in the absence of rugae. The presence of intratubal pathology during falloposcopy is also associated with a much worse prognosis for repair.

8. What is the best method for repair of distal tubal occlusion?

Both laparoscopy and laparotomy appear to have similar success rates for repair of distal tubal occlusion. The most important prognostic factor for achieving pregnancy appears to be the status of the tube—not the modality utilized for repair. There does not appear to be any benefit to laser or any of the newer modalities for opening the tube in regard to success rates. Distal neosalpingostomy and lysis of adhesions can be performed laparoscopically in most instances with the benefit of shorter recovery and hospital stay, less risk of de-novo adhesion formation, and less postoperative pain. Laparotomy, therefore, should be reserved for patients whose disease is not amenable to laparoscopic repair and who cannot afford in vitro fertilization (IVF). During an unsuccessful laparoscopy, the decision to convert to a laparotomy should be considered carefully in light of the excellent outcomes with assisted reproductive technology (ART) and the poor prognosis in patients with severe tubal disease.

9. Discuss the risk of ectopic pregnancy after tubal reconstructive surgery.
Ectopic pregnancy rates after tubal surgery are directly related to the etiology of the tubal disease as well as the status of the tubes. Patients with mild disease have a better chance of conception; the risk of an ectopic gestation is between 5% and 10%. As the severity of the tubal disease worsens, the percentage of ectopic pregnancies increases. Having an ectopic pregnancy usually indicates intrinsic tubal disease, and subsequent pregnancies are complicated by another ectopic gestation in approximately 12–15% of cases. Heterotopic pregnancies currently occur in 1 in 4–5000 pregnancies, although the majority of heterotopic gestations are due to superovulation associated with ART.

10. How big of a problem is infertility due to tubal or peritoneal factors?
Although individual clinics may see a skewed population of infertility patients due to expertise in specific areas, overall 25–30% of all infertile couples cannot conceive due to anatomic distortion and tubal occlusion. It is the most frequent finding in female infertility, accounting for over 50% of cases.

11. What is the most common cause for bilateral proximal tubal occlusions?
Spasm of the uterotubal sphincter is the most common reason for bilateral proximal tubal occlusion encountered during an HSG. Spasm can result simply from the increased intrauterine pressure in response to the injection of dye. The description of pain during the procedure should raise the suspicion that the inability of dye to enter the interstitial portion of the fallopian tube may be physiologic. This problem can be minimized by slow and gentle injection of dye into the uterine cavity, with care exercised to minimize the increase in intrauterine pressure. Alternatively, administration of a smooth muscle relaxant such as glucagon or oral valium 30 minutes before the procedure or an analgesic such as ibuprofen may reduce the incidence of spasm. Selective transcervical cannulation of the fallopian tube with injection of dye can also help to differentiate spasm from pathology.

12. What is the success of surgical intervention in cases of bilateral proximal tubal occlusion?
True proximal occlusion can be treated with transcervical balloon catheterization or direct hysteroscopic catheter insertion. Success rates for patency of at least one tube are as high as 90%, although pregnancy rates are usually much lower (20–40% after 1 year). Laparotomy for cornual resection and reimplantation for proximal tubal obstruction is a technically challenging operation to perform. The full-term pregnancy rate after surgery is historically very low, making it a procedure that is rarely performed when IVF is available.

13. Does tubal disease affect ART outcome?
Three randomized controlled trials have addressed this question with the conclusion that patients with sonographically visible hydrosalpinges have a significantly lower pregnancy and ongoing/live birth rate compared with patients without sonographically visible hydrosalpinges who undergo IVF for tubal factor infertility. Therefore, patients in whom hydrosalpinges are seen on ultrasound during the work-up for IVF or stimulation should be counseled to undergo salpingectomy or occlusion of the proximal tubal segment(s) of the affected tube(s) before replacing embryos into the uterine cavity. There was no significant difference in miscarriage or implantation rates between the two groups. Patients with tubal disease but without sonographically visible hydrosalpinges do not appear to benefit significantly from surgery prior to IVF.

14. What is salpingitis isthmica nodosa (SIN)?
SIN, as the name implies, is thought to be caused by an infectious process of the tubes that leads to hypertrophy and subsequent occlusion of the proximal fallopian tube. This diagnosis can

be made only histologically, but it may be suspected based on the finding of diverticula within the tubal lumen.

15. What are lead-pipe tubes?

The term *lead-pipe tubes* comes from pelvic tuberculosis, in which the tubes are fixed and rigid, giving the appearance of lead pipes on HSG. Confirmation should be made by purified protein derivatives (PPD) skin testing and an acid-fast bacilli staining of menstrual blood to look for active disease. Even after proper medical treatment, the prognosis for pregnancy is dismal, and IVF offers the only chance for conception if the uterine cavity is free of disease.

16. Which patients are not candidates for tubal surgery?

Patients who have had prior attempts at repair and patients with multifocal tubal disease have a very poor prognosis for success and therefore are not surgical candidates. Patients who have medical conditions contraindicating anesthesia and patients with severe tubal disease are also not candidates for tubal surgery. Although there is no age cut-off for surgery, patients who are 40 years or older have a significantly lower chance for success with restorative surgery. Because of the rapid decline in fecundity that accompanies advancing maternal age, IVF should be encouraged. A single cycle of IVF offers the same chance of conception as does surgery and waiting for 1 year.

17. What is the main reason for requesting tubal ligation reversal in the United States?

Approximately 13% of all patients who have undergone bilateral tubal ligation (BTL) regret their decision. The younger the patient at the time of BTL, the more likely she will later regret her decision. The incidence of regret was 20% for women 30 years of age or younger compared with 6% in women over age 30. Only 1% of women who have had a tubal ligation actually undergo reversal. The most common reason for requesting reversal of sterilization is the desire for more children with a new partner.

18. Which tubal ligation procedures are associated with the best likelihood of pregnancy after reversal?

Procedures that destroy the least amount of tube have the highest success rates after reversal. Clips or rings generally give the best chance for pregnancy after surgical repair, with an intrauterine pregnancy (IUP) rate of approximately 85%. Cautery, especially monopolar cautery of three contiguous areas, destroys the greatest amount of tube, is associated with a much lower success rate, and is less likely to be reversible.

19. What are the chances that tubal ligation reversal will be successful?

Tubal ligation reversal success rates are most importantly influenced by three factors: length of the fallopian tube following repair, location of the anastomosis, and age of the female partner (assuming no male factor is present). If < 4 cm of viable tube is available for anastomosis, the chances for reversibility are quite poor. If ≥ 5 cm of viable tube is present, the chance of success can be estimated by multiplying the length of the longest tube by 10 (e.g., 6 cm × 10 ≥ 60% success rate within 1 year). The location of the anastomosis also plays a role with isthmic-isthmic reanastomosis giving the best outcomes and ampullary-ampullary reanastamoses resulting in significantly poorer outcomes. The success rates also diminish as the discrepancy in diameter of the two segments to be reanastamosed increases. Longer than 4 years from ligation to anastomosis, associated tubal diseases, and overweight status may also decrease the likelihood of success.

20. What is the best way to perform BTL reversal?

Currently, laparotomy and magnification of 4× or 6× with either loupes or an operative microscope offer the best chance for successful reversal. Laparoscopic BTL reversal in the hands of an experienced surgeon with skills at laparoscopic suturing has resulted in pregnancies. Laparoscopic BTL reversal using the Davinci robot offers all of the advantages of laparoscopic surgery with the advantage of being able to use fine suture material (6–0 and 8–0), three-dimensional visualization, and greater magnification and has resulted in patency and pregnancies. The results with laparoscopic surgery are still preliminary and come from highly skilled laparoscopic surgeons. Further trials are needed.

21. What steps are required before and during the performance of BTL?
Consent must be clearly documented in the chart with the appropriate consent form signed and the required elapsed interval of time from consent to sterilization. The permanency of the procedure should be clearly discussed with the patient and documented. If the procedure is not done during the follicular phase of the cycle, a highly sensitive urine test should be done before administering anesthesia. During the procedure, fimbriae must be clearly identified to ensure that the structure being ligated is indeed the fallopian tube and not the round ligament. If an excisional procedure is to be performed, be sure to send the specimen to pathology and follow up on the pathology report to ensure that the tubes were indeed excised. If the tube cannot be definitively identified by visualizing the fimbriae, every attempt should be made to correctly identify the fallopian tube. Dye can be injected transvaginally to identify the tube, and excision of a segment of tube should be done to confirm that the fallopian tube was indeed obstructed. Postoperative HSG should be performed if surgical confirmation is not absolute.

22. What is the failure rate of tubal sterilization?
Five-year cumulative life-table analysis shows that the probability of failure of tubal sterilization is 1.3%. The younger a woman was at the time of sterilization, the more likely it will be that she will experience failure. Failure rates also differ by method of sterilization; 10-year failure rates are most common with the clip type procedures (52.1/1000) and bipolar coagulation in young women (54.3/1000) and least common with postpartum partial salpingectomy (7.5/1000). Another reason for failure of sterilization is that the patient has already conceived a pregnancy before undergoing the procedure. Interval sterilization should be performed in the early follicular phase before ovulation, and the use of a hormonal contraceptive agent or barrier method should be encouraged.

23. What method of BTL has the lowest failure rate?
The Uchida and Irving procedures, in which the proximal stump is buried, are associated with the lowest failure rate. However, they are also the most technically difficult to perform and are associated with the highest morbidity rate; hence they are the least commonly performed.

24. What is the ectopic pregnancy rate after tubal ligation?
The 10-year cumulative probability of ectopic pregnancy is 7.3/1000 procedures. The incidence varies depending on the type of procedure performed. Bipolar coagulation has the highest cumulative probability of 17.1/1000 procedures, whereas postpartum partial salpingectomy has the lowest at 1.5/1000 procedures. If a pregnancy test is positive after tubal sterilization, one-third of pregnancies are ectopic.

25. What is the incidence of ectopic gestation after BTL reversal?
If a pregnancy test is positive after tubal reconstructive surgery, the risk of ectopic pregnancy is approximately 2–4%. Any patients who conceive after tubal surgery should have close follow-up and monitoring for the probability of an ectopic gestation. Follow-up should include serial assessments of beta human chorionic gonadotropin (BhCG), baseline progesterone levels, and early transvaginal ultrasound examination when the BhCG value is > 1,500 IU/ml by an experienced sonographer.

26. What is the best energy source to use for tubal surgery and repair?
Many energy sources are available to cut and effect hemostasis. Currently the most popular methods to cut and coagulate include laser, electrical energy, harmonic scalpel, radiofrequency energy, and thermal coagulation. Some sources have a more finite spread of energy with less lateral destruction of tissue, and others offer better hemostasis; however, none appears to offer sig-

nificant advantages in regard to pregnancy outcome. The operator should use the method with which he or she is most familiar and feels most comfortable.

27. What new methods of sterilization are available?

Hysteroscopic placement of spring-loaded plugs into the proximal tubal ostia (Essure) has recently been approved by the U.S. Food and Drug Administration (FDA) as a method of sterilization. In Europe, no pregnancies have been reported after the correct placement of this device, and a 100% occlusion rate has been documented on HSG 3 months after the intervention. The device induces an endothelial reaction and subsequent occlusion of the proximal tubal segment. The need for an alternate method of contraception for 3 months after the procedure and the requirement by the FDA for a follow-up HSG to demonstrate complete tubal occlusion limit its desirability. Whether these devices are removable and whether the intrauterine portion of the device can affect subsequent success with ART if the patient desires pregnancy in the future are unanswered questions.

28. What evaluations should be performed before scheduling a tubal ligation reversal?

Since most patients requesting reversal have a new partner, a semen analysis should be performed to evaluate semen quality. The presence of a severe male factor is a contraindication for surgery because the couple will fare better with IVF and assisted fertilization. An evaluation of the endometrial cavity, whether by saline infusion sonography (SIS), hysterosalpingogram, or hysteroscopy, should be performed at the same time as the reversal procedure. Evaluation of ovulation can be done by menstrual cycle charting. In the presence of normal cyclic menses, no further evaluation for ovulation needs to be performed.

29. For how long should a couple attempt pregnancy after tubal surgery?

Most pregnancies occur within the first year after surgery. If pregnancy has not occurred by then, tubal patency should be evaluated by HSG. Surgery for reocclusion is not warranted because the success rates are extremely low. IVF in the presence of reocclusion offers excellent success rates, depending on the age of the female partner.

30. Can postoperative adhesions be prevented?

Adhesions arise within the peritoneal cavity in response to tissue injury (e.g., dessication, trauma). Reperitonealization of the damaged surfaces occurs by reformation of new mesothelium overlying the denuded areas and takes approximately 5 days. Thus, since healing occurs with the formation of new peritoneum, large defects heal as rapidly as small defects, and prevention of adhesions is limited to this early interval after surgery.

Various procedures and products have been evaluated in an attempt to reduce the complications of adhesion formation after pelvic reconstructive surgery. To date, there does not appear to be any benefit with regard to reducing adhesion formation or improving pregnancy rates with postoperative hydrotubation, instillation of fluids or dextran into the peritoneal cavity at the end of surgery, reperitonealization, placement of omental grafts, or second-look laparoscopy.

Interceed (oxidized, regenerated cellulose) is effective in reducing adhesion formation (de novo and reformation) after pelvic surgery, but the field needs to be hemostatic. Gore-Tex appears to be more efficacious in preventing adhesion formation than Interceed, but its usefulness in reproductive surgery is limited by the need to suture the material in place and the need for subsequent removal of the nonabsorbable material. The benefit of these products in reducing adhesion formation has been clearly demonstrated. With regard to pregnancy outcome, however, their efficacy has not been studied in a randomized, controlled trial. Limited evidence indicates that Sepra film (sodium hyaluronate and carboxymethylcellulose) reduces adhesion formation, but it is quite cumbersome to use and not readily amenable to laparoscopic placement.

31. Does tubal sterilization have any noncontraceptive health benefits?

It appears that patients who undergo tubal sterilization have a lower incidence of ovarian cancer (relative risk = 0.29–0.69) even after adjusting for age, use of oral contraceptives, and parity.

This finding is possibly due to decreased exposure of the peritoneal cavity to environmental toxins. There does not appear to be a decrease in the incidence of acquiring a sexually transmitted disease after sterilization. Interestingly, of couples in whom one partner has undergone sterilization, hysterectomy was 4–5 times more common when the woman was sterilized than when the male partner had undergone a vasectomy.

BIBLIOGRAPHY

1. American College of Obstetricians and Gynecologists: Benefits and Risks of Sterilization. ACOG Practice Bulletin No. 6. Washington, DC, ACOG, 2003.
2. Damewood MD: Tubal Reconstructive Surgery. In Adashi EY, Rock JA, Rosenwaks Z (eds): Reproductive Endocrinology, Surgery, and Technology. Philadelphia, Lippincott-Raven, 1996, pp 2091–2104.
3. Farquhar C, Vandekerckhove P, Watson A, et al: Barrier agents for preventing adhesion formation after surgery for subfertility. Cochrane Database of Systematic Reviews 3, 2003.
4. Hanafi M: Factors affecting the pregnancy rate after microsurgical reversal of tubal ligation. Fertil Steril 80:434–440, 2003.
5. Hillis SD, Marchbanks PA, Tylor LR, Peterson HB: Poststerilization regret: Findings from the United States collaborative review of sterilization. Obstet Gynecol 93:889–895, 1999.
6. Johnson NP, Mak W, Sowter MC: Surgical treatment for tubal disease in women due to undergo in vitro fertilization. Cochrane Database of Systematic Reviews 3, 2003.
7. Johnson N, Vandekerckhove P, Watson A, et al: Tubal flushing for subfertility. Cochrane Database of Systematic Reviews 3, 2003.
8. Johnson NP, Watson A: Postoperative procedures for improving fertility following pelvic reproductive surgery. Cochrane Database of Systematic Reviews 3, 2003.
9. Nardin JM, Kulier R, Boulvain M: Techniques for the interruption of tubal patency for female sterilization. Cochrane Database of Systematic Reviews 3, 2003.
10. Peterson HB, Xia Z, Hughes JM, et al: The risk of pregnancy after tubal sterilization: Findings from the U.S. collaborative review of sterilization. Am J Obstet Gynecol 174:1168–1170, 1996.
11. Rock JA, Katayana KP, Martin EJ, et al: Factors influencing the success of salpingostomytechniques for distal tubal occlusion. Obstet Gynecol 52:591, 1978.
12. Saravelo H, Li TC, Cook I: An analysis of outcomes of microsurgical and laparoscopic adhesiolysis for infertility. Hum Reprod 10:2887, 1995.
13. Shoysman R: Tubal microsurgery vs. IVF. Acta Eur Fertil 15:5, 1984.
14. Vazquez G, Boeckx W, Brosens I: Prospective study of mucosal lesions to fertility in hydrosalpinx. Hum Reprod 10:1075, 1995.
15. Watson A, Vanderkerckhove P, Liliford R: Techniques for pelvic surgery in subfertility. Cochrane Database of Systematic Reviews 3, 2003.
16. Westrom L: Incidence, prevalence and trends of acute pelvic inflammatory disease and its consequences in industrialized countries. Am J Obstet Gynecol 138:880, 1980.
17. Winston RML, Magara R: Microsurgical salpingostomy is not an obsolete procedure. Br J Obstet Gynecol 98:637, 1991.
18. Woolcott R, Fisher S, Thomas J, Kable W: A randomized, prospective, controlled study of laparoscopic dye studies and selective salpingography as diagnostic tests of fallopian tube patency. Fertil Steril 72:879–884, 1999.

V. Assisted Reproductive Technology

37. SPERM RETRIEVAL TECHNIQUES

Peter T.K. Chan, M.D., and Peter N. Schlegel, M.D.

1. Explain the acronyms TESA, PESA, MESA, and TESE.
TESA = TEsticular Sperm Aspiration.
PESA = Percutaneous Epididymal Sperm Aspiration.
MESA = Microsurgical Epididymal Sperm Aspiration.
TESE = TEsticular Sperm Extraction.

2. Why is it important to use these acronyms with precision and accuracy?
The acronyms for the common surgical sperm retrieval techniques can be confusing. However, each technique is significantly different from the others in terms of indications, yield, invasiveness, and complications. Hence, health care professionals should be careful in referring to each of the acronyms when they communicate with each other in order to avoid confusion.

3. Describe the techniques for TESA, PESA, MESA, and TESE.
TESA is a percutaneous procedure in which a needle of 18- to 25-gauge is inserted into the testicular parenchyma to sample the seminiferous tubules by aspiration (Fig. 1). Spermatozoa are obtained by rupturing the tubules as well as by removing the entire tubules.

PESA is a technique in which sperm is aspirated and sampled percutaneously from the epididymis, usually with a needle of 21- to 25-gauge (Fig. 2).

MESA is an open procedure in which the epididymis is exposed via a scrotal incision. Individual epididymal tubules are identified and isolated microsurgically. Micropuncture of an epididymal tubule is performed, and the fluid, which contains sperm, is aspirated with a micropipette (Fig. 3).

TESE is an open procedure in which the testicle is exposed via a scrotal incision. An avascular

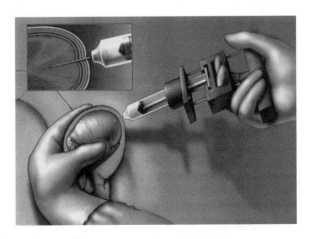

FIGURE 1. Testicular sperm aspiration (TESA).

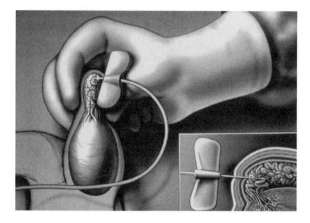

FIGURE 2. Percutaneous epididymal sperm aspiration (PESA).

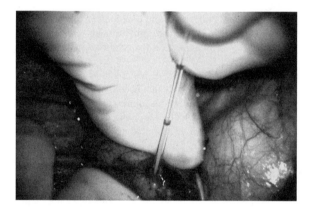

FIGURE 3. Microsurgical epididymal sperm aspiration (MESA).

area of the tunica albugenia of the testis is identified, preferably with the aid of an operating microscope, and incised to expose the underlying seminiferous tubules for sperm retrieval (Fig. 4).

4. What other surgical sperm retrieval techniques are available?

Seminal vesicle aspiration is generally performed transrectally under transrectal ultrasound guidance in men who have ejaculatory duct obstruction with dilated seminal vesicles. Like transrectal biopsy of the prostate, this procedure requires prophylactic antibiotic coverage. Complications, which are similar to those in prostate biopsy, include rectal bleeding, hematuria, prostatitis, and sepsis.

Electroejaculation is used in men who have a neurologic ejaculatory disorder, such as spinal cord injury or psychogenic anejaculation, without mechanical obstruction of the excurrent ductal system. Details of this procedure are covered in chapter 22.

Sperm collection from post-ejaculation urine is used in conjunction with electroejaculation or in men with isolated retrograde ejaculation. Details of this procedure are described in chapter 15.

Percutaneous testicular core biopsy. A biopsy gun of size 14-gauge or smaller (similar to the ones used for prostate biopsy) can be used percutaneously to obtain a core of seminiferous tubules for sperm retrieval (Fig. 5).

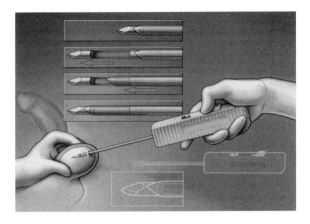

FIGURE 4. Testicular sperm extraction (TESE).

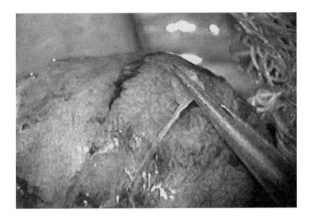

FIGURE 5. Percutaneous testicular core biopsy.

5. How is TESE different from biopsy?

Although in both cases, seminiferous tubules are removed, the two procedures are different in many aspects.

Comparison of TESE and Testis Biopsy

	TESE	TESTIS BIOPSY
Objectives	To find adequate amount of sperm for assisted reproduction and/or cryopreservation.	1. To sample one or few areas for histologic evaluation of the semineferous tubule. 2. To confirm the presence of spermatogenesis in suspected cases of obstructive azoospermia.
Anesthesia	Although local anesthesia is feasible, in nonobstructive azoospermic cases when longer operating time is necessary, regional or general anesthesia may be required.	Local anesthesia

Comparison of TESE and Testis Biopsy

	TESE	TESTIS BIOPSY
Incisions on tunica albugenia	A long incision is made on the tunica albugenia to extensively sample seminiferous tubules for sperm.	One or a few small incisions are made to obtain a small quantities of seminiferous tubules from one or more sites in the testicle.
Extent of testis exploration	Particularly with microdissection, virtually the entire testicular parenchyma can be explored and sampled.	Limited to the superficial seminiferous tubules accessible at the incisions.
Invasiveness	Larger incisions are made to the tunica albugenia.	Less extensive or invasive than TESE
Surgery time	In nonobstructive azoospermic cases, up to 3 hours per testi may be required for exploration.	Generally complete within 30 minutes
Selection of tissues	All tissues are initially examined intraoperatively by an embryologist microscopically to determine the extent of the procedure needed to find sperm.	Not necessary

6. What are the indications for PESA and MESA?

Generally, epididymal sperm aspiration with PESA or MESA should be performed only in men who have sperm in the epididymides. In other words, the man should have active spermatogenesis with passage of sperm to the epididymis. This indication includes all men with obstructive azoospermia, such as those who had previous vasectomy, failed vasovasostomy/vasoepididymostomy, congenital absence of vas, or ejaculatory duct obstruction. In addition to men with obstructive azoospermia, men who had ejaculation disorders, such as anejaculation or retrograde ejaculation, are potential candidates for PESA and MESA.

7. When should epididymal sperm aspiration (PESA or MESA) not be used?

PESA and MESA are contraindicated in all men without active spermatogenesis, because they generally do not have sperm in the epididymis. Thus, men with nonobstructive azoospermia or testicular failure should not undergo PESA or MESA for sperm retrieval.

8. How is MESA different from PESA?

PESA is a percutaneous procedure, whereas MESA is an open procedure that requires a surgical microscope. The differences between the two procedures are summarized below.

Comparison of MESA and PESA

	ADVANTAGES	DISADVANTAGES
MESA	Microsurgical procedure allows lower complication rate. Epididymal sperm has better motility than testicular sperm. Multiple vials of sperm with fewer contaminants (red and white blood cells) generally can be obtained in a single procedure. Sample can generally be cryopreserved for future use. Since it is performed under direct vision, it allows selection of regions of the epididymis with the best quality of sperm, possibly improving its survival after freezing-thawing during cryopreservation and limiting DNA damage by reactive oxygen species.	As an open procedure, it is more time consuming than percutaneous procedures. Although local anesthesia is feasible, regional or general anesthesia is preferred. Microsurgical skills are required to perform the procedure.

Comparison of MESA and PESA

	ADVANTAGES	DISADVANTAGES
PESA	No microsurgical skill required. Local anesthesia is generally adequate. This procedure is most appropriate in men with no previous scrotal procedure or pathology and with dilated and easily palpable epididymis.	Complications include hematoma, pain and vascular injury to testes and epididymis. Variable success in obtaining sperm. Generally smaller quantity of sperm obtained than with MESA; often not enough sperm for cryopreservation. Some series reported that 20% of obstructive azoospermic cases may fail to have sperm retrieved with PESA.

9. Where in the epididymis should PESA/MESA be performed?
Although in a normal, unobstructed epididymis, more mature sperm are found in the cauda than in the caput epididymis, the situation is somewhat different in an obstructed epididymis. In obstructive cases, the dilated cauda epididymal tubule contains mainly old and degenerated sperm fragments with macrophages and other inflammatory cells. On the other hand, more fresh and motile sperm can generally be found in the caput epididymis. Thus, PESA/MESA should preferably be performed in the proximal caput epididymis.

10. In cases of obstructive azoospermia, which is the better option: reconstruction (with vasovasostomy or vasoepididymostomy) or sperm retrieval (with MESA or PESA) for IVF/ICSI?
Both are feasible alternatives. However, various studies have suggested that reconstruction is a more cost-effective option than upfront sperm retrieval for IVF/ICSI. On the other hand, when a co-existing female factor requires the use of assisted reproduction, IVF/ICSI with surgical sperm retrieval is the preferred choice.

11. In cases of obstructive azoospermia, is surgical reconstruction feasible after previous epididymal sperm retrieval with MESA or PESA?
Yes. Within the caput, tubules from the efferent ductules may not have coalesced into a single tubule; thus, obstruction of one efferent ductile may not obstruct all sperm flow in the epididymis. Beyond the caput epididymis, the epididymal tubule is a singular continuous tubule. Surgical procedures such as PESA or MESA may cause scarring of the tubule, leading to permanent obstruction at the site of puncture. However, these patients may still undergo reconstruction with vasoepididymostomy at a site proximal to the puncture site, where sperm can be found. In fact, if the epididymal obstruction is minimal after PESA or MESA, sperm may still pass beyond the epididymis to the vas, and a vasovasostomy (in men with a previous vasectomy) can be performed.

12. What are the indications for TESA and TESE?
TESA and TESE are techniques for retrieving testicular sperm. Since testicular spermatozoa have not yet undergone epididymal maturation, they mostly are immotile. Nonetheless, they can be used for fertilization with assisted reproductive technology. Unlike PESA and MESA, which should be performed only in men with active spermatogenesis (e.g., men with obstructive azoospermia), TESA and TESE can also be used to retrieve sperm in men with nonobstructive azoospermia or testicular failure. Although TESA and TESE can also be used in men with obstructive azoospermia, the more mature epididymal sperm obtained by MESA may be preferable for immediate use in assisted reproduction.

13. Compare TESA and TESE.
TESA is a percutaneous procedure, whereas TESE is an open procedure that may require the use of a surgical microscope. The differences between the two procedures are summarized below.

Comparison of TESA and TESE.

	ADVANTAGES	DISADVANTAGES
TESA	No microsurgical skill required. Local anesthesia. Can be used for obstructive and nonobstructive azoospermia.	Immature or immotile testicular sperm. Yield of sperm is generally low, particularly in nonobstructive azoospermia. Complications include hematoma, pain, and vascular injury to testes and epididymis.
TESE	Since it is performed under direct vision, complication rate is low especially if performed microsurgically. Preferred technique for non-obstructive azoospermia. Multiple areas of seminiferous tubules can be sampled. Samples are often adequate in quantity for cryopreservation for future use. Since it is performed under direct vision, it is the procedure of choice in men with previous scrotal inflammation (epididymo-orchitis), scrotal surgery, (especially those with postoperative complications), or small testicles.	As an open procedure, it is more time-consuming than percutaneous procedures. Although local anesthesia is feasible, regional or general anesthesia is preferred.

14. What is microdissection?

Microdissection is an advanced version of TESE that applies microsurgical technique in the retrieval of sperm from seminiferous tubules. Often the seminiferous tubules from different areas of the testis may be associated with different states of maturation of spermatogenesis. In other words, in some areas the Sertoli cell-only pattern may be present, whereas other areas may have maturation arrest, hypospermatogenesis, or even normal spermatogenesis. Seminiferous tubules with more "active" or advanced states of spermatogenesis have a different appearance under an operating microscope from tubules with less spermatogenic activity. Hence, under $25\times$ magnification, retrieval of seminiferous tubules that appeared larger may lead to a higher chance of finding sperm.

When performing microdissection, the testis is opened extensively with a long transverse incision on the tunica albugenia to allow a thorough search of tubules in virtually the entire testis, including those lying deeply within the testis. The use of microdissection technique allows removal of a smaller quantity of seminiferous tubules by selecting only the ones that are likely to contain sperm and sparing the remaining tubules.

15. What are the advantages of using microdissection for TESE?

1. Unlike traditional TESE, in which a chunk of testis parenchyma is removed, microdissection removes only individual seminiferous tubules. Hence, there is a lower risk of damaging the androgen-producing Leydig cells located in the interstitium of the testis.

2. By providing a "cleaner" or "purer" sample of tubules that have a higher chance of containing sperm, microdissection allows the embryologist to find sperm more effectively.

3. A more thorough search of the entire volume of seminiferous tubules, including the ones lying deep to the testis, can be performed. Depending on the volume of the testis, a thorough microdissection may require up to 3 hours per testis to perform. With microdissection, it is not infrequent to find sperm in patients who have had a negative conventional TESE. On the other hand, after a negative microdissection, we do not know of any cases of positive sperm retrieval in subsequent procedures.

16. Summarize the success rates of the various retrieval techniques.

The success rate of finding sperm depends not just on the techniques used, but also significantly on the clinical profile of the patient. Generally, for obstructive cases, finding of sperm by PESA, MESA, TESA or TESE should approach 100%, since active spermatogenesis is present.

Success Rates of Sperm Retrieval with Various Techniques.

	OBSTRUCTIVE AZOOSPERMIA	NONOBSTRUCTIVE AZOOSPERMIA
PESA	~ 89–95%	Not indicated
MESA	~ 99%	Not indicated
TESA	~ 100%	11–60%
TESE	~1 00%	40–62%

However, in selecting the type of sperm retrieval technique, one should also focus on factors other than sperm retrieval success rates. Additional factors that should be considered include the quantity of sperm obtainable (MESA > PESA and TESE > TESA), possibility for cryopreservation for future use (MESA > PESA and TESE >TESA) , invasiveness and duration of the procedure (PESA > MESA and TESA > TESE), and expertise of the surgeon performing the procedure.

17. Can pooling of samples be done to acquire an adequate amount of sperm for intrauterine insemination instead of ICSI?

For intrauterine insemination, the minimum quantity of motile sperm required is generally 5–10 million. A single procedure of surgical sperm retrieval from the testis or epididymis generally does not provide such a high quantity of motile sperm. In the past, before the technique of IVF/ICSI was widely available, pooling of multiple retrieved sperm samples for IUI had been performed. However, in view of the invasiveness and cost of multiple retrieval procedures to obtain adequate quantity and quality of sperm, the cost for cryopreservation and storage of retrieved sample, the loss in sperm yield in using cryopreserved sperm, the lower success rates with IUI vs. IVF/ICSI, currently it is not advisable to pool multiple surgically retrieved sperm samples for IUI when IVF/ICSI is available.

18. How long should one wait before repeating a surgical sperm retrieval?

For open sperm retrieval procedures, particularly TESE or microdissection in which the testis blood supply within the tunica albugenia may be partly violated during the procedure, we recommend at least a 6-month period of recovery before repeating the procedure. The same recommendation generally applies to percutaneous procedures (PESA, TESA) also. Although in percutaneous procedures there is no skin incision, extensive blinded puncture to the testis and epididymis may nonetheless cause significant damage to the blood supply and/or scarring in the organs.

19. Is fresh sperm better than frozen sperm for assisted reproduction?

Most IVF centers prefer to use a fresh sperm sample because a significant proportion of sperm may not survive the freezing and thawing procedure, particularly in case of nonobstructive azoospermia. Some investigators reported that as few as 30–35% of testicular sperm samples from men with nonobstructive azoospermia will survive freezing-thawing. Loss of sperm from freezing and thawing is particularly problematic in cases of nonobstructive azoospermia because there is generally not a large quantity of retrievable sperm.

On the other hand, some experts believe that, even in cases of nonobstructive azoospermia, a frozen sample may be preferable because the sperm that "survive" the freezing/thawing cycle may be "better" sperm for fertilization. Although there is no argument that excess sperm from retrieval procedures should be cryopreserved for future use, in practical terms the use of cryopreserved sperm provides additional logistic convenience in that one may consider performing ovulation induction in the female partner only if testicular sperm are found for cryopreservation.

20. In obstructive azoospermia, what are the choices of sperm retrieval techniques?

In obstructive cases, we generally prefer retrieving sperm from the epididymis, where more motile and mature sperm can be found. MESA, in which a specific epididymal tubule is opened microsurgically, generally provides a cleaner sample of sperm with minimal contamination with blood. Furthermore, a larger quantity of sperm can be retrieved for cryopreservation for future use. PESA, on the other hand, is quicker and does not require a skin incision. However, because the needle puncture is a blinded procedure, the patient should be informed about the risk of bleeding, hematoma, and ischemic damage to the testis and epididymis.

In obstructive cases, testicular sperm may be retrieved for reproduction using TESA or TESE. When PESA is unable to retrieve good quantity and quality of sperm or when the surgeon does not have microsurgical expertise to perform MESA, retrieval of sperm percutaneously with needle aspiration or with a biopsy gun can provide an adequate amount of sperm. Open TESE may be used if the percutaneous procedure fails. In this setting, we recommend submission of a piece of testis for histologic evaluation to confirm the diagnosis of obstructive azoospermia.

21. In nonobstructive azoospermia, what are the choices of sperm retrieval techniques ?

As stated previously, unlike obstructive azoospermia, men with nonobstructive azoospermia have poor production of sperm from the testis. Thus, sperm retrieval from the epididymis (PESA and MESA) should not be attempted. Although percutaneous testicular sperm retrieval procedure with TESA may be attempted first, the yield is generally lower than TESE or microdissection. Hence, to avoid unnecessary injury to the blood supply of the testicular tunica albugenia from blind puncture with TESA, we recommend TESE or, preferably, microdissection for nonobstructive azoospermic cases. Submission of a piece of testis for histologic evaluation to confirm the diagnosis of nonobstructive azoospermia and to evaluate for intratubular germ-cell neoplasia should also be performed.

22. Can a biopsy be done to predict the success of retrieval?

In infertile men, the histologic state of spermatogenesis in the testis is usually not homogeneous. Thus, during a biopsy when only one or a few superficial areas of seminiferous tubules are sampled, even if they show a Sertoli cell-only pattern, it is impossible to predict absolutely whether additional foci elsewhere in the testis may have more advanced spermatogenesis and sperm can be found. Hence, in counseling individual patients, a diagnostic testicular biopsy is not necessary prior to sperm retrieval. That being said, the histologic pattern of the testis obtained from a biopsy can provide an estimate of the likelihood of finding sperm during retrieval by TESE. The percentages of successful sperm retrieval are ~ 80% for hypospermatogenesis, ~ 50% for maturation arrest, and ~ 25% for Sertoli cell-only pattern.

23. What are the complications of sperm retrieval?

In addition to complications related to anesthesia, specific complications of surgical sperm retrieval include wound infection, hematoma, and pain. Less frequently, ischemic damage to testis or epididymis, epididymal scarring/obstruction, hypogonadism, and testicular atrophy may occur.

24. What type of anesthesia is required for surgical sperm retrieval?

Surgical sperm retrieval is an outpatient procedure. When it is performed percutaneously, only local anesthesia is required. Local anesthesia can be achieved by infusion of anesthetic agents along the puncture area. In addition, a spermatic cord block should be done to provide effective anesthesia to the testis and epididymis and to avoid discomfort during the procedure.

If an open procedure is to be performed, local anesthesia may also be used. If the procedure is expected to last longer than 2 hours or if the patient may have difficulty remaining still, regional or light general anesthesia is preferred.

25. If a patient failed a previous surgical sperm retrieval, is it worth repeating the procedure?

Obviously, in a true obstructive azoospermic case, there is very little chance of failing sperm retrieval (except with PESA). If it does occur, repeating the procedure with an open technique, including MESA or TESE, should allow sperm to be found from the epididymides or testes, respectively.

In nonobstructive azoospermic cases, patients with a failed TESA should be re-explored with TESE, preferably using a microdissection technique for sperm retrieval. Likewise, as stated previously, patients with a failed limited TESE may have sperm found in a subsequent microdissection exploration.

26. How many times can sperm be retrieved ?
In obstructive azoospermic cases in which sperm production is normal, sperm can be retrieved multiple times. One should keep in mind that surgical sperm retrieval is an invasive procedure with a measurable risk of tissue damage and complications. Thus, we recommend cryopreservation of additional sperm from each procedure to reduce the need of repeating surgical procedure frequently.

In nonobstructive azoospermic cases, sperm retrieval can also be repeated multiple times. However, in such cases there is often only a limited number of foci where spermatogenesis is active. Moreover, once these foci are removed, they will not regenerate. Thus, at one point no sperm may be found in subsequent retrieval procedure despite previous successful retrieval. As in obstructive cases, we recommend cryopreservation of excess sperm for future use to avoid repeating the retrieval procedure.

27. Where are the safe areas in the testis for puncture or incision during TESA or TESE?
There are fewer arteries on the upper medial and upper lateral surface, which are safer for incision and suture placement. However, because of individual variation of the location of vessels, careful inspection, preferably with optical magnification, in areas where incisions are to be made is important to avoid damaging the arteries. In addition, since the blood vessels in the tunica albugenia of the testis run transversely, incision should be made transversely to avoid cutting across vessels.

28. What are some of the most challenging scenarios of sperm retrieval?
Generally, it is a challenge to find sperm during retrieval procedures in all cases of onobstructive azoospermia. Particularly difficult cases include patients who have severe defects in spermatogenesis, such as those with the Sertoli cell-only pattern from previous testicular biopsy and those who failed to have sperm retrieved in previous TESE.

29. What are the contraindications for sperm retrieval?
In general, sperm retrieval should not be performed in any patient who is not fit to undergo scrotal surgery. Examples includes men with active urinary tract or genital infection, bleeding diathesis, high risks of postoperative complications, or previous scrotal surgery within the past 3–6 months.

In cases with a low chance of success in finding sperm, proper counseling should be offered if surgical sperm retrieval is to be attempted. Examples include men with significant genetic abnormalities, such as complete deletion of the Y-chromosome in the AZF a or b (but not c) regions. Finally, surgical sperm retrieval should not be repeated in men who have had a previously negative sperm retrieval after a thorough microdissection because the chance of finding sperm is low.

30. In nonobstructive cases, if sperm is not identified intraoperatively in TESA or TESE, is it hopeless to find sperm?
Generally, samples retrieved during the sperm retrieval procedure should be evaluated by the embryologist immediately to indicate or estimate whether an adequate amount of high-quality sperm is available for immediate use or cryopreservation. However, a more thorough examination of all retrieved samples, particularly those from TESE or microdissection, may take hours to complete. Hence, even if intraoperatively no sperm is reported in the preliminary evaluation by the embryologist, sperm may subsequently be found after further processing, including mechanical and enzymatic dispersion of the retrieved sample.

BIBLIOGRAPHY

1. Chan PT: Azoospermia: Evaluations and treatments. J Male Sex Reprod Health 2(3): 113–118, 2002.
2. Chan PT: Genetic risks associated with advanced reproductive technology. J Male Sex. Reprod Health 2(4):161–164, 2002.
3. Chan PT, Palermo GD, Veeck LL, et al: Testicular sperm extraction combined with intracytoplasmic sperm injection in the treatment of men with persistent azoospermia postchemotherapy. Cancer 92: 1632–1637, 2001.
4. Chann PT, Schlegel PN: Curr Opin Urol 10:617–624, 2000.
5. Chan PT, Schlegel PN: Dagnostic and therapeutic testis biopsy. Curr Urol Rep 1(4):266–272, 2000.
6. Schlegel PN, Su LM: Physiological consequences of testicular sperm extraction. Hum Reprod 12(8): 1688–1692, 1997.
7. Schlegel PN: Testicular sperm extraction: Microdissection improves sperm yield with minimal tissue excision. Hum Reprod 14:131–135, 1999.
8. Su LM, Palermo GD, Goldstein M, et al: Testicular sperm extraction with intracytoplasmic sperm injection for nonobstructive azoospermia: Testicular histology can predict success of sperm retrieval. J Urol 161:112–116, 1999.

38. GENERAL EMBRYOLOGY

Lucinda L. Veeck, M.L.T., h.D.Sc.

1. Who takes care of the oocytes, sperm, and preembryos in an in vitro fertilization (IVF) laboratory?

Clinical embryologists. These laboratory scientists with training in tissue culture possess specialized skills in handling spermatozoa, oocytes, and preembryos.

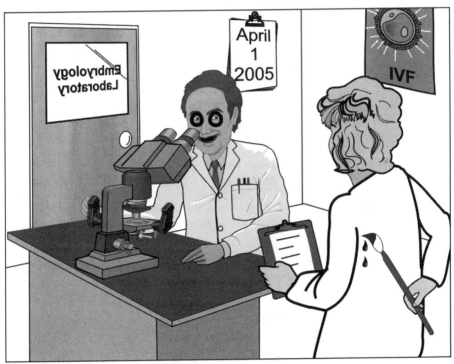

"They look OK to me"

2. How do embryologists keep the preembryos of different patients separate and safeguarded from mix-ups?

Responsible IVF teams have extremely stringent rules in place to prevent laboratory error. These rules include, but are not limited to, the following:

- Samples from only one patient are handled at any given time.
- Workspaces never hold specimens from more than one patient.
- Patient names are read aloud from all tubes or dishes containing oocytes, preembryos, or spermatozoa, often by two embryologists.

- Routine laboratory supplies are never reused; disposable materials are purchased and discarded after a single usage.
- Either the laboratory director or laboratory supervisor is required to be on site at all times whenever patient samples are handled.

3. Are there ways to protect the laboratory against malicious intent (by outsiders, patients, or others)?

Experienced laboratories have well-defined and regularly tested safeguards in place to prevent specimen damage in the event of equipment malfunction, hazardous environmental conditions (e.g., fire, temperature, toxic, or other disaster), or electrical outage. To safeguard against malicious acts by outsiders, one may choose to install laboratory motion sensors, videotape recorders, and/or sound-monitoring systems in order to monitor critical rooms around the clock.

4. At what phases of oogenesis are female gametes found in the ovary before puberty, after puberty, and at time of ovulation?

Before puberty. Oogenesis stops at prophase I (i.e., prophase of meiosis I). These gametes are called primary oocytes.

After puberty. Each month a few primary oocytes resume meiosis I. As a result of completing meiosis I, both a secondary oocyte and a first polar body are produced. At this stage oocytes are ovulated.

5. What are the components of a mature oocyte?

The diameter of a mature human oocyte is approximately 110–115 μm and is bounded by a plasma membrane called the oolemma. Surrounding the oocyte/oolemma is a glycoprotein envelope called the zona pellucida that protects the oocyte (Fig. 1). The presence of a first polar body indicates the oocyte has reached maturity and is capable of undergoing a normal fertilization process.

6. What are the morphologic differences between oocytes that are at metaphase II, metapahase I, and prophase I stages of maturation?

Metaphase II (MII): first polar body present, no germinal vesicle; inseminated or injected 3–5 hours after collection

Metaphase I (MI): no first polar body, no germinal vesicle; inseminated or injected 1–5 hours after extrusion of the first polar body

Prophase I (PI): germinal vesicle present (a prominent nucleus with large nucleolus); usually not inseminated or injected; if done, should be carried out 26–29 hours after collection if the first polar body has been extruded.

7. What are pronuclei?

Within a few hours of a sperm penetrating the oocyte, male and female pronuclei (Fig. 2) are formed from the sperm and oocyte chromatin. The stage at which pronuclei are visible is termed the *pronuclear stage,* and the specimen is defined as a *prezygote* or *ootid.* Pronuclei come in close contact, eventually lose their apposed pronuclear membranes, and enter into syngamy. This final event of the fertilization process involves the reorganization and pairing of maternal and paternal chromosomes and formation of the zygote.

8. What percent of oocytes and preembryos are estimated to be chromosomally abnormal?

The fact that many gametes are genetically abnormal must account for much of the failed fertilization observed in IVF programs. If we are to accept earnestly the many reports describing high percentages of chromosome abnormalities in sperm, oocytes, and developing preembryos, it seems a wonder that we are managing so well to overpopulate the earth. It is well documented that chromosomal abnormalities among first-trimester spontaneous abortions occur at a rate of about 60%. In addition, it has been estimated that more than one-fourth of oocytes that fail fertilization and up to 10% of spermatozoa carry a chromosomal aberration. A review of the literature

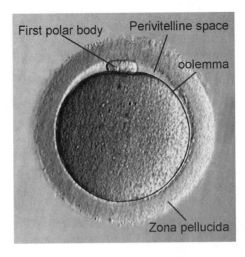

FIGURE 1. Fully mature oocyte at metaphase II (MII) of meiosis. (o, oolemma; p, perivitelline space; f, first polar body; z, zona pellucida).

has led some investigators to conclude that at least 50% of conceptuses developing after natural conception are chromosomally abnormal.

9. How are testicular biopsy specimens prepared for fertilization differently from ejaculated samples?

In the Cornell program, difficult testicular tissue samples are "digested" during processing, using enzymes such as collagenase to break down cellular bonds. This process ensures that bound spermatozoa are released from tissue components and can be isolated more easily.

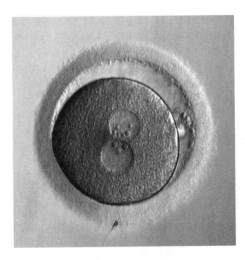

FIGURE 2. Oocyte in the process of fertilization displaying two pronuclei. A single spermatozoan is bound to the zona at a 6 o'clock position. The nucleoli within both pronuclei (female pronucleus above and male pronucleus below) are aligning at adjacent poles.

10. Are pregnancy results lower when microsurgically retrieved spermatozoa are used?
Results demonstrate that clinical pregnancy outcomes are not significantly lower for couples using microsurgically collected spermatozoa compared with couples using ejaculated spermatozoa.

11. Typically, what percentage of oocytes become fertilized normally after insemination or ICSI?
In the Cornell, program, three of four oocytes (75%) are expected to become normally fertilized after either insemination or intracytoplasmic sperm injection (ICSI) procedures are carried out.

12. How does an embryologist assess fertilization?
The embryologist must rely on the presence and number of pronuclei, assessed during one or two brief examinations, to determine whether normal fertilization is ongoing. Practical criteria for sperm penetration in living material include (1) observation of two pronuclei at 10–18 hours postinsemination, and (2) visualization of two polar bodies in the perivitelline space. Assessment of these two parameters is rapid and simple.

13. How accurate is pronuclei count in assessing fertilization?
Unfortunately, the identification of two pronuclei cannot ensure a normal fertilization process and does not guarantee that one pronucleus is of paternal and one of maternal origin. Evaluating second polar bodies is also potentially misleading because of polar body fragmentation. Yet another serious drawback to using a single observation to assess pronuclear number lies in the fact that counts have been observed to change during the pronuclear period. Most embryologists can relate instances of visualizing two pronuclei in an oocyte at an initial observation and one pronucleus (or three pronuclei) during a follow-up evaluation, or vice-versa. Although pronuclear and polar body determination are not ideal for the assessment of sperm penetration, they do provide the most useful and least time-consuming means of clinical evaluation.

14. If less than 50% of my eggs are fertilized normally, should I become concerned?
Absolutely not. Although statistics show us that normal fertilization occurs in three of four mature human oocytes, many couples experience fertilization results higher or lower than this average. Factors that influence fertilization include the proportion of oocytes that are indeed mature, proportion of oocytes that are truly healthy, and proportion of spermatozoa that are normal.

15. What are sequential media? Why are they now used so often in IVF laboratories?
Sequential media were developed in response to the need to culture preembryos beyond the 8-cell stage of development. These media mimic the nutrients found in the fallopian tube (phase I sequence) and the receptive uterine cavity (phase II sequence). Only with the development of sequential media have we been able to routinely grow viable blastocysts in IVF laboratories with some measure of confidence. By meeting the nutritional requirements of the preembryo as it develops and differentiates (including carbohydrate and amino acid gradients) and by reducing stress, one can support the development of highly viable blastocysts in culture.

16. What is the difference between an embryo and a preembryo?
These terms are often used loosely and interchangeably to describe the early conceptus from 2-cell to blastocyst stages. Technically, the **preembryo** represents the early cleavage stage before formation of the actual embryo. The preembryonic period ends at approximately 14 days after fertilization with development of the primitive streak. The true **embryo** then forms and persists until major organs are developed. Once the neural groove and the first somites are present, the embryo is considered completely formed. In humans, the embryonic stage begins at approximately 14 days after fertilization and encompasses the period when organs and organ systems are coming into existence.

17. What are the average developmental stages for preembryos on days 1, 2, 3, 4, and 5 after fertilization?

On a practical basis, two-cell conceptuses are observed at any time 20 hours after insemination, usually around 24 hours, and may persist until 42 hours after insemination. Viable four-cell preembryos are observed between 36 and 60 hours after insemination. Eight-cell stages are not generally seen until after 54 hours but usually before 72 hours. In normally fertilized specimens, retarded growth (no doubling in 24 hours) often indicates reduced viability, but accelerated cleavage (doubling in 12 hours) may not necessarily reflect a healthier conceptus. Occasionally pregnancies are established with slowly growing preembryos, even those found to possess only 6–8 blastomeres at 96 hours. In the Cornell program, intrauterine transfer is usually postponed whenever preembryos are observed to possess less than 5 blastomeres on day 3. If any further cleavage occurs over the next 48 hours, transfer is carried out; if no further cleavage occurs, transfer is cancelled.

If preembryos are cultured to the blastocyst stage (day 5 or 6 after fertilization), additional observations are carried out on days 4 and 5 and possibly day 6. One would expect to find appropriately compacting morulae on day 4 and cavitating blastocysts on days 5 and/or 6. (See Figs. 3–10).

18. What characteristics of the preembryo do embryologists note as favorable?

Few cytoplasmic fragments, equally sized blastomeres, and normal growth rate are considered good indicators of preembryo health.

19. Are cytoplasmic fragments within a preembryo considered to be detrimental to further development?

Because preembryos flushed from the uterine cavity after fertilization in vivo often exhibit cytoplasmic fragments, one can deduce that in vitro culture methods are not solely responsible for producing preembryos with this seemingly abnormal morphologic characteristic. Nonetheless, we observe that those exhibiting large numbers of anucleate fragments do tend to implant less frequently. This finding may be due to a reduction in the available cytoplasm necessary for normal cell division or may simply reflect that fact that numerous fragments interfere with the process of *compaction* by making intimate cell-to-cell contacts difficult.

20. What is "hatching"?

Hatching is the natural process by which the expanded blastocyst breaches and escapes through the zona pellucida, or shell, of the preembryo before implantation in the uterine cavity (see Figs. 11 and 12).

21. What is assisted hatching (AHA)? When should it be used?

Assisted hatching is a microsurgical procedure performed in the embryology laboratory on preembryos before intrauterine transfer. The procedure involves making a small hole in the zona pellucida, or outer shell of the preembryo, and theoretically facilitates the natural hatching process. Hatching from the zona pellucida is necessary before blastocyst implantation can take place in the uterine cavity. Excessive cytoplasmic fragments may be removed simultaneously during the procedure. Indications for assisted hatching are:

- Maternal age > 37 years
- Zona pellucida thickness > 17 ìm
- Other zona pellucida abnormalities, such as bilayering anomalies and odd shapes
- Greater than 20% cytoplasmic fragmentation
- Two or more previous failed IVF attempts

22. How are preembryos actually graded for quality?

As a result of the reported correlations between morphology and pregnancy, embryologists generally use some sort of grading scheme to document the presumptive quality of transferred

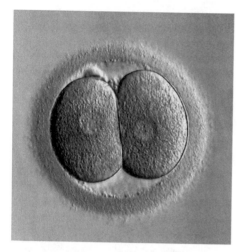

FIGURE 3. A two-cell conceptus. The first cleavage generally occurs at approximately 24 hours post-insemination.

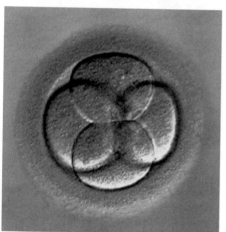

FIGURE 4. Four-cell conceptus exhibiting optimal morphology. The blastomeres are symmetrical and of equal size; two lie in one plane of focus and two others, with opposing polarity, lie in another. No cytoplasmic fragments are observed. The cytoplasm is clear and homogeneous. The zona shows normal morphology and is relatively thin.

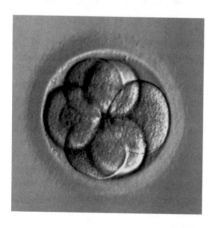

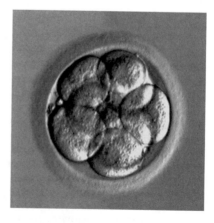

FIGURE 5. A preembryo with 6 blastomeres. Implantation of such a preembryo may lead to a healthy delivery.

FIGURE 6. Eight-cell conceptus.

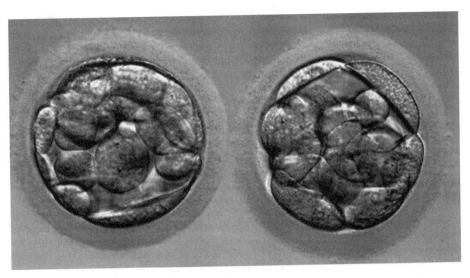

FIGURE 7. Two cavitating morulae approximately 96 hours after insemination.

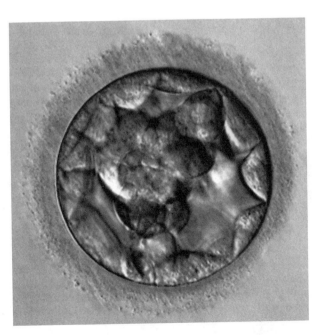

FIGURE 8. Cavitating morula on day 4. Cells inside are ICM cells, which are round in shape and are loosely aggregated. Cells located peripherally are trophectoderm cells, which show polarized alignment with one pole facing the zona pellucida while the other faces the blastocoele.

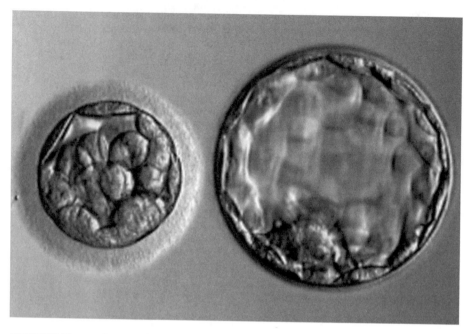

FIGURE 9. Blastocoelic enlargement. To the left, an early cavitating morula; to the right, an expanded blastocyst. Note the enlarging blastocoele and thinning zona pellucida as development advances.

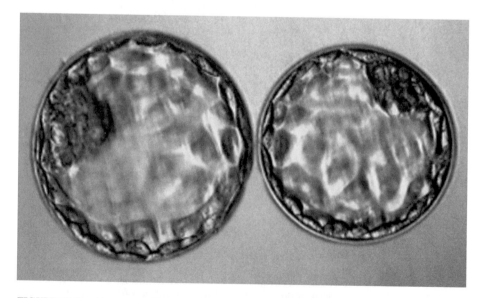

FIGURE 10. Two blastocysts with clearly distinguishable inner cell masses and confluent trophedtoderm.

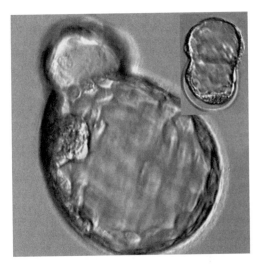

FIGURE 11. Initiation of hatching in a human blastocyst on day 6. In the human, the hatching site develops in close proximity to the ICM, while in the mouse hatching occurs in an area of the mural trophectoderm, opposite to the ICM (insert).

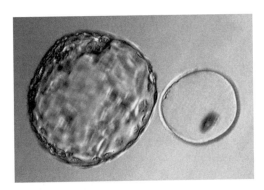

FIGURE 12. Hatched blastocyst. Note the increase in blastocyst size once the blastocyst is free of the zona pellucida.

preembryos. Most of these schemes are related to the extent of observed cytoplasmic fragmentation and growth rate, but some include other factors such as zona pellucida thickness or blastomere size or regularity. Usually, a grade is assigned to the transfer based on the morphology of the highest-graded preembryo in the group, with additional fractions added or subtracted for appropriate growth or for the concurrent transfer of other exceptional conceptuses. Some groups attempt to calculate an *average* score for the cohort of transferred preembryos based on the assigned grades of each individual preembryo, but these systems tend to be less informative when wide disparity exists between conceptuses, distorting the meaningfulness of an averaged final figure.

At Cornell, a day 3 grading system is used (1) to grade the morphology of cleaving preembryos and (2) to classify transfers according to the highest score in the cohort of conceptuses being replaced.

Grade 1: preembryo with blastomeres of equal size; no cytoplasmic fragmentation.

Grade 2: preembryo with blastomeres of equal size; minor cytoplasmic fragmentation covering <15% of the preembryo surface.

Grade 3: preembryo with blastomeres of distinctly unequal size; variable fragmentation.

Grade 4: preembryo with blastomeres of equal or unequal size; moderate to significant cytoplasmic fragmentation covering > 20% of the preembryo surface

Grade 5: preembryo with few blastomeres of any size; severe fragmentation covering > 50% of the preembryo surface

23. What does the grade of the preembryo mean?

We have observed that transfers with at least one grade 1 or grade 2 preembryo possess the greatest potential for establishing pregnancy. When data are normalized for the number of preembryos transferred, this trend still exists for all groups except single preembryo transfer, in which the number of replacements is too low for comparison and the group is highly represented by patients with poor ovarian response. Although a higher score (lower number in this case) is favorable, pregnancy is quite possible even in cycles with grade 4 or 5 morphology demonstrating blastomeres of unequal size and moderate-to-severe cytoplasmic fragmentation. Of interest is the fact that scores are remarkably repetitive for the same patient in succeeding cycles. The grading system used for blastocysts is described below.

24. What is a morula?

The morula is a developmental stage that occurs when the preembryo possesses approximately 8–16 blastomeres and begins to form intimate cell-to-cell contacts. At this stage, *compaction* begins and persists until the blastocyst is formed. The morula is commonly observed between 72 and 96 hours after insemination.

25. What does "compaction" mean in embryologic terms?

Compaction is a process through which a cleaving preembryo changes from a collection of individual cells into a more solid mass with indistinguishable cell membranes. Compaction results from the formation of tight intercellular junctions, which cause blastomeres to become closely apposed.

26. What is cavitation?

Cavitation is the process involving formation of the fluid-filled extracellular cavity within a compacted morula; this cavity increases in size to form the blastocoele of the blastocyst.

27. How are blastocysts graded?

Different grading systems have been proposed for scoring human blastocysts. One of the most popular was developed by David Gardner and his colleagues in the late 1990s.[1] In early 2000, we modified Gardner's 3-part grading system to fit the needs of the Cornell program. A blastocyst was defined as having a blastocoele filling greater than half the volume of the conceptus, and early stages must possess cells that suggest the formation of an inner cell mass (as opposed to *cavitating morulae,* which possess smaller blastocoeles and developing inner cell masses are unidentifiable). Briefly, our current system assigns to blastocysts a numerical score from 1 to 6 on the basis of their degree of expansion and hatching status:

1 = an early blastocyst (blastocoel filling greater than half of the volume of the conceptus) but without overall increase in size as compared with earlier stages.

2 = a true blastocyst (blastocoel filling greater than half of the volume of the conceptus) with slight expansion in overall size and some thinning of the zona pellucida.

3 = a full blastocyst (blastocoel filling greater than half of the volume of the conceptus) with overall size fully enlarged and a very thin zona pellucida.

4 = a hatching blastocyst (no biopsy, assisted hatching, or other artificial zona manipulation).

5 = a fully hatched blastocyst, completely removed from the zona pellucida (no biopsy, assisted hatching, or other artificial zona-manipulation).

6 = a hatching or hatched blastocyst resulting from manipulations that have created a substantial hole in the zona pellucida.

The development of the inner cell mass is assessed as follows: A, tightly packed, compacted cells; B, larger, loosely grouped cells or formation of a cellular bridge; C, no inner cell mass distinguishable; or D, cells of the inner cell mass appear degenerative. The trophectoderm is assessed as follows: A, many healthy cells forming a cohesive epithelium; B, few, but healthy cells, large in size, forming a loose epithelium; C, unhealthy, very large, or unevenly distributed cells, may appear as few cells squeezed to the side; or D, cells appear degenerative.

Using this system, transfers with at least one 1BD blastocyst (any real blastocyst by definition; 91% of cycles undergoing extended culture) result in a 75% clinical pregnancy rate and a 59% implantation rate. Transfers with at least one 3AA, 3AB, or 3BA blastocyst result in a 78% clinical pregnancy rate and 63% implantation rate. The fact that there is so little difference between cycles with "early" and "late" blastocysts indicate that *any* blastocyst on day 5 will lead to good pregnancy and implantation results. Only cycles without defined blastocysts on day 5 demonstrate significantly lower potential, although pregnancy and implantation are by no means negated (31% clinical pregnancy and 17% implantation).

28. Does maternal age play a role in pregnancy success after blastocyst transfer?

Shapiro et al.[4] studied the impact of maternal age in 300 women between the ages of 18 and 45 years undergoing blastocyst transfer. Fertilized oocytes were cultured up to 144 hours and subsequently transferred when at least one preembryo attained an expanded blastocyst stage. The rate of cycle cancellation before oocyte retrieval increased significantly with age, whereas the average number of oocytes per retrieval and the proportion of cycles with expanded blastocysts declined significantly. Although pregnancy rates per stimulation declined with age, pregnancy rates per transfer were approximately 50% across the entire age range. The decline in female fertility with age was concluded to be the result of reduced numbers of oocytes and the inability of fertilized oocytes to develop to the blastocyst stage. Implantation and pregnancy rates appeared to be unaffected by advancing age when blastocysts actually formed.

At Cornell, we have observed a similar trend toward higher clinical pregnancy rates in selected patients suitable for day 5 transfer over the age of 40 years. Nonetheless, the miscarriage rate, as reflected by a lower ongoing pregnancy rate in these women, is still higher than in younger women undergoing blastocyst transfer (see Tables 1 and 2).

Table 1. Results from All Day 5 Transfers, With and Without Actual Blastocysts Transferred

AGE (YRS)	NO. PATIENTS	NO. BL TR/TR	CLIN PREG/TR (%)	ONG PREG/TR (%)	MULT PREG/TR (%)	SACS/BL TR (%)
< 30	67	1.99 ± 0.12	72	69	37	59
30–33	104	2.04 ± 0.27	81	74	46	65
34–36	75	2.04 ± 0.26	68	57	32	53
37–39	53	2.11 ± 0.46	59	49	28	45
> 40	29	2.62 ± 0.67	66	41	17	37
Total	328	2.09 ± 0.38	71	62	36	55

BL = blastocysts, Sacs = gestational sacs by ultrasound examination.

Table 2. Results from All Transfer Cycles Involving at Least One True Blastocyst

AGE (YRS)	NO. PATIENTS	NO. BL TR/TR	CLIN PREG/TR (%)	ONG PREG/TR (%)	MULT PREG/TR (%)	SACS/BL TR (%)
< 30	64	1.98 ± 0.12	75	72	38	61
30–33	91	2.00 ± 0.21	86	78	52	71
34–36	71	2.03 ± 0.24	70	61	34	56
37–39	46	2.09 ± 0.41	63	52	30	48
> 40	26	2.65 ± 0.62	69	46	19	39
Total	299	2.07 ± 0.35	75	66	38	58

29. Are liveborn sex ratios skewed after blastocyst transfer?

The male:female live birth ratio for the U.S. and World is 1.05, or 51% males versus 49% females.[6] In our program, day 3 transfer has resulted in an expected male:female ratio of 51:49. The male:female ratio for day 5 transfer in our program is 56:44, an intriguing "mini-skew" that will be followed closely as numbers of children born after blastocyst transfer continue to grow.

30. Is the incidence of monozygotic twinning greater after blastocyst transfer?

Monozygotic (MZ) twinning results from the division of a single fertilized oocyte into two genetically identical preembryos, and is thought to occur in 0.42% of all deliveries from natural conception. Several studies have shown an increased risk for monozygotic twinning following day 5 transfer. Rates per clinical pregnancy range from 0% to 12.5%. The Cornell program has experienced a monozygotic twinning rate per clinical pregnancy of 0.49% for day 3 transfer (not significantly different from natural conception) and 3.4% per day 5 transfer (significantly higher than natural conception).

A synthesis of findings from various studies suggests at least three factors that are influential in monozygotic twinning among patients receiving infertility treatments: (1) ovulation induction, (2) certain IVF culture conditions, and (3) zona architecture/effect of micromanipulation. With these three variables occurring together so often in clinical infertility practice, the appropriate analysis to determine the specific contribution of each intervention has proved difficult to perform. If the natural rate of monozygotic twinning (0.42%) may be considered valid in settings of spontaneous conception and single implantation, the increase in the observed MZ twinning rate after blastocyst transfer may be partially explained by the increased number of implantations. Importantly, the clinical rarity of MZ twinning challenges the study of this phenomenon in the context of IVF, as relevant investigations require large samples ($> 10,000$ cases) to detect meaningful differences with suitable statistical power.[5]

31. Is blastocyst transfer really better than day 3 transfer?

Extended culture will not take a day 3 preembryo of poor quality and make it a better one. It is also unlikely that extended culture confers any special advantage to a woman with only one or two oocytes at harvest, at least not at this time. Our data show that in women exhibiting a good response to ovarian stimulation, transferring two embryos on day 3 serves the same purpose as transferring two blastocysts in terms of clinical pregnancy and reduction of high-order gestation. The value of blastocyst transfer arises from two factors:

1. In providing better selection criteria for determining exactly *which* conceptus should be transferred when numbers of fertilized conceptuses permit selection, and

2. In providing good chances for pregnancy with only one or two blastocysts replaced (thus lowering the multiple gestation risk).

32. What options are available to a couple persistently producing preembryos of poor quality (poor growth rates or poor morphology)?

- Change in ovarian stimulation protocol (medication type, dosages) or use of natural cycle
- Alteration in timing of hCG administration
- Change in fertilization method (ICSI or insemination)
- Change in culture media or protein supplementation
- Opportunity to culture fertilized oocytes on an autologous endometrial cell monolayer (co-culture)
- Application of assisted hatching
- Application of preimplantation genetic diagnosis
- Application of extended culture to determine whether or not preembryos arrest in culture
- Use of donor oocytes

33. What is coculture? Is it better than standard culture methods?

Coculture techniques appear to be helpful in encouraging preembryos to develop into viable fetuses. Fertilized oocytes are placed on a monolayer of cells during the culture period. Whether this monolayer imparts factors favorable to support growth,or whether the cells utilize unnecessary medium components and/or absorb toxins is not clearly defined. Probably coculture is helpful for both of these reasons, especially under conditions in which culture media or environmental factors are suboptimal. At Cornell, only autologous cell lines are used for coculture purposes in respect for patient safety and protection. Although autologous granulosa and cumulus cells have been utilized before, the current favored protocol involves the use of an endometrial cell line. Thus far, pregnancy rates have been highly encouraging for patients unsuccessful in previous attempts.

34. What are the differences among autologous, homologous, and heterologous coculture systems?
Autologous: derived from the same individual.
Homologous: derived from another individual in the same species.
Heterologous: derived from a different species.

35. How are autologous endometrial coculture cells prepared for use?
Briefly, endometrial cells are grown in culture after an endometrial biopsy. Once confluent, cells are frozen until the patient cycles for an IVF attempt, at which time the cells are thawed and plated. Three-fourths of a patient's fertilized conceptuses are placed on a monolayer of these cells on day 1 after harvest. Slightly enhanced growth and slightly improved morphology are noted for cocultured preembryos compared with controls.

36. Can any biochemical assays be used effectively to predict preembryo viability?
Recent studies have examined the relationship between preembryo nutrition and subsequent development in vitro.[2] It was determined that glucose consumption on day 4 by human preembryos was twice as high in those that ultimately formed blastocysts. It was also noted that blastocyst quality potentially affected glucose uptake, as evidenced by the fact that poor-quality blastocysts consumed significantly less glucose than top-scoring ones. Furthermore, there existed a significant spread of metabolic activities within a cohort of similarly graded blastocysts from the same patient. In another study looking at amino acids, it was found that depletion of leucine and formation of alanine (release into the surrounding medium on days 2 and 3) are positively correlated with normal blastocyst formation and implantation in the human.[3] These results suggest that assessing metabolic activity may prove a feasible means of determining conceptus "health."

37. When should preimplantation genetic diagnosis (PGD) be considered a management option?
To date, three major areas of PGD have been applied successfully. First, the sex of a preembryo can be determined reliably with fluorescence in-situ hybridization (FISH) techniques by using specific probes for the X and Y chromosomes or with specific sex chromosome sequence analysis by the polymerase chain reaction (PCR). In this manner, severe sex-linked disorders can be avoided. Secondly, by enumeration of chromosome composition utilizing fluorescence in situ hybridization (FISH), the exact ploidy of preembryos can be examined, concurrent with the diagnosis of certain common aneuploidies. For women of advanced maternal age, this option reduces or eliminates the risk of delivering a child with a chromosomal trisomy, such as Down's Syndrome (trisomy 21). FISH may also be used to detect structural chromosome abnormalities in cases of balanced translocations. Lastly, many single gene defects (e.g., cystic fibrosis, sickle cell anemia, Tay-Sachs disease) and other commonly occurring genetic disorders may be detected by PCR techniques. In the future, new DNA technologies, imaging systems, and chip technology may offer unimaginable possibilities for pinpointing single nucleotide variations within the entire human genome, thus allowing a precise prediction of preembryo genetic make-up.

38. What are stem cells? Why are they termed "pluripotent"?
Embryonic stem cells are cells with the ability to divide for indefinite periods in culture and

are able to give rise to the specialized cells and tissues of the body. These cells are generated from the inner cell mass of a blastocyst. Although stem cells can form every type of cell found in the human body, they cannot form an entire organism because they are unable to give rise to the placenta and supporting tissues necessary for development in the human uterus. These inner cell mass cells are therefore "pluripotent." Pluripotent stem cells undergo further specialization into stem cells that are committed to give rise to other cells with a particular function. These more specialized stem cells are termed *multipotent* stem cells. Examples of this include *blood stem cells,* which give rise to red blood cells, white blood cells, and platelets, and *skin stem cells* , which give rise to the various types of skin tissues.

39. What is genomic activation?

Genomic activation involves the transition of preembryonic development from control by maternally coded and stored messenger RNA in the oocyte to newly formed products of the preembryonic genome, including the paternally derived component. Genomic activation occurs at the 4- to 8-cell stage in human preembryos.

40. What is gene expression?

It is the full use of the information in a gene via transcription and translation, leading to production of a protein and, thus, the appearance of the phenotype determined by that gene. Gene expression is assumed to be controlled at various points in the sequence of events leading to protein synthesis. This control is thought to be the major determinant of cellular differentiation in eukaryotes.

BIBLIOGRAPHY

1. Gardner DK, Schoolcraft WB: In vitro culture of the human blastocyst. In Jansen R, Mortimer D (eds): Towards Reproductive Certainty: Infertility and Genetics Beyond 1999. Carnforth, Parthenon Press, 1999, pp 378–388.
2. Gardner DK, Lane M, Stevens J, Schoolcraft WB: Noninvasive assessment of human embryo nutrient consumption as a measure of developmental potential. Fertil Steril 76:1175–1180, 2001.
3. Houghton FD, Hawkhead JA, Humpherson PG, et al: Non-invasive amino acid turnover predicts human embryo developmental capacity. Hum Reprod 17:999–1005, 2002.
4. Shapiro BS, Richter KS, Harris DC, Daneshmand ST: Influence of patient age on the growth and transfer of blastocyst-stage embryos. Fertil Steril 77:700–705, 2002.
5. Sills ES, Moomjy M, Zaninovic N, et al: Human zona pellucida micromanipulation and monozygotic twinning frequency after IVF. Hum Reprod 15:890–895, 2000.
6. United Nations: Population Division. Available at http:/esa.un.org/unpp [panel 2].

39. EMBRYO TRANSFER

Lucinda L. Veeck, M.L.T., h.D.Sc.

1. How should physicians and patients decide how many preembryos to replace?
In deciding how many preembryos to transfer for a given patient, it seems most reasonable to weigh the risks of multiple pregnancy against age, previous history, preembryo morphology and development, desires of the couple, and the delivery and multiple gestation rates of a given clinic. Couples unwilling to consider selective reduction under any circumstance should never receive more than one or two conceptuses for transfer.

2. Which is better for transfer: a preembryo with 8 blastomeres or one with 14 blastomeres on day 3?
The ideal stage of development on the morning of day 3, approximately 65 hours after insemination or intacytoplasmic sperm injection (ICSI), is the 8-cell stage. Fewer than eight or greater than eight blastomeres by that time is associated with a lower incidence of blastocyst development, a finding closely confirmed by other investigators.

3. Which is better to replace: an 8-cell preembryo with 15% fragments or a 5-cell preembryo without any fragments?
The 8-cell preembryo, because a preembryo with up to 15% of its surface area filled with cytoplasmic fragments is not considered to be excessively compromised. Most embryologists prefer to replace the faster-growing conceptus.

4. Is a preembryo considered poor if it possesses an odd number of blastomeres?
No. In humans, 3-, 5-, 7-, and 9-cell preembryos are not uncommon, particularly when the examination is carried out during mitotic cell division. This sometimes asynchronous division persists throughout cleavage of the early healthy conceptus, and any number of blastomeres can be noted in a given observation.

5. If preembryos are graded very poorly, is it still worthwhile to carry out the transfer?
Because morphologic grading systems are subjective and imperfect, they can predict pregnancy potential only loosely. For instance, although pregnancy rates are shown to be lowest with the poorest grade within a grading system, pregnancy is not fully negated; neither is pregnancy an absolute certainty with the best grade of preembryos. For this reason, it is still reasonable to carry out transfer with preembryos exhibiting slow growth and/or moderate fragmentation.

6. Is it reasonable to replace fewer preembryos when morphology is extremely good?
It is not only reasonable, it is prudent to do so.

7. Should a "mock" transfer be carried out before the actual transfer?
A mock transfer involves passing an empty catheter through the cervical canal before preembryos are loaded in an effort to verify that the actual procedure can be performed easily and without trauma. Whether or not to carry out mock transfers is a clinic-specific choice. When done, mock transfers provide an element of safety and do not expose patients to increased discomfort.

8. Why is it important to carry out preembryo transfer under sterile conditions?
Bacteria and airborne toxins possess the potential to compromise preembryo viability. For this reason, transfers are carried out in operating rooms or clean-procedure rooms under sterile conditions. In addition, the introduction of any nonsterile instrument into the vaginal canal potentially exposes patients to avoidable health risks.

9. Why are powdered surgical gloves washed with sterile water before use in the embryology laboratory and operating room?

Studies done in the early 1980s demonstrated that the powder present on most surgical gloves is extremely toxic to mouse and human preembryos. It has become general practice, therefore, to use either powderless gloves or to rinse gloves with sterile water before use.

10. What should physicians and embryologists do when a patient presents with an allergy to latex products?

Patients with latex allergies must be protected from exposure to any latex product, either directly or through inhalation of airborne particles. When a patient presents with such an allergy, non-latex gloves are used throughout her treatment. In addition, she should be scheduled as the first oocyte harvest and first intrauterine transfer of the day so that airborne particles are reduced within the procedure room.

11. Is preembryo transfer painful to most women? Does it require anesthesia?

For the vast majority of women, preembryo transfer without anesthesia is painless and is carried out in an unexpectedly rapid manner. The occasional woman with a pain-sensitive cervix may experience some discomfort as the catheter passes into the uterine cavity, but usually not enough discomfort to require anesthesia.

12. Does the presence of blood and/or mucus on the transfer catheter impact subsequent results?

In our experience, when the soft and pliable Wallace catheter is used, blood and mucus are rarely observed. Nonetheless, analysis of transfer data indicates that the presence of blood on the outside of the catheter is not negatively associated with pregnancy success.

13. Is one transfer catheter better than another?

The choice of transfer catheter is highly clinic-specific. In the Cornell program, physicians prefer to use a very soft and pliable catheter as opposed to the more rigid types. It is believed that a softer catheter exposes the cervix to less trauma and reduces uterine contractility.

14. What can physicians and embryologists do when a transfer is extremely difficult?

With appropriate investigation beforehand, transfer difficulty can be anticipated and dealt with before the actual replacement. Women can have the cervix dilated in advance, transfers can be scheduled for an earlier day, or anesthesia can be considered. It is not unusual to attempt a mock transfer and/or dilation at the time of oocyte harvest while a patient is sedated. In addition, several options are available on the day of replacement: (1) use of a tenaculum to straighten the cervical canal, (2) minor dilation, and (3) ultrasound guidance. These efforts,however, are rarely required in an experienced program.

15. What options are available when a transfer is not possible on day 3 (e.g., because of patient illness, ovarian hyperstimulation, extreme cervical stenosis)?

The most common options are delaying transfer until day 5 or cryopreserving all preembryos for future replacement.

16. How long does it usually take to complete intrauterine transfer?

At Cornell, the average time that a patient spends in the procedure room is less than 15 minutes. During this time, she discusses her treatment with the attending physician and attending embryologist, is prepared for transfer (put into lithotomy position, with vaginal/cervical area washed), a mock transfer is done, and the actual transfer is carried out.

17. What exactly is in the catheter besides the actual preembryo?

Avery small volume of culture medium and, in the Cornell program, a small volume of the patient's own blood serum. We choose never to transfer any foreign protein to our patients.

18. Do patients ever run the risk of having foreign protein transferred into their bodies during preembryo replacement?
Some groups choose to transfer small amounts of commercially available serum or plasma products to the uterus because these products are components of their culture medium/culture system. At Cornell, where all media are prepared on site, we have chosen to use a patient's own serum in an effort to assure ourselves that patients are protected against any threat of homologous infective agents.

19. In the case of a woman using a gestational carrier, would one carry out transfer using the serum of the genetic mother or of the carrier?
The carrier's serum should be used, since she is the one having preembryos put into her body.

20. What is the approximate volume of culture medium transferred along with the preembryo?
Approximately 50 μl or 0.05 ml.

21. Do blastocysts require special handling at the time of intrauterine transfer?
Yes. Because they are fluid-filled (possess a blastocoel), they tend to float rather than sink when transferred to the more viscous medium that often has a high protein composition. This characteristic makes them a bit more difficult to be picked up within the catheter without drawing up excessive amounts of extra medium. In addition, the zona pellucida that surrounds an expanded blastocyst is very thin and fragile or may be absent altogether. Because these conceptuses are more highly prone to traumatic damage, special care must be exerted to handle them carefully and gently.

22. Can preembryos stick to the inside of the transfer catheter? If they do, is pregnancy still possible after a second transfer?
Preembryos can stick inside or be left inside a transfer catheter. For this reason, embryologists always return to the laboratory to inspect the catheter and rinse it thoroughly before a patient is released from the procedure room. If one or more preembryos are identified in the medium that is rinsed through the catheter, it/they can be washed and retransferred easily. Subsequent pregnancy rates do not appear to be negatively affected after a transfer/retransfer is carried out.

23. Is it better to perform preembryo transfer under ultrasound guidance?
Some groups experience improved pregnancy rates using ultrasound guidance during intrauterine transfer procedures, whereas others do not. In our experience, the use of ultrasound guidance is indicated for difficult replacements and has been found useful as a teaching tool.

24. How long should a woman stay in bed after transfer?
There are no published studies to indicate that any period of bed rest is necessary after intrauterine replacement. Nonetheless, most programs advocate a quiet period of approximately 30 minutes before patients are released.

25. Are there restrictions to physical activities after preembryo transfer?
Common sense dictates activities following the procedure. It is probably prudent to avoid overly strenuous activities for the first few days, remembering that implantation will occur about 1 week after oocyte collection. Beyond that, there are few specific recommendations other than the instructions given by the attending physician.

26. Can preembryos "fall out" or be expelled from the uterus after coughing or physical trauma?
No.

27. If a patient is given medications such as antibiotics or corticosteroids to take until pre-embryo transfer but still has some left when transfer is done, should she finish the medications or stop taking them?

Finish all medications as prescribed.

BIBLIOGRAPHY

1. Kojima K, Nomiyama M, Kumamoto T, et al: Transvaginal ultrasound-guided embryo transfer improves pregnancy and implantation rates after IVF. Hum Reprod 16:2578–2582, 2001.
2. Sallam HN, Agameya AF, Rahman AF, et al: Impact of technical difficulties, choice of catheter, and the presence of blood on the success of embryo transfer—experience from a single provider. J Assist Reprod Genet 20(4):135–142, 2003.
3. Spandorfer SD, Goldstein J, Navarro J, et al: Difficult embryo transfer has a negative impact on the outcome of in vitro fertilization. Fertil Steril 79:654–655, 2003.
4. van Weering HG, Schats R, McDonnell J, et al: The impact of the embryo transfer catheter on the pregnancy rate in IVF. Hum Reprod 17(3):666–670, 2002.

40. CRYOPRESERVATION OF PREEMBRYOS

Lucinda L. Veeck, M.L.T., hD.Sc.

1. When were the first clinical pregnancies established using cryopreservation techniques?

The first delivery after freezing and thawing a human preembryo took place in Australia in 1983. Subsequent to that event, the first child was born after freezing a human blastocyst in the United Kingdom in 1985.

2. Why is the cryopreservation procedure considered an important adjunct therapy during in vitro fertilization (IVF)?

Most IVF programs have embraced cryobiology to augment clinical pregnancy from a single cycle of ovarian stimulation. As ovulation induction protocols have improved, allowing the recruitment of multiple healthy oocytes, the need has grown to manage their numbers responsibly. It is usual today to harvest in excess of 10, or sometimes even 20, mature oocytes from a woman. Before freezing techniques were routinely used in the laboratory, a woman producing so many gametes would be forced either to limit the number inseminated or to risk having to discard healthy preembryos since only three or four could be transferred safely to the uterus after fertilization.

3. Is preembryo cryopreservation permissible in every country in the world?

Most countries embrace cryopreservation as a means of storing fertilized conceptuses for potential future transfer. But some countries, such as Germany, place strict limitations on the use of this technique. Although there is no explicit legal prohibition against cryopreservation in Germany, in practice, German guidelines permit freezing only at the pronuclear stage of development. Cryopreservation of preembryos is permitted only under special circumstances (e.g., in cases in which embryo transfer is not possible). A few other countries have published similar guidelines.

4. Which preimplantation developmental stage is optimal for cryopreservation (1-cell, 4-cell, 8-cell, or blastocyst)?

All developmental stages freeze and thaw well. However, depending on the protocols used for the procedures, a given reproductive center may experience better pregnancy rates with one stage over another. For instance, in the Cornell program, clinical pregnancy rates after freezing and thawing blastocysts are higher than those observed with earlier stages, but this may not be the case for all programs.

5. Does any evidence indicate that the method of ovarian stimulation affects survival or pregnancy after thawing and replacement?

Despite reports in the literature about poorer preembryo survival or lower pregnancy rates using various ovarian stimulation protocols, we have not been able to demonstrate significant differences in our results. In other words, the experience of a large IVF program using multiple methods to recruit oocytes has shown that once a preembryo or blastocyst is frozen, its chances for surviving thaw and implantation are stable across all modes of ovarian stimulation.

6. What are "cryoprotectants"? Why are they used?

Freezing techniques use cryoprotective agents to control ice crystal formation at critical temperatures. The formation of intracellular ice crystals can mechanically damage preembryos and blastocysts by disrupting and displacing organelles or slicing through membranes. It has been shown that when human cells are placed into a medium that contains an intracellular cryoprotective agent, intracellular water readily exits the cell as a result of the higher extracellular concentration of cryoprotectant. This form of dehydration protects the cell.

7. What is "seeding"? Why is it important during the freezing process?

Cryoprotectants are beneficial in their ability to lower the freezing point of a solution. Solutions may remain unfrozen at $-5°C$ to $-15°C$ because of *super cooling* (cooling to well below the freezing point without extracellular ice formation). When solutions super-cool, cells do not dehydrate appropriately because there is no increase in osmotic pressure from the formation of extracellular ice crystals. To prevent super-cooling, an ice crystal is introduced in a controlled fashion in a process called *seeding*. This process contributes to intracellular dehydration as water leaves the cell to achieve equilibrium with the extracellular environment. If the rate of cooling is too rapid, water cannot pass quickly enough from the cell, and as the temperature continues to drop, it reaches a point when the intracellular solute concentration is not high enough to prevent the formation of ice crystals.

8. Which cryoprotectants are optimal for different stages of development?

Membrane permeability by cryoprotectants varies between developmental stages. As such, it has been found that different cryoprotective agents are more suitable for freezing than others. Dimethyl sulfoxide (DMSO) and 1,2-propanediol (PROH) are frequently used for freezing early cleavage stage preembryos, whereas glycerol is commonly used for blastocysts. All three intracellular agents have fairly small molecules that permeate cell membranes easily. In addition, there are several extracellular substances that help dehydrate and protect cells. The most frequently used is sucrose, which possesses large, nonpermeating molecules and exerts an osmotic effect to aid in accelerated cell dehydration. Sucrose cannot be used alone but is often used in conjunction with standard permeating, intracellular cryoprotectants.

9. What is vitrification? Has this technique been used successfully for preserving human preembryos?

The idea behind vitrification is to protect cells by completely avoiding all ice crystal formation. To accomplish vitrification, cryoprotective solutes must be increased to 40% (weight/volume) or higher. DMSO is frequently used, but PROH, ethylene glycol, and other agents have been tested. Because high concentrations of these cryoprotectants are toxic at room temperature, specimens are generally exposed to them at $0°C$. Samples may be plunged directly into liquid nitrogen without needing to introduce a seed; the viscosity is so high that solutions solidify into glasslike states. Vitrified specimens must be thawed in ice water, which is fairly inconvenient. Although the procedure has been slow to gain acceptance for routine human cryopreservation, several live births have recently been reported.

10. Is it better to freeze in cryovials, straws, or cryoloops?

All three freezing vessels demonstrate highly satisfactory results after minor modifications are made in freezing protocols. The only concern with the use of cryoloops is the direct exposure of specimens to liquid nitrogen and the potential cross-contamination of microbes and/or viruses that may be in the liquefied gaseous solution.

11. Should one worry about cross-contamination of viruses or bacteria within liquid nitrogen storage tanks?

Cross-contamination has generated great concern for IVF programs because bacteria and viruses may remain viable under typical freezing conditions. Responsible programs minimize risks by providing quarantine storage tanks for preembryos from virally infected patients and by choosing methods of storage (storage vessels and vessel covers) that reduce the opportunity for infectious agents to spread.

12. How long does the actual freezing process take?

Typical cryopreservation protocols involve a 2- to 4-hour freezing process. Vitrification procedures, however, are carried out very rapidly.

13. Are preembryos usually frozen separately or in groups?

Depending on the number frozen, preembryos can be stored separately or frozen in groups of two to three per cryovial or straw. It is a common practice to freeze multiple preembryos together (usually two) in an effort to reduce total storage space.

14. What is the temperature of liquid nitrogen (the liquefied gas used to freeze and store preembryos)?

Liquid nitrogen is quite cold—approximately $-196°C$.

15. How are frozen preembryos stored to ensure their safety over long periods of time?

Under liquid nitrogen storage, preembryos remain frozen and safe. Cryostorage tank maintenance involves routine, documented checks to ensure that liquid nitrogen levels are adequate, that low-level alarm systems are in place and working properly, and that the physical storage tanks themselves are free from defects (e.g., they do not exhibit tank "sweating" or breaks in the vacuum seals).

16. How long can frozen preembryos be stored in liquid nitrogen?

During the storage phase, all chemical reactions within cells should be suspended. Under extremely cold liquid nitrogen storage conditions, it is estimated that it would take hundreds of years before background ionizing radiation could cause significant damage to stored cells.

17. Generally, what percent of frozen preembryos survive freezing and thawing?

Three out of four conceptuses are generally expected to survive the rigors of freezing and thawing. This proportion may be somewhat higher or lower in individual programs and may show some patient variability, but overall survival rates within any program should certainly be higher than 50%.

18. How does one know if a preembryo has survived freezing?

Fertilized oocytes. The morphology of thawed pronuclear oocytes is generally similar to pre-freeze appearance, but occasionally the cytoplasm is clearer and organelle accumulation around pronuclear structures is reduced. After thawing, nucleoli are often seen scattered within pronuclei despite their alignment at pronuclear junctions before freezing. Because it is single-celled, it is easy to determine whether or not the pronuclear oocyte has survived thawing; when its membrane is not intact, the cell appears flattened and usually dark in color. Left in culture for 15–24 hours, the healthy pronucleate oocyte enters into syngamy, completes the fertilization process, and proceeds to the first cleavage. Cell division is the true indicator of survival after thaw; fewer than 5% that appear healthy after thawing fail to follow this pattern.

Preembryos. Survival is sometimes difficult to evaluate because not all blastomeres survive freezing and thawing. Dying blastomeres may be present among living ones but can be removed easily during assisted hatching procedures. Generally, a preembryo possessing > 50% viable blastomeres upon thaw is considered a survivor.

Blastocysts. One uneasy task immediately after thawing is to determine that a blastocyst has indeed survived because it presents in a contracted state for up to several hours after reincubation in standard culture medium. In our experience, blastocysts that shrink appropriately in response to cryoprotective agents, exhibit contracted, healthy-appearing cells after thaw, and proceed to re-expand in a short time survive quite well.

19. How are frozen embryo transfer (FET) cycles monitored differently from fresh IVF cycles?

Most thawed preembryos are replaced in either natural (no exogenous medications) or programmed cycles (cycle controlled by drugs). Natural cycle replacement is considered the easier regimen and is suitable for women who ovulate regularly and normally. In natural cycles, blood is drawn daily from approximately day 10 of the menstrual cycle and tested for estrogen (E_2) and luteinizing hormone (LH); ultrasound scans may be performed on a daily or every-other-day basis to access follicle growth and ultimate follicle disappearance. On the other hand, programmed cycles usually involve downregulation of the cycle with agonists of gonadotropin-releasing hormone (GnRH), followed with E_2 replacement by means of injection or patch for a given number of days. Replacement in a programmed cycle is much more like undergoing a fresh cycle. Examples of typical replacement regimens carried out in the Cornell program are given below:

Natural cycle
- *Prezygotes:* Thaw on day of ovulation or next day (day after LH peak and/or day of E_2 drop); transfer on day after thaw.
- *Preembryos:* Thaw one day after ovulation (two days after LH peak and/or day after E_2 drop); transfer on day of thaw.
- *Blastocysts:* Thaw five days after LH peak; transfer on day of thaw.
- No progesterone unless indicated/previous failure.
- Methylprednisolone (16 mg/day for 4 days starting on day of LH surge) plus tetracycline (250 mg 4 times/day for 4 days, starting on day of LH surge).
- Progesterone (if indicated): 200 mg micronized P_4 vaginally 2 or 3 times/day; continued until negative pregnancy test 14 days after replacement or through week 12 if pregnancy occurs (weaned downward starting in weeks 9–10).

Programmed cycle
- Luteal suppression with 0.2 mg GnRH agonist; 0.1 mg starting on predetermined day 1 and maintained until day 15 (adequate suppression confirmed on day 2 of cycle).
- Transdermal estrogen patches (Climara, 0.1-mg patch):
- Days 1–4   0.1 mg every other day
- Days 5–8   0.2 mg every other day
- Days 9–10   0.3 mg every other day (depending on E_2 levels)
- Days 11–14   0.4mg every other day
- Days 15+   0.2 mg (two patches every other day for 7 weeks)
- 50 mg P_4 starting on day 15; continued until negative pregnancy test or through 12 weeks' gestation (weaned downward starting week 9–10, depending on serum levels).
- Tetracycline (250 mg 4 times/day for 4 days) plus methylprednisolone (16 mg/day for 4 days) starting on day 15.
- *Prezygotes:* Thaw on day 16; transfer next day.
- *Preembryos:* Thaw on day 17; transfer same day.
- *Blastocysts:* Thaw day 20; transfer same day.

20. Do thawed preembryos replaced in natural cycles do better than those replaced in programmed cycles using medications?
When replacements are carried out as outlined above, there appears to be no difference in clinical pregnancy results between natural or programmed cycles.

21. Do preembryos that have undergone ICSI survive freezing and thawing at the same rates as those having undergone insemination?
Yes.

22. Why is it important to freeze the pronuclear stage oocyte before it enters syngamy?
Because waiting to freeze the fertilizing oocyte after this event negatively affects results. It is thought that the lack of a spindle during this stage in large part explains its excellent potential for survival and implantation. However, the urgency to begin freezing before a designated time has proved inconvenient for some programs without adequate staffing.

23. If not all the blastomeres (cells) of a preembryo survive freezing and thawing, will this have a negative impact on subsequent implantation?
Although there is no convincing evidence that the loss of one or two blastomeres is overtly

detrimental to very early developing preembryos, it has been reported that fully intact preembryos demonstrate a higher implantation rate than partially intact ones.

24. Should degenerative blastomeres be physically removed from a preembryo before intrauterine transfer?

It is quite reasonable to remove degenerating or dying blastomeres because their presence may adversely affect living cells. Removal can be accomplished through a process called assisted hatching. A hole is made in the zona pellucida of a preembryo through which the dying cells are removed.

25. Do blastocysts frozen on day 5 of development (about 120 hours after insemination) implant at greater rates than those frozen on day 6 (about 144 hours after insemination)?

It is generally assumed that blastocysts that develop in a timely manner in vitro are of better quality than those that develop more slowly. However, a retrospective review of blastocyst thaw outcomes from Cornell demonstrates otherwise. In our program, blastocysts have been frozen on either day 5 or day 6 depending on their speed of growth in vitro. Blastocysts frozen on day 5 are thawed the day before transfer, whereas blastocysts frozen on day 6 are thawed in the morning when transfer is carried out.

In 2002, we analyzed pregnancy outcomes in 84 patients returning for thawed blastocysts over a 2-year period. Thirty-nine patients received a transfer from day 5 frozen-thawed blastocysts and 45 patients underwent transfer with day 6 blastocysts. There were no significant group differences in patient age (34.0 vs. 34.8 years, respectively), average number of blastocysts transferred (2.3 vs. 2.0), or morphology of the blastocysts after thawing. No significant differences were found in the post-thaw survival rates (73.4% vs. 80.5%), clinical pregnancy rates (63.2% vs. 63.4%), or ongoing pregnancy rates (55.3% vs. 53.7%), nor were differences observed in implantation rates (39.8% vs. 39.5%) between the two groups. Although it is logical to assume that preembryos reaching the blastocyst stage faster (on day 5) might be "healthier" than their day 6 counterparts, these data and the data of others suggest that rate of development may not be crucial to subsequent post-thaw success.

26. Why do blastocysts contract when they are placed in cryoprotective media?

Blastocysts with a high probability of survival after thaw act as perfect osmometers, shrinking, reexpanding, and swelling in accordance with their osmotic environment.

27. Do all blastocysts reexpand after cryopreservation and thawing? Is this process important?

In our experience, healthy blastocysts reexpand within a few hours of thawing, sometimes almost immediately. Those that do not are considered to be nonviable.

28. Can blastocysts be frozen successfully after they have hatched from the zonae pellucidae?

Zona-free blastocysts (either naturally or purposefully hatched) survive freezing and thawing without difficulty, indicating that the zona coat is not necessary for protective purposes during these procedures.

29. What does "cumulative" pregnancy mean in terms of cryopreservation and thawing?

A cumulative pregnancy rate includes pregnancies from both fresh and frozen/thawed replacements. This method assesses the total pregnancy potential from a single cycle with freezing and accounts for pregnancy achieved from either fresh or thawed attempts within a given population.

30. How are base fresh pregnancy rates and cumulative pregnancy rates calculated?

1. The **base** fresh pregnancy rate is defined as the number of clinical pregnancies established after the transfer of noncryopreserved preembryos divided by the number of noncryopreserved (fresh) transfer cycles: 250/500) $\times$ 100 = 50%.

2. The **cumulative** or "augmented" pregnancy rate is defined as the actual number of clinical pregnancies generated by the transfer of noncryopreserved preembryos *plus* the actual number of clinical pregnancies generated by the transfer of thawed preembryos in cycles failing to become pregnant with fresh transfer, divided by the total number of cycles with transfer: (250 + 125/500) × 100 = 75%. Using this method, cycles with fresh pregnancy only or thawed pregnancy only contribute equally to the final result; cycles with pregnancies in both fresh and thawed attempts are counted only once (e.g., as a cycle with pregnancy).

Cumulative pregnancy rates are apt to be greater than 85% for patient populations with at least one frozen/thawed preembryo, indicating a high clinical pregnancy potential in established programs with solid cryopreservation techniques.

31. Which is more important—age of the preembryo at the time of freezing or age of the patient at the time of replacement?

Clearly, maternal age of the patient or an oocyte donor at the time of freezing has a greater impact on subsequent results than does patient, donor, or recipient age at the time of thawing.

32. Does any evidence suggest that children born after freezing and thawing are at higher risk for congenital abnormalities?

Cryopreservation has no apparent negative impact on perinatal outcome and does not appear to adversely affect the growth or health of children during infancy and early childhood. The available data indicate no elevation in the congenital malformation rate for children born after freeze/thaw procedures.

33. What are a couple's options if they decide that they do not wish to continue storing frozen preembryos?

Three options are generally available to parents not wishing to maintain their frozen preembryos: (1) thaw them for destruction (thaw in such a manner that they are no longer viable); (2) donate them for approved research efforts; or (3) donate them to another infertile couple. The third option requires additional medical screening on the part of donors.

34. What generally happens to frozen preembryos that are abandoned by their parents?

In some countries, such as the United Kingdom, laws mandate destruction after a given period of abandonment. Abandonment is defined as no communication with parents over 5 years, no payment for storage fees, and no success in contacting parents after sincere, documented efforts to locate them. In the United States, there is no such mandate, and most programs are left to make their own regulations to cover these unfortunate instances.

BIBLIOGRAPHY

1. Cohen J, Simons RF, et al: Pregnancies following the frozen storage of expanding human blastocysts. J In Vitro Fertil Embryo Transf 2(2):59–64, 1985.
2. Trounson A, Mohr L: Human pregnancy following cryopreservation, thawing and transfer of an eight-cell embryo. Nature 305:707–709, 1983.

41. OVARIAN STIMULATION FOR ASSISTED REPRODUCTION

Owen K. Davis, M.D., and Zev Rosenwaks, M.D.

1. What are the indications for and limitations of natural cycle in vitro fertilization (IVF)?
The first successful, full-term human IVF pregnancy resulted from the retrieval of a single, endogenously selected oocyte in a spontaneous menstrual cycle. Subsequent clinical experience demonstrated a marked improvement in IVF success rates with the transfer of multiple embryos and led to the routine use of ovulation-inducing agents to effect controlled ovarian hyperstimulation (COH). Nonetheless, some assisted reproduction therapy (ART) centers continue to offer unstimulated, natural cycle IVF as an alternative strategy that may reduce the expense associated with gonadotropins and that essentially eliminates the risks of ovarian hyperstimulation syndrome (OHSS) and multiple pregnancies. In addition, unstimulated IVF may be considered in clinical circumstances in which the hyperestrogenic state resulting from exogenous stimulation of the ovaries is deemed to pose unique risks, as in patients with a history of breast cancer or thromboembolic disorders. These same patients may also experience increased risks with pregnancy, however, and should undergo appropriate pretreatment consultation and counseling. Finally, natural cycle IVF may also be considered in patients who fail to respond to COH and for whom exogenous hormones confer no additional benefit.

2. Can oral antiestrogens be used as single agents for IVF?
The use of clomiphene citrate (CC) as a single agent for ART is infrequent, owing to the recovery of only one or two oocytes per cycle. In addition, this approach entails a relatively high risk of cycle cancellation (25–40%) due to an inadequate response or premature surge of endogenous luteinizing hormone (LH). CC is typically administered orally at a dose of 100–150 mg for 5–7 days, commencing between the second and fifth day of the cycle. Cycle monitoring entails serial sonograms and serum estradiol and LH levels, often with frequent urinary LH measurements as follicular maturation becomes advanced. Oocyte retrieval is generally timed with the administration of exogenous human chorionic gonadotropin (hCG; 5,000–10,000 IU) once the lead follicle attains a mean diameter of at least 18 mm, with harvest 34–36 hours later.

Tamoxifen, a related oral antiestrogen, has recently been proposed for COH in breast cancer survivors undergoing ART, given that it can effect multifollicular recruitment and is deemed safe and, in fact, therapeutic in such patients. Again, the decision to attempt conception naturally or through fertility treatments in the setting of a history of breast cancer should be undertaken with appropriate consultation with the patient's oncologist and after discussion of the theoretical risks.

3. Can the response to oral antiestrogens be enhanced with gonadotropins in ART?
The coadministration of exogenous gonadotropins with CC was found to lead to a considerably more robust follicular response than CC alone, and this approach to COH was widespread before the popularization of pure gonadotropin protocols. CC and gonadotropins may be coadministered either concurrently or sequentially. Concurrent regimens entail administration of CC (50–150 mg) for 5 days in the early follicular phase, with coincident administration of gonadotropins (typically at doses ranging from 75 to 300 IU/day). In sequential protocols, the administration of CC precedes the initiation of gonadotropin stimulation, often with 1 or 2 days of overlap. As with CC-only regimens, hCG is administered once the lead follicles are 18 mm or larger. Before the introduction of gonadotropin-releasing hormone (GnRH) antagonists, the principal disadvantage of this approach was the relatively common occurrence of an untimely spontaneous LH surge. Although CC is currently not a mainstay of COH for ART, combined CC/gonadotropin protocols may still be useful in the empirical treatment of patients with a low response to more commonly used regimens.

4. Can ovarian stimulation be achieved by using gonadotropins alone?

Gonadotropin-only ART regimens were introduced on the premise that pure gonadotropins represent a more physiologic approach to COH, avoiding some of the potentially detrimental effects of CC on oocytes and endometrial development. At present, several gonadotropin preparations are commercially available, including urinary menotropins (human menopausal gonadotropin [hMG], purified urinary follicle-stimulating hormone [FSH]) and recombinant formulations (e.g., rFSH, rhCG). All are injectable, and most can be administered either subcutaneously or intramuscularly. Before the advent of GnRH agonists, gonadotropins were administered alone, starting on cycle day 2 or 3, in an effort to optimize the recruitment of follicles from the gonadotropin-sensitive pool. Such protocols used hMG and FSH, either alone or in combination, at an initial total daily dosage ranging between 150 and 300 IU/day for most patients.

5. What is the role of GnRH agonist (GnRHa) in ovarian stimulation for ART?

GnRHa blocks the release of gonadotropins from the pituitary gland. The use of GnRHa is considered the dominant approach to COH. This downregulation approach obviates the approximately 10% risk of cycle cancellation due to spontaneous LH surges associated with premature ovulation. In addition, evidence indicates that this approach leads to an overall enhancement of IVF success rates.

6. Describe the GnRHa downregulation protocol.

Standard GnRHa downregulation in the U.S. typically entails the initiation of daily subcutaneous leuprolide acetate, 0.5–1.0 mg daily, in the mid-luteal phase of the preceding menstrual cycle (e.g., day 21 of a 28-day cycle). Exogenous gonadotropin stimulation commences after the onset of menses (typically day 2 or 3, but initiation may be delayed), with continuation of the leuprolide until the administration of hCG, once the lead follicles have attained a mean diameter > 16 mm. Although routine luteal support with exogenous progesterone is the dominant practice pattern in ART, this approach is particularly advised in the setting of GnRHa downregulation, given the suppression of endogenous gonadotropins.

7. What are the disadvantages of GnRHa downregulation?

- Increased duration and total dose requirement for gonadotropins.
- Risk of oversuppression with a resulting low stimulation response, particularly in patients with unsuspected diminished ovarian reserve.
- Luteal initiation of a GnRHa may also result in baseline ovarian cysts due to the initial agonistic effects. For this reason; some clinics routinely pretreat with an oral contraceptive pill (OCP) to reduce the occurrence of functional cysts.

During COH, the initial daily gonadotropin dosage may remain fixed or be either increased or decreased ("step-up" or "step-down") according to protocol and individual patient response. We prefer a step-down approach with dosage reduction once initial follicular recruitment has been achieved, typically after 2–4 days of stimulation (e.g., at an estradiol level of 150–200 pg/ml). This strategy reduces the total gonadotropin dosage, thus reducing cost and risk of OHSS and possibly resulting in more synchronous follicular development.

8. What is hormonal luteal support ?

Routine exogenous hormonal luteal support for ART has gained widespread acceptance. This practice stems, in part, from concerns that the luteal phase is often shortened in gonadotropin-stimulated cycles and that the aspiration of follicles at the time of oocyte harvest may impair subsequent luteal phase steroidogenesis through the mechanical disruption of the granulosa cells. Most clinicians advocate luteal supplementation in protocols using GnRHa or GnRH antagonists, given the suppression of endogenous pituitary function. The importance of luteal support in general has not been unequivocally established, but one meta-analysis demonstrated an overall benefit in terms of IVF pregnancy rates.

9. How is hormonal luteal support achieved?

Most commonly, exogenous pure progesterone is administered, starting on the day after oocyte retrieval. We prefer intramuscular progesterone in oil, 25–50 mg/day, which is continued until at least day 28 and subsequently until documentation of fetal cardiac activity in conception cycles. Alternatively, progesterone may be administered via vaginal suppositories, capsules, or vaginal gels. Another approach to luteal support is the administration of additional hCG injections following embryo transfer. This approach is comparably effective but entails a higher risk of developing OHSS, particularly in patients with an exuberant response to COH.

10. Why is ovarian hyperstimulation important for ART?

Ovarian hyperstimluation is important for ART insofar as multiple oocytes and embryos can be obtained. The goal of COH for ART is to attain multiple mature oocytes, thus permitting an increased likelihood of fertilization and the availability of normally developing embryos, the replacement of more than one embryo in an attempt to optimize pregnancy rates, and a greater ability to select morphologically "optimal" embryos for transfer. In addition, multiple oocytes/embryos permit cryopreservation for future use and are important for ancillary procedures, including preimplantation genetic diagnosis (PGD). About 25–50% of embryos are expected to harbor the genetic abnormality in question.

11. How does individual patient response to COH vary?

Individual patient response to COH is highly variable. Patients can be broadly categorized as normal, high, and low responders. Consistent criteria for classifying response are lacking, although most clinicians agree that a cycle resulting in a peak estradiol level < 600 pg/ml and 5 or fewer oocytes constitutes a low response, whereas a cycle with a peak estradiol level > 2,000 pg/ml and 20 or more oocytes constitutes a high response. An abnormal response, whether deficient or excessive, can be problematic and presents a clinical challenge. Low responders attain fewer oocytes and embryos, and embryo quality frequently is reduced due to diminished ovarian reserve. High responders, on the other hand, are at increased risk for the development of severe OHSS, which can be life-threatening.

12. How can a patient's response to COH be predicted?

A given patient's response to previous COH attempts is invaluable in determining an optimal protocol for further treatment, and records of prior cycles should be reviewed. When a presenting patient is treatment-naïve, the choice of protocol is influenced by a number of factors, including age, results of ovarian reserve testing, and ovulatory status. Generally speaking, younger patients with normal ovarian reserve testing (e.g., day 3 FSH and estradiol levels, clomiphene citrate challenge testing, basal antral follicle counts) or a history of polycystic ovary syndrome (PCOS) tend to manifest a high (and potentially excessive) response to COH, whereas older patients and/or patients with abnormal ovarian reserve testing (e.g., borderline or elevated FSH) tend to manifest a lower and possibly inadequate response. The selection of the optimal stimulation protocol, therefore, depends on the patient's history and clinical (physical and laboratory) evaluation.

13. What strategies are effective in treating high responders?

Patients manifesting an excessive response to COH are at high risk for both OHSS and cycle cancellation in an effort to avert OHSS. Such a "PCO-like" response can be tempered by a "gentle" approach to COH. The use of GnRHa downregulation, in and of itself, does not attenuate the risk of an excessive response, nor is the choice of purified or recombinant FSH in lieu of hMG (which has primarily LH-like activity) advantageous. Rather, the most effective approach is a reduction in the dose of gonadotropins (e.g., initiated at 150 IU/day), in some cases combined with "dual suppression," consisting of an OCP for 21 or more days, overlapping with a GnRHa for continued downregulation. In our experience, dual suppression combined with low-dose gonadotropins is the most effective approach to treatment of the abnormal high responder. This strategy attenuates the peak estradiol response and optimizes the proportion of mature oocytes retrieved.

14. Can a COH cycle with an abnormally high response be salvaged?

In some cases, an excessive response cannot be predicted or occurs despite a modest stimulation protocol. Cycle cancellation (stopping gonadotropins and withholding hCG) prevents OHSS but requires retreatment at a subsequent interval. In some cases, particularly when the pre-retrieval estradiol level and/or number of intermediate size follicles is deemed to pose a moderately increased risk for OHSS, a reduced dose of hCG (3,300–5,000 IU) can be administered with cryopreservation of all embryos for transfer in a future cycle. Cryopreservation without embryo transfer reduces the incidence, severity, and duration of OHSS, given that the syndrome is exacerbated by pregnancy, due primarily to endogenous production of hCG. Similarly, a patient's clinical progression can be closely monitored in the interval between oocyte harvest and potential transfer. When the risk of OHSS is considered excessive (e.g., pain, weight gain, markedly enlarged ovaries, or significantly increased volume of free pelvic fluid determined by sonography), cryopreservation can be performed for all embryos.

15. What is "coasting"?

An alternative to cycle cancellation or primary cryopreservation in COH cycles manifesting an excessive estradiol response has been termed "coasting" and consists of withholding gonadotropins for 1 or more days while continuing pituitary suppression with the GnRHa. Our general practice is to consider coasting in the setting of mature follicles with a peripheral estradiol level exceeding 3,000–3,500 pg/ml or in the setting of smaller follicles (e.g., lead diameters of 13–14 mm) with excessive and rapidly increasing estradiol levels. Although the estradiol level typically rises during the first 1 or 2 days of coasting, a decline is generally seen within 2–3 days. HCG can then be administered (usually at a dose of < 5,000 IU), once the serum estradiol drops to a safer concentration (e.g., < 3,000).

In "coasted" ART cycles, fewer total oocytes generally are recovered in comparison with "noncoasted" cycles with upfront cryopreservation of all embryos, but pregnancy rates following fresh transfer are satisfactory with a comparably reduced incidence of OHSS. In essence, "coasting" can avoid the need for future "thaw" cycles using cryopreserved embryos. It should be emphasized that even with coasting, it is still essential that patients undergo close clinical monitoring to determine whether one should proceed with embryo transfer. Postretrieval cryopreservation may still be prudent if the risk of significant OHSS is nonetheless perceived to be high.

16. Discuss some of the pitfalls in choosing a protocol for the low responder.

Treatment strategies for stimulation of the low responder are generally less successful than those designed to attenuate the response of high-response patients. As a group, low-response patients tend to be older and are more likely to manifest clinical evidence of diminished ovarian reserve (i.e., diminished numbers and/or quality of oocytes). The relative efficacies of the available COH regimens for this poor prognosis population are difficult to assess rigorously, given the inconsistent definitions of what comprises a "low responder" in the published literature and the inherent heterogeneity of this population. Furthermore, there are exceedingly few randomized, controlled trials (RCTs) of different stimulation protocols; most reports use patients as their own historical controls, an approach compromised by phenomena such as "regression to the mean."

17. What strategies are frequently used for stimulation of the poor responder?

Although intuitively appealing, simply increasing the dose of administered gonadotropins beyond 300 IU/day is of limited benefit in treating low-response patients undergoing ART. Nonetheless, clinicians often prescribe 450 IU/day as a starting dose in such cases.

In marginally low-response patients (e.g., older women with normal ovarian reserve testing), reducing the GnRHa dosage in long suppression protocols may be beneficial (e.g., "low dose" leuprolide, initiated at 0.5 mg rather than 1 mg/day in the preceding mid-luteal phase and subsequently reduced to 0.25 mg/day with the commencement of COH).

Current, maximally aggressive COH strategies can be broadly divided into (1) GnRHa "flare" protocols and (2) protocols avoiding the use of a GnRHa altogether with the addition of a terminal course of a GnRH antagonist once follicular recruitment has been achieved with a high-dose gonadotropin regimen to avoid a premature LH surge. Other empirical strategies include combined clomiphene citrate with high-dose gonadotropins (see above) and, more recently, the adjunctive use of aromatase inhibitors such as letrozole.

18. What are GnRHa "flare" protocols?
Two flare strategies have been widely used in an effort to adequately treat poor-response patients undergoing ART.
One approach, variably called a "short," "flare-up," or "co-flare" GnRHa protocol, entails the administration of full-dose GnRHa commencing in the early follicular phase (e.g., leuprolide, 1 mg/day starting on cycle day 2) with addition of high-dose gonadotropin stimulation (e.g., 450 IU) on day 3 or 4. In the flare protocols, the agonist properties of the GnRHa preparation are exploited. This strategy allows utilization of the patient's initial endogenous gonadotropin surge to augment the ovarian response to achieve ovarian hyperstimulation.
The principal alternative flare protocol is the OCP/ "microdose agonist" or "microflare" regimen. The patient receives OCP pretreatment for 14–21 days, followed by twice-daily administration of microdose agonist (typically leuprolide, 40 μg twice daily) commencing on the third day after discontinuation of the OCP. High-dose gonadotropins are initiated on the third day of the microflare. Of note, this protocol requires dilution of the GnRHa by the dispensing pharmacy/clinic.
Proponents of the OCP/microdose strategy argue that the OCP reduces the likelihood of corpus luteum rescue and that the very low dose of GnRHa leads to a more sustained stimulation with less augmentation of ovarian androgen production than the standard flare strategy. Once again, randomized controlled trials are lacking, and the use of such protocols should be empirically tailored to the individual patient.

19. What is the role of GnRH antagonists in the treatment of the poor responder?
Apart from flare-type protocols, regimens incorporating one of the GnRH antagonists (e.g., ganirelix, cetrorelix) are the other dominant contemporary approach to the stimulation of the low responder. High-dose gonadotropin stimulation is initiated at the start of the follicular phase, with the addition of the GnRH antagonist once follicular recruitment has been observed (e.g., mean diameter of lead follicles exceeding 12 mm). This approach avoids any pituitary suppression until the point at which prevention of an endogenous LH-surge is desired. Available published data do not permit definitive comparison of the antagonist vs. flare protocols for poor response patients. One apparent advantage of the antagonist approach is the potential for fewer injections and a shorter duration of stimulation compared with the OCP/microdose agonist regimens.

BIBLIOGRAPHY

1. Benadiva CA, Davis O, Kligman I, et al: Withholding gonadotropin administration is an effective alternative for the prevention of ovarian hyperstimulation syndrome. Fertil Steril 67:724, 1997.
2. Licciardi FL, Liu H-C, Rosenwaks Z: Day 3 estradiol serum concentrations as prognosticators of stimulation response and pregnancy outcome in patients undergoing in vitro fertilization. Fertil Steril 64:991, 1995.
3. Muasher SJ, Oehninger S, Simonetti S, et al: The value of basal and/or stimulated serum gonadotropin levels in prediction of stimulation response and in vitro outcome. Fertil Steril 50:298, 1988.
4. Schoolcraft W, Schlenker T, Gee M, et al: Improved controlled ovarian hyperstimulation in poor responder patients with a microdose follicle-stimulating hormone flare, growth hormone protocol. Fertil Steril 67:93, 1997.
5. Scott RT, Hofmann GE, Oehninger S, et al: Intercycle variability of day 3 follicle-stimulating hormone levels and its effect on stimulation quality in in vitro fertilization and embryo transfer. Fertil Steril 54:297, 1990.

42. INTRAUTERINE INSEMINATION

Janet Choi, M.D., and Pak H. Chung, M.D.

1. What is intrauterine insemination (IUI)?

IUI is a procedure in which semen, often after a "washing" procedure to improve the quality and concentration of motile sperm, is placed into the woman's cervix (also known as intracervical insemination; Fig. 1) or uterus (Fig. 2) near the time of ovulation. This procedure is often recommended for couples who are infertile because the male partner has difficulties in depositing semen into the cervix/uterus through natural intercourse or mild-to-moderate impairment in semen parameters, particularly sperm density and motility. The pregnancy rate of IUI can be significantly improved if the female partner undergoes ovulation induction.

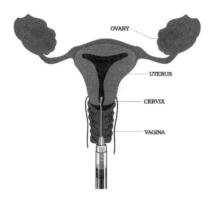

FIGURE 1. Intracervical insemination.

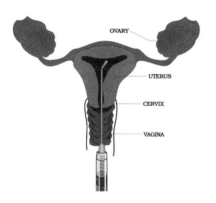

FIGURE 2. Intrauterine insemination.

2. How do you evaluate patients before starting a clomiphene citrate (CC)/IUI or gonadotropin/IUI cycle?

A basic work-up of both female and male patients should be performed to determine the cause of infertility. The female should undergo a thorough history and physical exam, with special attention to the menstrual history, prior pregnancies (if any), and any prior fertility treatment. Laboratory evaluations should include day 3 levels of follicle-stimulating hormone (FSH) and estradiol (E_2) to determine ovarian reserve; if these levels indicate compromised reserve, one may consider proceeding to IVF. Other lab tests include levels of thyroid-stimulating hormone (TSH) and free thyroxine (T_4) to rule out thyroid dysfunction, prolactin levels, cervical cultures to rule out gonorrhea and chlamydial infection, and liver function tests if history or physical exam suggests the presence of active liver disease. In addition, hysterosalpingography (HSG) helps to determine tubal patency. Because CC is relatively noninvasive and inexpensive, some physicians forego a complete infertility work-up before initiating CC treatment, waiting to finish the evaluation if the patient fails several CC cycles.

3. Who are candidates for CC treatment? Who may not respond at all to CC?
    CC can be used for ovulation induction in anovulatory or oligo-ovulatory patients or for superovulation in patients who regularly ovulate. Patients who best respond to CC tend to be relatively well estrogenized (positive progestin withdrawal bleed) and have normal gonadotropin levels. Other patients who may benefit from CC are those with luteal phase defects (stimulating multiple follicles may then stimulate more progesterone production in the luteal phase) and unexplained infertility. Patients who are hypogonadotropic or hypergonadotropic with low estrogen levels (severe hypothalamic dysfunction or ovarian dysfunction) generally do not respond to CC treatment.

4. What is the mechanism of action of CC?
    CC has combined estrogen antagonist and agonist effects. At the level of the hypothalamus, CC acts as a weak agonist, binding the nuclear estrogen receptors for weeks at a time (compared with native estradiol, which binds only for several hours), thus eliminating estrogen's negative feedback effect. Release of gonadotropin-releasing hormone (GnRH) is then increased, stimulating more gonadotropin release and resulting in the development of more follicles. In the genital tract (endometrium, vagina), the antagonistic effects of CC are more apparent; it can thin the endometrial lining and decrease vaginal cornification. CC may also decrease cervical mucus production.

5. How is CC usually dosed for IUI?
    CC is available as 50-mg tablets. The usual starting dose is 50–100 mg per day from day 3 to 7 or day 5 to 9. Dosage may be adjusted according to the body mass index (BMI) of the patient, and treatment can be initiated at half a pill (25 mg) per day. There is no significant difference in success rates in relation to which cycle day CC is started, so long as the treatment is initiated before dominant follicle selection is under way. Once ovulation is achieved with a certain dose, that dose should be maintained for several cycles before more aggressive treatment is attempted. If ovulation does not occur or if follicular development is poor (< 2), the dosage is increased by 50 μg for the next cycle. Generally, increasing CC dosage also increases the antiestrogenic effects on the endometrial lining and cervical mucus production. The maximum daily dose used is 200–250 mg. Note that 50% of CC conceptions occur at the starting dose, and 70% occur with doses $\leq$100 mg. For ovulatory patients who are trying to delay ovulation for religious reasons (e.g., Orthodox Jewish women), the physician may suggest taking the CC a little later in the cycle (cycle days 5–9 or even 7–11).

6. If patients do not respond to CC treatment but are not amenable to gonadotropin injections, are there any other alternatives?
    If a patient does not respond to maximal doses of CC, prolonging the duration of CC treatment from 5 to 8 or 10 days can be considered. Studies have shown that this approach may increase circulating estrogen levels, enhancing follicular development. In patients with polycystic ovary syndrome (PCOS), the use of metformin may enhance the responsiveness of the ovaries to CC.

7. Are any side effects associated with CC?
    The main side effects include hot flushes (10%), abdominal/pelvic discomfort (5%), breast discomfort (5%), nausea and/or vomiting (2%), headaches/mood changes (1.3%), visual changes (1.5%), and, rarely, hair loss or dryness (0.3%). Poor cervical mucus may also result from CC

treatment; the reported incidence ranges from 15% to 50%. Ironically, luteal phase defects can result from CC treatment, presumably from the antiestrogenic effects on the endometrium. In such cases, human chorionic gonadotropin (hCG) or progesterone supplementation can be used, or the patient can be advanced to gonadotropin therapy. Every patient who undergoes CC treatment should be advised of the 12–15% multiple pregnancy rates, consisting largely of twins.

8. How should a patient undergoing CC/IUI treatment be monitored?

Because CC is a first-line infertility treatment, it usually does not require extensive monitoring. If timed intercourse is anticipated, patients can start home monitoring of ovulation by urine detection of luteinizing hormone (LH), beginning on day 10 (given a 28-day cycle). The couple should have intercourse on 3 consecutive nights, starting with the evening of the surge. If no LH surge is detected by urine by day 14, the woman should be monitored in the office by vaginal ultrasound examination. HCG triggering is performed when the lead follicle is 18 mm or larger in diameter. If IUI is used, patients can either monitor ovulation by urine, as described above, or be monitored by ultrasound examination, starting on day 10. Once an LH surge is detected or the lead follicle reaches 18 mm when HCG is to be given, patients are scheduled for an IUI on the following morning.

9. If a patient fails CC, what do I do next?

Failure with the use of CC has to be defined as ovulation failure or conception failure. If a patient does not ovulate even with the highest dose of CC (200–250 mg/day), the physician has to resort to the use of gonadotropins. However, in cases of conception failure, the patient and physician should be aware that each treatment cycle with CC/IUI is associated with only an 8–12% pregnancy rate. CC/IUI should be repeated for up to 3–6 cycles (depending on the age and anxiety level of the patient) before treatment is escalated.

10. Infertility treatment follows the law of diminishing return. Explain.

Treatment of infertility at any level is usually most effective within the first 3–6 cycles. Beyond that point, pregnancy is less likely. There may be some factors prohibiting pregnancy that the particular treatment is not correcting. Patients should be counseled to consider more aggressive therapy. Prolonging treatment at any level without progression does not benefit patients. One would hate to see a 40-year-old patient, for instance, who failed 3 years of CC treatment.

11. What is the role of the use of metformin in ovulation induction?

For women with PCOS who are insulin-resistant (ratio of fasting glucose to fasting insulin < 4.5), the use of metformin (500 mg 2 or 3 times/day) in conjunction with CC may improve the success rates. Metformin, which decreases hepatic gluconeogenesis and increases insulin sensitivity, has been found to decrease hyperinsulinemia, free testosterone levels, and basal and stimulated LH levels in insulin-resistant women, thus helping to improve responses to CC. Some detractors question whether the improvement in fertility is due to the metformin or the weight loss that generally follows the start of metformin therapy. For patients with milder PCOS without insulin resistance, the addition of metformin to ovulation induction is more controversial.

12. Does dexamethasone have a role in ovulation induction?

In patients with high androgen levels, dexamethasone (0.5 mg at bedtime) helps blunt the nocturnal peak of adrenocorticotropic hormone (ACTH). It thus decreases the adrenal contribution to the androgen pool, and ovarian follicular androgen levels decrease as well. These actions may help sensitize ovarian response to CC. However, dexamethasone is associated with the usual steroid side effects and has to be used and monitored with caution. In current practice the ready availability of gonadotropins for patients who fail to respond to CC almost precludes the use of dexamethosone.

13. Is CC contraindicated in any patients?

Preexisting ovarian cysts, especially if large (greater than 15–20 mm at our center) generally preclude the use of CC and gonadotropins until the cysts resolve. The concern is that the medications may stimulate further cyst growth and ovarian enlargement. Some physicians, however, do not routinely screen for cysts at the beginning of CC treatment. Because CC is partly metabolized in the liver, patients with active liver disease should not undergo CC treatment. In addition, patients who have experienced visual disturbances in the past with CC should not use it again.

14. What is the cost of a CC/IUI cycle?
Five CC pills (50 mg each) cost about $50, whereas an IUI may cost anywhere from $250 to $400 (which includes the IUI and sperm wash). Doctor's fees may be additional.

15. What is the pregnancy rate per CC/ IUI cycle?
As previously stated, the monthly pregnancy rate is about 8–12%. The 6-month cumulative conception rate is about 60–75% in the indicated (anovulatory or unexplained infertility) patient population.

16. If patient does not become pregnant with an adequate trial of CC, gonadotropin therapy is indicated. What types of gonadotropins are available on the market?
Gonadotropoins are FSH and LH. They are either urine-derived or manufactured using recombinant DNA technology. The second process involves insertion of the human FSH or LH genes into Chinese hamsters cells, which then produce human gonadotropins. Available products on the market include pure FSH and combination FSH/LH.

	Pure FSH	**FSH + LH**
Urine-derived	Metrodin	Pergonal
	Fertinex	Repronex
Recombinant	Gonal-F	
	Follistim	

The above gonadotropins were available at the time of the writing of this book. Soon urinary products will be phased out and recombinant gonadotropins will predominate.

17. Is there a difference in efficacy between pure FSH and a combination of FSH/LH?
Theoretically they can be used interchangeably for ovulation induction as long as the total dosage is determined. However, in patients with PCOS and a low FSH/LH ratio, the use of pure FSH is usually advocated. In patients with hypogonadotropic hypogonadism, the use of both FSH and LH should be considered. In the setting of in vitro fertilization (IVF), certain patient populations will benefit from the addition of LH.

18. What are the side effects of gonadotropin therapy?
Gonadotropins are more potent stimulants of the ovaries than CC. Patients have to be counseled that the risk of multiple births is much higher. In general, there is a 20–25% chance of multiple births, largely composed of twins. But in younger patients, the potential risk of conceiving triplets or higher-order multiples is significant (5%). Therefore, intensive follicular monitoring is mandatory. If more than 3–4 mature follicles are detected in any treatment cycle, consideration should be given to canceling the cycle or converting to IVF if it is an option. Ovarian hyperstimulation syndrome (OHSS) is associated with gonadotropin therapy. Again, follicular monitoring is crucial to the avoidance of severe OHSS. Occasionally, the injection of gonadotropin can cause local irritation, redness, or swelling.

19. Given the potential serious side effects of gonadotropins, how do I monitor a gonadotropin/IUI cycle?
On cycle day 2 or 3, patients should have a baseline ultrasound (to rule out any ovarian cysts or other pathologies) as well as a serum check of estradiol (E_2), FSH, and LH. At our laboratory, if the E_2 is greater than 70 pg/ml or FSH is greater than 12 mIU/ml, indicating compromised ovarian reserve, we do not start treatment during that month. The starting dosage of gonadotropins is based on the patient's age, ovarian reserve, BMI (higher dosages for higher BMI), and past stim-

ulation history (if any). If a patient appears to have PCOS, we generally start on very low-dose gonadotropins (1 ampule or 75 units per day) because of the patient's sensitivity to these drugs. Otherwise patients are started with 150 units per day. Typically, patients return after 2–3 days of gonadotropin therapy to check an estradiol level. Ultrasonographic monitoring begins after 4–5 days of therapy with daily ultrasounds and estradiol checks once the lead follicles attain diameters of 12–13 mm. The dosage of gonadotropins is adjusted according to response. One word of caution about patients with PCOS: stimulation has to be slow. One should never rush to increase the dosage of medication if a patient does not respond. We usually increase by half an ampule of gonadotropin every 5–7 days of stimulation until a response is seen.

Normally, patients without PCOS require about 7–9 days of gonadotropin therapy before the follicles are mature enough (diameter of 16–18 mm) to be triggered for ovulation with exogenous hCG. About 34 hours after hCG administration, IUI is performed. Although textbooks maintain that luteal support is not necessary in cycles not using GnRH suppression, we tend to use some form of vaginal progesterone support starting 2 days after the IUI until 7 weeks of pregnancy or until the patient begins her next menstrual cycle.

20. In a treatment cycle using ovulation induction drugs, should an IUI always be performed?

In the absence of a male factor and antisperm antibodies, IUI is not necessarily required. However, patients have to be counseled about pregnancy rates of treatment with and without IUI. In a retrospective analysis of treatment for unexplained infertility, investigators found that pregnancy rates per cycle were as follows: CC/intercourse (IC), 5.6%; CC/IUI, 8.3%; gonadotropins/IC, 7.7%; and gonadotropins/IUI, 17.1%. In general, whenever gonadotropins are used, given the nature and involvement of the therapy, IUI is always recommended despite the absence of male factor infertility.

21. Is there a benefit to doing more than one IUI (i.e., 2 IUIs on 2 consecutive days) per treatment cycle?

Although some studies have reported increased pregnancy rates with IUIs 12 and 36 hours after hCG administration, a recent meta-analysis found no significant improvement in pregnancy rates with two IUIs versus one IUI. We encourage the couple to have intercourse on the day of or following the day of insemination. In certain patient groups for whom intercourse with resultant sperm ejaculation is not possible, such as lesbian couples, one can argue for the use of two IUIs following the hCG trigger.

22. What is the cost of a gonadotropin/IUI cycle?

Gonadotropins cost between $35 and $70 per ampule or 75 units. If a patient averages 2 ampules per day for 7–9 days, the cost of the medication approximates $1000. HCG costs about $30–40 per vial. Add the cost for monitoring and IUI, and the final cost may total about $2000–2500 per cycle for patients with no insurance coverage.

23. What is severe OHSS?

Severe OHSS occurs in 1–2% of stimulated cycles, although the incidence of milder forms can be as high as 20–30%. No one is certain of the exact pathophysiology of OHSS, but it is thought that high E_2 levels resulting from controlled ovarian hyperstimulation (COH) cycles triggered by ovulatory doses of hCG can induce OHSS in certain patients. Vascular endothelial growth factor (VEGF) stemming from ovarian granulosa cells also seems to have a role in OHSS, triggering the increased vascular permeability and third spacing of fluid found in OHSS. Risk factors associated with the development of OHSS include young age, low body weight, rapidly increasing E_2 levels, high follicle count, and PCOS.

One cannot always predict who will develop OHSS, however. Many patients with very high E_2 (> 3000 pg/ml) will not develop OHSS, whereas others with relatively low E_2 levels (< 1500 pg/ml) occasionally show signs and symptoms of OHSS. Most patients with OHSS present within a few days to 1 week of hCG administration, with another subset presenting at the time of increasing hCG levels associated with pregnancy. Signs and symptoms range from mild abdominal discomfort to nausea, vomiting, tense abdominal distention (from fluid third-spacing, ascites), ovarian enlargement (ovarian dimensions can range up to 15–20 cm in length in rare cases), and shortness of breath (either from abdominal fluid pushing up on the diaphragm or from hydrothorax). With the fluid shifts, hemoconcentration and hypovolemia can occur with a resultant increase in blood viscosity (and a possible increased risk of coagulation), hypotension, and decreased organ (such as renal or hepatic) perfusion. In the most extreme cases, renal failure and/or thromboembolism can occur. Fortunately, most cases do not reach such severity and can be managed on an outpatient basis with reassurances to the patient that symptoms usually resolve over 7–14 days.

Although severe OHSS requiring hospitalization is relatively infrequent, we monitor COH patients closely for developing OHSS. Anyone complaining of abdominal discomfort following a COH cycle with hCG is brought in at least for a baseline assessment. A thorough physical exam checking for hypotension, sudden weight gain (from fluid retention), respiratory distress, ascites, and deep venous thrombosis is performed. A vaginal ultrasound is done to check for free fluid in the pelvis as well as for ovarian enlargement (> 5–6 cm). Baseline laboratory assessment includes a complete blood count (checking for leukocytosis and/or hemoconcentration due to fluid shifts) and an electrolyte panel (to check for hyponatremia, renal or hepatic dysfunction). If symptoms are severe, prothrombin time and partial thromboplastin time are measured to assess the need for anticoagulation. If patients are found to have mild symptoms of OHSS but are able to tolerate oral intake of fluid and food and have normal laboratory values, they are generally managed on an outpatient basis. If the patient is unable to tolerate oral intake and/or manifests laboratory abnormalities such as a hematocrit > 50, hospital management is considered with strict monitoring of fluid input/output and coagulation prevention.

24. What are the criteria for canceling a CC or gonadotropin cycle?

If a patient fails to develop any mature follicles following a full course of CC or gonadotropins (up to 1–2 weeks), the cycle should be stopped. On the flip side, if the patient develops too many mature follicles (usually ≥4) with estradiol levels > 1500 pg/ml, treatment should also be cancelled, and no IUI or pregnancy attempt by intercourse should be done because of the increased risk of multiple pregnancies. (In this situation, the risk of multiple pregnancies needs to be weighed against the patient's age and likelihood that she would become pregnant at all). If conversion to IVF is a possible option, patients should be counseled. If the decision to convert to IVF is made, a GnRH antagonist should be administered to minimize risk of ovulation before oocyte retrieval.

25. Is there a role for natural cycle/IUI in treating some patients?

Natural cycle/IUI alone is indicated in young, regularly ovulating patients with a mild male factor. It may also be indicated in patients using donor sperm.

26. Does the use of ovulation induction medications increase the risk of ovarian cancer?

Although some early studies suggested an increased risk of ovarian epithelial cancer in patients previously treated with fertility drugs, these findings have been questioned. Many researchers believe that it is not the fertility drugs but rather patients' history of infertility that places them at an increased risk of developing ovarian cancer. A recent meta-analysis found no increased risk of invasive ovarian cancer with fertility drug use, although there was a small risk of borderline serous tumor development in nulligravid women using fertility drugs (OR = 2.43, 95% CI = 1.01, 5.88). In general, the use of ovulation induction medications is believed to be safe as long as there is an appropriate indication, monitoring is adequate, and the patient is fully counseled.

27. How is IUI actually performed?

After timing for IUI is decided, the male partner usually collects the sperm specimen at home or at the center. Sperm wash takes generally 30–60 minutes to prepare the sperm for IUI. IUI usually does not require analgesics or anesthesia. After the cervical mucus is wiped, the sperm pellet is drawn into a flexible plastic catheter, which is then inserted gently into the uterine cavity through the cervix. Caution must be taken to avoid pushing the catheter too hard and causing bleeding. A trick is to bend the tip of the catheter to avoid catching it within the crevices of the cervical glands. A smooth and easy IUI should be accomplished within 1 or 2 minutes. An important step before the actual IUI is to verify the specimen with the couple.

28. What is the risk of infection with IUI? Does it warrant the use of antibiotics?
The risk is fairly low; about 1 in 500 IUIs result in infection. Sterile preparation and handling of the specimen and a swift IUI are keys to preventing complications. Avoid contaminating the tip or portion of the catheter to be inserted into the uterine cavity.

29. How is the luteal phase managed in ovulation induction treatment cycles?
Progesterone supplementation is usually recommended empirically in both CC and gonadotropin cycles, despite the lack of clear evidence from a randomized, controlled trial to prove its superior efficacy compared with no supplementation. If progesterone is used, it is started two days after IUI. Progesterone formulations commonly used include vaginal suppositories, 200 mg at bedtime or twice daily, and micronized progesterone, 200 mg 3 times/day, applied vaginally. Intramuscular progesterone is seldom used in IUI cycles. Rarely, some physicians prefer the use of hCG for luteal support.

30. When do I perform a pregnancy test after IUI?
Fourteen days after IUI, serum hCG can be assessed to document IUI outcome. Even in the absence of pregnancy, menses may be delayed because of the use of progesterone. Therefore, a missed period is not a reliable way to determine pregnancy. If progesterone has been used, it should be continued for another 3 weeks until ultrasonographic evidence of a fetal heartbeat is established.

31. How do I calculate gestational age in IUI cycles?
If pregnancy is established, the day of IUI should be considered as two weeks' gestational age.

BIBLIOGRAPHY

1. Adashi EY: Ovulation induction: Clomiphene citrate. In Adashi EY, Rock JA, Rosenwaks Z (eds): Reproductive Endocrinology, Surgery, and Technology, vol. 1. Philadelphia, Lippincott-Raven, 1996, pp 1181–1206.
2. American Society for Reproductive Medicine: Guideline for Practice: Induction of Ovulation with Clomiphene Citrate. Birmingham, AL, American Society for Reproductive Medicine, YEAR?
3. American Society for Reproductive Medicine: Guideline for Practice: Induction of Ovulation with Human Menopausal Gonadotropins. Birmingham, AL, American Society for Reproductive Medicine, YEAR?
4. Cantineau AE, Heineman MJ, Cohlen BJ: Single versus double intrauterine insemination (IUI) in stimulated cycles for subfertile couples. Cochrane Database Syst Rev (1):CD003854, 2003.
5. Franks S, Hamilton-Fairley D: Ovulation induction:gonadotropins. In Adashi EY, Rock JA, Rosenwaks Z (eds): Reproductive Endocrinology, Surgery, and Technology, vol. 2. Philadelphia, Lippincott-Raven, 1996, pp 1207–1223.
6. Guzick DS, Sullivan MW, Adamson D, et al: Efficacy of treatment for unexplained infertility. Fertil Steril 70:207–213, 1998.
7. Ness RB, Cramer DW, Goodman MT, et al. Infertility, fertility drugs, and ovarian cancer: A pooled analysis of case-control studies. Am J Epidemiol 155:217–224, 2002.
8. Speroff L, Glass RH, Kase NG (eds): Clinical Gynecologic Endocrinology and Infertility, 6th ed. Philadelphia, Lippincott Williams & Wilkins, 1999.
9. Venn A, Watson L, Bruinsma F, et al: Risk of cancer after use of fertility drugs with in-vitro fertilisation. Lancet 354:1586–1590, 1999.

43. IN VITRO FERTILIZATION

Pak H. Chung, M.D., Gianpiero D. Palermo, M.D., and Zev Rosenwaks, M.D.

1. What is in vitro fertilization (IVF)?

IVF is an assisted reproductive technique wherein oocytes are surgically retrieved, inseminated, and fertilized outside the body. The resultant embryos are grown in culture media and subsequently replaced into the uterus for pregnancy.

2. What does in vitro mean literally?

In Latin, "in vitro" literally means "in glass," as in a test tube or Petri dish used in experiments. Hence offspring from in vitro fertilization have been known as "test-tube babies" in laymen's terms.

3. How many IVF procedures are performed in the United States per year?

According to the most recent report by the Centers for Disease Control and Prevention (CDC) and the Society for Assisted Reproductive Technology (SART), in 2001 over 100,000 ART procedures were performed in 384 reporting clinics in the United States, resulting in over 29,000 live births (deliveries of one or more living infants) and over 40,000 babies.

4. What are the indications for IVF?

IVF is indicated for but not limited to the following causes of infertility:
- Female tubal factor
- Male factor, including obstructive and nonobstructive causes
- Advanced maternal (female) age
- Endometriosis
- Idiopathic infertility for which traditional or conventional treatment methods have failed
- Antisperm antibodies
- Genetic abnormalities, for which genetic testing of embryos is used either to reduce miscarriages or prevent transmission of specific genetic diseases.

5. When should IVF be considered for women suffering from tubal factor infertility?

IVF was originally developed to bypass the need of a healthy fallopian tube, in which sperm and eggs meet for fertilization. Tubal disease accounts for 20–25% of cases of female infertility. Tubal obstruction can be caused by pelvic inflammatory disease, ectopic (tubal) pregnancies, previous tubal and/or pelvic surgery, abdominal infections (e.g., ruptured appendix, tuberculosis), endometriosis, and adhesion formation after any abdominal surgical procedure. The gold standard for detecting tubal obstruction is the hysterosalpingogram (HSG).

Currently, when tubal obstruction is diagnosed, treatment options include tubal surgery or IVF. If the patient is relatively young ($<$ 35 years old) and has never had tubal surgery, laparoscopic evaluation and possible tubal reconstruction can be considered. Hysteroscopic cannulation of the fallopian tubes may also be an option in some instances of proximal tubal obstruction. In making such decisions, prognosis must be compared with particular attention to the severity of tubal disease and the probability of success with each treatment option.

In women who are older than 35 years or in whom previous tubal surgery has failed, IVF should generally be the first choice of treatment.

6. When is IVF a better treatment option following a voluntary tubal ligation?

Tubal reversal or reanastomosis is a microsurgical procedure traditionally performed via a minilaparotomy, although laparoscopic approaches have been successfully used. Tubal reversal should generally be performed in young women ($<$ 35 years old) who have normal ovarian reserve (as assessed by a day-3 levels of follicle-stimulating hormone [FSH]and estradiol [E_2]) and who wish to have more than one child. Such procedures should be reserved for women who have an adequate proximal tubal stump and intact fimbria. If any of the above criteria are not met, IVF may be a more reasonable option, because it does not require general anesthesia or major surgery. When indicated, however, tubal reanastomosis is highly successful. Success rates approach 65–70% in the year after surgery but drop progressively thereafter. IVF can result in delivery rates exceeding 50% per attempt in young women (< 35 years of age).

7. When is IVF indicated for endometriosis?
Although the role of minimal or mild endometriosis as a cause for infertility still remains enigmatic, there is little doubt that moderate and severe endometriosis can lead to infertility. The underlying mechanism of endometriosis-associated infertility may be multifactorial. An obvious factor is pelvic adhesions with distortion of pelvic anatomy. Other less clear factors include activation of peritoneal macrophages (which may have an impact on egg, sperm, or embryo viability as well as on implantation), changes in reproductive hormones, and altered immune responses.

Conventional therapies for endometriosis entail surgical ablation and anatomic restoration as well as hormonal suppressive therapy. If infertility is the goal of treatment, expectant management after surgery and ovulation induction can be considered in young women (< 34 years). When conventional treatment is ineffective or for women ≥ 35 years of age, IVF should be the treatment of choice.

8. When should IVF be used for male factor infertility?
Currently, male factor infertility accounts for more than half of the cases of infertility in couples. It often coexists with female factor infertility. When subnormal semen profile parameters are found in the male partner (low sperm density, motility, and/or morphology), an evaluation by an experienced reproductive urologist is indicated with the aim of correcting the underlying etiology and any existing or coexisting disease.

When no further improvement can be achieved for the male partner, as in cases of "idiopathic" infertility, treatment options are dictated by the severity of infertility. An andrology laboratory experienced in sperm preparation techniques is essential to determine the optimal treatment approach. In general, when a motile sperm fraction of > 5×10^6 can be recovered, a trial with intrauterine insemination, generally with ovarian stimulation, should be considered. When intrauterine inseminations fail to achieve pregnancies or if the initial motile sperm recovery fraction is less than 1×10^6, IVF with intracytoplasmic sperm injection (ICSI) is indicated (see below).

9. What is the difference between swim-up and density gradient sperm selection methods?
Both methods are commonly used in IVF laboratories. Swim-up is particularly effective with good semen samples (adequate concentration and motility), whereas density gradients such as Percoll gradients are reasonably useful with most subnormal semen samples (e.g., oligozoospermic and oligoasthenozoospermic samples). Percoll is useful not only for increasing the population of motile and normal form of spermatozoa but also for eliminating seminal bacteria and reducing reactive oxygen species caused by lipid peroxidization.

10. Should older women undergo IVF as the first line of treatment for infertility?
Age of the female partner is a critical determinant of fertility potential and thus is a critical variable affecting fertility treatment outcome. Ovarian reserve, which often reflects the biologic age of the ovary, is another critical variable in determining fertility potential. Ovarian reserve can be inferred by measuring day-3 concentrations of follicle-stimulating hormone (FSH) and estradiol (E_2).

A high level of FSH is an indicator of diminishing ovarian reserve. This measurement may be quite important in evaluating how aggressively to treat women approaching the age of 40 and also in giving the woman a realistic idea of her chance for a successful pregnancy. A single elevated FSH level is an indicator of a poor prognosis despite normal subsequent FSH levels. A clomiphene challenge test may provide even more information about a patient's ovarian reserve than a day-3 FSH level.

Women who exhibit abnormal ovarian reserve at any age should be encouraged to undergo IVF sooner rather than later. Similarly, women presenting with infertility who are older than 36 or 37 years of age should be encouraged to pursue IVF, because it is the treatment with the highest fecundity rate.

11. Is IVF a reasonable treatment option for couples with unexplained infertility?

Idiopathic infertility is a diagnosis of exclusion. Such a diagnosis implies that with present evaluation techniques, *no* obvious factor of infertility is discovered. As such, treatment is largely empirical. Superovulation with intrauterine insemination is often attempted for several cycles. If pregnancy does not occur, it is appropriate to use IVF. IVF is not only therapeutic in such instances, resulting in high pregnancy rates, but it can also serve as a diagnostic tool, allowing direct evaluation of sperm and egg interaction as well as evaluation of the quality of the ensuing embryos. Thus, failure of fertilization may uncover a hitherto undiagnosable factor, as would the observation of poor embryo development in vitro. It is paradoxical that statistically couples categorized with "unexplained infertility" can expect high rates of success with IVF compared with couples with tubal factor infertility.

12. Can IVF technology be used to avoid the transmission of specific genetic abnormalities?

The advent of IVF and the ability to observe and examine preimplantation embryos in the laboratory have allowed clinicians and scientists to expand its use for nonfertility indications. One example is the application of preimplantation genetic diagnosis (PGD). Structural chromosomal abnormalities such as balanced translocations, robertsonian translocations, or numerical abnormalities (aneuploidy) related to advanced maternal age can be detected by fluorescent in situ hybridization applied to a single blastomere removed from the 3-day-old embryo. Molecular probes using PCR or other appropriate methods can detect specific gene defects, such as cystic fibrosis, sickle cell anemia, and others.

13. What is the minimal work-up necessary to prepare couples for IVF?

First and foremost, a thorough evaluation should ensure that IVF is the appropriate treatment for the specific cause of infertility. One must also ascertain whether ovarian reserve is normal, because donor eggs may be necessary when the ovarian reserve is poor. Documentation of a normal uterine cavity either by hysterosalpingogram or ultrasound is essential. Semen analysis determines whether standard insemination or intracytoplasmic sperm injection (ICSI) is to be used. We recommend mapping the cervical-uterine angle and assessment of the size of the cavity with a mock (trial) transfer; this technique ensures a smooth embryo transfer and proper placement of the embryo(s).

14. Describe how gonadotropins are used for ovarian stimulation in IVF.

Gonadotropins are most often used for ovarian stimulation in IVF for the purpose of recruiting multiple follicles. Currently several gonadotropin preparations are available in the United States, including (1) recombinant FSH, formulated in 75-unit ampules or in multidose vials for subcutaneous use, and (2) human menopausal gonadotropins (HMG), with combined action of FSH and leutinizing hormone (LH), formulated in ampules for either subcutaneous or intramuscular delivery.

In general, daily injections are started on cycle days 2 or 3, depending on the protocol. Adjustment of gonadotropin dosage may be needed, depending on ovarian response and follicle size as determined by ultrasound measurement. To prevent spontaneous ovulation before oocyte retrieval, many IVF centers choose to downregulate endogenous gonadotropins with a GnRH analog (especially in young women with normal ovarian reserve), beginning one week before the anticipated menstrual period. An alternative strategy is to use a GnRH antagonist during the mid-to-late follicular phase of the stimulation cycle. Human chorionic gonadotropin (HCG)—the surrogate LH surge—is used to trigger final oocyte maturation when at least 2 or 3 follicles reach an average diameter of 16–18 mm by ultrasound. It is highly recommended that each IVF center define its own follicle size criteria for HCG administration.

15. How is the dosage of gonadotropin determined for individual patients?

The dosage of gonadotropins should be tailored to the patient's specific needs. Variables to be considered must include age, ovarian reserve, body mass index, and, if available, the response to gonadotropins in previous stimulation cycles. Preparations to be used include hormonal medications with either FSH action alone or with combined FSH and LH action.

16. Can IVF be performed during a natural cycle without ovarian stimulation?

Historically, the first successful IVF pregnancy followed the retrieval of a single egg during a spontaneous, nonstimulated menstrual cycle. However, without stimulating for multiple oocytes, natural cycle IVF is associated with relatively low pregnancy rates— especially in older women, whose oocytes tend to be chromosomally abnormal and who have a relatively higher risk (30%) of retrieving no oocytes in a cycle. Natural cycle IVF minimizes the risk of ovarian hyperstimulation syndrome (OHSS) and multiple gestation. Natural cycle IVF has enjoyed a renaissance of sort, especially when used for patients who cannot be exposed to high estradiol levels due to cancer (breast cancer survivors) or other medical conditions.

17. Who was the first successful IVF baby?

Louise Brown in England.

18. How is oocyte retrieval accomplished?

Historically, oocyte retrieval was performed via laparoscopy. A needle was introduced into the visualized follicles. However, since only the peripheral follicles are visualized, follicles deeper in the ovaries are missed, resulting in relatively low ooctye yields.

Currently, oocyte retrieval is efficiently performed with transvaginal ultrasound guidance. Patients do not require endotracheal intubation or general anesthesia. Intravenous sedation is adequate for the procedure. After the needle is inserted into the follicle under ultrasound guidance, a negative pressure of 80–100 mmHg is applied to aspirate the follicular fluid, which is collected into tubes. Follicle collapse can be visualized on ultrasound, indicating successful retrieval of an ooctye. The tubes are then transferred to the adjacent laboratory for examination and identification of the oocytes. The needle is progressively introduced into successive follicles. Ideally, oocyte retrieval is best performed by aligning the needle in such a way that only a single or few punctures through the vaginal vault are needed per ovary.

19. Once the oocyte reaches the laboratory, how is fertilization accomplished?

The incubation of oocyte and sperm is carried out in vitro in suitable culture media, arranged in droplets supplemented with a protein source. The semen is usually obtained shortly before oocyte recovery. It is liquefied at room temperature and washed. Each oocyte is inseminated with approximately 150,000 to 500,000 motile sperm. The sperm and oocytes are incubated for 12–18 hours at 37°C in 5% carbon dioxide and 98% relative humidity. When severe semen profile abnormalities exist, ICSI is performed.

On the following day the oocytes are examined for fertilization, as indicated by the appearance of two pronuclei and extrusion of the second polar body. Normally fertilized oocytes (zygotes) are further cultured in vitro for up to 3 or 5 days, and quality checks are performed every 24 hours. Embryos are graded according to the number and size of the blastomeres, fragmentation, characteristics of the cytoplasm, and number of nuclei.

20. Is preincubation of oocytes in culture media before insemination beneficial?

Yes. The prefertilization incubation allows some extent of in vitro maturation and therefore enhances the fertilization rate. However, lengthening incubation time does not necessarily translate to a higher pregnancy and delivery rate.

21. What is the most common type of abnormal fertilization with IVF?
Tripronuclear (3PN) fertilization, which most likely is characterized by a dysfunctional cortical reaction. Embryos generated from tripronucleated zygotes need to be recognized. Transfer of embryos developed from tripronuclear zygotes may be responsible for trophoblastic degeneration.

22. When and how are embryos replaced into the uterus?
Embryo transfer typically takes place three days after oocyte retrieval, when the embryo has cleaved two or three times to the 6- to 8-cell stage. When several embryos are available, one can delay transfer until day 5 (at the blastocyst stage), permitting further selection of the best embryos. The transfer procedure usually does not require anesthesia. The number of embryos to be transferred is determined by the age of the female partner, her history, and embryo morphology (which correlates with embryo quality).

23. How do we support the luteal phase after IVF stimulation and retrieval?
In some women progesterone secretion may be deficient following IVF. This problem presumably occurs more frequently in women who are downregulated with GnRH agonists, since pituitary suppression deprives the corpus luteum of endogenous LH stimulationFurthermore, removal of granulosa cells along with the oocytes debulks the ovary of these progesterone-producing cells. Thus, it is customary to support the luteal phase with either progesterone or with additional HCG, which stimulates the corpus luteum to secrete progesterone.

Progesterone (P_4) treatment is started one day after egg retrieval either via intramuscular injection (25–50 mg/day) or by the vaginal route (e.g., 50-mg suppositories 3 times/day or 200-mg micronized progesterone capsules 3 times/day). We prefer to measure serum progesterone and estradiol levels 10, 12, and 14 days after retrieval to assess the adequacy of the hormonal milieu in the postimplantation period. Some IVF centers administer small doses of HCG either subcutaneously or intramuscularly to increase endogenous corpus luteum P_4 production, although this approach may increase the risk of OHSS.

24. How do we counsel patients about IVF success rates?
First and foremost, one must keep in mind what definition of "success" is used in a discussion. IVF success rates can be expressed as clinical pregnancies (demonstration of a gestational sac and fetal cardiac activity) or deliveries per cycle initiated, per oocyte retrieval, or per embryo transfer.

Success rates vary among IVF centers. An important variable of IVF success is the age of the female partner and her functional ovarian reserve. When counseling couples about success rates, age-specific results must be discussed. It is useful to report success rates by the following age groups: < 35, 35–37, 38–40, 41–42, and > 42 years of age, since these categories appear to be biologically distinct. Although for most patients the age-specific delivery rate per cycle is most relevant, for clinicians the best index reflecting IVF efficiency and the capability of a center are its age-specific implantation rates (fetal heart beats per embryo transferred).

25. What are some of the potential complications of IVF?
Although complications of IVF are relatively rare, couples should be clearly informed about OHSS, multiple gestations, and complications related to transvaginal oocyte retrievals, which can be associated with injury to other pelvic structures, bleeding, and infection. Carefully performed transvaginal ultrasound guided procedures are exceedingly safe.

26. Discuss the significance of OHSS.
OHSS is a potentially life-threatening condition that occurs only after an ovulatory stimulus (e.g., HCG) is administered to women who develop excessive numbers of follicles in response to gonadotropin treatment. The syndrome is associated with profound fluid shifts from the intravascular to extravascular spaces (e.g., peritoneal cavity, pleural compartment)—presumably sec-

ondary to increased inflammatory intermediates released by the ovulated follicles. The syndrome can be avoided by withholding the ovulatory stimulus (HCG) and by cycle cancellation. The key to avoiding OHSS is prevention. Most critically, prevention entails recognizing the patient at risk (young age, polycystic ovaries, and a history of OHSS) and tailoring the stimulation protocol accordingly.

Women at risk benefit from dual suppression with oral contraceptive pills overlapping with GnRH agonist downregulation, followed by the administration of low gonadotropin doses (150 IU/day or less).

27. Discuss multiple gestations as a risk of ART.

According to the U.S. National CDC-SART report in 2001, 36% of all live births were multiple pregnancies, with approximately 4% of live births being triplets or higher multiples. With the advent of the prolonged 5-day embryo culture, one can theoretically select the one or two best morphologically developed embryos, thus avoiding or minimizing high-order multiple gestations.

28. When should embryos be replaced back into the uterine cavity?

In the early days of IVF, embryos were transferred at the 2- to 4-cell stage on the second day after retrieval and insemination. Later it was realized that further in vitro evaluation allowed the selection of the most developmentally advanced embryos at the 6- to 8-cell stage, resulting in better success rates. Recently, the development of different sequential media has made it possible to efficiently culture embryos to day 5–6 after fertilization, allowing growth to the blastocyst stage. Blastocyst transfer, which may represent 25% of cases in some IVF centers, has resulted in high embryo implantation rates.

29. Does success after the transfer of cryopreserved/thawed embryos vary with embryo stage?

With contemporary methods of ovulation induction for IVF, it is not unusual to obtain more than 10 mature oocytes in young women. Considering that no more than two or three embryos are generally transferred during a fresh cycle, it is apparent that an efficient embryo cryopreservation program will maximize the cumulative chances for pregnancies.

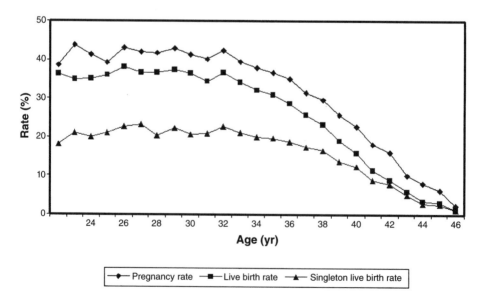

FIGURE 1. Effect of age on pregnancy and liver birth rates for ART cycles using fresh nondonor eggs or embryos. (Adapted from the 2001 CDC Assisted Reproductive Technology Success Rates National Summary.)

Although cryopreservation of zygotes and early cleaved embryos can attain reasonable pregnancy rates, recent improvements in cryopreservation of blastocysts (5–6 days after fertilization) have resulted in per embryo implantation rates exceeding 35% with pregnancy rates of approximately 50–60% per transfer of two embryos.

30. Does the female partner's age affect IVF success rates?
In general, monthly fecundity diminishes with advancing maternal age. Similarly, IVF pregnancy success rates are profoundly affected by age. Figure 1 from the CDC-SART national data for 2001 illustrates this phenomenon. Maternal age does not seem to affect the egg's ability to be fertilized but has a tremendous impact on the consequent embryo's ability to implant. The damage mainly occurs during the first meiotic division due to the malsegregation of the chromosomes. Advanced maternal age is also characterized by a reduced availability of oocytes due to the exhausted ovarian reserve.

31. How does paternal age affect IVF?
Paternal age, although claimed to be associated with a higher incidence of sperm chromosomal aneuploidy, does not appear to affect IVF outcome.

32. Do women who have previously conceived and given birth have higher success rates than women who have never conceived?
Women with proven fertility, who have previously delivered liveborn infants, appear to have a better chance of conceiving after IVF. However, women who have had previous miscarriages have success rates comparable to those of women who have never achieved a pregnancy.

33. What are the indications for intracytoplasmic sperm injection (ICSI)?
ICSI, a micromanipulation technique first reported in 1992, has significantly improved the

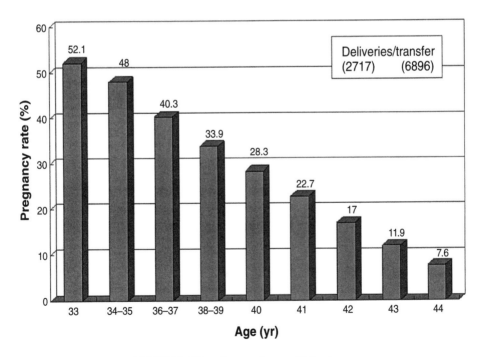

FIGURE 2. Effect of maternal age on ICSI outcome.

outcome of male factor infertility treatment. Although ICSI is most often used for male factor infertility, there are other instances when it should be applied. Indications are summarized below.

Male factor indications
- <500,000 motile sperm in the ejaculate
- <1% normal morphology
- Compromised motility
- Azoospermia: with surgically retrieved sperm (epididymal or testicular)
- Abnormal acrosomes in spermatozoa
- Antisperm antibodies
- Previous poor or failed fertilization

Female factor indications
- Too few oocytes
- Excessive thickness of zona pellucida
- Oocyte dysmorphism
- Abnormal cortical reaction

34. With are the most important factors affecting the outcome of ICSI?

The most important factor in determining the success rates after ICSI is the age of the female partner (Fig 2). In addition, sperm of poor quality, such as severe asthenospermia (poor motility) or teratospermia (poor morphology), appear to result in lower fertilization rates and decreased pregnancy outcomes.

BIBLIOGRAPHY

1. Barmat LI, Liu HC, Spandorfer SD, et al: Human preembryo development on autologous endometrial co-culture versus conventional medium. Fertil Steril 70:1109–1113, 1998.
2. Kligman I, Rosenwaks Z: Differentiating clinical profiles: Predicting good responders, poor responders, and hyperresponders. Fertil Steril 76:1185–1190, 2001.
3. Palermo GD, Takeuchi T, Neri QV, et al: Application of intracytoplasmic sperm injection in assisted reproductive technologies. Reprod Biomed Online 6:456–463, 2002.
4. Spandorfer SD, Chung PH, Kligman I, et al: An analysis of the effect of age on implantation rates. J Assist Reprod Genet 17(6):303–306, 2000.
5. Spandorfer SD, Goldstein J, Navarro J, et al: Difficult embryo transfer has a negative impact on the outcome of in vitro fertilization. Fertil Steril 79:654–655, 2003.

44. INTRACYTOPLASMIC SPERM INJECTION

Gianpiero D. Palermo, M.D.

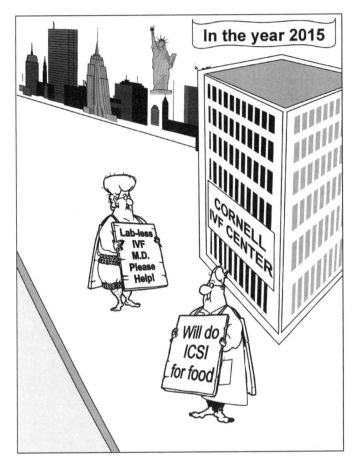

With time, the price of anything will come down, even in New York City.

A1 Intellectual Media

1. What is intracytoplasmic sperm injection?

Intracytoplasmic sperm injection (ICSI), developed by Gianpiero Palermo in 1991, is one of the most sophisticated micromanipulation techniques used for in vitro fertilization (IVF). ICSI involves puncturing the outer layers (zona pellucida and oolemma) of the egg and releasing a single spermatozoon into the cytoplasm by a glass microtool. Thus, unlike conventional IVF, in which a single oocyte is incubated with 150,000 to 500,000 motile sperm, in ICSI one spermatozoon is injected into an oocyte for fertilization.

ICSI is ideally carried out microscopically under ×400 magnification. Two types of glass microtools are used: a holding pipette for stabilizing the egg and a microinjection pipette for injecting the single sperm (Fig. 1). This technique bypasses the natural selection performed by the egg coat as well as membrane fusion between the two gametes.

2. Describe the fertilization steps with conventional IVF.

Spermatozoa are selected by different preparation methods and added to the culture medium containing the oocytes. The head of a spermatozoon containing the acrosome rich with enzymes, such as hyaluronidase, help the sperm cell to make its way to the cumulus corona cells surrounding the oocyte. Once the sperm head touches the zona, an acrosome reaction occurs and the spermatozoon reaches the perivitelline space by means of its own motility. Once there its postacrosomal segment fuses with the microvilli of the oolemma. After fusion, the fertilizing spermatozoon is entirely incorporated into the egg. This process also activates, through calcium oscillation, the oocyte that will be responsible for sperm decondensation and pronuclei formation. Fertilization is assessed by the presence of two clear pronuclei and two distinct polar bodies, also known as a zygote, approximately 16–18 hours after insemination.

3. What are the advantages of ICSI?

This technique bypasses many of the pathologic barriers that can result in infertility. Barriers in females include tubular obstruction, cervical environment hostile to sperm, excessive thickness of the zona pellucida, and oocyte dysmorphism. Barriers in males include abnormal ejaculation, azoospermia due to obstruction of the excurrent ductal system for sperm passage, and decreased quantity and quality of sperm. Especially with severe male factor infertility, ICSI is able to achieve fertilization and embryo cleavage independent of semen parameters, sperm origin, or presence of antisperm antibodies. The only requirement for a successful ICSI procedure is one viable spermatozoon!

4. What are the differences between ICSI and conventional IVF in terms of outcome?

Regardless of the paucity and/or maturity of available spermatozoa, ICSI has achieved consistently high fertilization and pregnancy rates that are comparable to those obtained with conventional IVF in couples with non-male factor infertility. In addition, pregnancy characteristics, neonatal outcome, and early development are also comparable between IVF and ICSI.

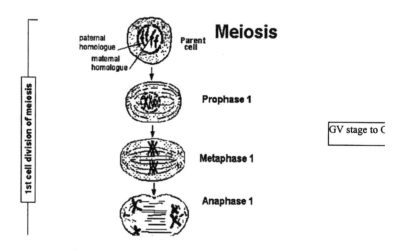

FIGURE 1. Intracytoplasmic sperm injection.

5. Describe the evaluation process of oocytes after ICSI.

After injection of the sperm, the eggs are incubated for 16–18 hours, then examined for possible damage from micromanipulation and for evidence that fertilization has occurred. Approximately 95% of the injected eggs survive the procedure. Eggs that are normally fertilized display two distinct spherical nuclear structures, one called the female pronucleus and the other the male pronucleus. Both are found in the center of the egg with an extrusion of a second polar body in the perivitelline space. These pronucleii contain the female and male chromosomes, which will come together a few hours later to form the early embryo. After a specified culture period, the resulting embryos can then be transferred back to the woman's uterus, with standard embryo replacement techniques, used for pre-implantation genetic diagnosis (PGD), or frozen for future treatment.

6. Does ICSI involve any risks?

Although ICSI is an effective fertility management option, since it bypasses many natural barrier of conception, there have been concerns about its safety and the offspring produced with this technique. Children born through ICSI using severely compromised spermatozoa are at risk to inherit genetic defects—for example, impaired spermatogenesis if a Y chromosome microdeletion is inherited from the father. This finding is largely due to the fact that infertile men have a higher incidence of peripheral chromosomal abnormalities as well as a higher frequency of aneuploidy in spermatozoa.

7. What genetic diseases in men with male factor infertility may be found in couples undergoing ICSI?

The frequency of Y chromosome microdeletions in men with severely compromised spermatogenesis is 5–15%. This deletion mutation is passed on to male, but not to female, offspring because only male offspring inherit the paternal Y chromosome. In addition, about 4% of men with severe male infertility have numeric or structural chromosomal abnormalities, such as translocations or inversions.

Congenital absence of the vas deferens (or CAVD) is characterized by an absent transport of spermatozoa from the testes to the urethra. Men with CAVD often have mutations in a gene associated with cystic fibrosis.

8. Are ICSI offspring at higher risks of having chromosomal abnormalities?

The technique itself apparently does not induce any chromosomal abnormalities; however, the severely infertile status of men treated by ICSI may be responsible for transmitting such defects.

9. Do children born after ICSI develop normally?

Recent studies have raised concerns in regard to the health and development of ICSI children. Bowen et al. postulated that at age 1 year ICSI children have a slower mental development. However, in our follow-up study of 5-year-old ICSI children, it appears that the psychological and motor developments of ICSI children are comparable to those of other children.

10. What is "rescue ICSI"?

Failure of fertilization occurs in about 10–25% of IVF cycles. Before ICSI became available, it was routine practice to reinseminate 1-day-old oocytes that had failed to fertilize. The outcomes of this practice, however, were poor. With the introduction of ICSI, it has been attempted to inject spermatozoon into oocytes had failed to fertilize with conventional IVF. This practice is generally known as "rescue ICSI."

11. In case of IVF failure, should rescue ICSI be performed?

Although several investigators reported successful rescue of 1-day-old oocytes by ICSI after fertilization failure, sperm injection into an oocyte that has been previously exposed to spermatozoa generally presents a poor developmental potential for resulting embryos. In addition, there is a higher incidence of chromosomal abnormalities in the resulting embryos. Rescue ICSI currently remains an experimental procedure. In the United Kingdom, in fact, the utilization of rescue ICSI has been banned.

12. Does ICSI successfully treat immunologically infertile cases?
Yes. Couples with positive antisperm antibodies of any class and any localization can be successfully treated by ICSI. At Cornell, no significant difference has been observed in terms of fertilization, pregnancy, and miscarriage rates between immunologically infertile patients and other patients.

13. Should ICSI become the standard insemination method to fertilize the oocyte?
Although ICSI was originally developed to treat mainly severe male factor infertility, its indications have been expanding. Currently, ICSI is used routinely in cases of limited numbers of oocytes, thickness of the zona pellucida, and recurrent polyspermia as well as when preimplantation genetic diagnosis is indicated. Finally, to ensure a more consistent fertilization rate, ICSI is now performed in large IVF centers such as Cornell at a rate of 75–80% of all assisted reproductive techniques.

14. How can we improve fertilization rates with testicular spermatozoa?
Although the fertilization rates obtained with surgically retrieved spermatozoa were satisfactory, they were significantly lower than the rates observed with ejaculates. The reason was attributed to a different constitution of the sperm membrane, presumably related to a higher lipid content, that appeared to benefit by a more aggressive immobilization procedure. This aggressive immobilization facilitates the release of a sperm cytosolic factor that is able to activate the oocyte by altering membrane permeabilization.

15. How is a single spermatozoon handled for ICSI?
Before injection, the sperm tail needs to be disrupted to enhance fertilization. This disruption is achieved by rubbing the tail against the bottom of the plastic dish with a microinjection pipette until the sperm cell is immobilized.

16. Does the injection technique affect ICSI outcome?
ICSI remains a highly sophisticated gamete micromanipulation procedure. Meticulous technique under the most optimal conditions is crucial for success. Skills and experience are required to obtain an optimal egg survival and a consistent fertilization rate. It has been reported that aggressive aspiration of cytoplasm is accountable for a compromised embryo development.

17. Do ICSI embryos develop as well as embryos from conventional IVF?
Preliminary reports suggested that embryos from ICSI are compromised and may carry a higher rate of aneuploidy. However, more recent and larger series have demonstrated a comparable blastocyst formation rate as well as implantation, pregnancy and delivery rates between the two methods of assisted reproduction.

18. What are the main concerns about the ICSI procedure?
There are several concerns about the ICSI technique, such as (1) mechanical disruption of the oolemma with the degeneration of the oocyte; (2) cytoskeletal damage, leading to possible chromosomal abnormalities from cell division; and (3) utilization of dysmorphic/dysfunctional spermatozoa that carry abnormal genetic traits.

19. Is there any indication for ICSI other than infertility?
In couples for whom a genetic analysis of the embryo is required, particularly for assessment of single gene defects, ICSI represents the ideal assisted reproduction method because it mini-

mizes the risk of contamination with spermatozoa that can interfere with the results of genetic evaluation of the embryo.

BIBLIOGRAPHY

1. Bowen JR, Gibson FL, Leslie GI, Saunders DM: Medical and developmental outcome at 1 year for children conceived by intracytoplasmic sperm injection. Lancet 351:1529–1534, 1998.
2. Chen HL, Copperman AB, Grunfeld L, et al: Failed fertilization in vitro: Second day micromanipulation of oocytes versus reinsemination. Fertil Steril 63:1337–1340, 1995.
3. Dozortsev D, Rybouchkin A, De Sutter P, Dhont M: Sperm plasma membrane damage prior to intracytoplasmic sperm injection: A necessary condition for sperm nucleus decondensation. Hum Reprod 10:2960–2964, 1995.
4. Fishel S, Aslam I, Lisi F, et al: Should ICSI be the treatment of choice for all cases of in-vitro conception? Hum Reprod 15(6):1278–1283, 2000.
5. Kuczynski W, Dhont M, Grygoruk C, et al: Rescue ICSI of unfertilized oocytes after IVF.Hum Reprod 17:2423–2427, 2002.
6. Morton PC, Yoder CS, Tucker MJ, et al: Reinsemination by intracytoplasmic sperm injection of 1-day-old oocytes after complete conventional fertilization failure. Fertil Steril 68:488–491, 1997.
7. Nagy ZP, Staessen C, Liu J, et al: Prospective, auto-controlled study on reinsemination of failed-fertilized oocytes by intracytoplasmic sperm injection. Fertil Steril 64:1130–1135, 1995.
8. Palermo G, Joris H, Devroey P, Van Steirteghem AC: Pregnancies after intracytoplasmic injection of single spermatozoon into an oocyte. Lancet 340:17–18, 1992.
9. Palermo GD, Takeuchi T, Neri QV, et al: Application of intracytoplasmic sperm injection in assisted reproductive technologies. Reprod Biomed Online 6:456–463, 2003.
10. Palermo GD, Neri QV, Hariprashad JJ, et al: ICSI and its outcome. Semin Reprod Med 18:161–169, 2000.
11. Palermo GD, Schlegel PN, Colombero LT, et al: Aggressive sperm immobilization prior to intracytoplasmic sperm injection with immature spermatozoa improves fertilization and pregnancy rates. Hum Reprod 11:1023–1029, 1996.
12. Park KS, Song HB, Chun SS: Late fertilization of unfertilized human oocytes in in vitro fertilization and intracytoplasmic sperm injection cycles: conventional insemination versus ICSI. J Assist Reprod Genet 17(8):419–424, 2000.
13. Takeuchi T, Colombero LT, Neri QV, et al: Does ICSI require acrosomal disruption? An ultrastructural study. Hum Reprod 19:114–117, 2004.
14. Yuzpe AA, Liu Z, Fluker MR: Rescue intracytoplasmic sperm injection (ICSI): Salvaging in vitro fertilization (IVF) cycles after total or near total fertilization failure. Fertil Steril 73:1115–1119, 2000.

45. IN VITRO MATURATION

William M. Buckett, M.D., and Seang Lin Tan, M.D.

DEFINITIONS AND TERMS

1. What is in vitro maturation (IVM)?

IVM is the development in vitro of immature oocytes (usually at the germinal vesicle stage) into mature metaphase II oocytes—with the extrusion of the first polar body and expanded cumulus ready for fertilization.

Although IVM has been used to describe the maturation of immature oocytes obtained in the course of conventional in vitro fertilization (IVF) with ovarian stimulation or in the course of natural-cycle or minimal-stimulation IVF, the main clinical application of IVM is the retrieval of immature oocytes from completely unstimulated ovaries and their subsequent maturation in vitro and fertilization. This approach allows the generation of embryos for transfer to the uterine cavity and possible pregnancy. It is, therefore, is an effective assisted reproductive treatment for infertility.

2. Define oocyte maturation.

Human oocytes are arrested at the prophase I stage of meiosis during fetal life until puberty. These immature oocytes can be found in the nongrowing follicles. As each cohort is recruited and follicular dominance is established at each cycle, the oocyte acquires the ability to reinitiate meiosis.

After resumption of meiosis, the nuclear membrane dissolves and the chromosomes progress from metaphase I to anaphase I and then to telophase I. The dissolution of the nuclear membrane is known as germinal vesicle breakdown (GVBD). After the completion of the first meiotic division and the extrusion of the first polar body, the second meiotic division starts and is arrested at the metaphase II stage (MII) until ovulation and fertilization. Immature oocytes (i.e., those which have not reached MII) are unable to undergo fertilization and subsequent embryo cleavage. Oocyte maturation, therefore, can be defined as the reinitiation and completion of the first meiotic division from the germinal vesicle (GV) stage to MII, with accompanying cytoplasmic maturation.

3. How is IVM different from conventional IVF?

In conventional IVF, the patient requires daily injections of exogenous gonadotrophins, often after pretreatment with analogs of gonadotropin-releasing hormone (GnRH), to generate more oocytes and therefore more good-quality embryos for transfer. In IVM the immature oocytes are retrieved without recourse to ovarian stimulation. They are then matured in vitro and used to generate the embryos for transfer. Therefore, women undergoing IVM avoid the ovarian stimulation associated with conventional IVF.

4. Where and in whom was IVM first performed?

The first time that human oocytes were successfully matured in vitro, leading to a live birth, was in Seoul, Korea. Immature oocytes were retrieved from women undergoing caesarean section as a source of oocytes for donation. The immature oocytes were matured in vitro and fertilized; the subsequent embryos were transferred to the prepared uterus of a woman with premature ovarian failure.

The first pregnancy and live birth following IVM without ovarian stimulation in a woman using her own immature oocytes was in Melbourne, Australia. The first successful cases in North America were in Montreal, Canada.

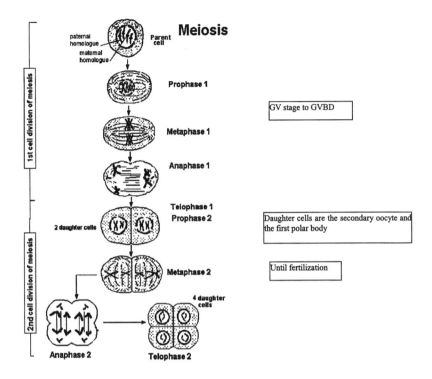

Meiosis. The relevant changes pertaining to the oocyte are shown on the right.

5. Is IVM better than conventional IVF?

So far, no prospective randomized clinical trials have compared implantation, pregnancy, and live birth rates with IVM and conventional IVF. Current clinical pregnancy rates, both in Montreal and Seoul, following IVM in women with polycystic ovary syndrome and without ovarian stimulation, are in the region of 30–40% per cycle. This rate compares with clinical pregnancy rates of 40–50% per cycle following conventional IVF. Case-controlled studies currently suggest that implantation rates are lower following IVM compared with conventional IVF.

Obviously, IVM has the advantages of avoiding the risks and costs of ovarian stimulation.

BENEFITS AND RISKS OF IVM

6. What are the disadvantages of ovarian stimulation for conventional IVF?

The disadvantages of the ovarian stimulation used in conventional IVF are threefold: Ovarian stimulation increases direct and indirect costs, has some side effects, and has some short- and possibly long-term risks.

Drug costs alone account for a significant proportion of the overall costs of conventional IVF—either directly to the couples undergoing treatment or to the healthcare systems providing the service. Women undergoing ovarian stimulation for conventional IVF also need ultrasound and endocrine monitoring. Monitoring necessitates increased time from work, travel, and other indirect costs of treatment.

Side effects of ovarian stimulation for conventional IVF include pain and irritation at the site of injection. Although this problem has been ameliorated by the subcutaneous use of more highly purified or recombinant preparations, the risk of allergic response still remains. Other commonly reported side effects include hot flashes, tiredness, breast or nipple tenderness, pelvic discomfort or pain, and emotional lability. Ovarian cyst formation is also well recognized and can further increase the length of ovarian stimulation and necessary monitoring.

7. What are the risks of ovarian stimulation for conventional IVF?
Ovarian hyperstimulation syndrome (OHSS) is the most serious complication of ovarian stimulation for IVF. The cardinal features of the syndrome are marked ovarian enlargement and acute third-space sequestration of fluid, mainly intra-abdominal ascites. Direct action of the excessive exogenous gonadotrophins accounts for the ovarian enlargement, but no studies have identified the cause of the fluid shift, although the human chorionic gonadotropin (hCG) given to initiate oocyte maturation and the rising hCG of early pregnancy (particularly when raised in multiple pregnancy) are implicated in the severity of the syndrome. The fluid shift can cause respiratory distress secondary to a splinting effect of the abdominal ascites on the diaphragm or directly as a result of pleural effusion or even pulmonary edema. The resultant hemoconcentraion can also lead to renal failure, stroke, and even death.

Patients with a pretreatment ultrasound diagnosis of polycystic ovary syndrome (PCOS) are at increased risk of developing OHSS, and treatment with GnRH analogs is also associated with a higher incidence of OHSS. Although there are a number of strategies to reduce the risk of OHSS, none is universally successful. The only way to prevent OHSS altogether is to avoid stimulating the ovaries with gonadotropins.

Over the past few years a number of studies have suggested that the incidence of ovarian cancer may be higher in women who have had multiple courses of fertility drugs. However, although the available data do not support a causal relationship, some women still prefer to avoid fertility drugs, if possible.

8. How are these risks overcome with IVM?
IVM avoids ovarian stimulation, thereby avoiding the increased cost, monitoring, side effects, and risks associated with ovarian stimulation for conventional IVF. Some monitoring for the possible development of a dominant follicle or a poor endometrial response is, however, necessary with IVM.

9. Is IVM safe for patients?
Women undergoing IVM still need immature oocyte retrieval and embryo transfer. Therefore, the small risks that are associated with oocyte retrieval and embryo transfer—namely bleeding and possible infection—are also present for women undergoing IVM.

Severe bleeding is extremely rare following either conventional IVF or IVM oocyte retrieval, although any bleeding diathesis is obviously a contraindication. Serious adnexal infection following oocyte retrieval occurs in about 1/1000 oocyte retrievals and is usually seen in association with severe endometriosis and endometriomas or with severe tubal disease and hydrosalpinges.

10. Are children born from IVM at increased risk of congenital abnormalities?
Among the few hundred babies born worldwide following IVM of immature oocytes, there has been no increase in the incidence of congenital or chromosomal abnormalities. Nevertheless, as with any new development in the field of reproductive medicine, continued neonatal and childhood surveillance is appropriate.

11. Is there any increased risk of miscarriage or pregnancy complications following IVM?
There has been no reported increase in the risk of miscarriage or of late pregnancy complications following treatment with IVM. Again, appropriate maternal and fetal monitoring is indicated at present.

12. How does IVM compare with natural-cycle IVF?
In natural-cycle IVF, conventional IVF is performed without ovarian stimulation or, in some circumstances, with minimal stimulation. Usually a maximum of 1–3 oocytes are obtained at

oocyte retrieval, and programs that offer natural-cycle IVF usually perform repeated oocyte retrievals in successive months. Pregnancy rates are usually low because there is a 20–30% possibility that no oocyte is retrieved, the oocyte does not fertilize, or the embryo does not cleave. Nevertheless, natural-cycle IVF avoids the risks and side effects associated with conventional IVF.

Although no randomized controlled trials have compared IVM with natural-cycle IVF, the pregnancy rates reported after IVM are higher than those reported after natural-cycle IVF.

INDICATIONS AND CONTRAINDICATIONS

13. What are the indications for IVM?

IVM should be considered in the following circumstances:

1. Women with PCOS who have failed to achieve a pregnancy after more than 6 cycles of ovulation induction.

2. Women undergoing IVF for any indication who are noted to have polycystic ovaries on ultrasound scan (namely, a total of more than 20 antral follicles from both ovaries).

3. Women who repeatedly produce a majority of poor-quality embryos during conventional IVF for no apparent reason.

4. IVM can be considered for oocyte donors, young women undergoing chemotherapy or radiotheapy, and young women wishing to preserve fertility in general. In such cases IVM avoids the increased time and monitoring needed for the ovarian stimulation associated with conventional IVF.

14. Which tests may be used to determine who may be better suited for IVM?

At present, measurement of the antral follicle count by early follicular-phase ultrasound (day 2–5) appears to be the best test to determine who will produce sufficient immature oocytes for IVM and who will ultimately generate good-quality embryos. In our program, an antral follicle count of over 20 (total) in both ovaries combined is considered sufficient to consider IVM.

Measurement of ovarian total volume, ovarian stromal volume, and ovarian stromal blood flow are also associated with IVM success; however, these factors are less reliable determinants than the antral follicle count. Measurement of endocrine and biophysical parameters has not shown to determine outcome with IVM.

15. How important are age and serum levels of follicle-stimulating hormone (FSH)?

Age remains an important determinant of pregnancy and live birth. Successful pregnancies and healthy births are less common in women over 40 years of age.

Elevated levels of FSH are related to poor IVM outcome in so far as the antral follicle count in patients with high FSH levels is generally low.

16. Can immature oocytes be cryopreserved?

Yes. Cryopreservation and subsequent survival after thawing of immature human oocytes is a relatively new assisted reproductive technology. A novel application of this technology is to preserve fertility in women about to undergo potentially sterilizing treatment (e.g., total body irradiation prior to bone marrow transplant for refractive leukaemia). IVM avoids the time needed to effect ovarian stimulation and, therefore, may be a more appropriate option without unduly delaying chemotherapy or radiotherapy. Moreover, the use of gonadotropins for ovarian stimulation may be contraindicated in some malignancies.

17. What are the contraindications to IVM?

As with conventional IVF, the contraindications for oocyte retrieval remain the same: severe systemic disease, bleeding diatheses, and current pelvic infection. However, because of the repeated ovarian puncture and the small ovarian size compared with stimulated ovaries, any condition in which oocyte retrieval may be particularly difficult or hazardous—such as the presence of large endometriomas—is a relative contraindication.

IVM PROCEDURE

18. How is an IVM treatment cycle managed?

Women with amenorrhea receive vaginal progesterone for 10 days to induce a withdrawal bleed. All women then undergo a baseline ultrasound scan on day 2–4 of menstrual bleeding to ensure that no ovarian cysts are present and to measure the antral follicle count in the two ovaries.

Transvaginal ultrasound is repeated between day 6 and day 10 to exclude the development of a dominant follicle. All follicles should be < 10 mm in diameter to proceed to oocyte retrieval, which is performed between days 9 and 14. In women with ovulatory cycles, immature oocyte retrieval is planned between days 8 and 11 to reduce the risk of observing a dominant follicle > 10 mm in diameter

All women receive an injection of 10,000 IU hCG 36 hours before immature oocyte retrieval. Transvaginal ultrasound-guided immature oocyte collection is performed using a specially designed 17-gauge, single-lumen aspiration needle with a reduced aspiration pressure of 7.5 kPa. Aspiration of all small follicles is performed using repeated ovarian puncture as necessary. Follicular flushing is not performed at our center, although some programs have used flushing with some success. Oocytes are collected in culture tubes containing warm 0.9% saline with 2 IU/ml of heparin.

The oocytes are evaluated for the presence of a germinal vesicle (GV) in the cytoplasm of the oocyte, after which the immature oocytes are transferred into maturation medium for culture. The immature oocytes are incubated in culture dishes containing 1 ml of maturation medium (TC-199) supplemented with 20% heat-inactivated maternal serum, 0.25 mmol/L of pyruvic acid, 50 mg/ml of penicillin, 5 mg/ml of streptomycin, and 75 mIU/ml each of FSH and luteinizing hormone (LH) at 37°C in an atmosphere of 5% carbon dioxide and 95% air with high humidity. After culture, the maturity of the oocytes is determined by microscopic examination at 24 hours and 48 hours.

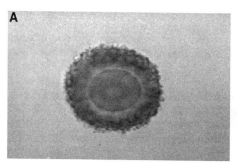 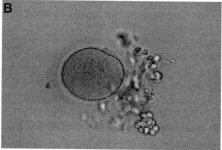

A, Immature oocyte, demonstrating germinal vesicle and compacted cumulus.
B, Mature MII oocyte, demonstrating the first polar body and expanded cumulus.

Oocytes that are mature are then denuded of cumulus cells and prepared for intracytoplasmic sperm injection (ICSI). A single spermatozoon is injected into each metaphase II (MII) oocyte. Fertilization is assessed 18 hours after ICSI for the appearance of two distinct pronuclei and two polar bodies. Embryos are transferred on day 2 or 3 after ICSI.

For endometrial preparation, women receive estradiol valerate, starting on the day of oocyte retrieval, depending on the endometrial thickness on that day. If the endometrial thickness is < 6 mm, a 10-mg dose is given; if it is > 6 mm, a 6-mg dose is given. Luteal support, provided by 200 mg of intravaginal progesterone or 50 mg of intramuscular progesterone, is started on the day of ICSI and continued, along with estradiol, until 12 weeks of gestation.

19. What techniques are used to maximize the retrieval of immature oocytes?

Immature oocyte retrieval in a woman with highly mobile polycystic ovaries, small antral follicles, and thick, dense ovarian stroma can be difficult. Good-quality transvaginal ultrasound is essential. If the ovaries are particularly mobile, application of abdominal pressure by an assistant can help "fix" the ovary while the initial ovarian puncture is made. To place the collection needle into the small antral follicle, it is essential that, prior to entry, the needle is at a 90° angle to the follicle wall. If not, the needle easily slips into the surrounding stroma. In women with PCOS there is often a dense echogenic stroma with the antral follicles found peripherally. Attempts to avoid going through large amounts of stromal tissue should be avoided because this technique can block the collection needle with the resultant loss of immature oocytes. Frequent removal of the collection needle, flushing in heparinized saline, and reinsertion in the appropriate plane are essential to maximize immature oocyte yield.

20. What anesthesia is given?

Initial series and trials with IVM used either general or spinal anaesthesia. This approach was thought to be important for two resons: (1) Any movements by the woman can make an already difficult retrieval even more challenging, and (2) the multiple punctures needed were likely to be quite painful. However, the use of local anesthesia in the upper part of the vagina and in a paracervical block in combination with patient sedation (as commonly used in conventional IVF) has reduced the need for spinal or general anesthesia.

21. How do embryo quality and embryo implantation compare with conventional IVF?

IVM treatment results in higher pregnancy rates when more than six embryos are produced, allowing the selection and transfer of good-quality embryos, with a high cumulative embryo score (CES). There is a trend toward decreased implantation rate of embryos derived from in vitro-matured oocytes with increasing patient age, which correlates with data from natural and IVF cycles. There is also a strong relationship between embryo quality, as characterized by the CES, and the chance of pregnancy. However, when CES and implantation rates in women undergoing IVM are compared in case-controlled studies with those from women undergoing conventional IVF, both are lower.

22. How is the endometrium synchronized with the embryonic stage?

As in women undergoing conventional IVF, the embryo is often transferred to the endometrial cavity ahead of the time of implantation. Because women with PCOS are anovulatory and those who have undergone IVM have not produced a mature oocyte in vivo and therefore have not produced the estradiol required before luteinization, a short course of estradiol steroid is necessary before progesterone luteal support is initiated (see question 18).

23. How is embryo transfer performed?

Embryo transfer should be performed in exactly the same manner as embryo transfer for women undergoing conventional IVF or oocyte recipients.

24. Since women undergoing IVM have not had GnRH analogs, is luteal support still necessary?

As detailed in question 22, all successful IVM programs give estradiol and progesterone support in the maturation and luteal phases. Certainly, women with anovulatory cycles need such steroids to synchronize endometrial development, and experience from oocyte donation programs suggests that continuation until 3 months of pregnancy is appropriate, although no studies to date have addressed this issue.

25. Can multiple cycles of IVM be performed? How soon after treatment failure can a second cycles be attempted?

Multiple cycles (up to 3) of IVM have been performed. As with any assisted reproduction technology, the decision to go beyond three cycles needs to follow appropriate counseling about the likelihood of success and other therapeutic options. Although it is unknown whether repeat IVM treatments can be performed in successive menstrual cycles, it seems prudent at this stage to wait for 2 or 3 months to allow any ovarian trauma to resolve.

26. Can embryos generated from IVM be cryopreserved?

As with conventional IVF, IVM treatment can generate embryos that are supernumerary to the index treatment cycle. These embryos can be cryopreserved and used in a later cycle. Pregnancies and live births have been reported following the cryopreservation and thawing of embryos generated from IVM treatment cycles.

27. Are IVM treatment cycles ever cancelled?

The presence of a dominant follicle on ultrasound at day 8 or day 10 is associated with a poorer immature oocyte yield and, therefore, ultimately with lower pregnancy and live birth rates. Although pregnancies have occurred in the presence of dominant follicles, because of the lower chances of success, cycle cancellation and IVM treatment in the subsequent menstrual cycle are indicated.

LONG-TERM CONSEQUENCES OF IVM

28. Is IVM associated with pelvic infection and adhesions?

At present, there have been no reports of pelvic infection or adhesions following immature oocyte retrieval for IVM treatment. Because both been reported as a rare consequence of conventional IVF, they may be a rare consequence of IVM also. It certainly does not seem that there is any increased risk over that associated with conventional IVF.

29. Are there any long term consequences of the progesterone and estradiol used?

There appear to be no long-term consequences of progesterone and estradiol used for luteal support during IVM. The doses of progesterone are identical to those used in conventional IVF. Although there are occasional progestogenic side effects, they resolve after pregnancvy and no long-term problems have been reported.

The dose of estradiol used for endometrial synchronization in IVM is less than that given for women using donated oocytes in an oocyte donation program or those undergoing hormone replacement prior to embryo transfer with cryopreserved embryos. At these doses, no long-term complications have been reported to date.

30. Can IVM be used for oocyte donation?

IVM allows potential oocyte donors the option of avoiding the time, cost, and risks associated with IVF, particularly those with polycystic ovary morphology. Pregnancies and live births have been reported using IVM for oocyte donation.

BIBLIOGRAPHY

1. Cha KY, Koo JJ, Ko JJ, et al: Pregnancy after in vitro fertilization of human follicular oocytes collected from nonstimulated cycles, their culture in vitro and their transfer in a donor oocyte program. Fertil Steril 55:109–113, 1991.
2. Chian RC, Buckett WM, Tan SL: In vitro maturation of human oocytes. Reprod Biomed Online 2003 [in press].
3. Chian RC, Buckett WM, Too LL, Tan SL: Pregnancies resulting from in vitro matured oocytes retrieved from patients with polycystic ovary syndrome after priming with human chorionic gonadotropin. Fertil Steril 72:639–642, 1999.
4. Tan SL, Child TJ, Gulekli B: In vitro maturation and fertilization of oocytes from unstimulated ovaries: predicting the number of immature oocytes retrieved by early follicular phase ultrasonography. Am J Obstet Gynecol 186:684–689, 2002.
5. Trouson A, Wood C, Kausche A: In vitro maturation and the fertilization and developmental competence of oocytes recovered from untreated polycystic ovarian patients. Fertil Steril 62:353–362, 1994.

46. PREIMPLANTATION GENETIC DIAGNOSIS

Kangpu Xu, Ph.D., and Peter T. K. Chan, M.D.

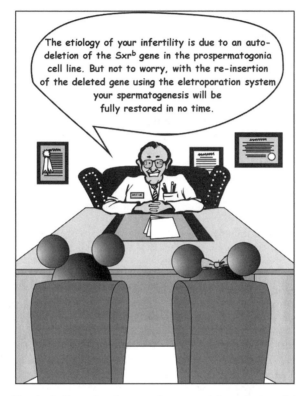

The etiology of your infertility is due to an auto-deletion of the Sxr^b gene in the prospermatogonia cell line. But not to worry, with the re-insertion of the deleted gene using the eletroporation system your spermatogenesis will be fully restored in no time.

Thanks to the extensive genetic research in rodent models

A1 Intellectual Media

1. What is preimplantation genetic diagnosis (PGD)?

PGD, whether it is done for chromosomal defects or for single gene disorders, is performed on cells or genetic materials (the polar body or blastomere) removed from an oocyte or an embryo in its preimplantation stage. Genetic analysis of these materials provides information about the "genetic status" of the embryos before their implantation in the uterus. PGD has been used for more than a decade. Nevertheless, the growth of knowledge and experience has been limited because PGD is offered by only a small numbers of centers worldwide. Education of patients as well as physicians is needed to use this technology more effectively. With the information derived from the Human Genome Project, genetic testing will continue to play an important role in reproductive medicine in the twenty-first century.

2. What are the advantages of PGD over prenatal diagnosis?

PGD offers a distinct advantage over prenatal diagnosis in that it allows detection of genetic anomalies in the conceptus in the embryo stage, ensuring that only embryos free of detectable anomalies will be transferred after in vitro fertilization (IVF). Anomalies that can be detected range from embryonic chromosomal aberrations to single gene mutations. Risk of miscarriages due to chromosomal aneuploidy may therefore be reduced. Equally important, the detection of single gene mutations allows replacement of only unaffected embryos for pregnancy. Parents who are carriers of severe genetic disorders can thus minimize the risk of carrying an affected fetus and greatly reduce the need to make the difficult decision of a therapeutic abortion. Finally, PGD provides additional features that are not applicable to prenatal diagnosis, including evaluation for late-onset genetic disorders (e.g., due to mutation[s] of cancer predisposition genes) and embryo HLA typing for later harvesting of cord blood for stem cells to be used for bone marrow transplantation.

3. What forms of genetic anomalies can be detected with PGD?

Theoretically, PGD is feasible for every genetic disorder for which the causative mutation(s) is clearly identified. With the limitation both in the available genetic technology and in our knowledge of the genetic basis of diseases, however, current techniques are reasonably reliable for the detection of only a limited number of genetic disorders only. The various forms of embryo genetic anomalies detectable by PGD include:

1. **Chromosome aneuploidy.** Assessment of chromosomes can reveal any numerical chromosomal anomalies in the embryo.

2. **Structural anomalies of chromosomes.** Structural anomalies such as translocation and deletions can also be detected.

3. **Gene mutation.** Currently, over 100 single gene disorders, including cystic fibrosis, sickle cell anemia, beta-thalassemia, and Tay-Sachs disease, can be detected with PGD. The list of detectable single gene defects is rapidly growing.

4. What are the main indications for PGD?

Because PGD is such a powerful tool and is under rapid development, the following list is far from complete. In the future, there will be more indications that we have not yet envisioned today.

1. **Chromosomal aneuploidy analysis or screening.** This indication accounts for more than half of the couples undergoing PGD in most centers. Aneuploidy evaluation particularly benefits two groups of patients: those who experience repeated miscarriages or failures of in vitro fertilization (IVF) and those of advanced maternal age.

2. **Carriers of balanced chromosome translocations.** PGD technology can detect embryos with unbalanced chromosomal materials to allow transfer only of balanced/normal embryos.

3. **Couples with X-linked disorders** such as hemophilia, muscular dystrophy, Lesch-Nyhan syndrome, adrenoleukodystrophy, and X-linked mental retardation. Sexing of embryos by PGD allows implantation of unaffected embryos.

4. **Carriers of single gene mutation(s),** such as cystic fibrosis and sickle cell anemia. PGD can potentially eliminate the risk of passing the mutation to the next generation. A related, though slightly different indication, is for the D antigen of the Rh blood group system (RhD). Maternal alloimmunization is the most common cause of fetal hemolytic disease. If the mother is RhD-negative and the father is heterozygous for RhD, PGD can allow selection of only RhD-negative embryos for transfer back to the uterus, thus avoiding an alloimmunized pregnancy.

5. **Late-onset diseases** (e.g., Huntington disease). This category may also include those at higher risk for developing familial cancer (e.g., breast cancer).

6. Patients who wish not only to have children free from a genetic disorder but also to provide **cord blood for harvesting stem cells for bone marrow transplantation** to save a sibling affected by the disorder. HLA typing can be performed in this scenario to match an embryo with the affected sibling.

5. What is the major limitation of PGD?

The most important limitation of PGD is that only when a sufficient number of embryos with good quality is obtained can an accurate genetic diagnosis and an effective selection be made.

Generally, the embryo yield is closely related to the woman's reproductive age and ovarian function. Furthermore, women of more advanced age usually have a higher proportion of aneuploidy embryos than younger women. Therefore, women at a more advanced reproductive age seeking PGD may not have enough materials for a proper PGD diagnosis to ensure implantation of normal embryos. Finally, current PGD procedure does not yet allow simultaneous analysis of chromosomal aberrations and single gene defects. Thus, even when an embryo tests negative (unaffected) for a specific genetic disorder, it may not be able to survive due to chromosomal anomalies that were not identifiable simultaneously. Nevertheless, active research in this area promises a breakthrough in the near future.

6. How accurate is PGD procedure?

The accuracy of PGD varies from one procedure to the other.While embryo gender determination by FISH appears to be the easiest and most accurate procedure, other more sophisticated procedures are prone to inaccuracy. In addition to technical limitations, other biologic factors may also affect the accuracy. Notably, embryo moscaicism and allele drop-out (see below) are responsible for several misdiagnoses reported in the literature.

It is estimated that accuracy of PGD ranges from about 90% for aneuploidy screening to close to 99% in for embryo sexing, with most of the other procedures somewhere between. It should be emphasized that the accuracy of PGD will never be 100%, since single cell genetic analysis in PGD faces more limitations than prenatal diagnosis procedures, for which hundreds or even thousands of cells are available for evaluation.

7. What specific factors can result in misdiagnosis with PGD?

Apart from human and technical errors, several specific factors may increase the risk of misdiagnosis:

1. **Background signals.** In fluorescent in situ hybridization (FISH), background fluorescence signals may interfere with correct interpretation of the labeling results, leading to misdiagnosis of chromosome patterns of the embryo.

2. **Allele drop-out** (ADO). ADO refers to the failure of amplification of one of the two alleles in a heterozygote during polymerase chain reaction (PCR). This problem can occur when the quantity of DNA is too low, as when genetic materials from only a single cell are available. ADO can result theoretically in misdiagnosis in 5–10% of cases. So far a misdiagnosis rate of about 1.8% has been reported. Tremendous efforts and progress are being made to reduce the rate.

3. **Embryo mosaicism.** This term refers to an abnormal phenomenon in the early preimplantation embryos. For example, in an 8-cell embryo, not all of the cells (blastomeres) necessarily have exactly the same genetic make-up. Variations of chromosome numbers among individual blastomeres in the same embryo are not uncommon. If the biopsied cell from the embryo happens to be different from the rest of the embryo with mosaicism, a misdiagnosis may occur. Biopsy of two cells from an embryo may reduce the risk of misdiagnosis significantly. However, it is not yet clear whether removal of two cells from an embryo, especially an embryo of suboptimal quality, will affect its viability.

8. How is PGD for embryo sexing performed?

Embryo gender determination is the most reliable procedure of all PGD indications. As in PGD for chromosomal aneuploidy, additional blood tests from the parents are not required. Blastomeres are biopsied on day 3 and fixed on a slide for FISH analysis with probes for X and Y chromosomes, along with an additional autosomal probe (e.g., for chromosome 18) as a positive control. Embryo sexing for medical reasons has been accepted largely by society. Sexing for family balance or social reasons is more controversial. More debate is needed to reach a consensus before most PGD centers will offer this service for family balancing or social reasons.

9. How is PGD for single gene disease performed?

Theoretically, PGD is able to detect any DNA sequence alterations, as long as detailed genetic information is available. As of June 9, 2003, there are 10771 entries of established genes or phenotype loci (10,143 autosomal, 550 X-linked, 41 Y-linked, and 37 mitochondrial genes) (see http://www.ncbi.nlm.nih.gov:80/Omim/). In practical terms, only a fraction of these diseases and many fewer of the mutations will be the targets of PGD. For example, one of the best characterized genes is the cystic fibrosis transmembrane conductance regulator (CFTR) gene, of which more than 1000 mutations have been identified so far. Many of the CFTR mutations may cause severe cystic fibrosis, and PGD is indicated for parents at risk of having affected children. PCR-based genetic testing, using the existing primers, is generally available for the most common mutation(s), such as the three base pair nucleotide deletion on exon 10 (also known as delta-F508). If the mutation is a less frequent or newly discovered one, newly constructed primers and modification of existing protocol may be necessary. The PGD laboratories can sometimes develop a new protocol for specific cases.

10. Is it possible to test for both aneuploidy and a single gene mutation with PGD?
It is obviously ideal to be able to test for both chromosomal anomalies and single gene mutations, particularly for women of advanced maternal age and/or at risk of having embryos with chromosomal anomalies. Although some investigators have reported the feasibility of this approach, current technology cannot yet provide adequate accuracy to achieve this goal routinely. Extensive research in this area is under way.

11. How long might it take to develop a PGD procedure for a specific couple?
Depending on the purpose of PGD and the type of PGD tests involved, there may be a necessary waiting time to allow preparation of the specific materials required for PGD for a specific couple.
1. PGD for embryo sex determination and aneuploidy screening can be performed using standard FISH procedure. Generally no waiting time is necessary.
2. For determination of chromosomal structural anomalies, a waiting period of a few weeks is necessary to allow confirmation of parental karyotype and testing for the probe combination to be used in FISH.
3. PGD for single gene mutations is a more complex situation. In specialized PGD laboratories, if the disorders and mutations are common and protocols have already been worked out, no waiting time may be necessary. However, if a new protocol is required for the recently discovered mutations, it may take longer, depending on the availability of the research support of the PGD laboratories. Generally, it may take from a few weeks to several months.

PATIENT PREPARATION FOR PGD

12. If the patient's doctor and genetic counselor suggest PGD, what is the next step?
Generally speaking, this means that the doctor or genetic counselor suspects or has confirmed a genetic condition in the patient or the patient's partner that can be passed to children. First, it is necessary to "genetically define" the condition. To this end, additional information beyond a clinical diagnosis, which is generally based on symptoms, signs, biochemical analyses, and imaging studies, is required. Analysis at the molecular level must be performed and the gene as well as its specific mutation(s) determined. For instance, if the condition is cystic fibrosis, the specific CFTR mutation(s) carried by the parent(s) should be determined.
Once such information is obtained, the patients should consult a PGD center/laboratory to check whether an existing protocol is available for the specific genetic condition. Generally, if the genetic condition is a common one, the laboratory is likely to have an existing protocol. Currently, however, only a few protocols exist for the various disorders that can be tested with PGD. Even when an existing PGD protocol for the disease of interest is not available to the specific laboratory, it is possible that the laboratory will be able to develop one, especially with the active development of more sensitive and generalized methods such as sequencing and gene chips.

13. Where is PGD performed?

In addition to advanced assisted reproduction, many reproductive centers in North America offer expertise in both embryology and genetic counseling. A genetic counselor generally suggests PGD for fertility treatment whenever it is indicated. Alternatively, patients who are considering or interested in PGD may initiate a discussion with a geneticist or genetic counselor. Because of the technical complexity of PGD, not many reproductive centers around world offer PGD "in house," although the number is growing. However, some centers can perform embryo biopsy and ship the tissue to special genetic laboratories that perform single cell analysis for PGD. Be aware that while some PGD laboratories specialize in chromosomal analysis, others may be offering only single gene mutation analysis. A few centers offer full PGD service. Thus, depending on the indications for PGD and the genetic conditions of interest, the physician or genetic counselor may refer the patient to specific laboratories that are appropriate.

14. Are additional genetic evaluations required for the parents before PGD?

The answer depends on the indication for PGD. For chromosome aneuploidy evaluation, additional genetic evaluation of the parent is not necessary. For specific genetic conditions, however, additional genetic tests are necessary for two purposes: (1) to re-confirm the presence of the genetic condition, even when previous genetic evaluation have established the diagnosis, and (2) to test the probes (in FISH study) or primers (in PCR) to ensure that an accurate single cell PGD can be performed for the condition.

15. Why does the patient need to go through prenatal diagnosis if the embryos have already been tested by PGD?

As discussed previously, PGD results are based on evaluation of only one or two cells removed from an embryo. Technical mistakes may occur, although the chance is very low. Another factor of concern is mosaicism in early preimplantation embryos. Embryo mosaicism is encountered not infrequently, especially in cases associated with more advanced maternal age. If the biopsied cell from the embryo happens to be different from the rest of the embryo with mosaicism, a misdiagnosis may occur. Hence, even after PGD confirmation, prenatal diagnosis is still necessary during pregnancy to minimize the chance of misdiagnosis so that a corrective decision can be made.

IVF, ICSI, AND RELATED ISSUES

16. Why is intracytoplasmic sperm injection (ICSI) needed for PGD when normal semen is used?

ICSI uses a micromanipulator to deliver a single sperm inside an oocyte (see chapter on ICSI) and is commonly used for the treatment of severe male factor infertility. For certain types of PGD procedures aimed at evaluating only chromosomal aneuploidy (such as FISH; see below), fertilization by routine in vitro insemination (i.e., non-ICSI assisted reproduction) can be used when semen quality parameters are adequate. However, when PGD for the evaluation of single gene disorders, which generally requires single cell DNA amplification by PCR, is to be performed, ICSI becomes a prerequisite. The reason is that with ICSI, a single sperm and single ovum are involved, resulting in one embryo for PGD, whereas with routine in vitro insemination a relatively large number of sperm are present. Therefore, the risk of "genetic contamination" for subsequent PGD will be too high.

17. Can PGD be done for a couple undergoing natural pregnancy?

Because cells from embryos in their preimplantation states are needed for PGD, it can be performed only as part of an in vitro fertilization (IVF). Pregnancies achieved naturally or by intrauterine insemination (IUI) are not candidates for PGD. For these cases, other forms of prenatal evaluations, including amniocentesis and fetal ultrasound, can be used to evaluate fetal malformations, chromosomal anomalies, or some other genetic disorders.

18. Why is blastocyst culture necessary for PGD?

To minimize any potential risks that may jeopardize the pregnancy outcome, current clinical PGD procedure is preferably, if not almost exclusively, based on fresh embryo transfer. Although live births have been reported from biopsied, frozen, and subsequently thawed embryos, viability of the cryopreserved biopsied embryos is significantly compromised. After embryo biopsy performed on day 3, genetic testing on the blastomeres generally takes about 24 to 48 hours. Meanwhile, the biopsied embryos are cultured in the incubator until results are ready and a decision about transfer can be made. During this incubation period, a healthy embryo continues to develop to reach the compact morula or blastocyst stage. Although prolonged culture periods may not be beneficial to all embryos, transfer of embryo cultured up to day 5 is a routine procedure in selected cases. In fact, some investigators believe that embryos capable of developing to day 5 may indicate that implantation is more likely to be successful.

19. What are the chances that after PGD no embryo is available for transfer?

Overall, no embryos are available for transfer in approximately 15% of patients undergoing embryo biopsy. The most important factors associated with a higher likelihood of no embryo to transfer are advanced female partner's age and poor ovarian reserve, which generally result in inadequate number of embryos in the treatment cycle for PGD.

In addition, the chance of having genetically unaffected embryos for transfer is also closely related to the type of PGD required. For example, among couples who are carriers (i.e., heterozygous) of recessive genetic disorders and are willing to accept transfer of carrier embryos, 75% of embryos will be transferable (25% homozygous noncarrier plus 50% heterozygous carrier). On the other hand, among couples with one partner affected with a dominant genetic disorder, 50% of embryos will be unaffected. Finally, couples seeking embryo HLA typing in addition to mutation screening for a genetic disorder (in the scenario of providing stem cells for bone marrow transplantation for an affected sibling), will have a much lower chance of having embryos that are both HLA-matched and unaffected by the genetic disorder.

20. How long does it take to have results for PGD tests?

Current PGD procedures are designed to meet the limited time frame (42–48 hours) for a day-3 blastomere biopsy followed by day-5 embryo transfer, with the exception of PGD on polar bodies. Results are usually ready around noon of day 5. However, delay may occur for various technical reason, and embryo transfer on day 6 may still be a viable option. If a delay is foreseen and day-6 transfer is not possible, embryos (at the blastocysts stage) may be frozen for subsequent transfer. In reproductive centers that do not perform PGD in house, biopsied embryo cells must be shipped as soon as possible to the specialized laboratory for PGD testing. Co-ordination between the reproductive centers and the PGD laboratories is critical to minimize delay. Although most transfers can be expected on day 5, there is a chance that the transfer will have to be cancelled if no "unaffected" or viable embryo is available for transfer.

EMBRYO BIOPSY

21. What is embryo biopsy?

Like gamete micromanipulation techniques used in assisted hatching or ICSI, embryo biopsy is carried out microscopically using a set of micromanipulators. An oocyte/embryo is first placed in a medium drop in a petri dish and covered with oil to prevent evaporation. The oocyte/embryo is held steady by a holding pipette on one side, and an opening on the zona pellucida is created on the opposite side by using one of the following methods: (1) mechanically with a needle, (2) chemically with acid Tyrode's solution, or (3) with a laser beam. A third micropipette is used to aspirate the polar body or one or two blastomeres, which are then fixed onto a slide for chromosome analysis or loaded into a small tube for DNA testing. Oocytes/embryos are returned to the culture medium.

22. When can biopsy take place?

Polar bodies are the products of the first and second meiotic divisions of an ovum. The first polar body biopsy is usually carried out within 6 hours of egg retrieval and the second polar body biopsy on the next morning. The more commonly performed blastomere biopsy is generally performed on the morning of day 3 after fertilization when the embryo has reached 6- to 10-cell stages. Occasionally, day-3 biopsy may be postponed to late afternoon if embryo development is delayed. Although day-4 biopsy is still possible, it is not generally advisable because the embryos at this stage undergo compaction—a specific process in which cells begin to adhere to each other because of the expression of specific cell surface adhesion molecules. More damage may result if biopsy is performed on a compacted embryo. On day 5 when a blastocoele is formed, the embryo, now called a blastocyst, has two distinct cell types: an inner cell mass and trophectoderm cells. The blastocyst can again be biopsied. As explained previously, if a day-5 biopsy is performed, only one day is available for PGD analysis since day 6 is the day on which embryos need to be inside the uterus so that implantation can properly take place.

23. What factors should be considered in deciding whether embryo biopsy for PGD should be performed?

Deciding whether embryo biopsy should be performed for PGD can be a complicated process. In addition to achieving the objective of identifying genetically unaffected embryos, various other factors must also be taken into consideration:

1. **Quality of embryos.** If the quality of embryos is poor (e.g., day-3 embryos with < 7 cells and significant amount of fragmentation), there may be marginal advantage to performing embryo biopsy for PGD. The embryos may not be of good enough quality (even if they are genetically unaffected by PGD) to be transferred successfully.

2. **Nature and severity of the genetic disorder in question.** The likelihood of passing the genetic disorders and the potential consequence should be evaluated for determining the risk-benefit ratio of performing embryo biopsy for PGD.

3. **Alternative options,** including chorionic villus sampling or prenatal amniocentesis, should also be considered.

4. **Psychosocial factors of the couple.** Couples who have experienced repeated miscarriage previously may have different emotional tolerance for experiencing additional adverse pregnancy outcomes. Their attitude toward therapeutic abortion, acceptance of genetically affected children, and availability of support are also factors to be considered.

24. What are the chances of damaging an embryo during biopsy?

Embryo biopsy is an invasive procedure in which one or two cells are removed from a 6- to 10- cell embryo on day 3 after fertilization. Numerous animal research data, which have been confirmed in some human studies, indicate a minimal detrimental effect on healthy embryos when a limited number of cells (1 or 2) is removed. In addition, evidence from human embryo cryopreservation indicates clearly that a healthy baby can be obtained from embryos in which up to half of the number of blastomeres are lost during freezing-thawing.

On the other hand, removal of cell(s) may be significantly harmful when embryo quality is marginal, as in embryos with lower cell numbers or with a high degree of fragmentation. In addition to embryo injury from removal of blastomeres, the other risk of embryo biopsy may come from accidental damage to the remaining blastomeres during the process of opening the zona pellucida by exposure of acid Tyrode's solution or with laser beam, the two most commonly used methods for embryo biopsy. For example, excesive release of acidic solution or the high temperature generated by the laser may create visible or invisible damage that can decrease implantation rate or adversely affect subsequent fetal development. Overall, however, the chance of embryo damage during biopsy is very low (< 1 %), especially in an experienced laboratory.

25. Are babies born from biopsied embryo healthy?

The specific risks of IVF and ICSI are still under investigation, even though it is accepted that both procedures are safe. Hundreds of thousands of babies are born worldwide from IVF and

ICSI. In comparison, only about a thousand babies have been born after PGD. It is somewhat assuring that no notable increase in rates of abnormalities has been observed in these babies. Further detailed analysis with much more extensive data is required to make a better assessment of the risk(s) caused by IVF/ICSI procedures and by the biopsy procedure for PGD.

FISH AND CHROMOSOME ANALYSIS

26. How is PGD performed for chromosomal aneuploidy?
Numerical aberrations of chromosomes (aneuploidy) are the most common cause of embryonic loss. The risk increases as the mother's age advances. At present, aneuploidy in embryos is evaluated by florescence in situ hybridization (FISH), using a panel of probes designed to screen chromosomes that are more commonly involved in aneuploidy. Examples include probes for chromosome X, Y, 13, 14, 15, 16, 17 18, 21, 22, and so forth. The panel of probes may vary according to the history of the parents or the laboratories where FISH is performed.

27. What is FISH?
FISH is a highly sensitive technique most commonly used in PGD for the detection of numerical or structural chromosomal defects. FISH can identify the number of a specific chromosome or a segment of a chromosome in a single cell (blastomere). This goal is achieved by using specific probes to label a specific chromosome or a specific segment of a chromsoome of interest to allow microscopic visualization.

28. What are FISH probes?
FISH probes are segments of DNA, labeled with fluorescent dye, that complement a specific region of a particular chromosome. The spectrum of fluorescent dyes may vary (e.g., red, blue, aqua, green, yellow). These probes can be used to label specific segments of DNA from known chromosomes (usually those that are frequently involved in aneuploidy or other anomalies, such as chromosome 13, 16, 18, 21, 22, X and Y). Thus a multi-colored FISH probe "mixture" allows evaluation of multiple chromosomes in one labeling procedure.

During PGD, when the probes are applied to a fixed nucleus of a cell or a blastomere, they bind, or hybridize, only to the complementary segment(s) of the chromosomal DNA on the specific location of a particular chromosome. For instance, a FISH probe complementary to chromosome 13 and labeled with red fluorescent dye will bind only to a specific region of chromosome 13. Likewise, a FISH probe complementary to chromosome 21 and labeled with green dye will bind only to a specific region of chromosome 21. After washing away any unbound probes, spot(s) of fluorescent color can be visualized under a fluorescent microscope and image(s) can be recorded with a sensitive camera.

The number of signals corresponds exactly to the number of chromosomes within the nucleus of the cell tested. If two red, two blue, two aqua, two green, and two yellow spots are seen under the microscope when a specific commercially available kit is used, these findings indicate that the blastomere has a normal number of copies (i.e., diploid) of chromosomes 13, 16, 18, 21 and 22. If three green spots are noted while all other colors show two signals, the cell is a trisomy 21, indicating the transfer of the embryo may result in Down syndrome. These colored signals can be washed away, and a second set of multi-color FISH probes can be applied to allow assessment of an even greater number of chromosomes.

29. In planning PGD for balanced translocation, is a repeated karyotype analysis for the parents necessary?
Whether or not PGD for balanced translocation is feasible for a particular couple depends on prior knowledge of what chromosomes are involved and the exact "break-point" on the chromosomes. Inaccurate karyotyping—i.e., incorrect determination of chromosome number or incorrect evaluation of the arms (short and long) involved—is possible. A repeated blood test in the PGD laboratory to verify the translocation status is important, because the results can influence the cor-

rect selection of FISH probe combination to determine the balanced status of involved chromosomes. This principle is especially true when telomeric DNA probes, which label the extreme ends of the arms of a chromosome, are used for evaluation of balanced/unbalanced status. In practice, we have identified inaccurate karyotyping reports in several cases. Thus, re-evaluation of parental karyotypes by an independent and proficient laboratory is generally recommended in planning PGD.

30. Is it certain that an embryo with normal morphology is free of chromosomal aneuploidy?

Data obtained in the past decade clearly indicate that numerical chromosomal abnormality is associated with various abnormal morphologic characteristics of embryos, such as multinucleation and/or fragmentation. Nevertheless, morphologic evaluation is not adequate to rule out chromosomal aneuploidy. In fact, a substantial proportion of "normal"-looking embryos on day-3 or day-5, when embryo transfer will take place, have missing or extra chromosomes. This proportion increases with the mother's age. Screening embryos before transfer and selecting embryos with the correct number of chromosomes for replacement, therefore, may benefit some patients despite the presence of "normal"-looking embryos. This is particularly true in couples at increased risk of having aneuploidy embryos.

31. How many chromosomes can be evaluated with FISH?

Ideally, all 23 pairs should be screened. However, because of the time limitation in a fresh embryo transfer cycle and the limitation in the available color spectrum of FSIH probes, current technology allows reliable screening of up to 9 chromosomes only.

32. What additional technologies can be used for PGD?

Exciting techniques such as comparative genome hybridization (CGH) have been developed in the past 10 years or so, and their future application in PGD appears to be promising. In CGH, all DNA from a test cell—for example, a blastomere from an embryo—will be amplified and labeled with red fluorescent color. This DNA will be mixed in a 1:1 ratio with DNA from normal cells, which is labeled with green color. The mixture will be hybridized onto normal metaphase chromosomes. If the color of a specific chromosome (e.g., chromosome 21) is yellow (a chromatic result of equal mixing of green and red labling), as recognized by a sensitive camera and image-processing program, the test sample is normal for chromosome 21. If more red-labeled DNA is picked up by the camera on chromosome 21, this finding will indicate an extra chromosome 21 in the test sample. With CGH all 23 chromosomes can be analyzed in each cell in one setting. More work is required to optimize the procedure before CGH can be applied clinically for PGD. A modified version of the technique, called micro-array CGH, may prove to be more effective.

33. Can PGD detect chromosomal translocation?

Chromosomal translocation is a common genetic anomaly. In addition to affecting fertility in the parents, offspring may have a higher risk of spontaneous abortion or congenital anomalies. PGD may detect embryos that carry unbalanced chromosomal segments and replant only balanced or normal embryos for pregnancy, hence reducing significantly the risk of miscarriage and adverse fetal outcomes. Translocation in the parents is detected first by karyotype analysis. However, for PGD purposes, the sensitivity of karyotype analysis, even with a high- resolution karyotype evaluation, may not be adequate to provide the diagnosis. Thus, PGD for chromosomal tranlocation must be performed with specific FISH probes for chromosomal structural analysis.

34. What are the limitations of FISH in dealing with chromosomal structural analysis?

Most FISH probes can label a region of a specific chromosome; however, the probe does not usually provide information about whether or not the chromosome is intact. In chromosome structural anomalies (such as deletion or translocation), in which a segment of a chromosome is missing or translocated to another chromosome, a conventional FISH analysis may appear normal. Thus, although FISH is a useful tool for numerical chromosome anomalies, it cannot be used reliably to rule out all chromosomal structural anomalies. Modified FISH technique using whole chromosome painting probes may reveal some of the structural aberrations if genetic materials can be obtained at metaphase, when chromosomes condense, from preconception or preimplantation stages.

35. What are the concerns of PGD for chromosomal anomalies in the embryo when the female or male partner has balanced chromosomal translocation?

Balanced chromosomal translocation carriers are common in the population (~1/500 live births). People with balanced translocations often do not present with significant health problems. However, they may experience difficulties in achieving pregnancy or recurrent miscarriages. Furthermore, there is also a chance of producing genetically abnormal babies because of the increased risks of chromosomal anomalies in offspring. For women with balanced translocation, PGD may allow preselection of normal embryos for transfer.

Several approaches can help to identify chromosomal anomalies in the embryos. For example, the chromosomal content of the polar body reflects the chromosomal content of the oocyte. Polar biopsy with whole chromosome-painting probes for FISH analysis may be performed to determine chromosomal anomalies in certain types of translocation. This technique is usually combined with a day-3 biopsy to identify chromosomal anomalies in the embryo. If the male partner has a balanced translocation, polar body biopsy of the eggs is obviously not informative.

For day-3 embryos, telomeric probes have been used successfully. They provide information about whether or not the embryo has normal/balanced chromosomes. The telomeric FISH does not allow the distinction of normal from balanced status. Babies born from this technique have either a normal karyotype or a balanced type like their mothers. If balanced translocation is on the male side, polar body biopsy of the eggs is not informative, and PGD should be performed only with a day-3 biopsy and telomeric FISH probes.

PCR AND MUTATION ANALYSIS

36. How much DNA is in a single blastomere ?

The amount of DNA in single blastomere is only about 6 picograms, which is far too little for direct genetic analysis with any current technology.

37. What is polymerase chain reaction (PCR)?

PCR is a revolutionary biochemical technique that forms the basis of many molecular genetic tests. PCR allows exponential amplification of a particular sequence of DNA, from a single copy to millions of copies, in a matter of hours.

To obtain multiple copies of a particular sequence of DNA of interest (target sequence), two DNA primers, which are short DNA sequences of complementary DNA that span the target sequence, are designed. In the presence of DNA, polymerase, nucleic acids (the building blocks of DNA), and the primers under specified sequential temperature cycling conditions that allow DNA denaturation, annealing, and extension, the minute amount of the target sequence DNA will increase exponentially over 40 to 50 amplification cycles. Therefore, PCR allows exponential amplification of a particular sequence of DNA from two copies in the single cell (blastomere) to millions of copies in a matter of hours. Through this highly specific and highly efficient process, sufficient amount of DNA can be obtained for further genetic analysis.

Although DNA amplification by PCR is an efficient process, it is prone to contamination. While applying PCR in PGD, strictly controlled laboratory environment must be set up so that high accuracy and sensitivity for PGD can be achieved.

38. Who invented the technique of PCR?

PCR was developed by Kary Mullis in 1983.

39. Discuss the future of PGD.

Overall, pregnancy rates in patients undergoing PGD are comparable to the rates in patients who undergo IVF without PGD. Clearly, in recent years, the number of PGD patients has increased steadily as PGD becomes more available. There is no doubt that with the pace of advances in genetic technology, the list of diagnosable genetic conditions will grow rapidly. Furthermore, improvements in efficiency, accuracy, time, and cost-effectiveness can be expected.

Despite the established benefits of PGD in its current state, many authorities agree that it should still be considered a quasi-experimental procedure. New areas of application of PGD include diagnosis for late-onset diseases (such as genes involved in cancer predisposition) and HLA-matching of embryo to sick siblings so that a rescuing cord blood transfer can be performed. Hence, we should also be prepared to face the clinical and complex ethical implications of PGD.

BIBLIOGRAPHY

1. American Society for Reproductive Medicine Ethics Committee: ASRM supports sex selection to prevent genetic diseases. Available at http://www.asrm.org/Media/Press/ethics1099.html.
2. American Society for Reproductive Medicine and Society for Assisted Reproductive Technology: A practice report: Preimplantation genetic diagnosis. June 2001. Available at http://www.asrm.org/Media/Practice/preimplantation.pdf.
3. Conference Report: Preimplantation genetic diagnosis: experience of 3000 clinical cycles. Reprod. Bio-Med. Online 3:49–53, 2001.
4. ESHRE PGD Consortium Steering Committee: Data collection III. Hum Reprod 17:233–246, 2001.
5. Handyside AH, Kontogianni E, Hardy K, Winston RM: Pregnancy from biopsied human preimplantation embryos sexed by Y-specific DNA amplification. Nature 244:768–770, 1990.
6. Kuliev A, Verlinsky Y: Current features of preimplantation genetic diagnosis. Reprod BioMed. Online 5: 294–299, 2002.
7. Munne S, Sanalinas M, Escudero T, et al: Improved implantation after preimplantation genetic diagnosis of aneuploidy. Reprod Biomed Online 7:91–97, 2003.
8. Verlinsky Y, Rechitsky S, Schoolcraft W, et al: Preimplantation genetic diagnosis for Fanconi anemia combined with HLA matching. JAMA 285:3130–3133, 2001
9. Winston RML, Hardy K: Are we ignoring potential dangers of in vitro fertilization and related treatments? Nature Cell Biol Nature Med [Fertil Suppl] June:S14-S18, 2003.
10. Xu KP, Shi ZM, Veeck LL, et al: First unaffected pregnancy using preimplantation genetic diagnosis for sickle cell anemia. JAMA 281:1701–1706, 1999.
11. Xu KP, Rosenwaks Z, Beaverson K, et al: Preimplantation genetic diagnosis for retinoblastoma: The first reported live-born. Am J Ophthalmol 137:18–23, 2004.

47. OOCYTE AND EMBRYO DONATION

Ina Cholst, M.D.

1. What are the indications for oocyte donation?

Oocyte donation is indicated primarily for a situation in which the female partner is unable to produce a viable oocyte. Examples include congenitally absent ovaries (as in primary ovarian dysgenesis and Turner's syndrome), iatrogenic ovarian failure (secondary to extensive surgery, chemotherapy, or radiation), and, most commonly, premature ovarian failure or incipient premature ovarian failure. Much more rarely, oocyte donation can be used to prevent transmission of a genetic disease.

2. Is it important to evaluate the recipient's uterine cavity?

Yes. A hysterogram or sonohysterogram is important before the cycle to detect any abnormalities of the uterine cavity. During the cycle, sonograms should be done to assess the thickness of the endometrium, with aggressive replacement in situations in which the endometrium is thin.

3. What tests are appropriate for the recipient's partner?

Obviously, a semen analysis should be performed before a donor egg cycle is initiated. In addition, the recipient's partner should be evaluated for recessive genetic traits (as indicated by the partner's ethnic background) and infectious diseases.

4. How should donors be recruited?

Donor recruitment should be low-key and noncoercive. Donor recruitment should be done in such a way that interested donors are able to present themselves. Compensation should be appropriate to time and effort involved, without undue inducement.

5. How should donors be screened?

Donors should be screened for general medical health, reproductive health, infectious disease, and genetic disease. In addition, all donors should be screened psychologically.

6. What genetic testing should be done?

Ideally, all potential donors should be evaluated by a genetic counselor or other health care provider specifically trained to identify risk factors for genetic diseases. Such an evaluation may identify certain donors who should be excluded on the basis of family or personal history alone. Genetic evaluation also facilitates the most individualized and specific laboratory evaluation.

At a minimum, prospective donors of all ethnic groups should be screened for the most common 25 mutations of cystic fibrosis. In addition, Mediterranean donors should be screened for beta-thalassemia, Southeast Asian and Chinese donors for alpha-thalassemia, donors of African descent for sickle cell anemia, and Ashkenazi Jewish donors for Tay-Sachs and Canavan disease. More complete genetic screening includes chromosome analysis, fragile X testing, all 87 presently identified mutations for cystic fibrosis, and a full Ashkenazi Jewish panel, including Gaucher disease, Niemann-Pick disease, Fanconi anemia, familial dysautonomia, and Bloom syndrome.

Obviously, this is a rapidly changing area of medicine in which any list of detectable genetic diseases becomes quickly outdated. The genetic screening policies of a donor egg program should be continuously reevaluated and updated.

7. What infectious disease tests should be done?

Prospective donors should be asked detailed questions about sexual habits and exposure to drug use to determine that they are at low risk by history. Specific serologic testing should be done for syphilis, hepatitis B and C, and HIV I-II. Cervical cultures should be done for *Neisseria gonorrhoeae* and *Chlamydia trachomatis*. These tests should be done at initial screening and then repeated as close to retrieval as possible. Additional testing may be dictated by local or state requirements.

8. Is quarantine required for donor sperm?
Yes. Current guidelines require that donor semen be quarantined for 180 days and the donor retested for infectious disease before the semen is released for use.

9. Why is quarantine required for donor sperm but not for donor eggs?
At present, it is not technically possible to reliably freeze donor oocytes. If the technology were to advance to a stage where oocyte freezing was technically practical, it is highly likely that the same guidelines would be applied. Obviously, guidelines for both could change as infectious disease screening improves or with the emergence of new infectious diseases.
Although embryo freezing and quarantine are technically feasible and may be offered to couples, it is quite different from gamete freezing. A number of practical, legal, and ethical considerations have precluded this requirement. For example, if a gamete donor does not return for retesting, the gametes can be destroyed. Once an embryo is created from the donor oocyte and husband's sperm, destruction of that embryo is more difficult ethically and legally. Although we hope that all egg donors will return for retesting, obviously, they cannot be required to do so. Financial inducements, such as withholding of compensation (for time and effort involved) until after retesting 6 months later, are also considered coercive and ethically questionable.

11. What is the rate of serious complications experienced by oocyte donors?
Sauer's recent review of complications in oocyte donors confirmed the low incidence of complication in these healthy young women. In a series of 1000 retrievals of oocyte donors, seven (0.7%) experienced complications serious enough to warrant hospitalization. Included were three patients with severe ovarian hyperstimulation syndrome, two with adverse reactions to anesthesia, one with intra-abdominal bleeding after aspiration, and one patient with bladder atony and hematuria after aspiration. Obviously, all donors must be carefully informed and provide consent in regard to these possibilities.

12. How old is donor egg technology?
Pregnancy using eggs from other individuals has been a widespread practice in livestock management for over 50 years. Indeed, whole strains of cattle have been introduced into Africa by superovulation of cows, insemination with sperm of highly desirable steers, lavage from the uterus, and freezing, transporting, and transplanting the desirable embryos into less commercially viable surrogates. The embryos of rare animals, such as zebras, have been transferred and successfully carried in the uteri of more common animals, such as horses. It was not until 1984, however, that the first report of a donor egg pregnancy in a human appeared (Lutjen in 1984). Thus, this widespread, well-established, and highly successful technology can be considered to be only 20 years old.

13. What is the window of implantation?
The window of implantation refers to the relatively short period between cycle days 20 and 24 when the endometrium is receptive to implantation by the developing embryo. In donor egg cycles, it is critical that synchronization be coordinated between the recipient's endometrium and the created embryo.

14. How is synchronization of donor and recipient achieved?
In general, in fresh transfer cycles the recipient is synchronized to the donor's cycle. Gonadotropin agonist or antagonist is used to suppress the recipient's cycle. Estrogen and progesterone are then used to prepare the endometrium and synchronize to the donor's cycle.
When cryopreserved donor embryos are used, synchronization is relatively straightforward. The recipient is prepared with exogenous estrogen and progesterone, with day 15 being the first day of progesterone administration. Embryos are thawed on cycle day 14.

15. How is the recipient prepared to receive a donor oocyte?

The recipient must be synchronized to the cycle of the donor, and the endometrium must be prepared to receive the fertilized oocyte. Recipients with completely absent ovarian function are prepared and synchronized using estrogen and progesterone replacement. Recipients with some residual ovarian function need to receive a gonadotropin-releasing hormone agonist or antagonist to shut down residual function before replacement.

16. What estrogen replacement regimens are successful?

Various hormone replacement regimens have been described. All have as their primary objective the mimicking of the natural hormonal cycle. In virtually all protocols, natural estradiol and progesterone are used in physiologic amounts.

The estradiol can be administered orally (as micronized estradiol), parenterally, by transdermal patch, or by vaginal ring. Estradiol concentrations should be assessed frequently and should rise during the follicular phase, reaching levels of approximately 200 pg/ml in the late follicular phase, at the time of donor retrieval. Doses should be decreased after retrieval, with concentrations maintained at approximately 100 pg/ml during the luteal phase.

Transdermal estrogen delivery results in relatively stable absorption kinetics and avoids the high estrone levels that follow oral administration (due to metabolism during the hepatic first pass). In one common protocol, estradiol transdermal patches are applied to deliver a dose of 0.1 mg/day on days 1 to 5, 0.2 mg/day on days 6 to 9, and 0.4mg/day on days 10 to 13. After donor oocyte retrieval, the dose is decreased to 0.2 mg/day and continued at that level during the luteal phase. Of note, with all replacement regimens the length of the recipient's follicular phase may be adjusted to permit synchronization with the donor.

17. How is progesterone replacement administered?

Progesterone can be administered either as intramuscular (IM) progesterone in oil or as a natural progesterone vaginal suppository. (Oral micronized progesterone seems to be less successful in achieving a receptive endometrium). IM progesterone is generally favored as giving a more consistent and reliable dose of progesterone. IM progesterone is, to varying degrees, a muscle irritant and some patients are unable to tolerate it. Occasional patients develop inflammatory reactions or even fever as a reaction to the IM progesterone. In such patients, progesterone should be given as intravaginal suppositories.

IM progesterone in oil is given at a dose of 25 mg on day 15 and increased to 50 mg from day 16 onward. Ideally, midluteal progesterone concentrations should be 20 ng/ml or higher. Replacement protocols frequently result in midluteal endometrium that displays glandular-stromal asynchrony, with glands lagging behind appropriately advanced stroma. When the stroma is in phase, pregnancy is not impeded.

18. What are the indications for embryo donation?

Couples are candidates for embryo donation if they have neither eggs nor sperm.

19. What is the source of embryos for donation?

Couples who have undergone in vitro fertilization, have cryopreserved embryos, and have now completed their families may donate embryos. Such couples may choose to discard the embryos or to donate them to research or to other couples. Embryos should not be created for the purpose of donation.

20. How should couples who wish to donate embryos be screened?

Embryo donors must provide a medical and genetic history. Testing should be done (at least 6 months after the cryopreservation of the embryos) for HIV I-II, hepatitis B and C, and syphilis. Appropriate genetic screening, if it has not been done previously, should be done at this time.

21. What is embryo adoption?

Embryo adoption is a term that can be used for embryo donation. It refers to the fact that the child will not be related to either rearing parent. It emphasizes similarities between traditional adoption and embryo donation. These considerations may be important for the couple contemplating embryo donation. However, there are obvious differences as well. For example, there is a biologic connection to the rearing mother through the pregnancy and, for the child there may be absence of psychological fantasies of rejection, sometimes associated with traditional adoption.

BIBLIOGRAPHY

1. American Society for Reproductive Medicine: Guidelines for oocyte donation. Fertil Steril 77(6 Suppl 5):S6–S8, 2002.
2. American Society for Reproductive Medicine: Guidelines for cryopreserved embryo donation. Fertil Steril 77(6 Suppl 5):S9–S14, 2002.
3. American Society for Reproductive Medicine: Appendix A: Minimal genetic screening for gamete donors. Fertil Steril 77(6 Suppl 5):S15, 2002.
4. Moomjy M, Cholst I, Davis O, et al: Donor Oocytes in assisted reproduction: An overview. Semin Reprod Endocrinol 13(3):173–186,1995.
5. Rosenwaks Z: Donor eggs: Their application in modern reproductive technologies. Fertil Steril 47(6): 895–909,1987.
6. Sauer MV: Defining the incidence of serious complications experienced by oocyte donors: A review of 1000 cases. Am J Obstet Gynecol 184(3):277–278, 2001.

48. MEDICAL AND SURGICAL COMPLICATIONS OF ASSISTED REPRODUCTIVE TECHNOLOGIES

Dan Goldschlag, M.D.

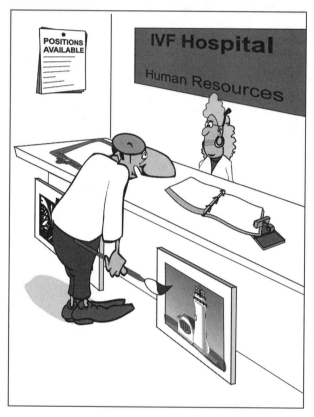

"But on the ad, it says a degree in ART !"

1. How are oocytes retrieved for in vitro fertilization treatments?

In the past, ooctyes were retrieved laparoscopically under anesthesia. Currently, oocytes are generally retrieved through transvaginal follicular aspiration. A vaginal ultrasound transducer is used to guide the aspiration. A needle is introduced into each follicle, and the follicular contents are aspirated.

2. What type of anesthesia is necessary for transvaginal follicular aspiration?

Local anesthesia, sedation, and regional or general anesthesia are options for transvaginal follicular aspiration. The choice depends on the experience of the physicians and the specific desire and needs of the patients. Generally, transvaginal follicular aspiration are performed under IV sedation as an outpatient procedure.

3. What complications can result from transvaginal follicular aspiration?

Ovaries are generally easily visualized through transvaginal sonography. This approach is relatively free of complications. Bleeding from the puncture sites of the vaginal mucosa is usually self-limited. Other rare complications include intra-abdominal bleeding, peritonitis, and infection. Prophylactic antibiotics are often administered just prior to follicular aspiration.

4. What are the advantages of transvaginal follicular aspiration over laparoscopic retrieval?

- Transvaginal follicular aspiration is a minimally invasive procedure and thus involves a lower risk of injury.
- No hospitalization is required.
- Even ovaries with adhesions are generally accessible to a vaginal approach.

5. When are oocytes retrieved?

Oocytes are aspirated before ovulation at approximately 35 hours after the administration of human chorionic gonadotropin, which is used to trigger ovulation.

6. List potential complications of in vitro fertilization.

- Ovarian hyperstimulation syndrome (OHSS)
- High-order multiple pregnancies

7. Define OHSS.

OHSS can occur with the use of ovulation induction agents. Multiple ovarian cysts develop in response to gonadotropin treatment. Large amounts of fluid can shift out of the intravascular space. The ovarian enlargement and the accumulation of third-spaced fluid can cause abdominal pain and shortness of breath. Complications include renal failure, shock, thromboembolic episodes, acute respiratory distress syndrome, and death.

8. What is the incidence of high-order multiple pregnancies?

Spontaneous triplet pregnancies occur at a rate of 1 in 6000 to 8000 births. With ovulation induction, the risk of twins pregnancies is reported to range from 0% to 40% and triplet pregnancies from 0% to 15%. Overall, the incidence of multiple pregnancies has risen over 400% between 1980 and 1997; 80% of high-order multiple pregnancies are believed to be due to the use of ovulation induction agents.

9. List complications of high-order multiple pregnancies.

- Pregnancy loss
- Preterm labor
- Preeclampsia
- Gestational diabetes
- Low birth weight

10. Why put patients at risk for multiple pregnancies? Why not simply transfer a single embryo?

Although single embryo transfer reduces significantly the risk of multiple pregnancies, it also results in a higher rate of failure to achieve pregnancy. The reason is that 75–80% of all conceptions are abnormal and end before 6 weeks' gestation. A balance among risk of multiple pregnancies, treatment costs, and patient satisfaction becomes a major factor influencing the number of embryos replaced.

11. Does a twin pregnancy from IVF carry a higher risk than one conceived naturally?

Outcomes are similar when one corrects for maternal age

12. What can be done for couples with a high-order multiple pregnancies?

The two main management strategies are (1) supportive care by maternal fetal medicine and (2) selective reduction.

13. When can selective reduction(s) of one or more conceptions be performed?

Apregnancy reduction is generally performed between 10 and 13 weeks. At the end of the first trimester, the fetuses are generally large enough for good visualization by abdominal ultrasound for selective reduction.

14. Explain autoreduction.

Autoreduction is a spontaneous process in which one or more fetuses arrest their development while at least one fetus remains viable. The majority of spontaneous fetal losses occur by the end of the first trimester; thus, one generally waits until that point to perform a selective reduction.

15. How is a selective reduction performed?

The chorionicity is determined before a selective reduction is performed. Transabdominal injection of a potassium chloride (KCl) solution is generally performed when multichorionicity is present.

16. How is a fetus selected for injection?

The fetus with the following features is generally selected for reduction:
- Easy accessibility of the fetus for injection
- Location away from the cervix
- Lagging crown-rump length, suggesting poor fetal development
- Smaller gestational sac than expected for fetal age
- Increased nuchal translucency, suggesting fetal anomalies

17. What is a blastocyst?

A blastocyst is an embryo that has continued to grow for 5 to 6 days in laboratory culture and has reached a stage with greater than 50 cells with other specific morphologic characteristics.

18. How does a blastocyst transfer reduce the risk of multiple pregnancy without decreasing overall pregnancy rates?

Blastocysts have a higher implantation rate than embryos in laboratory culture for only 3 days. By transferring in 1–2 blastocysts, one can prevent high-order multiple pregnancies without compromising pregnancy rate.

19. Is infertility a risk factor for ectopic pregnancy?

The incidence of ectopic pregnancy is higher in the infertility population. This finding may be related in part to the increased incidence of tubal abnormality in infertility patients

20. Is fertility treatment a risk factor for ectopic pregnancy?

Both ovulation induction with inseminations and IVF may be associated with increased risk of tubal, cervical, and interstitial pregnancies. This finding may be due to preexisting tubal disease or altered tubal/uterine function secondary to hormonal treatment. Preexisting tubal disease is probably the predominant factor leading to ectopic and heterotopic pregnancies

21. Are pregnancies conceived through assisted reproduction at high risk?

Not necessarily. Generally the increased pregnancy risks seen in infertility patients are related to specific patient-related risk factors (maternal age, primagravity, gynecologic and/or medical conditions). However, because many patients who undergo assisted reproduction therapy are older than 35 years of age and because multiple gestations are more commonly encountered, pregnancies conceived through assisted reproduction may require additional obstetric care.

BIBLIOGRAPHY

1. Ballabh P, Kumari J, Alkouatly HB, et al: Neonatal outcome of triplet versus twin and singleton pregnancies: A matched case control study. Eur J Obstet Gynecol Reprod Biol 107:28, 2003.
2. Berkowitz RL, Stone JL, Eddleman KA: One hundred consecutive cases of selective termination of an abnormal fetus in a multifetal gestation. Obstet Gynecol 90:606, 1997.
3. Centers for Disease Control and Prevention: Contribution of assisted reproductive technology and ovulation-inducing drugs to triplet and higher-order multiple births—United States, 1980–1997. MMWR 49:535, 2000.
4. Cohen J, Mayaux MF, Guihard-Moscato ML, et al: In vitro fertilization and embryo transfer: A collaborative study of 1163 pregnancies on the incidence and risk factors of ectopic pregnancies. Hum Reprod 1:255, 1986.
5. Evans MI, Goldberg JD, Dommergues M, et al: Efficacy of second-trimester selective termination for fetal abnormalities: International collaborative experience among the world's largest centers. Am J Obstet Gynecol 171:90, 1994.
6. Hillis SD, Owens BS, Marchbanks PA, et al: Recurrent chlamydial infections increase the risks of hospitalization for ectopic pregnancy and pelvic inflammatory disease. Am J Obstet Gynecol 176:103, 1997.
7. Keith LG, Oleszczuk JJ, Keith DM: Multiple gestation: Reflections on epidemiology, causes, and consequences. Int J Fertil Womens Med 45:206, 2000.
8. Sauer MV, Paulson RJ, Lobo RA: Pregnancy after 50: Results of 22 consecutive pregnancies following oocyte donation. Fertil Steril 64:111, 1995.
9. Tummers P, De Sutter P, Dhont M: Risk of spontaneous abortion in singleton and twin pregnancies after IVF/ICSI. Hum Reprod 18:1720, 2003.
10. Yaron Y, Bryant-Greenwood PK, Dave N, et al: Multifetal pregnancy reductions of triplets to twins: Comparison with nonreduced triplets and twins. Am J Obstet Gynecol 180:1268, 1999.

49. GENETIC COUNSELING

Jessica G. Davis, M.D.

1. What is a gene?
A Gene is a hereditary unit. In molecular terms a gene is a sequence of chromosomal DNA required for the production of a functional biochemical product.

2. What is a mutation?
A mutation is a permanent heritable change in the sequence of genomic DNA. Mutations can be de novo (sporadic) and/or familial.

3. What is a chromosome?
Chromosome is derived from the Greek words *chromo* (color) and *some* (body). Found in the cell nucleus, chromosomes are thread-like structures that contain genetic materials. Humans have 46 chromosomes (23 pairs). Pairs 1–22 consist of the **autosomes**, and one pair (XX or XY) is called the **sex chromosome**. Females have 46,XX chromosome complements and males have 46,XY chromosome complements.

4. What are the major patterns of inheritance?
- Autosomal dominant
- Autosomal recessive
- X-linked recessive
- X-linked dominant inheritance

5. What is multifactorial inheritance?
Many other traits are inherited in a more complicated fashion via a mechanism termed **multifactorial inheritance**. This mechanism is an imperfectly understood interaction between several genes (of maternal and paternal origin) and an unknown extrinsic factor(s) that occurs at a critical time in embryonic development or during an individual's life span. Examples of genetic problems that are thought to be due to multifactorial inheritance include birth defects such as cleft lip, cleft palate, clubfoot, and neural tube defects and common disorders of adult onset such as diabetes.

6. How many generations of family are needed to identify familial/genetic medical problems?
In general, the more information obtained, the more thorough an evaluation can be made. Taking a three-generation family history and constructing a pedigree can help identify a pattern of inheritance and/or susceptibilities for specific disorders.

7. List the goals of prenatal genetic diagnosis.
1. To allow couples at known increased risk for having a child with a specific birth defect/genetic disorder to begin a pregnancy with the knowledge that the presence or absence of the birth defect/genetic disorder can be diagnosed in the fetus by means of prenatal diagnosis.
2. To provide a range of options to pregnant women/couples at risk for having a child with a genetic disorder.

3. To offer reassurance and decrease anxiety, especially for those at high risk of a genetic disorder.

8. How has the availability of prenatal genetic testing made a difference to pregnant women and their partners?

Many couples at known risk for having a child with a severe genetic disorder have been able to have healthy children because of prenatal genetic testing. Others use the information obtained from prenatal genetic testing to prepare psychologically for the birth of a child with the genetic disorder in question and to obtain appropriate management/care for the birth of a child with a known genetic disorder.

9. Who is eligible for prenatal genetic diagnosis?

Pregnant women whose risk for fetal abnormality is equal to or greater than the risk of miscarriage from the diagnostic procedure itself are eligible.

10. What is the most common indication for prenatal genetic diagnosis?

Advanced maternal age, which is defined as a woman who is 35 years or older at the expected date of delivery (EDD).

11. Why is 35 years the cut-off point?

The age 35 years was selected as the cut-off point because the risk of the fetus having a chromosome problem is approximately equal to the risk of miscarriage associated with amniocentesis.

12. If a couple has a previous child with a de novo chromosome abnormality, should they consider prenatal genetic diagnosis for subsequent pregnancy?

Yes. Even though most parents of children with documented chromosome problems have normal chromosome complements (i.e., 46,XX and 46,XY), such couples are at increased risk for having a subsequent child with a chromosome problem. For example the age-related risk for a woman of having a child with Down syndrome (trisomy 21) at age 30 is 1/380. However, if the woman has had a child with Down syndrome in the past, she now has a risk of 1/100 for having a subsequent child with chromosomal abnormality.

13. Define chromosomal structural rearrangement abnormality.

Structural rearrangement indicates that there has been chromosome breakage, followed by reconstitution of the chromosomal elements involved in the break(s). Structural rearrangements can involve only a single chromosome or an exchange of chromosomal material between chromosomes.

14. Who is at risk for chromosomal structural rearrangement abnormality?

Persons who carry balanced structural chromosomal rearrangements are at increased risk of producing gametes with too many or too few chromosomes and therefore are at increased risk for having abnormal offspring with unbalanced chromosome complements. Thus, for couples in whom one or both members carry a structural chromosomal abnormality, prenatal genetic diagnosis should be provided.

15. What factors are important in determining the risk of having a child with a chromosomal abnormality if one parent carries a balanced chromosomal rearrangement?

The risk depends on the type of chromosomal rearrangement and sometimes on whether the translocation is carried by the mother-to-be or the father-to-be.

16. Is a positive family history for a single gene disorder another indication for prenatal genetic diagnosis?

Yes. Prenatal genetic diagnosis is an option if there is a family history of a genetic disorder that can be diagnosed in fetal cells/amniotic fluid by means of a biochemical genetic or molecular genetic (DNA) analysis. Most of these disorders are the so-called single gene disorders inherited in autosomal recessive, autosomal dominant, or X-linked fashion.

17. Discuss the role of maternal genetic testing in couples with a family history of an X-linked disorder for which there is no specific prenatal diagnosis test.
Even when no direct or alternative test is available, prenatal diagnosis allows the parents of a previous male child affected with a X-linked disorder to determine the fetal sex in a subsequent pregnancy. The information about the fetal sex may be used by the couple to decide whether or not to continue the subsequent pregnancy.

18. What are the other indications for prenatal genetic diagnosis?
Even in pregnant women who are not previously known to be at risk to have children with genetic abnormalities, when fetal abnormalities are detected by means of fetal ultrasound and/or the risk for fetal abnormalities is increased due to the results of routine maternal serum screening tests, it is necessary to discuss risks and options and to provide prenatal genetic diagnosis.

19. Can prenatal genetic diagnosis be used to test for all fetal abnormalities at the present time?
No. Although currently most chromosomal disorders and increasing numbers of single gene disorders can be diagnosed prenatally by means of amniocentesis or chorionic villous sampling, many other fetal abnormalities are not detectable at present.

20. What types of tests are available for prenatal genetic diagnosis?
Two major categories of tests are available: invasive and noninvasive.

21. List the available invasive prenatal genetic tests. Briefly explain each.
Amniocentesis is an outpatient procedure in which a sample of amniotic fluid is removed transabdominally by syringe under ultrasonographic guidance. The amniotic fluid contains cells of fetal origin that can be cultured for a variety of genetic diagnostic tests. The concentration of a fetal glycoprotein called alpha fetoprotein (AFP) is also measured in amniotic fluid. The concentration of AFP is generally elevated when an open neural tube defect (NTD) is present. Amniocentesis is generally performed at16 to 20 weeks of gestation.
Chorionic villous sampling (CVS) is also an outpatient procedure in which a biopsy of tissue from the villous area of the chorion frondosom is obtained using a transabdominal or transcervical approach under ultrasound guidance. The fetal cells obtained from this procedure can be cultured for a variety of diagnostic tests. Because no fluid is obtained, AFP levels cannot be assayed. CVS is generally performed between 10 and 12 weeks of gestation.
Cordocentesis is a procedure in which a sample of fetal blood is directly obtained from the umbilical cord under ultrasound guidance. The fetal cells obtained by means of this procedure can undergo various genetic diagnostic tests. Cordocentesis is performed at 19 to 21 weeks of gestation.

22. What are the risks of the invasive tests?
Amniocentesis: The major complication associated with mid-trimester amniocentesis is an 0.5–1% risk of inducing miscarriage.
CVS: The risk of fetal loss is approximately 1–2%. Also about 2% of CVS samples yield ambiguous results due to mosaicism or pseudomosaicism. Follow-up amniocentesis is recommended in order to determine whether the fetus has a chromosomal abnormality.
Cordocentesis: The incidence of fetal loss is 2–3%.

23. What noninvasive prenatal genetic tests are available?
1. **Assays in maternal serum.** Analysis of maternal serum for biochemical markers, including AFP, can be used to identify women at increased risk for having a child with Down syndrome, trisomy 18, and neural tube defects.

2. High-resolution ultrasound. High-resolution, real-time scanning is used for fetal assessment and for detection of varioius morphologic abnormalities. It is used to determine fetal age, identify multiple pregnancies, assess fetal viability, and monitor fetal growth.

24. Is maternal serum screening (MSS) a diagnostic test?
No. MSS in the first or second trimester is a screening test. MSS should ideally be offered to all pregnant women, especially those below the age of 35 years. MSS includes a panel of blood analytes designed to define the relative risk of various congenital conditions, such as neural tube defects or chromosome problems (e.g., Down syndrome). Interpretation of MSS is generally performed along with additional clinical studies. As an example, an MSS test for a pregnant women is termed a positive screen for Down syndrome if the estimated risk is equivalent to or greater that the risk for having a Down syndrome fetus in a 35-year-old woman.

25. If a women screens positive on her MSS test, what should be done?
Genetic counseling and more invasive prenatal genetic testing, including amniocentesis, should be offered.

26. What does a negative MSS screen mean?
The risk of having a child with Down syndrome, trisomy18, or a neural tube defect is reduced in women who screen negative on the MSS test. Their risks, however, are not zero.

27. How is ultrasonography used as a noninvasive prenatal test?
High-resolution, real-time scanning is used for fetal assessment and for detection of various morphologic abnormalities. It is used to determine fetal age, identify multiple pregnancies, assess fetal viability, and monitor fetal growth.

28. What types of ultrasound are used to assess the fetus?
Transabdominal ultrasound is the traditional method. However, transvaginal ultrasound is used with increasing frequency.

29. Is nuchal fold translucency (NT) a useful marker for fetal aneuploidy?
Yes. This measurement quantifies the subcutaneous translucency between the skin and the soft tissue overlying the cervical spine. NT can be increased because of an abnormal accumulation of fluid in the region behind the fetal neck at 10–14 weeks of gestation. The risk for chromosomal aneuploidy correlates with the degree of NT. Increased NT can also be seen in other genetic syndromes or at times if an underlying cardiac defect is present.

30. What role does preimplantation genetic diagnosis (PGD) play in prenatal testing?
This new technology uses molecular genetic or cytogenetic techniques to select embryos free of a specific genetic/cytogenetic conditions for transfer to the uterus during in vitro fertilization (IVF). Micromanipulation techniques can be used to biopsy a single cell from a 6- to 8-cell blastomere after IVF. Some programs biopsy the polar body. Some chromosome abnormalities can be identified using fluorescence in situ hybridization (FISH). Molecular genetic analysis for an ever expanding number of single-gene disorders using the polymerase chain reaction can also be performed. The type of tests undertaken depends on the genetic problem under consideration.

31. What is genetic counseling?
Genetic counseling is a major component of medical genetic practice that focuses on the patient as well as on past, present, and future members of the patient's family. It is concerned with informing the patient and family and with providing psychological counseling and support to help individuals and their families adapt and adjust to the impact and implications of the disorder in question, including recurrence risks.

32. What are the common indications for referral to a medical geneticist/genetic counselor?

- Family history of a hereditary condition such as neurofibromatosis, cystic fibrosis, Marfan syndrome, sickle cell anemia, thalassemias, mental retardation, and diabetes, to name a few
- Consanguinity
- Previous child with multiple congenital anomalies and/or an isolated birth defect such as cleft lip or palate or congenital heart disease
- Previous child with developmental delay, mental retardation, or autism
- Reproductive loss: two or more spontaneous abortions with or without a stillbirth.
- Infertility
- Follow-up for a positive newborn test, such as phenylketonuria
- Follow-up for a positive genetic diagnostic or screening test, including a poitive carrier test
- Prenatal diagnosis for advanced maternal age
- Pregnancy exposed to a teratogen, such as alcohol
- Before undertaking genetic testing or after receiving genetic test results, particularly with later-onset disorders such as cancer and neurologic disorders

33. Is genetic screening at the population level the same as testing for affected individuals or carriers within families?

No. Population screening is a public health activity whose purpose is to examine all members of a designated population, regardless of family history.

34. What are the best-known public health genetic screening programs?

Newborn screening programs. Population screening of all newborns is used to identify infants with genetic disorders for which early treatment can prevent and/or ameliorate the consequences of their disorders.

35. What are the criteria for newborn screening?

The stringent criteria for newborn screening include the following:

- Treatment is available.
- Early institution of treatment before symptoms appear will reduce or eliminate the severity of the illness.
- Routine observation and physical exam will not reveal the disorder in the newborn.
- A rapid economical, highly sensitive, and reasonably specific test is available.
- The condition is frequent and serious enough to justify the expense.
- An infrastructure is in place to inform parents and physicians about the screening test results, to confirm the test results, and to institute appropriate treatment and counseling.

36. What genetic disorders are included on the newborn screening panel in all states?

The number of tests on the newborn screening panel varies from state to state. However, some conditions are on the screening panel in all states, including phenylketonuria (PKU), galactosemia, and hypothyroidism.

37. What is a carrier?

A carrier is a healthy person who carries a single copy of a recessive (mutated) gene as well as a copy of its nonmutated partner gene. Another term for a carrier is heterozygote.

38. What is the purpose of carrier screening?

Currently carrier screening is performed to identify women/couples who are at risk for having children with severe autosomal recessive disorders.

39. Why do carrier screening programs focus on particular ethnic groups?

Some conditions are more prevalent in certain ethnic groups. The frequency of the disorder in the group targeted for screening must be high enough to justify screening. Examples of carrier screening include heterozygote screening for Tay-Sachs disease and Canavan disease in the

Ashkenazi (Eastern European) Jewish population, beta-thalassemia in persons whose ancestors came from the Mediterranean region, and sickle cell anemia in African Americans. Cystic fibrosis carrier testing is currently offered to all pregnant couples.

40. List the criteria for an effective carrier (heterozygote) screening program.
- Use a dependable inexpensive test.
- Use tests with very low false-positive and false-negative rates.
- Couples who screen positive should have access to genetic counseling.
- Prenatal diagnosis should be available.
- Participation should be voluntary but readily available to couples who are at risk.

41. What are the current ethical issues in medical genetics?
1. Privacy of genetic information
2. Misuse of genetic information
    - Discrimination in employment based on an employee's history or genetic test result
    - Discrimination in health insurance underwriting
    - Discrimination in life insurance underwriting.
3. Stigmatization.
4. Voluntary nature of genetic testing.
5. Testing children for adult-onset, genetic disease, carrier status, and/or genes that predispose to late-onset genetic disorders (not performed at this time)

42. Which chromosomal disorders are known to be associated with infertility?
- Klinefelter syndrome. Males with a 47,XXY chromosome make-up.
- Turner syndrome. Females with a 45, XO chromosome make-up.
- Deletions of the X chromosome. Women who have deletion of the p arm of the X chromosome involving the Xp11 region as well as Xp21 region will be infertile.
- Deletions involving the q arm of the X chromosome generally result in ovarian failure if they involve the proposed critical region of Xq13-q26.
- Women with X chromosome/autosome translocations whose break points are within the Xq13-q26 region.
- Men with microdeletions of the Y chromosome.

43. Which single gene disorders are associated with ovarian infertility?
- Fragile X syndrome: Women who carry FMR-1 premutations or a premutation gene of 50–200 repeats are at increased risk for developing idiopathic ovarian failure.
- Swyer syndrome or 46,XY gonadal dysgenesis: Patients with this condition have sexual infantilism, normal vagina and uterus, and streak gonads. Some patients have been found to have mutations in the SRY or sex-determining region on the Y chromosome.

44. Which single gene disorders are associated with male infertility?
- Androgen resistance (also known as testicular feminization, complete or incomplete): People with this autosomal recessive condition have complete or incomplete androgen receptor deficiency, resulting in a female phenotype, gonadal dysgenesis, or gender ambiguity. Their chromosome complements are 46,XY. They are azoospermic.
- Cystic fibrosis: This autosomal recessive condition is associated with congenital bilateral absence of the vas deferens. The absence of the scrotal vas blocks the transport of spermatozoa from the testis or the epididymis to the distal genital tract. Specific mutations in the cystic fibrosis transmenbrane conductance regulator gene cause this condition (see chapter on CBAVD).

45. Can infertility in women with nonclassic 21-hydroxylase deficiency be reversed?
Yes. Nonclassic 21-hydroxylase deficiency is an attenuated late-onset form of adrenal hyperplasia. Glycocorticoid treatment is effective in suppressing adrenal androgen production.

Women with postmenarchal 21-hydroxylase deficiency resume menses and exhibit improvement with respect to the clinical signs of androgen excess. Reversal of infertility has been reported.

BIBLIOGRAPHY

1. Harper PS: Landmarks in Medical Genetics Classic Papers with Commentaries Oxford, Butterworth Heinemann, 2004.
2. March of Dimes Resource Center. www.marchofdimes.com.
3. Rose P, Lucassen A: Practical Genetics for Primary Care. Oxford, Butterworth Heinemann, 1999.

50. PSYCHOLOGICAL ISSUES IN REPRODUCTIVE DISORDERS

Linda D. Applegarth, Ed.D., and Elizabeth A. Grill, Psy.D.

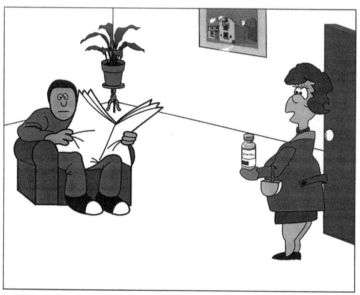

"The doctor said the only treatment for what I have is placebo".

A1 Intellectual Media

1. Why is infertility considered a life crisis?

Infertility not only has a significant impact on the emotional status of the affected person but also places stress on the relationship between partners. For many individuals and couples, the ability to conceive and give birth to a child is paramount to lifelong notions of femininity and masculinity, gender identity, and ultimately the meaning of life. Bearing children and parenting are often among the foundations on which a couple builds a relationship.

It is not only frustrating but also devastating for many couples who want to have children but cannot. According to Becker, parenthood appears to be a pivotal stage of the human life cycle and, more than marriage, symbolizes full responsibility as an adult. Ultimately, for most people, the goal of having children is profoundly intertwined with higher-level goals of fulfillment and happiness.

The inability to conceive or give birth to a healthy child clearly threatens gender identity, calls one's values and motivations for parenthood into question, and forces the couple to re-evaluate the meaning of their relationship. The individual and the couple are thrust into a crisis—a state of *emotional disequilibrium*. Those who lack adequate coping mechanisms to deal with the crisis often experience a loss of self-esteem and self-confidence, and the relationship between partners can suffer from blame, guilt, frustration, and disappointment.

2. What are the common emotional responses to the infertility crisis?

Most symptoms described by patients faced with infertility can be generally categorized as depression, guilt, isolation, and anger.

Depression. The depression resulting from infertility may manifest itself in a variety of ways. Women and men describe feelings of sadness and despair, tearfulness, persistent fatigue, sleep or eating disturbances, anxiety or irritability, and pessimism. Each of these symptoms can be indicative of a depressive state. Although some women experience long periods of profound depression, most more commonly describe short but recurrent episodes. Often they are precipitated by the onset of menses; social events such as baby showers, family holidays, and reunions; or the announcement of a friend's or family member's pregnancy. Certainly depression is a normal response to the emotional pain and loss associated with infertility; however, severe ongoing depression can result in feelings of hopelessness, an inability to function in daily living, severe anxiety or agitation, and suicidal ideation or behavior. This condition requires immediate mental health intervention.

Guilt. Feelings of guilt also often result from the infertility experience. Women tend to assume that they are the cause of the infertility. If the assumptions prove true, they may begin (often fruitlessly) to search for a cause. They reproach themselves for past "misdeeds" and may even offer to divorce their husbands to free them to have children with another partner. The attempt to determine how and why the infertility happened can assume an obsessional quality. As the condition persists, many patients feel increasingly out of control and powerless. Men may also experience guilt feelings, particularly if they have a diagnosed male factor. They seem often reluctant, however, to express these feelings as well as those of disappointment and grief to their partner. Their reluctance may rest in the notion that they will only contribute further to the emotional distress that they couple already experiences. Guilt feelings as well as a general sense of inferiority may be exacerbated by the overt and covert demands and expectations of family and friends. The infertile couple may experience overwhelming guilt and sorrow about disappointing or denying grandparents-to-be or potential aunts and uncles. The couple may also be consumed with guilt about being unable to fulfill their duties and responsibilities related to "carrying on the family name" or providing an heir.

Isolation. Feelings of isolation and social separateness begin to develop when the couple realizes that others seem to conceive and bear children effortlessly. They at once feel different and alone. This sense of isolation may develop when the couple is continuously questioned or teased about their childlessness. The need to insulate oneself from the emotional pain brought on by others' curiosity or by social celebrations such as baby showers, christenings, and family events is acute. To avoid this pain, many infertile individuals and couples tend to withdraw, to isolate themselves from family and friends with children, or to avoid activities that include children. The resulting feeling of isolation can significantly affect self-esteem. The infertile individual or couple thus feels different, impaired, and prohibited from being part of a larger, childbearing society.

Anger. Some men and women who experience infertility describe feelings of anger, often at life, because it has treated them unfairly. This generalized anger and feeling of helplessness, however, can be displaced onto the self (resulting in depression), one's partner, family members and friends, and medical staff. Anger often seems to be a direct consequence of the sense of powerlessness. Despite their best efforts, the couple cannot do what others can accomplish so easily. Although these patients can be difficult for medical professionals to deal with, their angry feelings and behavior usually mask anxiety, fear, and emotional anguish. Most people confronted with infertility have historically been able to feel a sense of control in their lives; they know how to succeed at most things in life. The infertility experience carries no recipe for success. Despite their best efforts, the couple may be faced with month after month of failed cycles and no guarantee of success. Without sufficient strategies for dealing with this crisis, many patients are left feeling hurt, frustrated, and angry.

3. Is it common for couples who are undergoing infertility treatment to experience depression and anxiety?

Several studies have shown that the inability to conceive or to give birth damages self-esteem and is often associated with deep feelings of depression, guilt, and anxiety. Infertility can be one of the most distressing life crises for a couple to face. The sadness that hits every month when a couple discovers that they are not pregnant can be profound and paralyzing. Several studies have shown that there are significantly more infertile women with current depression or a history of depression than fertile women and that the most depressed women have typically been trying for 2–3 years and have been diagnosed with a causative factor for their infertility. Overall, research has shown that women with long-term infertility are more anxious, more depressed, display more hostility, and report more health complaints than fertile women. One study showed that women without children were a subgroup particularly vulnerable to the stress of failure. Furthermore, predisposition toward anxiety, depressive symptoms prior to in vitro fertilization, and fertility history were the most important predictors of emotional response.

In fact, one study showed that infertile patients were just as depressed and anxious as patients who had cancer, heart disease, or HIV-positive status. These results suggest that the psychological symptoms associated with infertility are similar to those associated with other serious medical conditions. Therefore, some experts suggest that psychosocial interventions aimed at reducing depressive symptoms that are applied to serious medical illnesses should also be used to treat infertility patients. One study indicated that the diagnosis of infertility and its treatment was more effectively dealt with by women who had a good personality disposition and a high level of self-esteem, who were satisfied with their job and relationship with their husband, and who were willing to adopt a child as a last solution.

4. What are the symptoms of depression?

The Mental Health Professional Group of the American Society for Reproductive Medicine (ASRM) describe specific symptoms that can lead to minor or major depression. More than five symptoms are considered major depression, which can usually be relieved with mental health intervention. The ASRM recommends that if patients experience any of the following symptoms over a period of two weeks or longer, they should also seriously consider talking with a mental health professional as soon as possible.

- Loss of interest in usual activities
- Depression that doesn't lift
- Agitation and anxiety
- Marital discord
- Strained interpersonal relationships with your partner, friends, family, or colleagues
- Difficulty thinking of anything other than infertility
- High levels of anxiety
- Diminished ability to accomplish tasks
- Difficulty concentrating
- Change in sleep patterns (difficulty falling asleep, staying asleep, or waking up early n the morning)
- Change in appetite or weight
- Increased use of drugs or alcohol
- Thoughts about death or suicide
- Social isolation
- Persistent feelings of pessimism, guilt, or worthlessness
- Persistent feelings of bitterness or anger

5. Why are infertility and infertility treatment often described as an "emotional roller coaster ride"?

The experience of infertility seems to be constantly fraught with highs and lows, hopes and losses—many of which are inexorably tied to the menstrual cycle. Initially, the infertility is probably not the primary focus of the couple's life, and hopes of a pregnancy remain high. As time

---

From Mental Health Professional Group of the American Society for Reproductive Medicine: Frequently Asked Questions—The Psychological Component of Infertility. Available at <www.asrm.org>.

passes, however, the hope diminishes and the world narrows. As pointed out in *Resolving Infertility*, life becomes an endless cycle of hormones and intimacy on demand. Gradually, the couple has difficulty remembering what life was like before the infertility. The quest for a baby requires complete dedication and commitment. As life feels more out of control, the roller coaster ride of hope and despair accelerates. Couples often begin a cycle of feeling optimistic and hopeful about the possibility of a pregnancy. When the menstrual period begins at the end of the cycle, grieving begins. Along with the losses involved in the inability to conceive, friendships are also lost as peers conceive and add second and third children to their families. The belief that life treats one fairly is also lost. With each month that goes by without a successful pregnancy, grief, pain, and anxiety can intensify. For most couples, until some sense of resolution is achieved, it is difficult to get off this emotional roller coaster. It is often the role of the mental health professional to assist couples to set limits on treatment and find meaningful ways to resolve the infertility.

6. Why is fertility treatment viewed as all-consuming?

For many patients and their partners, the infertility experience becomes part of every waking moment. Women, in particular, describe their infertility treatment as a "fulltime job." The desire to achieve a healthy pregnancy becomes extremely powerful, and many patients can think of little else. This obsessional response to infertility appears to stem from an effort to contain anxiety. Many patients, in fact, note that they constantly fear that their efforts to conceive or carry a healthy pregnancy will never be realized. The lack of control over treatment outcomes is key to this anxiety. Rumination and worry become constants, and many women become preoccupied with the body's failure to conceive. Ultimately, infertility treatment can dictate decisions about employment, household spending, vacations, and holiday and family gatherings. In addition, because treatment is often quite costly with limited or no insurance coverage, many couples worry endlessly about how they will pay for it. Financial concerns are then added to fears about treatment outcomes.

7. Why is infertility treatment so stressful?

Individuals and couples experience high levels of stress as they attempt to manage the physical, emotional, and financial concerns related to infertility. When diagnosed with infertility, many couples may no longer feel in control of their bodies or their life plan. Infertility can be a major crisis because it threatens a couple's life goal of achieving parenthood. Most couples are accustomed to planning their lives. Many times previous life experiences, together with the messages provided by Western culture, have taught them that anything is possible if they work hard enough. With infertility, this may not be the case and many infertile persons may experience intense frustration and may even refuse to entertain the possibility that they will not be rewarded for their unrelenting efforts and numerous sacrifices to create a child.

Infertility testing and treatment can be physically, emotionally, and financially stressful. Physically, couples may have to learn to properly mix medications and give injections. Women are required to go to their doctor's offices several times a week for monitoring. Often men must endure painful surgical procedures to aspirate sperm. The hormone levels that rise and fall every month further exacerbate the emotional roller coaster of rising hopefulness and sinking despair. Often insurance does not cover the cost of treatment and/or medications, which quickly becomes exorbitant. Anxiety over the expense of treatment further contributes to increased levels of emotional strain. The infertility experience challenges relationships. A couple's intimacy is often reduced to scheduled intercourse. Being around female friends and family who have children may be difficult. Trying to juggle medical appointments and medicine regimens with job responsibilities can also increase pressure on infertile couples and may jeopardize careers.

8. Do stress and depression affect infertility and treatment outcomes?

Research has shown that infertility causes stress, but one of the most pressing questions is whether stress causes infertility. Most experts say that little evidence indicates that stress directly causes infertility, but nearly all agree that the two are somehow related. High levels of stress may affect a woman's levels of estrogen and progesterone, hormones necessary for reproduction, and may also cause irregular ovulation. Prolonged stress may also cause fallopian tube spasms in women. Stress also affects men. Studies show that men with previously normal sperm counts are eight times more likely to have low sperm counts after a year or two of infertility.

The cycle of rising hopefulness and sinking despair with each month can create enormous levels of chronic stress that in turn can make it more difficult to conceive. This type of stress, which thas been found to cause or exacerbate infertility, is defined by Alice Domar as a combination of the physically damaging depression, anxiety, and isolation that infertile women relentlessly feel when they fail to get or stay pregnant year after year. Several studies using anxiety as a measure of stress have had mixed results. Some report that anxiety does influence infertility, and others suggest no relationship. However, recent studies that measure depression suggest that it plays a strong part in fertility. Several studies indicate that depressed women exhibit lower pregnancy rates than nondepressed women. For example, one study found that women with a history of depressive symptoms were nearly twice as likely to report subsequent infertility than women who were not depressed.

Several studies of infertile women undergoing a behavioral treatment program designed to elicit relaxation responses found statistically significant decreases in anxiety, depression, anger, and fatigue. In one study, 42% of women diagnosed with infertility who participated in a mind/body program conceived within 6 months of completing the program. Another study that placed women in either a mind/body group, a support group, or a control group showed that the women in the mind/body group were significantly less depressed 6 months later than the women in the support and control groups. Within a year, 54% of the support-group participants conceived pregnancies that resulted in a baby, compared with only 20% of the control group. The investigators recommend behavioral treatment that includes stress management and relaxation training for infertile patients who are overwhelmed by difficult decisions, show symptoms of anxiety, depression, or anger, or feel a need for more control in their lives.

9. How can patients cope with the stress of infertility?

It is important for couples to develop coping strategies to help mange the stress of infertility and its treatment and to restore a sense of control to their lives. As the feelings of anxiety and depression lift, couples find that they are better able to make important decisions to resolve their infertility and choose the type of treatment that makes sense. Beyond maintaining good eating habits and getting regular exercise, the first step in coping with a diagnosis of infertility is to learn about it and research all of the available treatment options. Being informed can help couples make better decisions about their care.

Research has also shown that mind/body approaches, particularly those utilizing the relaxation response and patients' negative beliefs, can reduce and counteract the effects of stress on physical, mental, and emotional health. Some studies even suggest that a behavioral treatment approach might be efficacious in the treatment of the emotional aspects of infertility and may lead to increased conception rates. Although relaxation techniques alone may not necessarily increase a patient's chances of getting pregnant, if practiced regularly, these techniques can help people manage inevitable stressors in a healthier way. Stress management techniques can help patients regain some control over their bodies and minds and can help people remember their lives beyond infertility. These benefits may help people feel more empowered as they find the tools to decrease anxiety, increase a sense of control, and restore a feeling of hope for the future.

One reason that women going through infertility tend to feel so depressed and anxious is that they feel unentitled to basic pleasures. Time is of the essence, marriages are strained, medical procedures are difficult, and a sense of hopelessness underlies daily events. Remembering the things that used to bring pleasure and then making it a point to do one of them once a day can help restore a sense of personal well-being. Pleasure may mean buying flowers, eating a favorite food without guilt, listening to a favorite song, buying a scented candle, getting a massage, reading a book unrelated to infertility, going to the movies, trying a new restaurant, or pursuing a hobby. Although this approach may seem difficult when couples are concerned and consumed with infertility treatment, taking a break to carve out some personal time can help to recharge the emotional and physical energy that has been depleted.

Lastly, infertility is often the first life crisis that drives couples to seek counseling with a mental health professional. Men and women may choose individual or couples' therapy to help them cope with the emotional roller coaster. Research has also shown that group support can help people diagnosed with infertility to feel better. Support groups provide men and women with a place where they can discuss their concerns related to medical and emotional experiences. In a confidential group atmosphere, individuals and couples can share practical advice and helpful tips. Group members have the opportunity to meet and talk with others undergoing similar experiences, share their feelings, learn helpful ways to manage emotional distress, and gain support during this difficult time. Many individuals coping with infertility also explore complementary therapies such as relaxation techniques, massage, acupuncture, and yoga.

The American Society for Reproductive Medicine recommends the following tips for stress reduction:

1. Keep the lines of communication open with your partner
2. Get emotional support so that you don't feel isolated. Individual or couple counseling, support groups, and books on infertility can help validate your feelings and help you cope.
3. Learn stress reduction techniques such as meditation or yoga
4. Avoid excessive intake of caffeine and other stimulants
5. Exercise regularly to release physical and emotional tension
6. Have a medical treatment plan that both of you are comfortable with
7. Learn as much as you can about the cause of your infertility and the treatment options available.

10. How does infertility affect self-image and self-esteem?

Infertility is an emotionally painful experience for most people. Because motherhood is seen by most women as a primary role in life, many women who fail to conceive or carry a pregnancy may also feel like a failure as a human being. It is common for some infertile women to describe themselves as "defective" or "damaged goods." Clearly this self-perception can lead to depression and loss of self-confidence and competence as well as fears of abandonment by loved ones. For many men, masculinity and fertility are deeply intertwined. If a male factor is diagnosed, self-esteem and self-image may also be negatively affected. An inability to impregnate his partner may strike heavily at a man's view of himself as "whole" and as virile and masculine. In sum, the inability to bear a child—such a basic part of life —can strike at the essence of the individual's sense of self and chip away at feelings of self-worth.

11. Why is infertility described as a loss?

The infertility experience involves many types of losses, real or potential. First, couples may anticipate the loss of a dream or the hope of fulfilling an important fantasy (parenthood). For many, the advent of another menstrual period or an early miscarriage may symbolize the loss of the longed-for child. Other losses may include the loss of a sense of being whole and healthy, loss of self-esteem and self-confidence, or loss of a loving, supportive relationship with one's partner or with family and friends. The childless couple may also feel a loss of status or prestige among their community of family and friends. Each of these types of losses can trigger depression and anxiety. The experience of infertility is ultimately the experience of loss.

12. How can patients manage negative thoughts while going through infertility treatment?

Women coping with infertility often complain that they get caught in a barrage of negative thoughts that become difficult to turn off. These thoughts and beliefs can have an adverse affect on mood, physical health, and behaviors. Cognitive therapy provides a treatment model for dealing with negative, self-defeating thoughts and irrational beliefs. It provides a way to recognize that stress is often caused by negative thoughts and that these thoughts create moods or emotions that, in turn, can affect physical symptoms and behaviors. Cognitive restructuring interrupts this negative cycle and helps women identify their negative thoughts, question their validity, and then replace them with new thoughts that are more balanced. Journaling can also help make sense of negative thoughts and facilitate emotional catharsis and insight.

13. How does infertility affect the couple/marriage relationship? Do other types of relationship problems develop from the infertility?

For many marriages, the dream of having a child is central to the relationship, and for some couples the failure to conceive may lead to absence of a purpose in the marriage or even a purpose in living. In general, research has revealed that marital adjustment and sexual satisfaction are stable across the first two years of treatment but then deteriorate after the third year. Regardless of when this breakdown may occur, most couples feel that the very foundation of the relationship is shaken as they are challenged to cope with stress and vulnerability, the loss of a dream, a sense of powerlessness, and feelings of guilt as well as blame.

Infertility often results in typical symptoms of depression such as moodiness, loss of interest in favorite activities, fluctuations in weight, sleep problems, energy loss, feelings of worthlessness or inappropriate guilt, difficulty concentrating, and thoughts of death or suicide that can further stress a marriage. It may be difficult to connect with a spouse who is frequently withdrawn, depressed, and lethargic and seems uninterested in you and the things that both of you used to enjoy doing together. In fact, spouses commonly complain that they no longer recognize the person that they married and may fear that they will never get him or her back.

Coping with infertility places many demands on a couple. Couples must learn how to give injections and master the terminology and nuances of reproductive medicine. Socially, they may find creative ways to avoid baby showers, christenings, and baby namings. In addition, sexual dysfunction or dissatisfaction may place tremendous strain on the marriage. Ultimately, couples' conversations, sex lives, work responsibilities, social events, vacations, and important decisions about the future begin to revolve around infertility and treatment plans.

14. Is infertility a frequent cause of couple separation or divorce?

It is encouraging to note that few couples separate or divorce as a result of infertility. Although the difficulties surrounding efforts to conceive or carry a child can be extremely stressful for most couples, many ultimately feel that the experience brought them closer together and led to the development of more effective coping skills. For some couples, however, infertility can serve as a catalyst for causing partners to become further alienated or withdrawn from one another. In such cases, it is likely that the relationship already had problems that were vague or poorly defined. The stress of infertility can exacerbate alcoholism or substance abuse, infidelity, verbal and physical abuse, and so on. When the infertility occurs, these relationships may not be able to withstand the physical and emotional pressures and strains inherent in this crisis.

15. How does infertility affect the couple's sexual relationship?

Sexual dysfunction may be either a cause or a consequence of infertility. Infertile couples have reported sexual problems ranging from lack of desire, pleasure, or spontaneity to sexual dysfunction. Infertility may rob couples of the sensuality and spontaneity of making love, and sex may become solely associated with the mechanical action of trying to conceive. Couples are given specific guidelines for when they can and cannot have sex. Their sex lives are quickly taken from the intimacy of the bedroom to the control of a doctor or a clinic or an ovulation kit. A constant barrage of shots, blood tests, and surgical procedures can leave women feeling physically and emotionally exhausted, which may further contribute to their disinterest in engaging in any type of sexual contact. In addition, many woman begin to associate sex with failure and avoid it whenever possible.

Men may begin to feel as though their wives have lost interest in sex, especially when they express interest in making love only in midcycle when they are fertile. This feeling may add more pressure for men who feel that the pleasure and enjoyment that were once intrinsic to lovemaking have shifted to the responsibility of performing on demand (e.g., during ovulation, postcoital tests, producing semen samples). Thus, many couples begin to feel that they are letting each other down, and those feelings of inadequacy can interfere with desire and performance in the bedroom.

It is clear that the stress, psychological demands, and physically intrusive procedures associated with infertility treatment can affect sexual self-image, desire, and performance. For many couples, making love is one of the best ways to connect emotionally, and when their sex lives are associated with failure, frustration, anger, and resentment, a crucial avenue of emotional expression disappears.

Couples who experience sexual difficulties or dissatisfaction caused by emotional or marital problems, stress, lack of knowledge, or infertility treatment may wish to consider professional counseling with an infertility counselor or sex therapist to help them develop and maintain a more positive, enjoyable sexual relationship during infertility treatment. Medication, surgery, or devices to treat anatomic problems may also be suggested to treat physical causes of sexual dysfunction.

16. Do men and women experience and respond to infertility differently?

Research about gender differences in psychological responses to infertility indicates that overall women experience greater levels of psychosocial distress than their male partners on global measures of anxiety, depression, hostility, and cognitive disturbances as well as on measures of stress and self-esteem. A woman's desire to have a baby tends to resonate at a biologic and emotional level much differently from a man's experience of infertility. Even when the problem is a male factor, women must endure the physical and emotional strains of infertility treatments. The woman must bear the brunt of the medical interventions and show up for regular monitoring. Although the man may find it easier to distract himself with work or other obligations, the day-by-day struggle of injections, side affects, periods, pregnancies, miscarriages, and D&Cs is happening inside the woman.

On the other hand, research has shown that men's responses to infertility closely approximate those of women if the infertility is attributed to a male factor and that men with male factor infertility exhibit more anxiety and somatic symptoms as well as feelings of stigma, loss, and poor self-esteem. Women may not understand the shame a man who associates potency with manliness may feel when he cannot "make" his wife pregnant, or the anxiety and degradation that men report when forced to provide a sperm sample for an IUI or IVF cycle.

The expectations and dynamics between a couple are also challenged. For many women, as efforts to have a child go unrewarded, thoughts about the infertility as well as the need to discuss it sometimes reach obsessional proportions. A failure of any kind has the potential to throw her into days of depression. The husband, on the other hand, may feel overwhelmed with his wife's despair and her constant desire to talk about the infertility He may either respond with calm, reason, and optimism in an effort to comfort his partner and be "the strong one," or he may begin to feel like a failure because he cannot fix the problem. In general, studies have shown that men tend to cope with the emotional stress of infertility by using denial, distancing, avoidance, and withdrawal, which may lead the female partner to believe that the man is callous and disinterested.

The man's behavior, in turn, may cause the woman to feel that her partner does not care about her distress or does not really want a child. Women tend to have more difficulty with staying optimistic and react to the infertility by expressing themselves emotionally. The woman may begin to resent her husband's ability to function effectively at work or to distract himself from the problems. It is typical for the woman to want her husband to be more emotional and for the man to want his wife to be more rational. As a result, partners may begin to doubt the stability of the relationship and may withdraw from one another, feeling angry, hurt, and alone.

Although there appear to be clear gender-specific responses to infertility, research has shown that overall both male and female patients with infertility are significantly more distressed then the average fertile couple. Although these diverse responses to the infertility crisis may provide some balance in the relationship, there may be periods in which the couple is unable to work through differences with respect to treatment decisions, parenting options, and so forth. In any case, the couple may benefit from counseling that is aimed at helping them develop more effective communication skills, respect their different coping styles, and ultimately get back on track together.

17. How do race, culture, and religion affect the individual's or couple's experience of infertility?

Race, culture, and religion can have a significant impact on the infertility experience. In some cultures, for example, the expectation that the couple will bear children as soon as possible is quite profound. The couple experiencing infertility in this environment feels shame and guilt and may shroud themselves in secrecy. Such an experience isolates the couple and leaves them devoid of a social support system. Some highly traditional or less-developed societies may, in fact, encourage the husband to leave his wife so that he can bear children with someone else, especially when social status and the family's welfare depend on the number of children produced. Many of these cultures are deeply entrenched in religious traditions that strongly influence how couples approach infertility diagnosis and treatment. Health care providers must understand and be sensitive to cultural differences that influence patients' understanding and reaction to infertility. For example, a patient who decides to wait on God, pray for a child, or consult a traditional healer may be interpreted as noncompliant or too passive by the medical community. Some individuals may also be reluctant to seek out infertility treatment, however, because it violates cultural norms and values. More specifically, certain medical assessment techniques and treatments are considered unacceptable and can create religious and moral conflicts for some groups. Lastly, differences among racial and ethnic groups also influence how infertility treatment is approached. Asians, for example, may view diagnosis and treatment as intrusive or immodest, whereas African-Americans may see the ARTs as unnatural or devoid of spirituality. In addition, clear economic barriers may prevent some racial or ethnic groups, such as African-Americans or Hispanics, from pursuing or following through with infertility treatment.

18. What issues should be considered for single women and lesbian couples?

For both single women and lesbian couples, the idea of motherhood by choice has only recently been widely acknowledged by physicians and other health professionals. Women who present to infertility clinics are not necessarily infertile or known to be infertile. Instead, they have chosen to have the assistance of medical professionals rather than conceive via sexual intercourse or self-insemination. As Jacobs has noted, the motivations for parenting given by single women or lesbian couples do not differ for those of married women. Many of these women state that they have always wanted to have children or hope to fulfill the expectations of family. As a result, single women and lesbians should not be asked to convince medical practitioners of their desire for children more clearly than married women do. Jacob also notes that currently few or no data indicate that children of single mothers by choice or lesbian couples are less well adjusted or mentally healthy than children of heterosexual couples.

Nonetheless, although many of these women tend to be thoughtful and deliberate in their decisions to conceive, others may make this decision impulsively and/or have not discussed the issue with family or friends. It may be helpful for those who wish to move forward with this decision to meet with a mental health professional. The purpose of this meeting is to review the ability to manage financially (as a single parent), ensure that they have a solid support system, and explore their own uncertainties and fears about this life-changing event. In addition, it is important that these women consider how they will tell the child about his or her conception through the use of donor insemination. The decision to use a known sperm donor has benefits; however, the potential social and legal ramifications should be considered. Such ramifications usually do not arise with the use of an anonymous sperm donor. If the lesbian couple has not come out to family members, work colleagues, and so on, it is critical that they give careful thought to what it may be like for a child to carry the burden of this secret. Lesbian couples wishing to have a child together should complete the process of coming out as part of their preparation for parenthood. As noted above, meeting with a mental health professional can be very helpful to single women and lesbian couples who have not fully processed their decision to become parents.

19. What issues are relevant to older couples who have delayed childbearing?

Many older couples who have delayed childbearing will face infertility. This unique circumstance requires not only understanding but also active support on the part of health and mental health professionals. Decisions about treatment or other family-building options should be made with care and sensitivity to the particular needs and concerns of the patient. Older couples may also have to be encouraged to be more aggressive in their treatment protocols, and any ambivalence that they feel about becoming parents should be explored early in the process.

Guilt is often a highly salient component of the emotional response to infertility in older couples. Because they have postponed childbearing or ignored the biologic clock, many patients become aware of a "missed opportunity." This awareness can lead to self-recrimination, regret, and depression.

Whether or not couples have delayed having children or only recently found one another as suitable partners, it is important that this unique patient group consider parenthood in the context of their lifestyles and age. Older couples who are emotionally and financially stable may be in an excellent position to parent; however, they must also consider the physical and emotional costs of being parents at this life stage. Motivations for parenting should also be explored since the reasons for wanting a child can change over the life cycle. As Applegarth and Kingsberg and Rosenthal have pointed out, it may be important for both partners to understand the longer-term implications for themselves as well as a child of being older and, as a result, at higher risk for death or age-related disability. From an ethical standpoint, controversy can arise as to whether to provide older infertile couples with limited medical resources such as ovum donation — or to do in vitro fertilization when the chances of success are negligible.

20. What are the unique issues and concerns for couples experiencing secondary infertility?

For many couples, the emotional impact of secondary infertility can be just as severe as it is for those who have never been able to have a child. Couples with secondary infertility describe themselves as experiencing the joys of parenthood while also feeling profoundly deprived because now it eludes them. The couple who already has a child (or children) often find themselves in the paradoxical position of being a biologic parent and also being infertile. They may feel confused and incredulous — grateful for the child that they have but also yearning for another. They may also delay seeking medical treatment because the previous pregnancy came easily and they assume that it will eventually happen again. When a pregnancy does not occur, women suffering from secondary infertility paradoxically chide themselves for not having sought treatment sooner.

Some patients with secondary infertility may feel resentful of those who are easily able to have a second or a third child or feel guilty and disappointed about being unable to give their child a sibling. Most of these couples maintain an active parenting role but also tend to feel different or apart from those whom they perceive as a "normal" family. Secondary infertility often creates a unique emotional dilemma: couples feel a societal pressure to have more than one child but may also be told by friends and family that they should "just be thankful for what they have." It is often difficult to reconcile the two positions, which leads to internal conflict and ambivalent feelings. As with primary infertility, secondary infertility often results in depression and anxiety. Many of these patients benefit greatly from individual or couples' counseling or from patient support groups aimed at assisting couples who are experiencing secondary infertility.

21. Why is it helpful for patients and practitioners to redefine the meaning of success for patients undergoing infertility treatment?

Most medical personnel and patients tend to view "success" as the achievement of a healthy, ongoing pregnancy. This notion is further reinforced by the understandable requirement on the part of infertility clinics to report publicly pregnancy statistics and ART success rates. Unfortunately, however, not all patients meet these criteria for success. For many, to have "failed" in treatment is interpreted as failure as a healthy, capable person. Similarly, most medical personnel are deeply invested in assisting couples to achieve healthy pregnancies and may also experience the failure to do so as a personal disappointment or loss. Treatment options and opportunities now seem limitless, making it increasingly difficult for patients to know when to end treatment. As the medical technology continues to develop, it is especially important to reframe and redefine "success" with a broader meaning. It must mean more than walking away from treatment with a genetic child, especially in light of the tremendous emotional risks that infertile patients take on a daily basis in their journey toward parenthood. The notion of "success" should be expanded to include the feeling that, regardless of outcome, the treatment experience helped to bring closure to a prolonged and painful life experience. Couples who leave treatment and turn to other family-building options or to "childfree" living must also be encouraged to feel comfortable with their decisions.

If health professionals in infertility and ARTs can reconstruct their ideas of success, they, too, may be more effective at dealing with their own anxieties and burnout. The infertile population is relentlessly persistent, demanding, and needy. Assisting some of these patients in their decisions to end treatment and helping them reformulate their personal definitions of success may be one of the greatest successes that any medical professional can achieve.

22. How does infertility affect relationships with family and friends?

Infertility can often cause a tremendous amount of strain on relationships with family and friends. Although some families and friends are supportive, others seem to add more stress to the process, often triggering anger and causing couples to withdraw into isolation. Couples may feel jealous of friends and relatives who conceive and deliver healthy babies with ease. Friends and relatives often aggravate the situation by repeatedly asking when the couple is planning to have children or by talking endlessly about their own or others' children.

Many couples openly share the details of their treatment with family and friends only to find that the constant questioning and advice offered by others greatly increases the levels of stress. Couples are often interrogated about the cost and procedures, which are then minimized with comments such as, "If you would just relax, take a vacation, have a glass of wine, and calm down, you would get pregnant." Or they may blame the couples' infertility on the woman's career and urge her to quit her job or limit her responsibilities in an attempt to avoid more stress.

There are many families who want to help but simply do not know what to do or say— there are families who simply do not seem interested in trying. Many parents feel uncomfortable discussing infertility because they associate couples' attempts to have a baby with sex. At other times, older generations are ignorant about modern technology's methods of conception. Most older people grew up during a time when women had few medical options and made the decision to adopt or live childfree. In some instances, religious beliefs and conservative ideologies can stand in the way of family support. Siblings and friends may shy away from the subject because they fear that infertility will affect them too, or they may flaunt their own fertility intentionally because of a competitive streak or unintentionally because of ignorance.

When couples feel this lack of understanding, they become reluctant to go home for holidays and deal with nieces and nephews and pregnant family members. When friends are getting pregnant easily, couples often feel that they are being left behind and begin to avoid baby showers, baby namings, and christenings. Consequently, couples begin to sacrifice their social networks when they need the support more than ever. It is usually healthier to temporarily limit contact with insensitive family members and friends and seek support from other people (e.g. therapists, groups, other friends and family members) who are better able to provide it.

23. What are some ways to cope with family and friends during this difficult time?

Couples often struggle with whether or not they want to disclose the details of their treatment. If they decide to tell, they must decide to whom. Often couples are disappointed because the people that they thought would be supportive turn out to be insensitive and hurtful. Friends and family members who may have been there for couples in the past might not necessarily be the ones to help them thorough this crisis; therefore, couples should be open to others who may be able to help them more.

In some cases, friends and family members need to be educated not only about infertility and its treatments but also about the ways in which they can provide support. To educate them, couples can lend books or point them in the direction of helpful websites. Couples usually expect friends and family members to know intuitively how and when to offer support, but couples should plan to communicate with others about what is helpful and what is harmful. They should form a united front and create a plan for social events or holidays when someone may be announcing a pregnancy. Couples should tell family and friends how and when they would like to be told the news so that they have a sense of control over the process.

Usually friends and family members want to support couples through this difficult time but might not know how. If, after educating and communicating with others, they still do not understand, it may be more appropriate to stay away from such people. Sometimes, couples feel guilty if they do not want to socialize with friends or family members who are pregnant or who have new babies. They often feel great relief once given permission to stay away from baby stores or from friends and family who are insensitive. Keeping infertility a secret may be the right decision for some, whereas selective avoidance of some family members, friends, events, and situations that bring about intense pain may feel more comfortable for others. Experts agree that couples should make decisions on a case-by-case basis while being sensitive to their own needs and careful not to isolate themselves completely from those who can provide the support that they need.

24. How can family members and friends support the infertile couple?

As Burns and Covington observe, involuntary childlessness is an intergenerational crisis that has the ability to strain or damage family relationships by impairing communications and interactions. When infertility interrupts the normal family life cycle, it is not uncommon that a family's unique flaws precipitate negative behaviors such as parental favoritism, poor communication, and/or unhealthy coping strategies. As a result, family (and friends) can sometimes be the infertile person's greatest challenge. They say insensitive things ("I think you're just too stressed and need a vacation.") or pry into the couple's personal lives ("Any big news this month?"). Many family members and friends, in fact, truly struggle with how to support the couple experiencing infertility. Support and interest are usually much appreciated by the infertile couple; however, advice is not. In an effort to be helpful, some family members talk of "miraculous pregnancies" that they have heard about, cut out articles, or suggest treatments or physicians. This type of behavior is usually unwelcome because it implies that the couple is incapable of making their own decisions.

Burns and Covington offer the following suggestions for family and friends:

1. Acknowledge infertility as a medical and emotional crisis with a wide variety of losses, disappointments, and costs.

2. Be sensitive to the pain, stress, and emotional pressure of childlessness or the inability to expand one's family as desired.

3. Ask the couple how they would like to be supported.

4. Emphasize the importance and value of the couple as family members and friends.

5. Keep lines of communication open, and stress the importance of honesty, candor, tact, and diplomacy in interactions.

6. Respect the boundaries that the couple sets regarding their infertility.

25. How can patients address infertility concerns and treatment issues in the workplace?

As couples attempt to juggle the demands of careers with the inconveniences of infertility, they struggle to maintain their performance on the job and often contemplate whether to continue working. The unpredictability of some medical treatments can limit both the husbands and the wife's ability to travel for work and to schedule appointments. Infertility treatment often requires that women have blood work and ultrasounds early in the morning. Husbands have to be available to provide sperm and often are responsible for helping their wives with daily injections that must be given at certain times. Couples struggle with whether to tell bosses and coworkers the truth about their tardiness and days off. They may feel pressured to tell in order to prevent rumors from spreading but may fear that telling could prevent them from receiving important assignments because of a lack of confidence. The increased stressors involved with infertility treatment often result in poor job performance, which may further affect the man or woman's self-esteem, especially when he or she has always taken pride in being a conscientious employee with a strong work ethic.

Some contemplate quitting their jobs either because they feel that infertility is a full-time commitment or because, as their priorities shift, they no longer feel fulfilled at work. Those who work long hours or travel a lot for business may even be concerned that the stress from the job is causing the infertility. Some begin to feel trapped as they lack the energy to perform a job search and worry that if treatment is successful, a new boss will not appreciate a pregnant new employee who will need time off for maternity leave. Couples may also struggle with whether the man or woman can even afford to quit with the increasing costs of treatment. It is strongly recommended that if people quit their jobs, they should make sure they have something other than infertility treatments to do.

26. When is counseling a necessary part of helping an individual or couple cope with infertility?

Many individuals and couples faced with the crisis of infertility can benefit from counseling. Depression and anxiety are often significant side effects of infertility. At various points in the experience, the individual or couple may also be thrust into a more intense crisis, i.e., a failed ART cycle, pregnancy loss, or bad news about future treatment options. When these situations occur, it is often advisable that patients obtain psychological counseling to help cope with such powerful and painful losses. Although the counseling is often intense and short-term, it can be especially constructive and helpful in re-establishing a sense of emotional equilibrium. This is true for distressed couples' relationships as well as for individuals.

Because infertility diagnosis and treatment can be prolonged, it is common for patients to feel that their lives are "on hold" as they await some form of resolution. The inability to move on with life can lead to depression. Although depression and anxiety are understandable responses to this highly uncertain and emotionally painful experience, some individuals are emotionally more fragile or prone to depressive episodes. Ongoing depression can result in feelings of hopelessness, inability to function in daily living, severe anxiety or agitation, and even suicidal thoughts or behavior. This condition requires immediate mental health intervention.

27. What different treatment approaches can be effective in counseling infertile individuals and couples?

A wide variety of psychotherapeutic treatment approaches can be highly effective in working with infertile patients—both as individuals and as a couple:

- Psychodynamic psychotherapy
- Cognitive-behavioral therapy, including stress management
- Brief strategic/solution-focused therapy
- Crisis intervention
- Grief counseling

The above psychotherapy approaches target different aspects of psychological functioning for change. The duration of treatments can be from hours to years, depending on the psychotherapist's theoretical orientation as well as the patient's request for treatment, financial resources, description of the problem(s), clinical diagnosis, and mental health status.

It appears that infertile patients primarily seek short-term or brief counseling or psychotherapy to relieve painful psychological symptoms resulting from the experience. Others may choose longer term treatment to deal not only with their involuntary childlessness but also with psychological issues and conflicts that may impede decision-making, relationships with family and friends, and ability to cope with the many aspects of daily living.

All infertility counselors can apply several specific tasks when meeting a new client for the first time. These tasks can serve a variety of important purposes and can be critical to the effectiveness of the work done between client and therapist. They include (1) forming a positive working relationship; (2) finding a treatment focus; (3) negotiating criteria for a successful outcome; (4) distinguishing clients from nonclients; (5) identifying patient motivational levels and tailoring interventions accordingly; and (6) doing something that makes a difference immediately.

Finally, Applegarth stresses that any given treatment approach is only as effective as the therapist who employs it. The psychosocial needs of those who struggle to build families are compelling and require clinical expertise and a clear understanding of the underlying emotional issues involved.

28. What are some ways to locate a psychotherapist with experience in infertility counseling?

Locating a psychotherapist to assist infertile patients with the emotional aspects of their condition can be done in several ways. First, many fertility clinics keep a list of referrals to mental health professionals who specialize in infertility counseling and understand its unique aspects. Some programs, in fact, have an in-house mental health professional to assist patients in dealing with the many emotional aspects of infertility. In addition, The Mental Health Professional Group of the American Society for Reproductive Medicine (www.asrm.org or 205-978-5000) also maintains a list of infertility counselors who practice throughout the United States as well as in other countries. Similarly, RESOLVE, the National Infertility Association (as well as other consumer support organizations) provides infertility counselor referrals through its local chapters around the country (www.resolve.org).

29. What should a couple know about third-party reproduction?

Couples considering third-party reproduction must mutually agree that their best alternative to genetic parenthood is the use of donated sperm, eggs, or embryos and must address the emotional consequence of reproductive failure as individuals and as couples. This process usually entails the couples' conscious decision to stop current medical treatment, redefine family, and grieve the biologic, genetically shared child they had hoped for. For most couples, this difficult and emotionally painful process can raise intense feelings of loss and force couples to confront their feelings about the preservations of their own genetic continuity.

Donor egg and sperm programs allow couples to preserve the genetic continuity of one partner. Egg donation offers the opportunity for both partners to participate in the creation of their child—one through the genetic connection, the other through a biologic one. The other participants in third-party reproduction are the sperm and oocyte donors who facilitate parenthood for infertile couples. Preparation of gamete donors varies across the different programs who participate in third-party reproduction. There tends to be more variation in anonymous sperm donation, with preparation primarily focused on medical screening. In contrast, oocyte donors usually receive more extensive assessment and preparation because the donation process is more medically intrusive and demanding. This process typically entails psychological assessment, genetic testing, physical examination, blood screening, and a psychoeducational discussion about possible feelings and questions that may arise in the future. Embryo donors are usually infertile couples who relinquish cryopreserved embryos or extra embryos from a current IVF cycle that they do not plan to use themselves. Preparation of embryo donors usually involves assessment of the donating couple and discussion of the social, legal, and psychological implications of donation.

Couples embarking on the path of third-party reproduction must think about what it means to be a parent and how parenting a child who is not genetically connected to both of them may be different from parenting a child who is genetically connected to only one of them. Couples who feel strongly about their genetic lineage may view donor sperm, egg, or embryo as severing their ancestral ties. Most couples fantasize about what their children will look like, what talents they will possess, and the kind of personality they will have. Couples who are considering donor gametes must face feelings of sadness about not being able to see some of the mother or father's traits reflected in their children. No matter how closely a donor resembles the mother or father, parents cannot ignore the fact that the donor still exists as a real and different person involved in the reproduction process.

Couples must decide whether they feel more comfortable pursuing an anonymous donor or known donor (e.g., family member) and their level of openness about the child's conception. For example, many couples worry that if their family knew about the donation, the child would not be loved or accepted in the same way as a full genetic child.

In addition, they must think about how the addition of a third party, known or unknown, will affect their feelings about themselves, the relationship between partners, and most importantly, the parents' relationship with the child. The man or woman who is unable to use his or her own gametes may wonder if he or she is capable of loving "someone else's child." Most recipient mothers wonder how they will feel carrying another women's genetic child and whether they will bond to that child in utero, after birth, and throughout his or her lifetime. For some couples this process brings up thoughts and feelings about adultery, and they must work toward separating the act of lovemaking from the act of procreation. Others fear that the biologic and genetic inequality of donor sperm or donor egg may eventually threaten their marriage.

Because of the complex emotional, ethical, and practical issues, the American Society for Reproductive Medicine in its 1993 *Guidelines for Gamete Donation* recommends that referral for evaluation and counseling be made available to couples before they attempt to conceive through gamete donation to avoid adverse emotional and psychological consequences.

30. What significant psychological issues are related to gamete donors?

In addition to protecting the emotional well-being of gamete donors, it is imperative to assist them in understanding as fully as possible the meaning and long-term implications of deciding to donate their genetic material to another individual or couple. To date, however, little research is available about the long-term psychological impact of being a gamete donor. Similarly, there appear to be no firm conclusions about whether donors should have access to information regarding the donation outcome, want to have access to information about the offspring or recipients, or want to have information about themselves disclosed to the other party. The lack of well-designed social research precludes any conclusions about deeper psychological motives for donating sperm, ova, or embryos.

An area of interest regarding gamete donation has to do with what we do know about the donors' motivations as well as understanding the reasons for the psychological screening of donors. The extent to which financial compensation is a motivating factor in providing gametes should be explored. The monetary rewards that result from the donation may contribute to the donor's denial or minimization of the longer-term implications of the donation. Novaes points out that if financial compensation were not available, the donor would feel compelled to consider the meaning that he or she attributes to the altruistic component of the donation. In essence, monetary reward for donating may be an "unethical means of obtaining the donor's consent."

However, because financial compensation for time, effort, and medical risk is an intrinsic part of gamete donation in the United States, it is one responsibility of the mental health professional to help donors understand the meanings and implications of the donation and to protect them from making inappropriate decisions about becoming a donor. This principle should apply to sperm donors as well as ovum and embryo donors; however, it does not appear that sperm donors are psychologically evaluated as carefully as ovum donors. This difference may, in part, be the result of a cultural "double standard" that suggests that ovum donors need protection more than sperm donors. At the same time, the medical risks taken by ovum donors is always an important consideration as well as the notion of informed consent regarding the complexities of the donation. In any case, the mental health professional acts as the donor's advocate.

31. What significant psychological issues are related to recipient couples of gamete donation?

Of utmost importance for recipient couples of gamete donation is to mourn appropriately the loss of a genetic offspring that is related to both partners. The inability to acknowledge such a loss often makes it difficult (and sometimes impossible) for the couple to feel comfortable and accepting of gamete donation. The ultimate loss of the ability to create a child can create a powerful emotional crisis as well as feelings of sadness, anger, and bereavement. The losses grieved during infertility often include the loss of hopes, future plans, marital satisfaction, self-esteem, and a loss of a sense of health and well-being. This grief can be experienced by both partners, regardless of whose fertility is lost.

It is advisable that couples meet with a mental health professional to discuss and explore their feelings and appropriately mourn the loss of a genetically related "dream child." The couple may also need assistance to identify and accept gamete donation as a viable family-building option. Couples often carry many fears and fantasies about gamete donation, including concerns that the donor will try to reclaim the offspring or that the child will wish to seek out his or her "real" mother or father. It is the role of the mental health professional to help the recipient couple explore and understand these fears, which may reflect ambivalence or unresolved grief regarding the inability to conceive and parent a genetic child.

Lastly, although the decision to use donated ova or sperm is private, the issue of disclosure of this decision to others or to the resulting offspring often creates anxiety, questions, and uncertainty for the recipient couple.

32. Discuss the main differences between choosing a known vs. an anonymous donor.

The decision to use a known or unknown donor is only one of the many decisions that affect all parties involved, including the potential offspring. Anonymous ovum donors are much more scarce than anonymous sperm donors. Some couples may wish to maintain privacy about the donor decision and therefore strongly desire anonymous donation, whereas others come to the process with additional losses because they do not know anyone who would be appropriate as a donor. Most couples who choose anonymous donation feel protected by the anonymity and believe that it creates a psychological barrier between them and the donor, enabling them to feel more secure as a family. Anonymous donation provides couples with privacy that gives them control over the information about their child's conception. The emphasis on the part of recipient couples on using an unknown gamete donor is often based on the need to feel that the child will never be confused about who his or her parents are.

The scarcity of anonymous donors is one of the main reasons that many recipient couples turn to known ovum donation. Another reason is that couples feel more comfortable in having control over the source of the gametes as well as the knowledge of medical and social histories. Recipients of known ovum donation often feel that they are more involved in the process and more in control of their lives after years of feeling helpless and out of control as a result of infertility. If the donor is a relative, the couple is also able to maintain a sense of genetic continuity. Couples who prefer a nonrelative as an ovum donor may feel comforted by knowing first hand the donor's personality, temperament, and physical attributes and may feel relieved with not having to deal with the social and relational confusion inherent in familial donation. Some choose a close friend, whereas others fear that ovum donation may jeopardize their relationship if something goes wrong, if they do not become pregnant, or if the donor becomes attached to the child and views it as hers. In some cases, known donors also give the child the option of knowing his or her genetic parent—an option that some donor recipient parents feel may help facilitate a more secure identity for their children.

33. Are emotional functioning and child development normal in families created through assisted reproduction?

Although the research in this area is somewhat limited, overall family functioning and child development in families who have participated in assisted reproduction are normal. According to the studies conducted by Golombok et.al., the overall quality of parenting in families with a child conceived by assisted conception is superior to that in families with a naturally conceived child. In one study, mothers of children conceived by assisted reproduction expressed greater warmth toward their child, were more emotionally involved with their child, interacted more with their child, and reported less stress associated with parenting than mothers who conceived their child naturally.

Similarly, fathers who participated in assisted reproduction were found to interact more with their child and to contribute more to parenting than fathers with a naturally conceived child. With respect to the children themselves, no group differences were found for either the presence of psychological disorder or children's perceptions of the quality of family relationships.

34. What factors should be addressed for couples considering adoption vs. gamete donation?

For some couples, the choice between adoption and gamete donation is quite straightforward. For others, the options are less clear and fraught with a wide range of feelings. Sometimes partners in a couple have different viewpoints and feelings about these options. Psychotherapeutic work in such cases includes not only assistance with decision-making but also couples counseling. Many couples ultimately feel comfortable moving on to adoption with the understanding that parenting a child(ren), regardless of his or her biologic origins, is the primary goal. Additionally, the adoption choice places both partners on equal footing with respect to the nonbiologic relationship to the child.

Other couples feel strongly that there must be a biologic or genetic connection to the child on the part of at least one parent so that they can feel more "connected" emotionally to their offspring.

Not infrequently the couple may choose gamete donation in lieu of adoption in an effort to hide their infertile status from others. Although every couple's privacy should be respected and maintained, it is also important that this issue be processed by the couple. Any parenting option chosen out of shame rather than comfort and commitment may delay a sense of resolution and readiness to parent.

It should be emphasized that in the cases of gamete donation or adoption, couples should be given at least 6 months to process emotionally their options after receiving a final recommendation to discontinue treatment or consider donated gametes. A rush to "fix" the infertility and avoid pain can easily lead to anxiety, panic, ambivalence, and conflict in the relationship at a later date. To move forward with a parenting option prematurely also may ultimately impact a parent's relationship with the child(ren). Additionally, options that initially seem unacceptable may—with time—begin to feel right and comfortable as the couple considers their feelings and processes their pain and loss.

35. How can infertile patients obtain information needed to make informed decisions about treatment and/or other family-building options as well as remaining "child-free?"

Many infertility clinics have mental health professionals to assist couples with tough decisions about treatment as well as other family-building options such as third-party reproduction and adoption. After years of treatment disappointments, some couples may also wish to consider a life together that does not include becoming parents. The last alternative can be especially challenging since the decision not to parent is not irreversible—unlike the decision to have or adopt a child. Couples choosing to remain "child-free" often need help in rebuilding their lives as a family of two. It is not a decision of default. The transition to focusing on the partnership alone, however, can take time and may feel awkward. Patient support organizations (e.g., Resolve: The National Infertility Association) provide not only information but also emotional support for couples who are attempting to determine which treatment or parenting option feels right for them. Resolve also provides support and information for couples considering "child-free" living.

36. How can infertile patients best prepare for ART procedures, including third-party reproduction?

Because it is virtually impossible for patients and professionals to control ART outcomes, patients can do a number of things to feel more prepared to deal with the procedures. Despite an awareness on the part of patients of the success rates of ART procedures, there is often a distorted idea of achieving a healthy, ongoing pregnancy—with unrealistically high expectations of success. Nonetheless, every stage of an ART cycle creates new fears and tensions for the patient. The failure to achieve pregnancy may cause significant grief reactions because, at the outset, individuals imagine themselves pregnant and develop lively fantasies about the pregnancy and the wished-for child. Strategies for preparing and coping with ART procedures include:

- Obtaining accurate and adequate information about medical, financial, emotional, and logistical aspects of the procedure
- Consulting with the physician and nursing personnel
- Meeting with the mental health professional for stress management or joining a support group
- Obtaining information and referrals for parenting options other than ARTs

In addition to the above strategies, couples preparing for third-party reproduction will find that the selection or matching of a suitable donor is also a significant aspect of the protocol. Grieving the loss of fertility, voicing fears and concerns about this alternative, and exploring fantasies about future lives as a family are intrinsic parts of preparing for third-party reproduction.

37. What psychological issues are involved in pregnancy loss?

For couples who may have spent years of anticipation, time, energy, and money to conceive a pregnancy, pregnancy loss or the death of a newborn is especially cruel. Pregnancy loss (whether spontaneous or planned) can be an emotionally traumatic experience involving varying degrees of grief, diminished self-esteem, and marital distress. Research has shown that the intensity of grieving is more closely related to the psychological attachment than the length of gestation. Each partner's experience of the grief is unique based on the psychological fantasies, hopes, and wishes that each person had for the unborn child as well as for his or her own future.

Spontaneous loss, miscarriage, stillbirth, or infant death comes at a time when the couple is already vulnerable and may have little time to prepare for it. This type of loss can result in acute grief, clinical depression, and/or the re-emergence of unresolved past losses. Because of the profound fluctuations in hormones, women may experience psychological and physical symptoms such as emotional sensitivity, difficulty sleeping, nightmares, lethargy, or the experience of producing milk, which may serve as constant reminders of the loss.

Planned terminations are often grieved and mourned in the same manner as spontaneous losses, although the social stigma associated with abortion may increase isolation and guilt about the chosen loss of a longed-for child. In either case, the loss of a pregnancy, whether it is spontaneous or planned, can be treated by others as a nonevent that may be glossed over or minimized. The couple has few socially acceptable avenues (e.g., funerals, rituals, cultural traditions) that can help them acknowledge loss and facilitate mourning. If the couple is unable to acknowledge or discuss the loss, a deep sense of shame and personal failure may become intensified.

The goal of all interventions after a pregnancy loss is to facilitate positive grieving. Grieving a perinatal loss can take longer than most people anticipate—from a few months to several years. In the case of stillbirth or infant death, evidence indicates that supportive interventions such as seeing, touching, and spending time with the baby may help facilitate the grief process by helping parents acknowledge the reality of the loss. It is also important for couples to understand that feelings of sadness may resurface during the anniversary date of the conception, birth date, death date, and holidays such as mother's and father's day. Closure or resolution usually occurs when the loss has been integrated into the person's life, which may coincide with a subsequent birth. However, women should be encouraged to allow sufficient time to heal physically and emotionally before attempting another pregnancy.

Interventions after Perinatal Loss

Medical
- Choice of induction/delivery plan
- Seeing, touching, spending time with the baby or viewing products of conception
- Naming the baby
- Taking pictures (if pictures are declined by parents, they should be stored in records for later availability)
- Providing mementos (e.g., lock of hair, wrist bad, foot/hand prints, length/weight certificate, symbolic representations, sonograms)
- Planning for disposition of body/tissue
- Funeral or memorial service
- Choosing room assignment off obstetrics floor or discharge planning
- Providing written material on perinatal grief and support resources
- Interim phone call from staff before follow-up visit

Psychological
- Creating a memory box or album (e.g., photographs, sonogram pictures, laboratory reported, IVF petri dish, cards, toy or item of clothing)
- Memorial activities (e.g., planning a tree, selecting a garden statue, donation to special charity, books for support groups, items for neonatal intensive care unit or high-risk unit)
- Self-care activities (e.g., regular exercise, proper diet, avoidance of alcohol/drugs, following a schedule/routine)
- Keeping a journal, diary, or audiotape describing the loss and grief
- Writing a letter or poem of goodbye to baby
- Planning a memorial service, private or with others
- Reaching out to a support group or family/friends

From Covington SN: Pregnancy loss. In Burns LH, Covington SN (eds): Infertility Counseling. Pearl River, NY, Parthenon Publishing Group, 1999, p 235, with permission.

38. What is involved in counseling couples about issues related to planned termination or multifetal reduction?

Multiple gestation is considered a high-risk pregnancy often associated with more nausea and vomiting, anemia, fatigue, weight gain, heartburn, lack of sleep, financial difficulties, depression, and marital discord. In many instances, multifetal reduction may be advised for the health of the mother and to improve the chances of a successful pregnancy. This is a painful irony for couples who have invested an enormous amount of money, time, and energy in pursuing pregnancy. Unfortunately, selective reduction is too often viewed as a quick solution to a potentially problematic situation, with little forethought and preparation given to the psychological implications.

Research has shown that dealing with the decision of whether to undergo multifetal pregnancy reduction can be a traumatic experience. Studies indicate that couples experience the events surrounding the reduction as chaotic and emotionally disturbing. Couples often struggle with extreme ambivalence while facing the loss of some of the babies and risk of loss of the entire pregnancy. Feelings of remorse are often associated with the couples' decision to eliminate one or more fetuses as well as a sense of fear that the children who are born may harbor unresolved feelings of guilt from being the fetus(es) to survive. Some couples experience multifetal reduction as the loss of another child, which may complicate the grieving process for those who have already experienced a previous miscarriage, stillbirth, or chemical pregnancy. Multifetal reduction is a loss that usually occurs in isolation without the support or knowledge of family and friends and within a social context of stigma and censure regarding pregnancy termination. Despite these potential psychological complications, research has shown that when pregnancy outcome is successful, multifetal reduction does not put women at significant risk for affective illness or elevated levels of psychiatric symptoms.

Research indicates that couples believe avoidance of high-order pregnancies should be of primary importance. Many patients are ignorant of the fact that multiple gestation is a potential outcome. Because the issue of pregnancy termination is politically sensitive and highly emotionally charged, few resources are available to couples. Experts suggest that couples should understand that multiple fetal reduction is a distinct possibility and may be medically advised, but it involves medical risks to the fetuses and mothers. Couples' long struggle with infertility usually precludes them from this possibility, and often psychological counseling is not suggested or required by the medical clinic. It is recommended that couples considering multifetal reduction undergo professional counseling before and immediately after the procedure.

39. How can parents be assisted in coping with a stillbirth or a severely disabled child?

Stillbirth, perinatal death, and birth of a severely disabled child are devastating life events for any couple, regardless of their previous fertility status. This profound loss is life-changing, and the natural course of mourning may take years. These types of losses are quite different and must be grieved in different ways. With a stillbirth or perinatal death, the loss is discrete, and although grief and mourning are profound, the couple has the opportunity to achieve closure and move on. Having a severely disabled child, however, is a lifelong loss that affects a wide range of family members and alters family dynamics.

In both cases, however, couples must be assisted in managing not only their grief but also the guilt that they may feel. Women especially describe ongoing guilt and distress. They may be preoccupied with thoughts and feelings that they did something during pregnancy to cause the problem.

Although individual psychotherapy can be helpful in the short term, many couples find that support groups dedicated to assisting with bereavement related to a stillbirth or perinatal death can be immensely useful. Similarly, institutions and organizations that work with the disabled have special support and resources for both parents and siblings. Many couples who experience a perinatal death or give birth to a disabled child find that only others who share this profound type of loss can truly understand its power and complexity. In either case, it is important for couples to receive psychological support and assistance as soon as possible. Most hospital social service departments have referrals available to couples and other family members.

BIBLIOGRAPHY

1. American Fertility Society. Guidelines for gamete donation. Fertil Steril 59:S1, 1993.
2. American Society for Reproductive Medicine and Infertility: Patient Fact Sheets. Birmingham, AL, American Society for Reproductive Medicine and Infertility, 1996.
3. Applegarth LD: Ethical issues in infertility nursing practice. Infertil Reprod Med Clini North Am 7:611–621, 1996.
4. Applegarth LD: The psychological aspects of infertility. In Keye WR, Chang RJ, Rebar RW, Soules MR. Infertility: Evaluation & Treatment. Philadelphia, W.B. Saunders, 1995.
5. Applegarth LD: Emotional implications. In Adashi EY, Rock JA, Rosenwaks ZR: Reproductive Endocrinology, Surgery, and Technology. Philadelphia, Lippincott-Raven, l996.
6. Becker G: Healing the Infertile Family: Strengthening Your Relationship in the Search for Parenthood. New York, Bantam, l990.
7. Berg BJ, Wilson JF: Psychological functioning across stages of treatment for infertility. J Behav Med 14:11–26, 1991.
8. Bergh C, Moller A, Nilsson L, Wikland M: Obstetric outcome and psychological follow-up of pregnancies after embryo reduction. Hum Reprod 14:2170–2175, 1991.
9. Bringhenti F, Martinelli F, Ardenti R, La Sala GB : Psychological adjustment of infertile women entering IVF treatment: differentiating aspects and influencing factors. Acta Obstet Gynecol Scand 76:431–437, 1997.
10. Burns LH, Covington, SN (eds): Infertility Counseling: A Comprehensive Handbook For Clinicians. Pearl River, NY, Parthenon Publishing Group, l999.
11. Cook R: The relationship between sex role and emotional functioning in patients undergoing assisted conception. J Psychosom Obstet Gynaecol 14:31–40, 1993.
12. Cooper SL, Glazer ES: Choosing Assisted Reproduction. Indianapolis, IN, Perspectives Press, 1998.
13. Covington SN, Burns LH: When infertility strikes the family. In Family Building—Resolve, Inc. Vol. 1(3), Spring, 2002.
14. Domar AD, Kelly AL: Conquering Infertility. New York, Viking Penguin, 2002.
15. Domar AD, et al: The impact of group psychological interventions on pregnancy rates in infertile women. Fertil Steril 73:805–811, 2000.
16. Domar AD, et al: The impact of group psychological interventions on distress in infertile women. Health Psychol 19:568–575, 2000.
17. Domar A, Dreher H: Healing Mind, Healthy Woman: Using the Mind-Body Connection to Manage Stress and Take Control of Your Life. New York, Dell Publishing, l996.
18. Domar AD, Zuttermeister PC, Friedman: The psychological impact of infertility: A comparison with patients with other medical conditions. J Psychosom Obstet Gynecol 14:45–52, l993.
19. Domar AD, Broome A, Zuttermeister PC, et al: The prevalence and predictability of depression in infertile women. Fertil Steril 58:1158–1163, 1992.
20. Domar AD, Zuttermeister PC, Seibel M, Benson H: Psychological improvement in infertile women after behavioral treatment: A replication. Fertil Steril 58:147–155, l992.
21. Domar AD, Seibel MM, Benson H: The mind/body program for infertility: A new behavioral treatment approach for women with infertility. Fertil Steril 53:246–249, 1990.
22. Garcia CR, Freeman EW, Rickels K, et al: Behavioral and emotional factors in treatment responses in a study of anovulatory infertile women. Fertil Steril 44:478–483, 1985.
23. Golombok S, Brewaeys A, Cook R, et al: The European study of assisted reproductive families: Family functioning and child development. Hum Reprod 11:2324–2331, 1996.
24. Golombok S, Cook R Bish A, Murray C: Families created by the new reproductive technologies: Quality of parenting and social and emotional development of the children. Child Devel 66:285–298, 1995.
25. Hynes GJ, Callan VJ, Terry DJ, Gallois C: The psychological well being of infertile women after a failed IVF attempt: The effects of coping. Br J Med Psychol 65(Pt 3):269–278, l992.
26. Jansen R, Mortimer D: Towards reproductive certainty: Fertility and genetics beyond 1999. In Plenary Proceedings of the 11th World Congress on In Vitro Fertilization and Human Reproductive Genetics. London, Parthenon Publishing Group, 1999.
27. Kedem P, Mikulincer M, Nathanson YE, Bartoov B: Psychological aspects of male infertility. Br J Med Psychol 3 (Pt 1):73–80, 1990.
28. Klonoff-Cohen H, Chu E, Natarajan L, Sieber W: A prospective study of stress among women undergoing in vitro fertilization or gamete intrafallopian transfer. Fertil Steril 76(4), 2001.
29. Link PW, Darling CA: Couples undergoing treatment for infertility: Dimensions of life satisfaction. J Sex Marital Ther 12:46–59, 1986.
30. Lalos A, Lalos O, Jacobsson L, von Schoultz B: Psychological reactions to the medical investigation and surgical treatment of infertility. Gynecol Obstet Invest 20:209–217, 1985.

31. Leiblum S (ed): Infertility: Psychological Issues and Counseling Strategies. New York, John Wiley & Sons, 1997.
32. McKinney M, Downey J, Timor-Tritsch I: The psychological effects of multifetal pregnancy reduction. Fertil Steril 64:51–61, 1995.
33. Meller W, Burns LH, Crow S, Grambsch P: Major depression in unexplained infertility. J Psychosom Obstet Gynaecol 23:27–30, 2002.
34. Nachtigal RD, Becker G, Wozny M: The effect of gender-specific diagnosis on men's and women's response to infertility. Fertil Steril 57:113, 1992.
35. Newton CR, Hearn MT, Yuzpe AA: Psychological assessment and follow-up after in vitro fertilization: Assessing the impact of failure. Fertil Steril 54:879–886, 1990.
36. Novaes SB: Giving, receiving, repaying: Gamete donor and donor policies in reproductive medicine. Int J Technol Assess Health Care 5:639–657, 1989.
37. Resolve, Inc: Resolving Infertility: Understanding the Options and Choosing Solutions When You Want to have a Baby. Oxford, MD, Amaranth Press, 1999.
38. Schinfeld JS, Elkins TE, Strong CM: Ethical considerations in the management of infertility. J Reprod Med 31:1038, 1986.
39. Thiering P, Beaurepaire J, Jones M, et al: Mood state as a predictor of treatment outcome after in vitro fertilization/embryo transfer technology (IVF/ET). J Psychosom Res 37:481–491, 1993.
40. van Balen F, Trimbos-Kemper TC. Long-term infertile couples: a study of their well being. J Psychosom Obstet Gynaecol 14(Suppl):53–60, 1993.
41. Wright J, Duchesne C, Sabourin S, et al: Psychosocial distress and infertility: Men and women respond differently. Fertil Steril 55:100–108, 1991.

51. PATIENT PERSPECTIVES
Joanne Libraro, RN, BSN

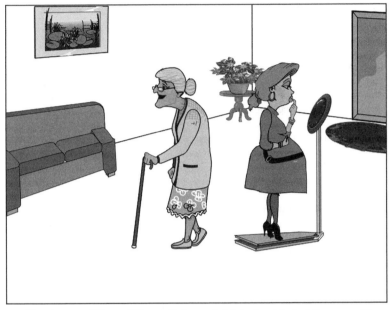

"Don't worry! You will lose all the weight during his toddler years!"

1. During a cycle of in vitro fertilization (IVF), do I really need to come into the office every day for monitoring?

The daily office visit is an integral part of a successful IVF cycle. The ability of reproductive endocrinologists (REs) to frequently monitor patients' response to fertility drugs allows a more specific adjustment of the stimulation protocols throughout the cycle. Frequently, practitioners base their stimulation protocols on a "step-up vs. a step-down" philosophy, depending on the response of the patients to the medications. A more frequent monitoring schedule allows adjustment of daily dosage of medications that are tailored to the need of the individual patient. For instance, in some settings the medications may need to be cut or "tailored" to as little as one-half of an ampule.

2. I have done IVF twice before. Why do I need to go to an IVF orientation class again?

Many fertility centers require the couples to attend an IVF orientation class in order to be assured that they understand the dynamics of the cycle at a particular center. Many significant differences can be noted when one goes from one center to another. A couple's comfort level at the center, along with their understanding of the differences in program philosophy, can contribute significantly to the success of fertility treatment. Furthermore, specific issues such as medication reconstitution, variation in the consent procedure, and availability of various services such as genetic counseling and preimplantation genetic diagnosis, vary significantly from center to center.

3. The doctor said I need a day-2 and day-3 blood test. Why?

Frequently patients are asked to have a baseline day-2 and day-3 blood test, which involves the measurement of serum levels of estradiol, follicle-stimulating hormone (FSH), and luteinizing hormone (LH). The assessment of estradiol and FSH are of particular prognostic values because both hormones are directly related to the natural ovarian response to the pituitary gonadotropin stimulation. These values are used to assess ovarian reserve and function, to allow an estimation of the potential response that a patient may have to hormonal ovarian stimulation for IVF, and to help design a medication protocol for stimulation.

4. During an IVF cycle, how many days will it take until my eggs are retrieved?

Normally in an IVF cycle, stimulation with medications is continued for days, followed by administration of human chorionic gonadotropin (hCG), which functions like LH to induce ovulation. Many factors affect the number of days of stimulation required for a patient before oocyte harvest. After a careful assessment of individual medical history, the physician prescribes a medication plan, or protocol, specific to the needs of the patient. However, frequent monitoring is required to determine the response of the patient to the protocol and the right time for egg retrieval. Therefore, there is no "absolute" number of days that a patient will be on stimulation. The average stimulation period, however, tends to be 8 to 14 days.

5. I have an infertility issue. Why are you putting me on birth control pills?

The use of oral contraceptives in an IVF cycle is confusing to many patients. Oral contraceptives are generally used for cycle timing and suppression of hyperstimulation, particularly in patients with polycystic ovary syndrome. It can also help to downregulate patient's cycles and assist with anovulatory/amenorrhic patients. For patients with a history of poor response to stimulation, some physicians may use birth control pills, in combination with varying doses of Lupron and gonadotropins, in a "flare" protocol to increase ovarian response to stimulation.

6. Do I need to be on total bed rest after the embryo transfer?

Absolutely not. Bed rest does not increase the implantation rate of embryos. In general, the feeling among practioners is that bed rest does not have an effect on overall pregnancy rates. However, modified activity and lifestyle adjustments are encouraged. The usual suggestion made to patients is to adjust their lifestyle appropriately and to know that they have done everything necessary to feel comfortable with their activity level. I generally ask patients to "do what makes you comfortable putting your head down on the pillow at the end of the day."

7. Are any support groups available for the infertility couples?

There are many support groups for patients to attend and use as resource or support. The American Infertility Association and Resolve are organizations that are highly effective in offering supportive lectures and group meetings for infertility couples. These national organizations are geared to provide infertility patients with education, advocacy, and support. Similarly, local support groups and private sessions are genereally available directly through the reproductive center. In addition, most reproductive centers have psychologists specializing in infertility for individuals and couples who have special needs or support.

8. Can I exercise when I am cycling?

Although exercise is permitted when a patient is actively in cycle for IVF, most REs at Cornell recommend that patients refrain from strenuous physical activity when follicular development is confirmed. There is also concern of ovarian torsion from high-impact exercise in which some patients may wish to participate.

9. Should I change my diet while I am cycling?

Basically no. The general recommendation is to treat yourself as though you were pregnant during the stimulation program. We suggest that patients refrain from using alcohol and limit the intake of caffeine while on the stimulation protocol, as in pregnancy. It is usually recommended that the patient modify the dietary intake of caffeine progressively and not abruptly; abrupt change can create physiologic complaints such as headache and fatigue. Some nutritionists may suggest that patients modify their diet to allow high intake of protein and calories for pregnancy. Additionally, a nutrionist may provide patients with a list of foods to be avoided. This list may include tuna and fishes with high mercury levels, unprocessed cheese, high-fat foods, and foods with high-carbohydrate content and concentrated sugar.

10. Do I need to start prenatal vitamins?

Prenatal vitamins are an important part of the preparation portion of an IVF cycle. The general recommendation is to start taking prenatal vitamins once you begin treatment for IVF.

11. Do my partner and I need to abstain before producing a semen sample for IVF?

Generally 2–4 days of abstinence from ejaculation for the male partner is recommended for the couple planning to do an IVF cycle with or without intracytoplasmic sperm injection (ICSI). An abstinence period shorter than 2 days may yield a sample with a lowered count, while longer than 4 days may yield a sample with lowered motility. For men with known male factor infertility, such as oligospermia (sperm count < 20 million/ml), alternative recommendations may be made.

12. My partner and I have frozen sperm samples. Can we use them for IVF?

Even for men who can produce sperm from ejaculation, having a frozen sperm sample prior to a fresh IVF harvest is always an advantage. In fact, some fertility centers require couples to cryopreserve a sperm sample before egg retrieval, particularly in the following situations:

- Couples that anticipate difficulty in ejaculation "on demand" at the time of IVF harvest
- Known subnormal semen or sperm quality, as in many cases of male factor infertility
- Uncertainty of the availability of the male partner at the time of IVF harvest, as seen in many couples who undergo IVF at a center not in their hometown

13. My partner had a vasectomy many years ago. Can I still do IVF?

Yes. Many men explore the option of assisted reproduction following vasectomy, often because they remarried with a childless female partner or have a change of hearts and want more children. In addition to offering various fertility options such as assisted reproduction, a vasectomy reversal may be recommended. Others options for obtaining sperm for reproduction may include surgical sperm retrieval with testicular or epididymal sperm aspiration (TESE), either freshly for immediate use or cryopreserved for future use. Some patients were counseled at the time of the vasectomy to cryopreserve sperm as a back-up for future use.

14. Is donor sperm an option for me?

Donor sperm is always an option for a patient/couple wishing to use it. Generally, to avoid cancellation of the entire IVF procedure, patients are offered donor sperm as a "back-up" on the day of IVF oocyte harvest in case sperm from the male partner is not available. In addition, in certain situations the patient/couple may choose to use frozen donor sperm upfront. Examples include single women without a male partner and women with a male partner with genetic abnormalities or azoospermia, particularly those who failed to undergo surgical sperm retrieval.

15. How do I choose donor sperm?

Generally, reproductive centers can refer patients to specific counselors affiliated with the individual cryopreservation bank to guide them in the selection process for a sperm donor. Particulars of the donor, such as physical characteristics, eye color, hair color, and ethnicity, are usually available to help make the selection. In addition, we strongly suggest that the couple/patient seek the support and guidance of a psychologist specializing in fertility.

16. How much donor sperm should I order?

Donor sperm are generally kept in the cryopreservation bank in divided portions or vials. Generally, the bank limits the quantity of donor sperm sent to the reproductive center for the couple. For back-up use, generally 2–4 vials are adequate. Unused portions of the donor sperm are kept for future use. In addition, we generally recommend that couples reserve additional samples from the same donor at the bank for additional future treatment. Availability of additional samples from the same donor for future reproductive use allows biologically related siblings, which many patients prefer.

17. My partner has no sperm in the ejaculate. We are planning for surgical sperm retrieval with TESE for an IVF cycle. Why does the doctor want him to produce a semen sample before the surgery?

Generally, for men who do not produce sperm in the ejaculate, surgical sperm retrieval with TESE (see sperm retrieval chapter) is required to obtain sperm for assisted reproduction. However, some of the "azoospermic" patients occasionally have rare sperm in the ejaculate that can be found by a more thorough search than a routine semen analysis. These rare sperm can sometimes be used for assisted reproduction, making surgical sperm retrieval unnecessary. Thus, in selected patients, a semen sample should be thoroughly evaluated prior to a planned TESE. In fact, cryopreservation of the semen sample can also be performed to preserve these rare sperm for future reproductive use.

18. My partner has low sperm production that requires surgical sperm retrieval by TESE. If I order donor sperm, will they use the donor sperm or the TESE sperm?

All attempts are made to use the male partner's sperm before the use of donor samples is considered. The fact that the couple has arranged donor sperm "back-up" should not affect the extent of tissue processing of the TESE specimen in looking for sperm.

19. Do I have a lower chance of pregnancy using TESE sperm?

Many patients do get pregnant with TESE sperm. However, the fact that TESE is required generally means that the male partner has poor sperm production; hence the quantity and quality of available sperm are poor. In other words, they have more severe forms of infertility. In fact, in approximately 30–50% of patients requiring TESE for sperm retrieval, no sperm are found at all. Even if sperm are found, their quantity and quality, along with the reproductive status of the female partner, are the most important factors affecting the success of fertilization.

20. If surgical sperm retrieval is required, does my cycle have to be coordinated?

Definitely. Whenever possible, the nurses at the reproductive center time the female cycle stimulation to coordinate with the date of surgical sperm retrieval. Frequently, this approach requires incorporating birth control pills and/or other means of intervention. The timing and fine-tuning of the date of the cycles should be well coordinated, without affecting the outcome of the cycle or causing unnecessary inconvenience to the patients and health care team.

21. I live in another town. After oocyte harvest and embryo transfer, can I do the follow-up bloodwork in my hometown?

Absolutely. Any blood tests for monitoring after the transfer can be done from the patient's home town. The nurses can provide patients with the necessary requisition forms to have all testing done outside and to arrange for results to be forwarded to the reproductive center. This approach is more convenient for patients and provides equally close follow-up for post-transfer monitoring.

22. I have an irregular work schedule. How to I maintain a close communication with the reproductive center during my reproductive treatment?

We generally encourage patients to continue with their daily activities as much as possible, including their work schedule, as long as they do not interfere with the fertility treatment. To maintain a close monitoring schedule during a treatment cycle, patients are asked to provide us with their cell phone numbers, home and/or work numbers, and e-mail address. When an answering machine or voice mail is to be used for leaving messages, the nursing staff ask the couple to leave an identifying greeting to ensure that staff are leaving the instructions at the appropriate location.

23. My partner and I are Sabbath observers. What if my transfer occurs on a Saturday?

Like most health institutions, many reproductive centers have special arrangement for patients of certain religious groups. For instance, if the embryo transfer falls on a Saturday, a Shabbus elevator may be available for patients coming into and out of the hospital. In addition, prior to embryo transfer, arrangements can be made for the couple to stay at a local hotel and avoid commuting from home. The presence of representatives of religious group during some procedures may also be arranged if the patient desires.

24. How can I schedule myself as a Sabbath observer to avoid a Saturday harvest?

Despite various arrangements to accommodate the special needs of patients, commonly many religious patients may prefer to undergo IVF oocyte harvesting not on certain days of a calendar. For instance, to avoid conflict with the Sabbath, nurses may arrange to have the patients begin their stimulation medications on a Friday. Typically the patient's retrieval day will be on a Monday or Tuesday instead of a Saturday. The timing of the retrieval is a significant concern to many religious patients. Nurses should make all efforts to address and acknowledge the patient's concerns.

25. Will I be able to get to the Mikvah before my harvest?

Mikvah may be a significant concern for some religious patients preparing for infertility treatments. Mikvah occurs 7 days (sunsets) following the last sight of any vaginal bleeding. For religious patients, this "timing" issue is of concern because the male partner is not allowed to provide a semen sample before Mikvah for assisted reproduction, since the couple is not permitted to have sexual relations until after Mikvah. If the cycle of the female partner progresses rapidly and the need for oocyte harvest arises before the scheduled Mikvah, many religious couples may choose to cancel the IVF cycle. Communication of such a concern between couples and nurses in charge is therefore important to allow adjustment of the cycle to avoid religious conflicts resulting in cancellation of reproductive treatment.

26. I have had my fallopian tubes removed. How can I do IVF?

Aclear advantage for patients undergoing IVF with preexisting tubal factor/disease is that the procedure eliminates the need for tubal involvement. Gonadatropin stimulation allows follicular growth and development. Oocytes are then harvested for fertilization to take place in vitro. This approach eliminates the need for tubal fertilization seen in a natural pregnancy. IVF, therefore, allows patients with infertility due to tubal issues to pursue pregnancy treatment.

27. After a failed IVF cycle, should I be doing IVF again with my own eggs?

The answer depends on oocyte yield, quality of fertilized embryos, embryo growth and development, and quality of the embryos at the time of transfer. Once these factors are assessed, the future plan can be better discussed with REs. They can make a more specific suggestion whether to include your own eggs or, alternatively, consider the incorporation of donor oocytes for future cycles. The decision to use donor oocytes is never an easy one. Counseling and guidance from doctors, staff psychologist, family, and, in some situations, religious representatives can be extremely helpful.

28. The doctor changed my protocol this time. Why would he do that?

After completing an IVF cycle, whether it was successful or not, the RE reviews the stimulation results and findings from the endocrine and embryology laboratories. If a future IVF cycle is desired, the patient and her partner can then discuss with the RE any suggestions of protocol modification. Generally, if the previous cycle was unsuccessful, future cycles will adopt a modified medication protocol. For a previous successful cycle, there is generally little change necessary. However, slight modification of the protocol may still be implemented to optimize outcome. When changes are made in the protocol, the REs may re-evaluate the hormonal profile, including a repeat day-2 and day-3 blood test, to reassess hormonal needs in a future stimulation cycle.

BIBLIOGRAPHY

1. Garner CH: Principles of Infertility Nursing. Boca Raton, FL, CRC Press, 1991
2. James CA: The nursing role in assisted reproductive technologies. NAACOGS Clin Iss Perinat Womens Health Nurs 3:328–334, 1992.
3. Spencer C: Assisted reproductive technology: A dilemma for the nursing profession. Contemp Nurse 4(4):174–177, 1995.

52. NURSING PERSPECTIVES OF FERTILITY PATIENT CARE

Joanne Libraro, RN, BSN

1. What are reproductive endocrinologists?

In North American and many other countries in the world, reproductive problems, especially those requiring the use of assisted reproduction such as in vitro fertilization (IVF) or intracytoplasmic sperm injection (ICSI), are generally managed by reproductive endocrinologists, who are gynecologists with special expertise in advanced assisted reproductive technologies.

2. What other health care professionals in a reproductive center are involved for the care of fertility patients?

Embryologists are specialists in charge of the evaluation of sperm and oocyte quality, performing IVF procedure, and evaluation of the quality of embryos. In addition, many embryologists are also actively involved in the cryopreservation of sperm, eggs, and embryos.

Andrologists/urologists are physicians specializing in male infertility. Like reproductive endocrinologists, they are involved in the overall reproductive health of the couple, with special attention to the male partners. In addition, they are in charge of the retrieval of sperm or other surgeries, including vasectomy reversal, to optimize the overall reproductive status of couple.

Reproductive nurses are specialized health care professional actively involved in the management of the couple's reproductive treatment. Generally, patients undergoing the reproductive treatment are in close contact, often on a daily basis, with the reproductive nurse in charge of their IVF cycle. In addition to providing answers to specific questions, reproductive nurses serve as a liaison between physicians or embryologists and patients. They generally have a thorough knowledge of the mechanisms of the particular reproductive center and are resourceful in providing additional care for patients who have special needs based on cultural, religious, or social background.

Genetic counselors are physicians specializing in perinatal or neonatal genetics. Their role is to provide counseling for couples who are at risk for having genetic disorders or passing them to offspring.

Psychologists are often needed because reproductive treatment can be a stressful process. In addition to providing special support for the emotional needs of patients, psychologists are also resourceful in providing help and counseling to patients with special needs, such as use of donor sperm or eggs or adoption.

3. Are patients able to administer their own injections of medication?

Most fertility centers incorporate injection education into their orientation process. These classes are intended to teach patients and their partners the correct method and technique for medication reconstitution and administration, including injection. Couples are encouraged to be independent for all medications administration. Injection may be performed intramuscularly (IM) or, as preferred by most patients, subcutaneously (SQ). Most IVF medications available today can be administered by subcutaneous injection. In fact, most of the medications today are so "user-friendly" that patients often do not even need the assistance of a partner to given the daily medications.

4. Are medications that require IM injection better than those that allow SQ injection?

Basically, no. The newly developed recombinant preparations, which can be administered subcutaneously, are as efficient for ovarian stimulation as the conventional medications that require IM injection. Most patients find SQ injection easier to administer than IM injection. The easier the administration, the better the compliance, which may translate ultimately to better success rates. Hence, some programs prescribe only SQ preparations, and others use them in combination. Ultimately, however, the patient's response to ovarian stimulation is what matters. No evidence suggests that one form of drug administration is better than the other.

5. Can SQ medications be injected into the thigh and abdomen?

Definitely. Patients have the flexibility of administering SQ medications into the abdomen or the thigh. This option allows the flexibility of administering the medications in a more comfortable and independent manner, which may increase patient satisfaction and compliance.

6. Should ice be applied to the injection site before injecting?

Although ice application or cold compress can have an anesthetic effect by "numbing" the nerves, hypothermia from application of ice, whether before or after the injection, can result in contraction of smooth muscle of blood vessels, leading to local vasoconstriction. Vasoconstriction may inhibit absorption of the medication. Thus, this practice is discouraged. We strongly suggest that patients use warm, moist compresses instead of cold application.

7. When should patients obtain and fill their medication prescriptions?

We generally encourage patients to obtain and fill all necessary medical prescriptions before starting the cycle. After completion of the consultation and evaluation with the reproductive endocrinologist, an IVF protocol specific to the individual patient is established with details about the medication regimen. Before actually beginning the IVF cycle, all new patients should meet with an IVF nurse for an orientation and protocol review. This meeting gives the patient the opportunity to ask further questions about the cycle, review the prescriptions, and prepare for the cycle.

8. When a patient is on a gonadotropin stimulation protocol, why is it necessary to continue leuprolide?

During ovarian stimulation for assisted reproduction, the use of subcutaneous leuprolide acetate (Lupron) on a daily basis is a standard in many protocols. While the exogenous gonadotropins serve to stimulate oocytes development, the addition of leuprolide serves to inhibit or downregulate naturally produced gonadotropins. This protocol lowers the chance of an untimely release, or surge, of luteinizing hormone (LH), a gonadotropin, which can result in premature ovulation. Thus the addition of leuprolide in gonadotropin stimulation protocols allows optimized oocyte recruitment and at the same time limits the risk of premature spontaneous ovulation.

9. Is there clinical difference between IM progesterone and vaginal preparations?

Progesterone, which can be administered intramuscularly or transvaginally, is more commonly used for intrauterine insemination than for IVF. Physicians generally prescribe the preparation of progesterone that they believe works best based on their experience. Intramuscular progesterone, compounded in oil and given in 25 to 50 mg doses daily, is a more commonly used form. Progesterone delivered intramuscularly allows serum levels to be determined and monitored to adjust the dosage. The disadvantages of this form of administration include the need for intramuscular injection and the systemic side effects of progesterone.

Progesterone administered transvaginally in the form of gel or suppositories acts directly on the endometrium during the luteal phase. Unfortunately, in this form of progesterone administration, serum progesterone levels cannot be used to adjust the dosage, because of the uterine first-pass effect. Additionally, some patients find the local side effect of vaginal discharge bothersome. Systemic side effects, however, are not as frequent as in the intramuscular form.

10. If a patient required preimplantation genetic diagnosis (PGD) for her IVF cycle, what exactly needs to be done differently?

For patients with genetic risks, PGD is an important part of the IVF pregnancy (see chapter on PGD). Special coordination with the PGD laboratory is required in planning the IVF cycle. This coordination includes arranging additional blood tests to allow the PGD laboratory to create biochemical probes for the specific PGD testing, preparing the patients for special consent procedures for PGD, and arrangement of genetic counseling with a specialist.

11. What is involved in the consent procedure?

IVF is a sophisticated form of management for infertility. Hence, proper consents must be obtained from all patients for all procedures involved in the entire process. Most reproductive centers provide the couple with a set of consent forms when they present for the initial consultation. Many reproductive centers have treatment and procedural consent forms that are center- and patient-specific. Generally, the physicians of the center provide counseling and answer all questions before obtaining consent for treatment. Additional questions or concerns can be raised by patients at any time, either with the treating physicians or the nurses in charge.

12. How do we help patients who speak limited English?

As American society becomes more and more multicultural, many reproductive centers in North America handle a significant volume of patients whose first language is not English. Most centers generally have personnel who are fluent in languages used by most major ethnic groups. In the rare cases when a specific translator is not readily available, we advise patients to bring in family members or relatives to provide translation for the consultation. Additionally, during the treatment period, we advise patients to identify friends or family members who may be available to interpret the daily instruction or other messages left on an answering machines.

13. If a patient is going to get her period over a holiday weekend, what arrangement needs to be made?

Depending on the natural cycle of the patient, upon ovarian stimulation for IVF the oocyte retrieval day may fall on a weekend or holiday. For most reproductive centers that handle a large volume of patients, this scenario is generally not a problem because often they are fully staffed even on weekends or holidays. Alternatively, other centers may choose to "time" patient cycles, with the use of oral contraceptive pills, to minimize the possibility of weekend retrievals. This approach ensures the availability of all necessary personnel when oocyte retrieval is to be performed.

14. If frozen embryos are available, is it preferable to use them for subsequent pregnancy or to start a fresh IVF cycle?

In the event of an unsuccessful fresh attempt at IVF, the general recommendation is to use frozen embryos rather than start a fresh IVF cycle. Physicians can offer patients either a natural or a programmed (i.e., medicated) frozen embryo transfer cycle. The advantage of this approach over initiation of another fresh cycle is that there is no need for additional ovarian stimulation or ova retrieval; hence the risks and costs of the procedure are reduced. However, this decision should also be based on the evaluation of the quality of the remaining frozen embryos, the age of the patient, and the underlying cause of the couple's infertility.

15. When using frozen embryos, what is the difference between a natural and a programmed cycle?

As opposed to a natural cycle, a programmed IVF cycle using frozen embryos requires the use of medications for hormonal suppression and replacement. In the natural cycle, the patient is guided to come in on cycle day 7–10, depending on the length of the cycle, to begin monitoring. The doctors assess the patient's menstrual cycle with ultrasound and serum progesterone levels in the luteal phase to determine whether she will qualify for the natural cycle. Once the ultrasound evaluation and the blood results indicate that the patient is near or at ovulation, the decision to thaw the patient's embryos for transfer is made.

Alternatively, in a programmed cycle the patient is first downregulated with leuprolide in the previous cycle. Once menses start, the patient is given estrogen over several days at increasing dosages to build and support the endometrial lining in anticipation of embryo implantation. Monitoring with ultrasound to assess the endometrial lining and measurement of serum estrogen levels are required. Once the situation is optimized, progesterone is started and then tapered gradually. The embryos are then thawed and transfered.

Note that for both natural and programmed frozen embryo cycles, the exact timing of the embryo transfer depends also on whether the "embryos" are preembryos or blastocysts, which in turn determines the day on which the embryos were initially cryopreserved.

16. Is one method better than the other?

Clinical pregnancy rates of both methods are comparable. However, for patients who are young, with regular menstruation and no other pathology, there is probably no need to utilize a programmed/medicated cycle. On the other hand, for patients who are anovulatory, preparation with oral contrceptive pills and leuprolide may be necessary. Hence a programmed cycle may be necessary. Additional factors that may influence the choice of a natural vs. a programmed cycle include the couples' working schedule, travel needs, and other personal factors.

17. In a frozen embryo transfer cycle, how many embryos are thawed and transferred?

The decision about the number of embryos to thaw and transfer is made by the embryologist and the patients' attending physician, based on patient age, quality of the embryos, and how they were frozen. Additionally, the patient's prior history of pregnancy and other clinical history contribute to the decision.

18. What is the main advantage of a frozen embryo cycle for most patients?

One of the clear advantage of undergoing a frozen embryo cycle with programmed or medicated cycle is the flexibility of timing of the procedure. This flexibility is particularly practical for patients who live out of town or have work commitments or other family/children issues.

BIBLIOGRAPHY

1. Garner CH: Principles of Infertility Nursing. Boca Rotan, FL, CRC Press, 1991
2. James CA: The nursing role in assisted reproductive technologies. NAACOGS Clin Issu Perinat Womens Health Nurs 3:328–334, 1992.
3. Queenan JT Jr, Ramey JW, Seltman HJ, et al: Transfer of cryopreserved-thawed pre-embryos in a cycle using exogenous steroids without prior gonadotrophin-releasing hormone agonist suppression yields favourable pregnancy results. Hum Reprod 12:1176–1180, 1997.
4. Sathanandan M, Macnamee MC, Rainsbury P, et al: Replacement of frozen-thawed embryos in artificial and natural cycles: Aprospective semi-randomized study. Hum Reprod 6:685–687, 1991.
5. Spencer C: Assisted reproductive technology: A dilemma for the nursing profession. Contemp Nurse 4(4):174–177, 1995.

53. PREGNANCY AFTER INFERTILITY

Laura Josephs, Ph.D.

1. How does pregnancy after infertility differ from other pregnancies?

The woman who is pregnant after infertility carries with her the shadow of her infertility history. She probably began her quest for pregnancy with reasonable optimism in regard to conceiving and carrying to term a healthy baby. During her struggle with infertility, her positive outlook has been replaced with negativity and fears. Her image of herself as successfully bearing a child has been damaged. Thus, she approaches the pregnancy with trepidation.

Obstetricians may notice that patients with infertility histories are more fearful than other patients. The fears of postinfertility patients may not be commensurate with their actual obstetric status; a good prognosis for the pregnancy from a medical point of view may not prevent the patient from foreseeing a negative outcome. In fact, although many pregnant women with an infertility history may look forward to a successful full-term pregnancy, as a group women who are pregnant following infertility show a higher rate of complications and pregnancy loss. This perhaps makes the pessimistic outlook of this group of patients more understandable.

2. Describe the psychological experience of the woman who is pregnant after infertility.

The typical initial response of women whose infertility experience and treatment culminate in pregnancy is relief and joy. Her diminished hopes finally have borne fruit. However, this excitement can be short-lived. Infertility has served as a trauma in which the quest for a baby has been met with one disappointment after another. Early anticipation of a successful pregnancy has been thwarted; the patient has been hit with "bad news" and negative outcomes month after month. Thus, it is natural that, despite her ongoing pregnancy, she expects more bad news. She goes to the bathroom expecting to see blood; she goes to her doctor's office bracing herself for a problem. She may or may not be at "high risk" from a medical point of view; her own point of view is almost always more negative than that of her obstetrician.

Postinfertility pregnant patients sometimes literally cannot believe that they are to give birth. Many will not buy maternity clothes until they are literally popping out of their regular outfits. Discussions of maternity leave are dismissed. Baby furniture and clothing are often purchased at the last minute. Although quickening is initially reassuring, monitoring fetal movements can become a painful obsession, fraught with anxiety.

3. What is the "premium pregnancy"?

The premium pregnancy is is viewed by the parents as one that will be near-impossible to replicate. It is a pregnancy seen as having great value. In fact, such pregnancies—having resulted from assisted reproductive technology—are often extremely costly from a monetary point of view. More importantly, patients feel that they have invested tremendous time and emotional energy in these pregnancies.

The premium nature of a pregnancy can affect decision-making during pregnancy. A patient who has achieved pregnancy after years of infertility may be extremely hesitant to undergo any prenatal testing that puts the pregnancy at risk (e.g., amniocentesis).

4. What emotions and psychological issues do women who are pregnant after infertility share in common?

Women who are pregnant after infertility are nearly always more fearful than the average obstetric patient. Postinfertility patients often are vigilant about monitoring symptoms of pregnancy and highly reactive to any perceived diminution of such symptoms. During pregnancy, such patients are not only experiencing a crucial life transition as they progress toward motherhood; they are also attempting to work through the painful sense of loss created by their struggles with infertility.

5. What identity issues do such patients face?

Most infertility patients began their quest to conceive a child with some optimism about their capacity to conceive and bear a healthy baby. This optimistic belief is tied to a positive image of oneself as a woman. During the struggle with infertility, the feminine self-image sustains damage, as the infertility patient now begins to see herself as a woman who is incapable of conceiving and carrying a healthy baby. Although pregnancy can help heal some of the wounds of infertility, the self-image is not magically repaired. In terms of identity, there is still an infertile woman inside the pregnant woman. She sits in her obstetrician's waiting room with other patients who look just like her, yet she does not feel like she belongs there. Patients must confront the wounds to self as they revise the self-image to allow for the psychological experience of pregnancy and, ultimately, motherhood.

6. What is the typical interpersonal experience of the pregnant woman with an infertility history?

The pregnant woman with an infertility history typically finds that others do not share her perspective. Interpersonally, others tend to approach the pregnant woman from a rather concrete, literal-minded point of view. People in her life who have been aware of her fertility problems assume that now she is pregnant her prior problems are over—her infertility experience erased, as it were. There is often little understanding of or patience with any fears or doubts that she expresses. To the degree that these interpersonal contacts felt that the now-pregnant woman leaned on them emotionally during her infertility, they may feel that they have given enough and possess little sympathy for her current situation. All of these dynamics may be heightened in relation to friends or contacts who themselves are (still) going through infertility. From the point of view of infertile friends, the patient is now on the other side of a great divide; it may be difficult for them to relate to her, to empathize with her worries, or to "be happy" for her. On the other hand, people who have not known about her infertility assume that she and her partner made a decision to get pregnant and were successful in conceiving naturally. Thus, the postinfertility pregnant woman often feels quite alienated from others.

7. How are the marriages of such patients affected by pregnancy?

Pregnancy, at long last, can help initiate a necessary healing process. Just as the woman's self-image has suffered as a result of the infertility, her partner's image of their marriage/intimate relationship is also affected by infertility. What begins as a natural quest to conceive a child together becomes a seemingly futile joint effort in which the marital relationship itself seems touched by failure and thus flawed. Again, pregnancy can begin to quell the doubts and fears about the marriage that were engendered by infertility.

On the other hand, marital problems can arise when the man's experience and the woman's experience of the postinfertility pregnancy diverge too widely. In particular, when the woman feels that her partner fails to understand some of her continuing anxieties and negative feelings, discord may result.

8. What husband-wife dynamics are commonly found in such marriages?

In traversing the experience of infertility and assisted reproduction, women often believe that they feel the psychological pain inherent in the process more acutely. Of course, it is the woman who achieves pregnancy (or fails to achieve pregnancy), and women in most cultures have been socialized to pursue pregnancy and motherhood with great vigor. During infertility, whatever their own private suffering, men often assume the role of the emotionally "strong" protector—the one to be leaned on, the one who keeps going no matter what. Obviously, this role is highly consistent with socialization of males in many societies. This common gender difference in response to infertility can result in problematic relationship dynamics. Women may believe that their male partners do not understand or empathize with their feelings, and men fear that their female partners are "falling apart" or "obsessed" with fertility issues.

For many men, the experience of a successful pregnancy following infertility can serve as a signal to "let go" of painful negative feelings, and they may desire that their partners do the same now that there is a "happy ending." Faced with this attitude, women may feel misunderstood, and in fact their negative or fearful feelings may increase, leading to a significant gap in the emotional experiences of the male and female partners.

9. How does infertility history affect the pregnant woman in the first, second, and third trimesters?

Because the first trimester is characterized by the highest risk of loss (miscarriage), the previously infertile woman typically experiences her highest level of anxiety during this time. Because pregnancy symptoms may be mild or imperceptible, she has no reassurance of an ongoing pregnancy and feels great trepidation between obstetrical appointments. In contrast, a minority of patients deny the possibility of loss, in a form of magical thinking. Having waited so long for a pregnancy, it is as though, once pregnant, nothing bad can possibly happen.

Getting past the first trimester and into the second is naturally seen as reassuring. Nonetheless, most patients with infertility histories continue to fear bad news. At quickening, the ability to feel fetal movements is comforting to patients. However, this experience also can become a source of anxiety, as patients obsessively monitor the movements, worrying that they are not frequent or strong enough.

The anxiety of the third trimester is of a devastating tragic loss—that having come so far, and, presumably, having attached oneself to the pregnancy and even relying on its culminating in the birth of a healthy child, tragedy will strike.

10. How do previously infertile patients approach prenatal testing?

Prenatal testing can be greatly feared. The infertile patient probably has undergone many tests during her experience of infertility. On many of these tests, the results have been disappointing or even traumatic. Naturally, at an underlying emotional level she anticipates that tests during pregnancy also will prove problematic.

Prenatal testing for the previously infertile patient must be understood in a context of a pregnancy that is highly valued. Any risks to the pregnancy posed by testing loom large for the woman who has worked hard and suffered to achieve pregnancy.

11. Explain denial of pregnancy.

Brezinka and colleagues have identified the syndrome of pregnancy denial. In contrast to pseudocyesis, in which a nonpregnant woman maintains that she is pregnant and experiences physical symptoms of pregnancy, a pregnant woman in denial maintains that she is not pregnant. It is fairly typical for postinfertility patients to show some denial of pregnancy. Patients view their pregnant state with disbelief and make no adjustments to this state; preparations for motherhood and the arrival of the baby are long delayed. The vast majority of patients realize that they are emotionally distancing themselves from the pregnancy due to fear of loss. In extreme cases, there may be an actual break with reality, in which the patient truly believes that she is not pregnant and will not accept appropriate obstetric care nor practice appropriate behaviors to safeguard the pregnancy.

12. How can the previously infertile patient navigate the emotional tasks of pregnancy?

For any obstetric patient, successful negotiation of the life-stage of pregnancy means an expansion of self-concept to enable the woman to become a mother and/or to mother this particular child. For the previously infertile patient, traversing this life-stage also entails gradually altering the self-concept to let go of the image of herself as infertile. Patients should not feel compelled to abruptly alter their self-images, nor should they succumb to external pressures to do so. Enduring change is most apt to occur more slowly.

Although patients have limited influence over their basic emotional responses to pregnancy following infertility, they can be encouraged to address other sources of life stress, wherever possible. Reducing baseline stress level can help patients cope with the stress of pregnancy. Relaxation techniques can be useful, and the physician can also help patients develop a program of physical exercise appropriate to the pregnancy.

A tiny percentage (probably less than 1%) of patients who become pregnant after infertility end up terminating the pregnancy in the absence of fetal anomalies. Although this phenomenon is uncommon and has not been well studied, clinical experience suggests that in the aftermath of infertility, some patients cannot cope with the actuality of pregnancy and prospective parenthood. It is speculated that a few patients have grown so focused on the all-important goal of "conquering infertility" that the prospect of having a child becomes distant and abstract.

13. What anxieties may be felt by the woman who has suffered one or more pregnancy losses?

The survivor of pregnancy loss deeply fears that her current pregnancy will end in the same manner. This anxiety seems to increase directly with the number of prior losses. Women who have endured pregnancy losses have experienced trauma in the context of pregnancy, and a new pregnancy ushers in fears of retraumatization. For such women, pregnancy does not represent a cause for celebration but rather a trigger for fear.

14. How does a new pregnancy affect the woman with a history of pregnancy loss?

Because a new pregnancy portends further trauma, the patient does not relax in response to the positive pregnancy test but instead braces herself for another traumatic loss. For some patients with loss histories, there is real (medical) reason to be concerned that the prior problem will repeat itself. For other patients, the prior loss or losses have been random and not likely to recur; thus, from a rational point of view there is no reason to be particularly fearful. But the unconscious mind does not distinguish between one pregnancy and another; at a deep level of the psyche there is a painful association of pregnancy with loss. This association is very difficult for patients to break.

15. What is the relevance of the point of loss (i.e., the time in the pregnancy when the loss occurred)?

For many patients, it is emotionally critical that they reach and then go beyond the point of the prior pregnancy loss(es). Anxiety is painfully heightened leading up to the point of loss, and passing this point frequently leads to some relief. Patients often believe that, once they pass this point in the pregnancy, they will let go of their anxieties; in actual practice, however, worries can diminish but rarely disappear.

16. What are the psychological complications of multiple pregnancy?

Multiple pregnancy, a frequent complication of assisted reproductive technology, engenders a variety of reactions. Prior to pregnancy, infertility patients typically feel that they would unambivalently welcome a multiple pregnancy, especially twins. In fact, this is often the initial reaction to the finding of twins or triplets. Having waited and struggled for such a long time, the prospect of bearing more than one child can feel like a sort of "bonus" for all the hard work and pain. Patients can experience a multiple pregnancy as an opportunity to "catch up" in terms of family building—both with peers who have had children easily and with their own original timetable, which has been sidetracked by fertility problems.

But these positive reactions can be joined by—or even replaced with—negative responses. Particularly in higher-order multiple pregnancies, patients must contend with the immediate question of fetal reduction, at best a painful prospect for patients who have been working so hard to achieve pregnancy. Beyond this thorny issue, patients understandably fear potential complications in the pregnancy and feel overwhelmed by the prospect of giving birth to and raising more than one child. When one partner has been more motivated to have a child than the other partner, the prospect of more than one child can feel like the realization of one partner's fears and can cause problems in the relationship. In addition, in a complex irony, patients may experience a multiple pregnancy not as evidence of enhanced fertility but as a sign of infertility (i.e., of the use of gonadotropins and/or reproductive technology), now revealed to the world.

Any negative response to multiple pregnancy can occasion great guilt on the part of fertility patients, who at bottom feel that they should be grateful for what they have. They well know that not long ago they would have given anything to be in this position.

17. How are patients affected by third-party reproduction?

Third-party reproduction is never a first choice. Interestingly, patients in same-sex relationships have had to confront and accept the inability to conceive a child with the loved one. For heterosexual single women, third-party reproduction often involves mourning the loss of a hoped-for relationship within which they had originally hoped to conceive a child. Heterosexual couples set out to conceive a child within their relationship. The path that leads to third-party reproduction is usually characterized by severe disappointment and great loss. Whether donor egg or donor sperm is used, both partners must grieve the inability to biologically create a child together. The partner whose genetic material will not be represented in the child may experience a sense of imbalance in the relationship.

18. What is the pregnant patient's experience of the sperm donor?

A central aspect of the pregnant patient's experience of the sperm donor is the fear of the impact on the pregnancy (i.e., on the baby). Normal anxieties about the as-yet-unseen infant's health and well-being can be intensified, as the patient fears giving birth to a monstrous creature of alien provenance. For heterosexual couples, both women and men fear that, without a genetic link, the man will be unable to bond with his child.

Fortunately, clinical experience and research have demonstrated that patients' fears surrounding gamete donation are unfounded. Findings have been reassuring, with one notable study showing that children conceived with sperm donation have closer parent-child relationships than their naturally conceived peers.

19. What is the pregnant patient's experience of the egg (oocyte) donor?

As in sperm donation, the pregnant donor egg recipient sometimes fears that the donor will adversely affect her pregnancy and that the baby will emerge as some bizarre, unknown creature that she will be unable to love. It is, nonetheless, truly reassuring for the donor egg patient to experience herself as carrying the child in the pregnancy and therefore as biologically (although not genetically) linked to the child. In addition, perhaps because patients are well aware of all that the oocyte donor needs to go through at a physical level to donate her eggs, it is not uncommon for patients to experience a sense of gratitude toward the egg donor, both during pregnancy and after the baby is born.

20. What are the particular challenges for the older mother?

By definition, the woman who is pregnant following infertility is an older mother than she had hoped to be, and this is a painful legacy of and reminder of her infertility after motherhood has arrived. For the mother who is significantly older than average, there is the additional difficulty of not feeling that she possesses much in common with other mothers around her, of feeling different or even abnormal. These feelings can replicate the infertility experience. Some older mothers report that people assume that they have had fertility problems and that they have used technology or even third-party assistance to conceive a child. Thus, there is a sense of being "exposed" as infertile, even after the achievement of parenthood.

A special issue for older parents is concern about their own health status and mortality. Obviously, an older parent is more likely than a younger parent to become ill and/or die at an earlier point in the child's life. Facing infertility means making a conscious decision about childbearing, and most older parents who have gone through infertility have considered the issue of their age. Studies of those most affected by the issue of older parenting—the children—indicate an awareness of both benefits (increased maturity and patience, desire to focus on child-rearing) and liabilities (decreased energy, less ability to be physically active, and potential compromised health).

21. What useful psychological interventions can the obstetrician offer to the pregnant patient with a history of infertility or reproductive loss?

Many obstetricians recognize that such patients possess anxieties that are not commensurate with their actual medical status. Such patients usually require reassurance that is beyond what other obstetric patients seem to need. Physicians can remind patients that, even though their fears are understandable in light of their emotionally traumatic histories, the psychological validity of their fears is distinct from any medical validity. As the patient gradually transfers her sense of trust from the reproductive endocrinologist who assisted her pregnancy to the obstetrician who will deliver her baby, the obstetrician can recognize his or her own importance in personally responding to the patient's questions and concerns.

22. Are patients with an infertility history more likely to experience postpartum depression?

Although a relationship between infertility history and subsequent postpartum depression has not been clearly documented, it has been found that stressful life events as well as chronic health problems are sometimes associated with postpartum depression. This finding suggests that infertility—understood both as a chronic health problem and a stressful life event—may well be a factor to consider in evaluating risk for postpartum depression. Bartlik and associates have pointed out that infertility patients may also be at risk for posttraumatic stress disorder (PTSD) after delivery. The infertility, assisted reproductive treatment, and the high-risk nature of pregnancy constitute the psychological trauma for such women.

23. What signs and symptoms during pregnancy predict a greater likelihood of postpartum depression?

An important predictor of postpartum depression is depression during pregnancy. A degree of anxiety is normal. But all patients who present with significantly diminished capacity to experience interest and pleasure in their daily lives, whose everyday functioning is impaired, who show hopelessness or suicidal ideation, or whose mood is frequently depressed should be carefully evaluated. As the pregnancy nears term, a slight degree of emotional distancing linked to lingering fears about the outcome must be distinguished from outright failure to form an emotional bond with the (soon-to-be-born) child. Depression before delivery is likely to worsen after delivery. Other important risk factors in terms of postpartum depression include prior history of depression or affective disorder as well as lack of social support.

24. When is psychological/psychiatric consultation advisable?

Although a degree of stress and anxiety is normal, when anxiety or other symptoms of distress become immobilizing, mental health consultation is recommended. Evaluation is advisable when anxiety or depression significantly interferes with a patient's daily functioning or with her ability to form an anticipatory bond with her baby. Intensity and frequency of symptoms also determine whether psychopharmacological consultation is recommended.

25. How can counseling help such patients?

Of course, the ultimate "fix" for the fearful postinfertility obstetric patient is to give birth to a healthy baby, but counseling can help the patient cope with a notably anxious time. Therapeutic empathy with the patient's feelings can help her better understand and accept herself, at the same time that confrontation of some of her irrational and self-defeating beliefs can help her be reassuring to herself. Although the patient, in her own fearfulness, may never acknowledge that the therapist—in his or her more rational and realistically optimistic perspective—is bound to be right about the safety of the pregnancy, ongoing psychotherapy can help the patient gradually internalize a more benign and hopeful world-view.

26. What community resources are available for patients who are pregnant after infertility?

RESOLVE is a well-established support organization for people with fertility problems, providing information, education, group counseling, and links to medical and mental health professionals. RESOLVE provides support groups as well as referrals for individual/couples therapy for patients who are struggling with psychological difficulties secondary to postinfertility pregnancy.

Because it can greatly benefit patients to speak with others who have already traversed this terrain, RESOLVE also offers a peer support network.

27. What about the experience of parenting after infertility?

Mental health professionals have speculated that because of the premium nature of postinfertility pregnancies, such parents will be more inclined toward overprotectiveness of children. Although studies have indeed found some excessive degree of protectiveness, the news in general is heartening for people who have become parents following infertility. Golombok and colleagues intensively studied the "children of infertility," that is, children conceived through assisted reproductive technology, gamete donation, and adoption. Results have been generally reassuring. In particular, the parent-child relationships were determined to be quite positive, with some findings showing that children conceived with assisted reproductive technology had better relationships with their parents than naturally conceived children.

BIBLIOGRAPHY

1. Bartlik B, Greene K, Graf M, et al: Examining PTSD as a complication of infertility. Medscape Womens Health 2:1, 1997.
2. Brezinka C, Huter O, Biebl W, Kinzl J: Denial of pregnancy: Obstetrical aspects. Psychosom Obstet Gynaecol 15:1–8, 1996.
3. Chaaya M, Campbell OM, El Kak F, et al: Postpartum depression: Prevalence and determinants in Lebanon. Arch Women Ment Health 5:65–72, 2002.
4. Covington SN, Burns LH: Pregnancy after infertility. In Infertility Counseling: A Comprehensive Handbook for Clinicians. New York, Parthenon, 1999, pp 425–448.
5. Dziechciowski M, Klimek R, Tomaszewska, B, Wicherek F: Threatened and recurrent abortions after treatment of infertility. Early Pregnancy 5:45–46, 2001.
6. Edozien L: Why do some women undergo termination of pregnancy after successful IVF treatment? Hum Reprod 13:2377–2378, 1998.
7. Golombok S, Murray C, Brinsden P, Abdalla H: Social versus biological parenting: Family functioning and the socioemotional development of children conceived by egg or sperm donation. J Child Psychol Psychiatry 40:519–527, 1999.
8. Murata A, Nadaoka T, Morioka Y, et al: Prevalence and background factors of maternity blues. Gynecol Obstet Invest 46:99–104, 1998.

54. FERTILITY AND CANCER IN WOMEN

Kutluk Oktay, M.D., and Erkan Buyuk, M.D.

1. What is the most common reproductive-age cancer requiring fertility preservation before initiation of chemotherapy?

Breast cancer. Of the 18,000 new cases in the U.S., 15% occur under the age of 45 years (reproductive age).

2. What class of chemotherapeutic agents is the most gonadotoxic and associated with the highest incidence of ovarian failure?

Alkylating agents. Women using alkylating agents have an odds ratio of > 4 for developing ovarian failure compared with controls. Platinum drugs are mildly toxic, with the odds ratio of approximately 1.5 for ovarian failure. Antibiotic class (e.g., adriamycin), antimetabolites (e.g., methotraxate), and vinca alkaloids (e.g., vincristine) do not appear to have a significant toxic effect on germ cells.

3. Which alkylating agent is most commonly associated with chemotherapy-related gonadal failure and infertility?

Cyclophosphamide. For example, if a 40-year-old women is treated with regimens including cyclophosphamide, her chance of ovarian failure is 40–80%.

4. How does chemotherapy result in premature ovarian failure?

Chemotherapy, especially alkylating agents, induces apoptotic cell death in primordial follicle granulosa cells. Because > 90% of the ovarian reserve is made up of primordial follicles, loss of these follicles is associated with premature or immediate ovarian failure.

5. Why are young women less likely to suffer from ovarian failure due to chemotherapy?

Primordial follicle reserve is established during fetal life, and the number of primordial follicles declines with age. Younger women have a larger number of primordial follicles and hence tolerate chemotherapy-related follicle loss better than older women. Nevertheless, immediate menopause can occur even in prepubertal cancer patients if high doses of chemotherapy or pelvic radiation are used.

8. Can agonists of gonadotropin-releasing hormone (GnRH) protect gonads against chemotherapy-induced germ-cell damage?

Primordial follicles do not express receptors for follicle-stimulating hormone (FSH); thus, suppressing FSH production by GnRH agonists should not have a protective effect. A randomized study demonstrated no benefit from GnRH analogs in prevention of chemotherapy-induced amenorrhea.

9. List the current and experimental strategies for fertility preservation.

Embryo, oocyte, and ovarian tissue cryopreservation has been practiced in women. In men, cryopreservation of sperm and, in rare cases, testicular tissue can be performed.

10. Is in vitro fertilization (IVF) safe in patients with breast cancer?

Breast cancer is an estrogen-dependent tumor, and undergoing ovarian stimulation for the purpose of embryo cryopreservation could in theory aggravate breast cancer. IVF may not be safe even in the estrogen receptor-negative breast cancer because of possible presence of estrogen receptor-positive cell subpopulations.

11. Is it safe to conceive after receiving chemotherapy?

Clinical studies found no increase in the incidence of anomalies in children of women who conceived years after receiving chemotherapy. However, a recent rodent study showed that the incidence of fetal loss and anomalies increases if pregnancies occurred immediately after chemotherapy. This finding is probably due to the presence of damaged growing follicles. For this reason, it is recommended that at least 6 months elapse after completion of chemotherapy to allow the damaged follicles to be replenished by cells that initiated growth after the completion of chemotherapy. Follicle growth from the primordial follicle stage takes longer than 3 months in humans.

12. Is there a time limit for cryopreservation of embryos, oocytes, or ovarian tissue?

At a temperature of $-180°C$, the only factor that may result in a time-associated deterioration is background radiation. Typically this amount of exposure is not significant during the life span of a human; thus, there is no practical limit on the length of storage of reproductive tissues.

13. Is there a "safe" way to perform IVF in patients with breast cancer?

Recently, an ovarian stimulation scheme using tamoxifen was reported to perform IVF in breast cancer patients. Tamoxifen reduces breast cancer occurrence and recurrence and at the same time is an ovulation induction agent. Tamoxifen stimulation resulted in a 2.5-fold increase in the embryo yield without an increase in cancer recurrence rates. In the study protocol, tamoxifen was used at doses of 60 mg, starting on cycle day 2 or 3, for 5–12 days.

14. What is oophoropexy?

In cases of pelvic radiation, ovaries can be surgically positioned outside the pelvis, as high in the abdomen as possible. Recently, a laparoscopic technique was reported, in which the utero-ovarian ligament is transected and ovaries are sutured to the anterior abdominal wall. However, due to kinking of ovarian vessels, ovarian torsion and premature ovarian failure can occur. Overall, the short-term success rate of oophoropexy appears to be around 50%.

15. What is the threshold dose of radiation that causes gonadal failure?

Age of the patient, field of treatment, and fractionation schedule of the total dose are important in the degree and duration of radiotherapy-induced testicular damage. A dose of 6 Gy may result in menopause in women over 40 years of age, whereas significantly higher doses (20–30 Gy) are required to induce ovarian failure in young women and children.

16. Can fertility be preserved in young women with invasive cervical cancer?

In addition to protecting ovaries against pelvic radiation by oophoropexy and ovarian cryopreservation, the uterus may be preserved by trachelectomy in early-stage cervical cancer. One large series reported 70% pregnancy rate after this procedure.

17. Can fertility be preserved in early-stage endometrial cancer?

There have been reports in which well-differentiated stage I endometrial cancer has been treated either with high-dose medroxyprogesterone acetate or megestrol acetate and gonadotropin-releasing hormone analogs. Around 88% success rates and pregnancies after the treatment have been reported with both modalities.

18. Can fertility be preserved in early-stage ovarian cancer?

Stage 1 epithelial ovarian cancer has been successfully treated with fertility-sparing surgery with or without adjuvant chemotherapy. Survival rates of 98% at 5 years and 93% at 10 years have been achieved with full-term deliveries after treatment. Fertility-sparing surgery should be considered as a treatment option in women with stage I epithelial ovarian cancer who desire further childbearing.

OVARIAN TISSUE CRYOPRESERVATION

19. How is ovarian tissue cryopreservation (OTC) done?
Typically, one ovary is removed laparoscopically, and the ovarian cortex is isolated. The cortex is cut into strips that are 10 mm long by 5 mm wide and 1 mm in thickness. These strips are then incubated in cryoprotectants and frozen with a slow-freeze protocol, using a programmable freezer.

20. What is the best protocol for OTC?
The slow-freeze, rapid-thaw protocol has been shown to be better than other freeze-thaw procedures.

21. Which cryoprotectants are used for OTC?
Propanediol, ethylene glycol (EG), and dimethyl sulfoxide (DMSO) are the most frequently used cryoprotectants for ovarian tissue freezing.

22. What is the mechanism of action of the cryoprotectants?
Cryoprotectants are solutions with high solute concentrations that dehydrate the cell and help prevent ice formation inside the cell. Intracellular ice damages organelles and cell membrane unless cryoprotectants are used.

23. Which cryoprotectant is best for OTC?
EG, DMSO, and propanediol have similar success rates. Survival of frozen-thawed tissue is significantly less with glycerol compared with EG, DMSO and propanediol.

24. What percentage of follicles is lost during the cryopreservation procedure?
According to Baird et al., 7% of follicles are lost during the freezing and thawing procedure.

OVARIAN TRANSPLANTATION

25. What are the techniques of ovarian transplantation?
Ovarian tissue can be transplanted either in the pelvis (orthotopic) or at a subcutaneous site (heterotopic). In the pelvis, ovarian cortical pieces are either placed retroperitoneally or implanted in the preexisting menopausal ovary. With the heterotopic technique, pieces are typically implanted beneath the forearm skin.

26. What are the advantages and disadvantages of orthotopic and heterotopic ovarian transplantations?
With orthotopic ovarian transplantation, in theory at least, the patient may become pregnant naturally. But the procedure requires general anesthesia, and, in the case of IVF, ovarian monitoring is more difficult compared with heterotopic transplantation. Heterotopic transplantation, on the other hand, is technically easier and can be done under local anesthesia. Ovarian tissue can be monitored more closely, but the patient always needs an IVF procedure in order to conceive.

27. Is there any contraindication to autologous ovarian transplantation?
The incidence of metastasis to ovaries is high in leukemias and neuroblastomas. Therefore, due to high risk of reseeding cancer cells, autologous transplantation is relatively contraindicated in such patients.

28. What is the risk of reseeding cancer cells with ovarian autotransplantation?
There is a concern that when ovarian tissue is cryopreserved while a patient has active cancer, the specimen may harbor cancer cells. However, most cancers do not involve ovaries unless there is systemic involvement and other metastasis. On the other hand, in acute leukemias, presence of blastic cells in the circulation is a real concern.

Risk of Metastasis to Ovaries in Different Types of Cancers

HIGH	MODERATE	LOW
Leukemia Neuroblastoma	Breast cancer (stage 4) Adenocarcinoma of the uterine cervix Adenocarcinoma of the colon	Breast cancer (stages 1–3) Ewing's sarcoma Hodgkin's lymphoma Non-Hodgkin's lymphoma Nongenital rhabdomyosarcoma Squamous cell carcinoma of the uterine cervix

29. What is the best way to detect ovarian metastasis before transplantation?
Although many immunochemical and molecular biological techniques have been suggested to detect tumor cells in biopsy specimens, routine histologic evaluation is still the most widely used procedure to detect cancer cells in the ovaries before transplantation.

30. What is the longest duration of survival of a transplanted human ovary?
To date, there have been few cases of ovarian transplantation. The longest duration of function is nearly 3 years.

31. What percentage of follicles is lost during the revascularization period?
Approximately 65% of the follicles are lost during the revascularization process after ovarian transplant.

32. What measures can be taken to prevent follicle loss during revascularization?
Vascular endothelial growth factor administration in animals was unsuccessful, and gonadotropin injections in humans have been used with limited success to improve revascularization of the transplanted ovaries.

33. Has ovarian transplantation been successful in humans?
There have been handful of ovarian transplant procedures in humans, and all resulted in ovarian endocrine function of 9 months to 3 years. However, no pregnancies have been reported yet. Pregnancies have been reported in rodents and sheep after ovarian transplantation.

OOCYTE CRYOPRESERVATION

34. Why is oocyte cryopreservation not as effective as sperm cryopreservation?
The mature oocyte is extremely fragile due to its large size, water content, and chromosomal arrangement. The spindle apparatus is easily damaged by intracellular ice formation during the freezing and thawing procedure.

35. What is vitrification?
Vitrification is the process of cryopreservation using high concentrations of cryoprotectants to solidify the cell in a glass state without the formation of ice.

36. Is vitrification superior to standard oocyte cryopreservation procedures?
Preliminary studies suggest that vitirification may be superior to standard oocyte cryopreservation techniques. In particular, the use of a nylon loop inside the cryovial demonstrated fertilization and blastocyst development rates that were equal to those of fresh oocytes.

37. What is the live birth rate per frozen oocyte?
The live birth rate following fertilization and insemination of frozen oocytes is 3–4%.

BIBLIOGRAPHY

1. Baird DT, Webb R, Campbell BK, et al: Long-term ovarian function in sheep after ovariectomy and transplantation of autografts stored at – 196°C. Endocrinology 140:462–471, 1999.
2. Bines J, Oleske DM, Cobleigh MA: Ovarian function in premenopausal women treated with adjuvant chemotherapy for breast cancer. J Clin Oncol 14:1718–1729, 1996.
3. Dargent D, Martin X, Sacchetoni A, Mathevet P: Laparoscopic vaginal radical trachelectomy: A treatment to preserve the fertility of cervical carcinoma patients. Cancer 88:1877–1882, 2000.
4. Goodwin PJ, Ennis M, Pritchard KI, et al: Risk of menopause during the first year after breast cancer diagnosis. J Clin Oncol 17:2365–2370, 1999.
5. Gougeon A: Dynamics of follicular growth in the human: A model from preliminary results. Hum Reprod 1(2):81–87, 1986.
6. Haie-Meder C, Mlika-Cabanne N, Michel G, et al: Radiotherapy after ovarian transposition: ovarian function and fertility preservation. Int J Radiat Oncol Biol Phys 25:419–424, 1993.
7. Hankey BF, Miller B, Curtis R, Kosary C: Trends in breast cancer in younger women in contrast to older women. J Natl Cancer Inst Monogr 16:7–14, 1994.
8. Higgins S, Haffty BG: Pregnancy and lactation after breast-conserving therapy for early stage breast cancer. Cancer 73:2175–2180, 1994.
9. Hovatta O: Cryopreservation of testicular tissue in young cancer patients. Hum Reprod Update 7:378–383, 2001.
10. Imai M, Jobo T, Sato R, et al: Medroxyprogesterone acetate therapy for patients with adenocarcinoma of the endometrium who wish to preserve the uterus-usefulness and limitations. Eur J Gynaecol Oncol 22(3):217–220, 2001.
11. Lane M, Gardner D K: Vitrification of mouse oocytes using a nylon loop. Mol Reprod Dev 58(3):342–347, 2001.
12. Lushbaugh CC, Casarett GW: The effects of gonadal irradiation in clinical radiation therapy: A review. Cancer 37(2 Suppl):1111–1125, 1976.
13. Meirow D, Epstein M, Lewis H, et al: Administration of cyclophosphamide at different stages of follicular maturation in mice: Effects on reproductive performance and fetal malformations. Hum Reprod 16:632–637, 2001.
14. Oktay K, Buyuk E: The potential of ovarian tissue transplant to preserve fertility. Expert Opin Biol Ther 2(4):361–370, 2002.
15. Oktay K, Newton H, Mullan J, Gosden RG: Development of human primordial follicles to antral stages in SCID/hpg mice stimulated with follicle stimulating hormone. Hum Reprod 13:1133–1138, 1998.
16. Oktay K, Buyuk E, Davis O, et al: Fertility preservation in breast cancer patients: In vitro fertilization and embryo cryopreservation after ovarian stimulation with tamoxifen. Hum Reprod 18:90–95, 2003.
17. Schilder JM, Thompson AM, DePriest PD, et al: Functional studies of subcutaneous ovarian transplants in non-human primates: Steroidogenesis, endometrial development, ovulation, menstrual patterns and gamete morphology. Hum Reprod 17:612–619, 2002.
18. Stehman FB, van Nagell J: Outcome of reproductive age women with stage IA or IC invasive epithelial ovarian cancer treated with fertility-sparing therapy. Gynecol Oncol 87:1–7, 2002.
19. Tulandi T, Al-Took S: Laparoscopic ovarian suspension before irradiation. Fertil Steril 70(2):381–383, 1998.
20. Wallace WHB, Shalet SM, Crowne EC, et al:. Ovarian failure following abdominal irradiation in childhood: Natural history and prognosis. Clin Oncol 1:75–79, 1989.
21. Wang CB, Wang CJ, Huang HJ, et al: Fertility-preserving treatment in young patients with endometrial adenocarcinoma. Cancer 94:2192–2198, 2002.

55. FERTILITY AND CANCER IN MEN

Peter T. K. Chan, M.D.

1. Why is cancer an issue in male infertility?

First, approximately 1 % of men with infertility harbor significant, potentially life-threatening underlying medical conditions that were not previously diagnosed. Among the various undiagnosed conditions is cancer. In fact, the incidence of testicular cancer (most commonly, seminoma) was estimated to be 16-fold higher in men who present with infertility compared with the general population. Thus, a thorough investigation in all men with infertility is mandatory.

Secondly, many men with cancer at a younger age may not have started or completed their family. Often cancer treatment (surgery, chemotherapy, radiation therapy) may have a significant negative impact on fertility. Hence, cancer survivors represent a subgroup of infertile patients who require special attention.

2. What types of cancers are commonly seen in cancer survivors seeking fertility treatment?

Testicular cancer, lymphoma, and leukemia are the common cancers in male survivors who seek fertility treatment. The reasons are threefold: (1) these cancers are more commonly seen in young men who have not started or completed their family; (2) the survival rates of these cancers with modern therapy have improved tremendously, with over 70% expected to be long-term survivors; and (3) survivors often have a good quality of life.

3. What are the psychological concerns of fertility in cancer survivors?

Recent studies suggest that the majority of young cancer survivors consider having children or completing a family. However, it is easily conceivable that they have complex biopsychosocial dynamics. Specific concerns of cancer survivors related to issues of fertility include fear of dying, fear of not being to procreate, fear of passing diseases to offspring, fear of genetic defects after chemotherapy that lead to health risks in offspring, and fear of not being able to see their children grow.

4. How does surgical treatment for cancer affect male fertility?

An example of the severe effect of surgical treatment on fertility is seen in testicular cancer. The affected testis is removed. Needless to say, lost of one gonad can significantly affect the man's reproductive health. In some cases of testis cancers, an additional surgery known as retroperitoneal lymph node dissection is required. Retroperitoneal tissues around the spine, into which the lymphatic system of the testis drains, are removed. Since the nerves controlling ejaculation run along the same area, ejaculatory disorders such as anejaculation and retrograde ejaculation are known complications after this surgery. Modern techniques with the application of optical magnification and modification of the extent of retroperitoneal dissection have significantly reduced the incidence of these complications.

5. What is the threshold dose of radiation that causes gonadal failure in men?

Radiation treatment affects postmeiotic spermatogenesis. The degree and duration of radiotherapy-induced testicular damage depend on the age of the patient, the field of treatment, and the fractionation schedule of the total dose. In men, doses as low as 0.1–1.2 Gy may damage dividing spermatogonia and disrupt cell morphology, resulting in oligospermia. Recovery may be possible but generally takes at least 3 months. Azoospermia may be permanent after single-fraction irradiation with 4Gy. At high radiation doses (> 20 Gy) endocrinologic function from Leydig cell is also affected.

6. What chemotherapy agents are commonly used in treating cancer in young men?
- **Hodgkin's lymphoma.** Commonly used combination chemotherapy protocols include the MOPP (mechlorethamine, vincristine, procarbazine, and prednisone) and ABVD (doxorubicin, bleomycin, vinblastine, and dacarbazine) protocols.
- **Non-Hodgkin's lymphoma.** Commonly used protocols include CHOP (cyclophosphamide, doxorubicin, vincristine, and prednisone) and COPP (cyclophosphamide, vincristine, procarbazine, and prednisone).
- **Testis cancer.** The BEP (bleomycin, etoposide, and cisplatin) protocol and its modification are commonly used.
- **Acute lymphocytic leukemia.** The commonly used protocol includes prednisone, vincristine, and daunorubicin L-asparaginase or cyclophosphamide.

Combination chemotherapeutic regimens greatly reduce the toxicity of the individual agents because they require lower doses of each agent. This approach reduces damage to spermatogenic stem cells and increases the possibility of eventual restoration of fertility after treatment.

7. Describe the effect of chemotherapy on male reproductive health.
The impact of chemotherapy on reproduction varies significantly, depending on the chemotherapy dose, duration of treatment, type of drugs used, the pretreatment reproductive status (semen and hormonal profile), and severity of the cancer.

The cytotoxic effects of chemotherapy primarily affect the actively proliferating type B spermatognoia. If partial or complete destruction of type A spermatogonia (the stem cell spermatognoia) occurs, sustained or irreversible loss of spermatogenesis can be expected.

Some chemotherapy protocols, such as MOPP, can result in 70–100% incidence of post-treatment azoospermia persisting over 10 years. Other regimens, such as BEP for testis cancer, result in long-term azoospermia in less than 20% of patients.

8. Discuss the importance of quality of sperm in cancer patients before therapy.
Even before toxic treatment such as chemotherapy, the semen quality of patients with cancer may not be normal. For example, three-fourths of men with testicular germ cell cancers and up to two-thirds of men with Hodgkin's lymphoma have subnormal baseline semen parameters at the time of diagnosis. Factors that may be associated with the subnormal quality/quantity of sperm include:
- **Systemic illness.** Systemic illness leading to cachexia can be seen in many cancers at advanced states. Organ failure, abnormal hormonal profile, and spermatogenesis failure can be expected in these settings.
- **Psychological stress.** Even in the absence of physical debilitation from the primary cancer, the diagnosis, treatment, and expectation of outcomes pose severe psychological stress. Spermatogenic failure may result from psychological stress.
- **Coexisiting abnormalities in spermatogenesis.** Particularly in men with testis cancer, semen parameters may be abnormal due to the presence of malignancy in the gonad. In addition, undescended testes, which are associated with inherently poor spermatogenic function, are generally seen in these patients. Even in the normally descended contralateral testis, suboptimal spermatogenic function have been reported.
- **Age.** Many of these cancer patients are young men. In adolescents, semen parameters may not be normal according to the reference values based on adult parameters simply because spermatogenesis is not fully mature.

9. What are the effective means to preserve fertility in men before cancer treatment?
- **Sperm cryopreservation.** By far the most important and practical means is sperm banking before the initiation of chemotherapy. This appoach allows sperm to be stored for future use after cancer treatment, especially if spermatogenesis does not recover.
- **GnRH suppression.** Preliminary investigations have addressed the use of analogs of gonadotropin-releasing hormone (GnRH) to prevent gonadal damage from chemotherapy.

This approach is based on the theory that reduction of the release of gonadotropins will result in suppression of active germ cell division in the gonad and thereby reduce the risk of chemotoxic damage. This approach is currently under investigation.

10. Why do a significant proportion of male patients fail to cryopreserve sperm before cancer therapy?

1. **Physician failure to discuss thoroughly the need for this option.** Often, in dealing with life-threatening illness such as cancer, the health care team, the patient, and the family may focus all their efforts and energy in fighting cancer. As a result, sperm cryopreservation may be overlooked or ignored intentionally. In addition, treating physicians who are unfamiliar with the sperm-banking procedure may be not comfortable enough to discuss the issues. For these reasons, it is generally advisable to have a health care professional who is knowledgeable in reproductive medicine to provide specific counseling before cancer treatment.

2. **Time limitation.** Generally, the time between the diagnosis of cancer and the decision to begin therapy is only a matter of days. As a result, the decision and arrangement of sperm cryopreservation must be made promptly. Since many cancer patients have abnormal semen parameters even before the initiation of cancer treatment (see question 8), more than one semen production, with preferably 2–3 days of abstinence, may be required to obtain adequate quantity and quality of sperm for preservation.

3. **Severity of the illness.** When the prognosis is poor, patients and physicians may choose to omit sperm banking. However, knowing that it is not possible to predict the outcome of treatment for all patients and that sperm cryopreservation is a relatively simple procedure, the decision to defer sperm cryopreservation should not be made without prudent consideration.

4. **Age of patients.** In the preteen population, spermatogenesis may not have begun. Even in young adolescents, it may be awkward to ask for a semen specimen by masturbation (see question 15). In addition, the need for sperm preservation for future procreation may not occur to paients who are not involved in a relationship. Finally, patients who are older, particularly those who have had completed a family and desire no further children, may decline sperm cryopreservation.

5. **Lack of fertility facility.** Although sperm cryopreservation service is readily available in most urban areas and can be arranged with relatively short notice, such may not be the case in many remote areas.

6. **Refusal by patients.** Generally patients experience significant psychological stress when dealing with cancers. Depression, pessimism and lack of proper counseling may lead the patient to decline sperm cryopreservation before cancer treatment. Although the true incidence remains to be fully evaluated, many patients who survive cancer often regret not having preserved sperm before treatment.

11. What percentage of patients with cancer bank their sperm before treatment?

Studies in the 1990s estimated that less than 30% of cancer patients choose to bank sperm. With the increasing availability of advanced assisted reproductive technologies and the increasing survival rate of patients with cancer, this figure is expected to increase in the future.

12. What factors influence the rate of sperm banking before cancer treatment?

By far the most important factor in influencing the rate of sperm banking in patients with cancer is a counseling session focusing specifically on the fertility impact of treatment. For various reasons, not all patients with cancer desire sperm banking even after a proper counseling session. However, sperm banking should not be omitted because treating physicians fail to inform patients properly about the impact of cancer treatment on reproductive ability or about the availability of sperm banking, which is a simple and inexpensive procedure that allows more options in the future.

13. What should be discussed when young men are counseled about sperm banking before cancer treatment?

This complex discussion is generally better handled by health care professionals who are knowledgeable in reproductive medicine. Areas that should be covered in the counseling include:

- Risks of impairment of reproductive health.
- Need for using assisted reproduction technologies.
- Process of cryopreservation, including cost, the need of more than one banking session, and the risk of decreased sperm yield from the freezing and thawing process.

Keep in mind that patients and their family are generally overwhelmed by the diagnosis of cancer and the treatments involved. Counseling for sperm banking should aim at providing an adequate amount of information to patients and clear answers to specific questions. Additional details such as the cost and risks involved if advanced assisted reproduction is required in the future may not be pertinent to all patients at the time of cancer treatment and may generate unnecessary stress for patients and their family.

14. Describe the sperm-banking protocol for patients who are about to undergo cancer treatment.

As discussed in question 8, semen parameters in patients with cancer may be subnormal even before treatment. No sperm cryopreservation protocol is universally accepted for patients with cancer. Unlike sperm banking in healthy men, which requires a 2- to 3-day period of abstinence, for patients with cancer it may be necessary to collect sperm once a day for a few consecutive days to collect any sperm available for cryopreservation and to avoid any delay in treatment.

15. In dealing with young adolescents, is sperm banking advisable?

This important issue should be handled on a case-by-case basis. Many youngsters may not have thought about future family or children. The discussion of future fertility with youngsters and their parents should be done by a dedicated fertility specialist to avoid generation of additional anxiety.

In addition, there may be concerns about asking young adolescents to provide semen specimen by masturbation. In reality, depending on the cultural background of the patients, many young adolescents may be able to or comfortable with providing a semen sample by masturbation. However, it is prudent to provide proper counseling to both patients and parents before requesting sperm cryopreservation.

In some cases, retrieval of sperm by surgical technique or electroejaculation may be considered. The advantage of this approach is that masturbation is not necessary. Disadvantages include the need for anesthesia and the risks of complications associated with the procedures.

16. Can spermatogenesis be preserved in prepubertal boys scheduled to receive cancer treatment??

Few mature spermatozoa are available before puberty. Even if sperm may be found in the ejaculate, requesting a semen specimen by masturbation in prepubertal patients is often difficult or inappropriate. Cryopreservation of sperm obtained by penile vibration, rectal electrostimulation or even surgically retrieved spermatozoa from testes has been proposed and attempted. However, performing an invasive surgical procedure may further delay chemotherapy, particular if a complication such as hemorrhage or infection occurs. Furthermore, in prepubertal boys only immature germ cells may be found. Experimental research has evaluated the feasibility of future reimplantation of the immature germ cells into the seminiferous tubules to allow recovery of spermatogenesis. Although some promising attempts have been made in experimental animals, restoration of active spermatogenesis is not yet successful. Furthermore, as in the case of ovarian tissue (see Chapter 63), there is a risk of reseeding malignant cells during germ cells r-implantation, especially in hematologic malignancies such as lymphoma and leukemia.

17. Do patients who did not bank sperm before treatment and who remain azoospermic after treatment have any chance of fathering genetic children?

Yes. In a retrospective analysis of men who had undergone chemotherapy and remained azoospermic for an average of over 16 years, sperm was found in approximately 50% during surgical testicular sperm retrieval. Using intracytoplasmic sperm injection (ICSI), one-third of such men were able to achieve clinical pregnancy in their partners, and 20% of pregnancies resulted in delivery of healthy babies. The success rate was similar to that in other men with nonobstructive azoospermia due to reasons other than cancer and its treatment. Despite these encouraging results, the authors still advocate sperm cryopreservation before the initiation of cancer therapy.

18. Is sperm from men treated for cancer associated with an increase in genetic risks?
Based on limited studies in the literature, no evidence suggests higher genetic risks, including congenital malformations, neonatal mortality, or other genetic disorders, in offspring from parents who have had previous chemotherapy. Nonetheless, some studies have reported an increased proportion of genetically abnormal sperm in men who have had previous chemotherapy, particularly within the first year after treatment. Thus, some physicians advise patients to attempt procreation only after a minimum of 1 year after chemotherapy.

Certainly, for cancer survivors who had been treated with chemotherapy, who desire further children, and whose reproductive function has recovered, attempting to conceive naturally should be encouraged. On the other hand, if reproductive function has not recovered and advanced assisted reproductive technologies such as ICSI is required, it is uncertain whether using previously cryopreserved sperm that were not exposed to chemotoxic agents offers lower genetic risks to the offspring. In this setting, it is crucial to provide genetic counseling for patients, focusing on the potentials genetic risks involved.

BIBLIOGRAPHY

1. Brinster RL: Germline stem cell transplantation and transgenesis. Science 296:2174–2176, 2002.
2. Chan PTK, Palermo GD, Veeck LL, et al: Testicular sperm extraction combined with intracytoplasmic sperm injection in the treatment of men with persistent azoospermia post chemotherapy. Cancer 92:1632–1637, 2001.
3. Nudell DM, Monoski MM, Lipshultz LI: Common medications and drugs: How they affect male fertility. rol. Clin North Am. 29:965–974, 2002.
4. Zapzalka DM, Redmon JB, Pryor JL: A survey of oncologists regarding sperm cryopreservation and assisted reproductive techniques for male cancer patients. Cancer 86:1812–1817, 1999.

VII. Legal and Ethical Issues

56. ASSISTED REPRODUCTION

Elizabeth Grill, Psy.D., Laura Josephs, Ph.D., and Melissa B. Brisman, J.D.

1. Does one partner have the right to use the frozen embryos created by the couple during a relationship after divorce or death?

Over the years most courts have agreed that the right to use embryos created during a relationship must be based on mutual consent at the time of the embryo transfer procedure. The trend in the law is not to allow a person to procreate with embryos that are composed of gametes from one person who objects to their use.

A.Z. v. B.Z., 725 N.E.2d 1051 (Mass. 2000) concerned a wife who wanted to use the embryos of the couple to procreate after divorce. The court stated that, even if the husband and wife had entered into an unambiguous agreement between themselves regarding the disposition of the frozen preembryos, it would not enforce an agreement that would compel one donor to become a parent against his or her will: "As a matter of public policy, we conclude that forced procreation is not an area amenable to judicial enforcement."

Davis v. Davis, 842 S.W. 2d 588 (Tenn. 1992) did not allow the creation of life against the ex-husband's wishes since it would impose unwanted parenthood, "with all of its possible financial and psychological consequences."

2. Discuss the wife's right to request surgical retrieval of sperm from her husband who just died.

In Britain, unless permission has been obtained from a man prior to his death, the government prohibits extracting sperm posthumously: "Our unregulated approach contrasts greatly with the system in England, where the Human Fertilisation and Embryology Authority, a Government agency, passes judgment on which fertility techniques are beyond the pale." Britain does not allow the use of a dead man's sperm without his prior consent.

In the United States, no official body overlooks fertility techniques, and no federal law prohibits posthumous conception. As such it is possible to extract a man's sperm without his consent when he is on his deathbed and then impregnate someone with his sperm (see Andrews LB: The sperminator. *New York Times,* March 28, 1999). Certain states have attempted to pass legislation preventing this occurrence, but most laws are in a state of flux. As long as the state in which the operation is performed has not passed a law against retrievial of sperm without consent, after death one is legally permitted to extract sperm from a deceased man and use it to impregnate his living wife. However, the American Society of Reproductive Medicine's opinion on posthumous reproduction states the following: "A spouse's request that sperm or ova be obtained terminally or soon after death without the prior consent or known wishes of the deceased spouse need not be honored." Without prior consent of the deceased individual one enters a quagmire of ethical dilemmas that cannot be easily solved.

3. Is a child conceived posthumously entitled to survivor and disability benefits under the Social Security Act?

Courts have ruled differently in different states on this issue. In *Gillett-Netting v. Barnhart, D.Ariz., No. CV-02-014,* for example, twins conceived by a widow via in vitro fertilization with her deceased husband's sperm 10 months after his death were not entitled to Social Security survivor benefits.

The Massachusetts Supreme Court, however, ruled differently in *Woodward ex rel. Estate of Woodward v. Commissioner of Social Sec., 435 Mass. 536, – N.E.2d –, 2002 WL 4289 (Mass. 2002)*:

> In certain limited circumstances, a child resulting from posthumous reproduction may enjoy the inheritance rights of 'issue' under the Massachusetts intestacy statute. These limited circumstances exist where, as a threshold matter, the surviving parent or the child's other legal representative demonstrates a genetic relationship between the child and the decedent. The survivor or representative must then establish both that the decedent affirmatively consented to posthumous conception and to the support of any resulting child. Even where such circumstances exist, time limitations may preclude commencing a claim for succession rights on behalf of a posthumously conceived child. Because the government has conceded that the timeliness of the wife's paternity action under our intestacy law is irrelevant to her Federal appeal, we do not address that question today.

These two cases illustrate once again the uncertainties in the law as it relates to reproductive matters.

4. What is the difference between a gestational carrier and a surrogate mother?

A surrogate mother is a woman who carries a child for another couple that is composed of her own egg and the sperm of the intended father or a sperm donor. In most cases, the surrogate mother is artificially inseminated to achieve pregnancy. A gestational carrier is a woman who carries for another couple and/or individual a child that bears no genetic tie to the gestational carrier. The egg, which comes either from the intended genetic mother or from a third-party ovum donor, has been fertilized with the sperm of the intended father or a sperm donor.

5. What is the state of the law regarding compensation of gestational carriers?

State laws vary on whether gestational carriers can be legally compensated. For example, New York does not allow gestational carriers to be compensated by statute. Other states permit courts to issue prebirth parentage orders allowing the genetic parents to be listed on the birth certificate of a child delivered by a gestational carrier without an adoption even if the gestational carrier was compensated. These orders implicitly endorse the right and legality of the carrier's compensation. Massachusetts, Maine, Connecticut, and Pennsylvania are among the few the states that have allowed such orders, but no statute directly addresses the legality of compensation in these states.

6. How can a patient maximize insurance coverage in a gestational carrier arrangement?

As gestational carrier programs become more popular, insurance companies are becoming more aware of the expense of such pregnancies, especially when they involve multiple births. Many companies now add exclusions for gestational carrier or surrogate pregnancies. Therefore, patients must be aware that if they are using a gestational carrier, a reproductive lawyer must make sure that their gestational carrier's insurance policy contains no exclusion for a gestational carrier's pregnancy. These exclusions are often buried in fine print or placed in the controlling legal document. When patients request the governing document, they are often given only a summary, and without a trained legal eye they may not be aware that the document provided is not the overriding insurance policy.

7. How much can an ovum donor be paid to donate her eggs?

Almost all states in the U.S. allow ovum donors to be compensated, and compensation varies widely by area of the country. Some programs compensate donors with $2,000, whereas in 2003 the average compensation in the New York City area was $7,500. The American Society of Reproductive Medicine states that sums of $5,000 or more require justification and that sums beyond $10,000 are inappropriate. But the American Society of Reproductive Medicine standards are only guidelines; they are not legally binding. Donors have received as much as $50,000 in compensation if they possess certain IQ levels and have certain bodily characteristics. The Ivy League schools have been targets of increasing advertisements for "a special woman" who meets a client's goals and specifications. As advertisements of this nature increase, it is likely that legislatures will set some ground rules, but without such laws the sky is the limit.

8. How can patients in a surrogacy, ovum donation, embryo, or sperm donation contract protect their legal rights?
Most state laws are unclear about the enforceability of such arrangements. Courts on the whole, however, are more likely to enforce the rights of either party when each party had adequate counsel and the terms of the arrangement were drawn up in a contract.

9. Can a gestational carrier abort the intended parents' fetus against their will?
Yes. A gestational carrier has complete control over her body despite what any legal agreement between the parties might state. Certain elements and rights of United States law cannot be contracted away. As long as the abortion is legal at that point in the pregnancy, the pregnant woman has the absolute right to choose [see *Roe v. Wade, 410 U.S. 113 (1973)*]. If, however, the gestational carrier tries to abort the fetus in the third trimester when the life is viable and the abortion procedure itself is illegal, she cannot legally do so. The reverse is also true in this case and perhaps even more troublesome, especially when a severe fetal defect is at issue. No court would force a woman to have an abortion that was legally permissible. If the contract with the couple states that the carrier will abort and she refuses, the only possible remedy for the couple in U.S. courts is monetary damages—not specific enforcement. It is not possible to compel the carrier to abort. If the child is the couple's biologic child, unfortunately they may be left with the serious consequence of bringing to life a biologic child with serious mental and physical handicaps.

10. Who is legally responsible for medical complications experienced by an egg donor?
This issue is governed by contract and is one of the legal pitfalls that many clinics in the United States have not adequately addressed. Many of the consent forms used by clinics make the couple legally liable for medical complications experienced by the egg donor; however, there should be a monetary limit to the couple's liability and a time limit after which the egg donor can no longer claim that the complication was a result of the ovum donation. Psychological complications should not be included after a certain date. Clinics also would be wise to require intended parents to purchase donor insurance. Donor insurance is a new product offered by some insurance companies to cover many of the complications that may result from an ovum donation; as with anything else, however, the policy must be scrutinized carefully. A fair balance must be achieved in protecting the donor from injuries sustained from the donation and limiting the couple's legal and financial liability resulting from the ovum donation.

11. How can we assure an embryo donor recipient that she will be considered the legal parent of any child she delivers?
Embryo donation is uncharted territory in almost every jurisdiction. Although increasingly more common, the procedure has no legal roadmap. The presumption in the United States is clear: if there is no law against it, the procedure can be undertaken. But it is not without serious legal risk. Undoubtedly, because of the circumstances that led to the donation itself, the likelihood is that the procedure will create biologic siblings of children already born. It is unclear whether the embryo recipient will be considered the legal mother without a formal adoption.

However, most courts would not know how to handle a case of adoption in this matter because most people do not know where the embryo came from. In addition, the presumption in every state is that if a woman gives birth to the child, she is the child's mother. Without any legal papers stating otherwise, she becomes the child's legal mother on his or her birth record. How can you then go to court asking to adopt what is already yours? The court is at a loss how to handle the matter, and legislatures have provided no remedy.

What about the rights of the siblings? Someday the courts will be forced to grapple with people who want to know where their biologic siblings have been raised. Embryo donation is one of the riskier reproductive alternatives and should be undertaken only with the aid of an experienced reproductive lawyer.

12. Define bioethics.

McCullough and Chervenak expand on Reich's definition of bioethics as the disciplined study of the morality of health care. They describe morality as "concern[ing] the beliefs and practices of human beings and social institutions about right and wrong behavior and about good and bad character" and note that the morality of health care includes the morality of physicians, patients, institutions, and policy makers. Simply put, medical ethics relates to what is right or wrong in the practices and decisions of health care practitioners in their treatment of patients. What is ethically acceptable relates to but is distinct from what is legally acceptable.

13. What are the major ethical issues raised by assisted reproduction?

Applegarth delineates the key ethical issues associated with infertility treatment:

1. Infertility and its treatment unfold within a psychosocial—not a purely physiologic—context.

2. Informed consent is a complex issue, especially as it relates to patients' genuine appreciation—or lack thereof—of the risks involved in reproductive treatment and the chances of success. Specifically, because of the often desperate desire to have a child, many patients may underestimate the physical and emotional impact of undergoing treatment while overestimating their own likelihood of succeeding in treatment and thus may approach decision-making from a skewed point of view.

3. Advances in reproductive technology have brought the process of creating a child some distance from nature, enabling physicians to offer patients a variety of permutations in terms of conceiving and carrying offspring. Women can be stimulated to produce multiple oocytes, resulting—among other things—in multiple births that otherwise would not have occurred. Patients can receive gametes—eggs and/or sperm—to create children who (from a genetic point of view) would not otherwise have been created. Patients (whether egg donor recipients or gestational carriers) can carry children whose genetic make-up has nothing to do with their own.

It should be noted that the assisted reproductive technologies are of benefit not only to patients/parents who have successfully received treatment but also to the children who otherwise would not have existed. Nonetheless, ethicists have pointed out that, because of the powerful coming together of patient demands with medical aspirations, reproductive technologies tend to be put into practice without full longitudinal study of their medical and psychological consequences.

14. Is artificial reproductive assistance for infertile couples unethical?

One of the most fundamental arguments brought against assisted reproductive technologies is whether artificial insemination, gamete or embryo donation, and in vitro fertilization are unnatural practices. For example, the development of in vitro fertilization has made it possible for one child to have as many as five different "parents," including an ovum donor, a sperm donor, a gestational carrier, and the two rearing parents. Furthermore, successful cryopreservation of sperm and embryos has enabled people to preserve their potential fertility almost indefinitely. These new parental configurations raise profoundly difficult and often disturbing ethical questions and have forced the people working in the field of reproductive medicine to confront whether specific technologies should be used for assisted reproduction simply because they exist.

Many experts argue for procreative liberty, asserting that, since the U.S. Constitution affords people the right to procreate coitally, it also gives individuals the right to procreate noncoitally. Others argue that helping couples to become parents through the use of reproductive technology supports autonomy, beneficence and justice, the three principal components of medical ethics. It supports autonomy when couples are given the power to make decisions about their treatment based on all of the information pertaining to their situation. It supports beneficence when couples are able to achieve their long-sought goal of parenthood. It supports the concept of justice if all

Cooper SL, Glazer ES: Choosing Assisted Reproduction. Indianapolis, IN, Perspectives Press, 1998.
Ryan KJ: Ethical and legal implications. In Adashi EY, Rock JA, Rosenwaks Z (eds): Reproductive Endocrinology, Surgery, and Technology. Philadelphia, Lippincott-Raven, 1996, pp 1941–1951.
McCollough LB, Chervenak FA: Ethics in Obstetrics and Gynecology. New York, Oxford University Press, 1994.

who are in need are able to use the technology, although for some people the rising cost of treatment and the lack of insurance coverage in many states may interfere with this principle. At times, autonomy may also collide with beneficence, especially when a patient requests a particular treatment that his or her provider believes may do harm to the patient or potential child. In such cases, one principle must be compromised for the sake of the other.

What is ethical may vary depending on the social, spiritual, and religious community from which one arises and in which one chooses to live. For example, the Vatican proclaimed that all forms of assisted reproduction that substitute for coitus within marriage are morally wrong. The Vatican noted that it is permissible to treat the reproductive system itself, such as by opening a blocked tube or relieving anovulation, but it is not morally correct to help a couple overcome infertility with gamete donation, artificial insemination, in vitro fertilization, or embryo transplant. Thus, the idea of forcing conception when otherwise it would not occur is unacceptable to some people holding strong religious or spiritual beliefs. Some religious followers believe that using artificial means may have negative effects on the marriage, family, and resulting children.

To date, however, no compelling arguments justify that assisted reproduction has detrimental consequences for the children and/or parents. On the contrary, infertile couples typically act responsibly after years of trying to achieve a planned pregnancy. In fact, others argue that unwanted and often unplanned natural conceptions may result in greater harm, such as abortion or potential abuse.

15. Should there be limits on access to in vitro fertilization?

Assisted reproductive technology is a unique area of medicine because patients request treatment to fulfill an often long-term quest to have a child even though the medical treatment may not be required to prevent harm or alleviate physical pain. Although historically physicians have an obligation to honor refusals of treatment, they do not have an obligation to honor all requests for treatment. Physicians may deny treatment based on the potential risks to the patient and even risks to the prospective offspring.

Often the decision whether to treat patients depends on the attitudes of the clinic staff at the various centers that provide assisted reproductive technology. Access to these services may be denied because of the presence of behaviors or conditions in the patient that the provider finds problematic for ethical or other reasons. Decisions to deny treatment may result from concerns about a patient's psychological or social history, prospective ability to parent, or perceived medical risks. Because of limited information about the long-term risks to women using fertility drugs, some professionals feel that there should be a limit on the number of cycles that women are allowed to pursue, whereas others feel that a patient's informed consent is enough to provide ongoing treatment. Some practitioners draw the line with patients who abuse alcohol, use illegal drugs, or have a history of abusing children, whereas others refuse treatment to unmarried couples or single women. Some countries have legislation against treatment of certain patients, such as unmarried women. In the United States, however, few laws address these issues, leaving many of the decisions in the hands of practitioners who often rely on the American Society for Reproductive Medicine guidelines.

In a study of the opinions of clinic directors at 184 assisted reproduction clinics in the United States, a large percentage of providers noted that they would like to restrict treatment in some situations, even though their clinic policy did not restrict access. Most dramatic in this regard were providers' opinions about the age limitations in the male partner of couples undergoing assisted reproduction. Overall, clinic policies appear less restrictive than opinions of their individual providers. One possible explanation for this discrepancy is patient autonomy, which is supported by many experts as well as the ASRM Ethics Committee (although the committee also recognizes the right of individual providers to choose not to treat patients in some cases). Another potential explanation for this difference is providers' fears of litigation based on claims of discrimination.

Applegarth LD: Ethical issues in infertility nursing practice. Infert Reprod Med Clin North Am 7:611–621, 1996.
Stern J, Cramer C, Garrod A, Green R: Attitudes on access to services at assisted reproductive technology clinics: Comparisons with clinic policy. Fertil Steril 77(3), 2002.

16. Should there be limits on embryo technologies that make it possible to select a child's physical and mental characteristics?

Preimplantation genetics, a procedure that examines embryos for genetic defects before they are transferred to the uterus, is currently offered to couples who are carriers of a genetic disease that they do not wish to pass to their offspring. Although scientists have not yet mapped the entire human genome, with the advances in the understanding of human genetics couples may soon be able to choose other characteristics of their unborn children. Genetic engineering would allow parents not only to select the sex of their child but also to determine the physical, intellectual, and perhaps even emotional and social characteristics of their offspring.

Some have argued that this technology is essentially eugenics disguised as new technology. Although many people support the use of preimplantation genetic selection for couples who are carriers of diseases, many do not support this technology for couples who wish to have a child of a particular sex or create a child who is tall or has a predisposition for music or sports. Many proponents of procreative liberty believe that people have a right to select the child that they want, whereas others see inherent dangers in society if couples are allowed to choose the specific characteristics of their offspring.

17. When reproductive technology is performed using third parties, it is ultimately the donor, surrogate, or gestational carrier who assumes many of the medical risks. Is this appropriate despite informed consent regarding the many aspects of the procedures?

Assisted reproductive technology is not without medical side effects or risks, and people who are desperate for children and require assistance from third parties may not be in the best position to objectively evaluate or explain these risks to others who may be involved. Since technology has made it possible to separate the various components of motherhood, ovum donors and/or surrogates who are not the intended parents are subjected to medical and psychological risks. Many argue that those who are infertile have the right to choose a procedure that involves potential physical and psychological harm, but that it is morally unacceptable to subject a young, fertile woman to the same risks when she is not the intended parent.

Experts question whether donors, especially those who have not yet experienced parenthood, truly understand the long-term emotional implications of their donation. Furthermore, questions are raised about whether it is ethical to subject healthy young fertile women, who in some cases may not have started or completed their own families, to the possible risks of treatment, including the potential risk of becoming infertile. Many argue that third parties, like infertility patients, are also entitled to autonomy when it comes to decisions regarding their bodies. Others argue, however, that there is always inherent coercion (financial or personal) for donors, surrogates, and carriers that cannot be dismissed and that can amount to exploitation.

There are concerns that the ever-increasing financial incentives to third parties may lead them to ignore potential harms. Some question what level of financial compensation to donors is fair and just as well as noncoercive and does not support a policy that encourages poor women to sell their eggs to women who are financially able to pay for them.

Further complicating the issue is the concern that the donor/surrogate who is a sister or friend may not truly be capable of consenting freely when her decision may seem critical to the future happiness of a much-loved individual. Professionals recommend careful medical and psychological counseling for all of the parties involved so that everyone may thoroughly consider the potential medical and psychological risks before deciding to move forward.

18. Should people be allowed to donate gametes to family members?

Gamete donation has made it possible for participants to cross generational lines and has raised many complicated ethical issues. Fathers can donate sperm for their sons. Although extremely rare,

Applegarth LD: Ethical issues in infertility nursing practice. Infertil Reprod Med Clin North Am 7:611–621, 1996.
Cooper SL, Glazer ES: Choosing Assisted Reproduction. Indianapolis, IN, Perspectives Press, 1998.

mothers may donate to their daughters when they are fertile enough to donate to a daughter who is old enough to have a child. It is possible for daughters and sons to donate gametes to their parents. In the cases of children donating to their parents, mental health clinicians usually feel strongly that because most children feel indebted to their parents to some degree, they are not truly free to say no to their parent's request in the same way they are free to say no to anyone else. In addition, many experts feel that the nature of the relationship may be violated as children are providing for their parents while the parents are still competent. In the case of a parent donating to a son or in some cases to a daughter, some professionals feel more supportive, because the concept of a parent giving to their child is already built into the parent-child relationship.

Often couples may ask a sister to donate, and others may ask another relative such as a cousin or a niece. Sister-to-sister or brother-to-brother donations may appear to be ideal on many levels because of their similar genetic make-up and continuity of the bloodline, but the practice is only as good as the health of the relationships between the two siblings and their respective spouses. If couples choose a sibling to donate, old patterns of sibling rivalry may be stirred up. In addition, many social and emotional entanglements may occur in the family—for example, if the child has an aunt who is her genetic mother and a cousin who is her half-sibling. When third parities are involved in family building, especially when they are a family member, recipient parents may fear that their children are likely to form a stronger attachment to the donor than to them. Some fear that if the donor were a sister, for example, the child may face the additional confusion of not knowing whether to relate to her as an aunt or as a mother. When a family gamete cycle fails to result in pregnancy, all involved are extremely disappointed, and as family members search for an explanation, old family dynamics may be re-enacted, resulting in blame or feelings of guilt.

Before such unique family-building scenarios are undertaken or endorsed, specific psychological issues need to be systematically addressed by the infertility counselor. Experts agree that it is necessary to assess the relationship between the participants to establish whether the reproductive plan is in the best interests of all involved, including the potential child. Infertility counseling must look for coercion, in which one party feels obligated to the other. Sometimes the counselor needs to help one party say no to an uncomfortable request. In child-to-parent donations, the counselor must address the imbalance of power and the inherent boundary violations that may leave the family system or the relationships vulnerable and at risk. The infertility counselor must also consider a son or daughter's relationship with the step-parent to make sure that there are no sexual overtones. It is critical for all of the parties involved to have a clear understanding of boundaries and to think through scenarios that may challenge these arrangements in the future. All parties should be in agreement regarding disclosure to others as well as to the potential child. Ultimately, the donor should feel comfortable allowing the recipients to make all decisions related to disclosure, the pregnancy, and the upbringing of the potential child. The infertility counselor must help all of the parties involved explore their motivations, concerns, expectations, wants, hopes, and fears regarding the process.

19. Should parents of third-party reproduction disclose to the child, family, or friends the genetic origins and gestational ties of their offspring?

Whether children conceived using donated gametes should be told about their genetic origins remains one of the most disputed ethical issues raised by the practice of assisted reproduction. The question of openness vs. secrecy is a complicated one, involving profound ethical, legal, religious, and psychosocial issues. Historically, parents have generally not been encouraged to tell others or their children that the family originated through nontraditional means. However, this trend appears to be slowly changing as people have come to recognize the hazards of secrecy. A growing body of opinion argues that it is not justifiable to keep such information secret, either be-

Gordon ER, Barrow RG: Legal and ethical aspects of infertility counseling. In Burns LH, Covington SN (eds): Infertility Counseling. Pearl River, NY, Parthenon Publishing Group, 1999, pp 491–512.

cause children have an inherent right to know about their genetic/gestational beginnings or because of concern about the effect of secrecy on family relationships. A family created as a result of reproductive technology will undoubtedly have hurdles to face.

The debate between disclosure and secrecy has its historical roots in the traditions of sperm donation and adoption. The first cases of artificial insemination using a donor was documented by William Pancoast, who claimed to have performed the procedure in secret. Thus began a trend of secrecy that has continued for 100 years for most couples choosing donor sperm. Male infertility is often associated with impotence or a lack of virility and thus carries with it a shameful stigma that is seldom discussed openly among health professionals. Consequently, many professionals may not address the overwhelming sadness that infertile men and their partners feel on learning their diagnosis, nor do they explore the psychological implications that using donor sperm may have on their relationship and on their family.

Most of the research that indicates an association between secrecy about genetic parentage and negative outcomes for children has stemmed from research on adoption. Research has shown that adopted children benefit from knowledge about their biologic parents and that children who are not given such information may become confused about their identity and at risk for emotional problems. Parallels have been drawn between adoption and assisted reproduction, and it has been suggested that lack of knowledge of, or information about, the donor may be harmful for the child.

There are also differences in regard to disclosure between those who use donor sperm vs. donor egg. Most ovum recipients, even though they may worry whether they will feel like the real mother, gain confidence that they will bond with the child that they carry. The biologic connection that the mother shares with the developing fetus is quite different from the infertile man whose wife conceives with donor sperm. In the latter case, the man must wait until after the birth to establish a relationship with the child. In addition, women for the most part are socialized to be more open about their personal lives. They are accustomed to sharing problems with friends and family and looking to others for mutual support and advice.

There are many reasons why a couple may choose not to tell family, friends and/or the child. Shame often fuels a nondisclosure stance. Unfortunately, shame is a byproduct of secrecy, which only increases the couple's feelings of inadequacy and may decrease their ability to form close relationships with the child. Couples may hold fast to the illusion that if they do not tell, they will remain protected from the sadness of not having a family by traditional means. However, families who protect secrets develop a complicated system of interpersonal relationships with taboo-like undercurrents that children often sense. This system of secrecy can inadvertently promote family estrangement and create unhealthy alliances between those who know and those who do not know and may also undermine the trust that is vital to a healthy parent-child relationship. When parents choose not to tell their children, they often live in fear that they may find out about their origins and that the bond of trust that children have with their parents will be threatened.

The decision to tell or not to tell a child about his or her genetic origins is compelling, and infertility counselors should be responsible for providing a forum for patients to safely explore their thoughts and feelings about disclosure. Couples should be encouraged to think through the different ways in which a child may have access to information in the future, such as the availability of DNA testing in more commonplace settings. It should also be stressed that legal aspects of sperm and ovum donation may be challenged in the future, thus changing the climate of openness vs. secrecy in the public domain. Other countries have already sought to establish open donor registries to protect the rights of the potential child. In addition, medical emergencies, such as the need for an organ or bone marrow transplant, may arise in the future and open the door for children to discover that they are not a direct match to their mothers or fathers. There are arguments both for and against disclosure, and each couple should be allowed to decide, with the help of infertility counselors, which choice is best for them and their child(ren) within the context of these issues.

If couples choose to disclose the information to their children, they should also understand the distinctions between openness and privacy. Couples still have the right to discern who will know, how they will find out, and when they will share the information. Because the decision to undertake gamete donation has lifelong implications for an entire family, the role of the mental heath professional and self-help organizations should not be underestimated. Experts agree that the more the recipient couple feels comfortable and prepared for this parenting option, the more likely it is that they will be fulfilled as parents and will make decisions that are in the best interest of the child.

20. How do medical practitioners/mental health professionals help determine when treatment should be stopped—in other words, when "enough is enough"?

Physicians are always obliged to inform patients, to the best of their ability, of the chances of success. Patients must wrestle with these numbers and come to a decision based on their own personal assessment. What is a "reasonable" chance of success? For some people, a 40% chance of successful pregnancy per cycle may feel insufficient to justify the medical risk and the emotional and financial strain of treatment. For others, numerous successive cycles with a likely success rate of 5% or less may feel acceptable, given the ferocity of their desire for a biologic child.

It is always difficult for patients to stop assisted reproductive treatment, even when the chances of success are very low. It is natural enough for any of us to believe that we will be the one who "defies the odds." Nonetheless, often patients on their own will come to a decision that coincides with the beliefs and recommendations of the physician. Conflicts in the doctor-patient relationship are most likely to arise when patients wish to persist in treatment, despite vanishing chances of succeeding. Given a particular patient's age, history, and so on, if there is no likelihood—or virtually no likelihood—that an assisted reproduction procedure will result in success, most practitioners would decline treatment, on the basis that it is medically inappropriate to subject a patient to risk with (virtually) no potential benefit. When the chance of success is small but exists, some practitioners leave the final decision to patients, as long as the patients are fully aware of the risk-benefit ratio. Other practitioners do not feel comfortable providing a medical procedure for which they feel the risk-benefit ratio is skewed and in such cases decline to provide assisted reproduction procedures. Mental health professionals can help patients to make choices about their treatment that are based on a realistic appreciation of risks and likelihood of success. Mental health professionals can also help patients cope adaptively with loss and identify potential self-defeating patterns in individuals and couples as they traverse the difficult and painful terrain of infertility and reproductive treatment.

21. How old is too old to participate in infertility treatment?

Medical, psychological, and ethical factors weigh heavily in the decision to have a child at any age. Despite the few sensationalized stories, it is well known that fertility in women, and less so in men, declines with age. However, reproductive technology has enabled many women and men past traditional reproductive age to conceive and, in many instances, carry a pregnancy to term. For example, oocyte donation to older women makes pregnancy feasible in virtually any woman with a normal uterus, regardless of age or ovarian function. Thus, women in their 50s and 60s can successfully gestate and birth a baby created from sperm and a donated egg.

Gordon ER, Barrow RG: Legal and ethical aspects of infertility counseling. In Burns LH, Covington SN (eds): Infertility Counseling. Pearl River, NY, Parthenon Publishing Group, 1999, pp 491–512.
Cooper SL, Glazer ES: Choosing Assisted Reproduction. Indianapolis, IN, Perspectives Press, 1998.
Golombok S., Murray C, Brinsden P, Abdalla H: Social versus biological parenting: Family functioning and the socioemotional development of children conceived by egg or sperm donation. J Child PsycholPsychiatry 40:519–527, 1999.

Several difficult but important ethical questions are the byproduct of reproductive technology. One question is whether the use of technology that extends a women's reproductive life is appropriate, and, if so, whether limits should be recommended for its application. Age minimums and maximums in reproductive practice have been an area of dispute. Ethicists question how old is too old. If there is an age that would be considered "too old", who should determine that age?

Some believe that the medical and psychological risks for both the older recipients and the children that they are hoping to bear far outweigh the benefits. Others believe that considering age limits for people to become parents is a form of ageism. Similarly, some find age limits a form of sexism since society has not had as dramatic a reaction to older men becoming fathers as it has had to older women becoming mothers.

22. Summarize the argument for reproductive rights for older women

The American Society for Reproductive Medicine noted that arguments in favor of oocyte donation to postmenopausal women are based on societal practices, gender equality, and reproductive freedom. Some believe that their right to procreative liberty or the moral right of everyone to reproduce does not depend on age and that this principle outweighs all other arguments. Proponents argue that individuals with life-limiting illnesses are not necessarily prohibited from reproduction based solely on their shortened life expectancy. It is also deemed medically safe, in most cases, for postmenopausal women in good health to carry a child using a younger woman's eggs.

Furthermore, in many cultures and in our society, it is not uncommon for children to be raised by grandparents who take on most of the parenting role and often bring more experience, patience, time, and economic stability to the family unit. Therefore, there is no reason to assume that society will be harmed by allowing older individuals who, in most cases, are clearly motivated to procreate. Based on this notion, there is also no reason to assume that older women and their partners lack the physical and psychological stamina for raising children. In addition, denying women an alternative for reproduction at ages equivalent to men is considered by some to be sexist and prejudicial, especially as women generally live longer than men.

23. Summarize the argument against reproductive rights for older women.

One major argument against oocyte donation to postmenopausal women is that it is unnatural to transcend biologic limits in terms of reproductive capacity.

One of the most frequently raised concerns with older people using technology to reproduce tends to be whether older women and men are being irresponsible or selfish by having children based on the increased risk of parental death or age-related disability. Questions are raised as to whether their offspring will be at too much risk to be abandoned or left to care for disabled elderly parents. Conversely, because of social stigma, children may be adversely affected psychologically and socially by having parents old enough to be grandparents. Another issue is whether older parents will have enough energy or physical stamina to properly interact with young children. Because parenting is both an emotionally stressful and physically demanding experience, older women and their partners may be unable to meet the needs of a growing child and maintain a long parental relationship.

Lastly, risks such as maternal fatality, hypertension, diabetes, preterm labor, pre-eclampsia and other complications of pregnancy and childbirth are increased in older women. In addition, there may be fetal problems, including retarded fetal growth, stillbirths, chromosomal abnormalities, and perinatal mortality. Although the use of donated oocytes from younger women can prevent chromosomal abnormalities, there are increased risks to both the mother and fetus due to an increased chance of multiple gestation, and/or prematurity due to maternal medical conditions.

24. How young is too young for someone to donate his or her gametes?

Donors are typically recruited on the basis of age, with younger donors often being more desirable than older ones. Many programs look at the age of majority as a reasonable requirement for younger donors, although the idea of having an enforced maximum age remains in question. The ASRM guidelines include an age range of 18–40 for sperm donors and 18–34 for oocyte donors, with recipients being informed if the donor is over 34. In the cases of known donation, women may be older than 35.

Many egg donation programs and sperm banks recruit donors from colleges and universities. Although younger donors are preferable for success rates, a moral question that seems to resurface is whether gamete donors in their 20s, who may not have a child of their own, can give psychological informed consent. Some argue that younger women and men are not at a sufficient point in their adult development, particularly as it pertains to reproduction, to be able to give true informed consent to donate their gametes.

It is recommended that a mental health counselor be an active part of helping donors contemplate whether they are certain that they are undertaking donation for reasons that are right for them now and in the future. They must give serious thought to how they feel about donating genetic material to help create a child with whom they may have no contact in the future. They must understand the differences between the genetic, gestational, and rearing aspects of motherhood. Those who have not started or completed their families must try to imagine how they would feel about having genetic children in the world if they become infertile themselves. Others must consider the meaning of anonymity and how they feel not knowing the outcome of their donation and whether a child(ren) was created with their help.

25. Should couples be allowed to choose the sex of their child for reasons other than to prevent the transmission of serious genetic diseases?

Technological advances in reproductive medicine have made sex selection a tangible reality; however, whether this technology should be made available to couples for nonmedical reasons has sparked an ethical debate within practices of assisted reproduction.

26. Summarize the arguments for preconception gender selection.

Proponents of gender selection typically believe that reproductive rights belong solely to the individuals or couples who seek to have a child and that gender selection is included as part of these rights. Arguments for gender selection also involve personal and social issues such as gender balance or distribution in a family with more than one child. For example, couples with one or more child of a particular gender may strongly prefer to have a child of the different sex. In other cases, they might have such a strong preference for a specific gender or a first-born child's gender that they might resort to abortion or be unhappy with children of the undesired gender or not reproduce at all unless preconception methods are available.

27. Summarize the arguments against preconception gender selection

Arguments against the use of gender selection appeal both to the immediate and inherent negative aspects of this technology and to the longer-term social consequences. One major concern is that this technology allows parents an inappropriate amount of control over characteristics that are considered nonessential. There is also a concern that this technology will increase or reinforce gender discrimination, either by allowing more males to be produced as first children or by encouraging parents to focus more on gender itself. Furthermore, there is a concern for the psychological welfare of children born as a result of gender selection, who may be expected to act in certain gender-specific ways when the technique succeeds and who may disap-

American Society for Reproductive Medicine Ethics Committee Reports and Statements: Ethical Considerations of Assisted Reproductive Technologies: Oocyte Donation to Postmenopausal Women. American Society for Reproductive Medicine, 1977.
Gordon ER, Barrow RG: Legal and ethical aspects of infertility counseling. In Burns LH, Covington SN (eds): Infertility Counseling. Pearl River, NY, Parthenon Publishing Group, 1999, pp 491–512.
Cooper SL, Glazer ES: Choosing Assisted Reproduction. Indianapolis, IN, Perspectives Press, 1998.

point parents' expectations when it fails. One of the longer-term societal concerns is that, if widely practiced, gender selection could lead to sex ratio imbalances similar to what has occurred in other parts of the world because of female infanticide, gender-driven abortions, and a one-child family policy. This type of practice may only reinforce gender bias in society as a whole as well as create an unbalanced emphasis on a child's genetic characteristics rather than his or her inherent worth. Lastly, there is concern that such techniques are an unnecessary medical, financial, emotional, and physical burden for parents and that it may lead physicians to use their skills for nonmedically indicated purposes, thus diverting medical resources from more important uses.

Gordon ER, Barrow RG: Legal and ethical aspects of infertility counseling. In Burns LH, Covington SN (eds): Infertility Counseling. Pearl River, NY, Parthenon Publishing Group, 1999, pp 491–512.

Ethics Committee of the American Society for Reproductive Medicine: Preconception gender selection for nonmedical reasons. Fertil Steril 75(5), 2001.

Ethics Committee of the American Society for Reproductive Medicine: Sex selection and preimplantation genetic diagnosis. Fertil Steril 72(4), 1999.

57. ADOPTION

Anne F. Malavé, PhD

1. What is adoption? How does it differ from foster care and guardianship?

Adoption is a *permanent* family-building option with complete transfer of all legal rights and responsibilities from the birthparent/s to the adoptive parent/s, who are then responsible for raising and parenting the child. Adoption does *not* include either foster care or guardianship (both of which are usually intended to be temporary) or "informal adoptions" (a common practice in some cultures, in which relatives other than the biological parents, often extended family members, raise children). Inherent in the above definition are both social and legal meanings of adoption. Many (but not all) infertility and adoption professionals also use the word in its social meaning to describe third-party reproduction (see questions 16 and 18).

2. How many people in the United States adopt and are adopted?

Currently there are estimated to be 5–6 million adoptees (people who have been adopted) in the United States. Although there is no complete record of how many people adopt, in 1992 the National Center for State Courts estimated that 118,779 people were adopted *domestically* (within the U.S.) that year. About half of these were relative adoptions, and half were nonrelative (i.e., "stranger") adoptions. There are approximately 30,000 infant adoptions in the U.S. each year.

3. How many international adoptions are there in the U.S.?

Preliminary data from the U.S. Department of State report that the total number of international adoptions reached 20,000 for the first time in 2002; the top sending countries were China, Russia, Guatamala, and Korea.

4. Describe some of the recent changes in adoption.

Adoption—a complex subject highly affected by sociocultural, psychological, and legal factors—has changed enormously in the past 10–20 years. One of the biggest changes is the decreased stigmatization of single mothers, which has led to the availability of fewer babies for adoption in the U.S. This development has led to more international adoptions, including more transracial and transethnic adoptions (see question 29) as well as more domestic adoptions from the foster-care system. Another consequence is a shift toward "openness" in adoption (see question 24), which has radically changed both the process and the practice of adoption.

5. What are the most common types of adoption?

The most common type of adoption is the relative, grandparent, or step-parent adoption. But when most people think of adoption, they usually mean nonrelative adoptions (there is no biological link between the adopted child and the adoptive parents).

6. What are the common reasons for adoption?

The most common reason for nonrelative adoption is infertility. These adoptive parents are known as "traditional adopters." Other categories include people who choose to adopt but are able have children biologically (known as "preferential adopters").

7. What percentage of adoptive parents are infertile?

Although there are no exact statistics, Berry, Barth, and Needell (1996) found in their research that a majority of subjects (86% of private agency adopters, 80% of independent adopters, and 49% of public agency adopters) reported that they adopted because they were unable to have a child biologically.

8. When is the right time for patients undergoing infertility treatments to consider adoption?

In the past it was generally considered best to wait until infertility treatments were finished and infertility feelings were resolved before starting to explore adoption. But now most professionals agree that it is wise for people to start to investigate adoption *while* they are pursuing infertility treatment. There are several reasons for this shift. In the first place, it is now accepted that the resolution of feelings about infertility is not a discrete process but rather continues over the course of a lifetime. Furthermore, there are many more medical options than before, which makes the decision to end treatment much more difficult. The area of adoption is complex; it consists of distinctly different avenues and is often experienced as overwhelming. This complexity makes it important for people to begin to familiarize themselves with the territory while they are still pursuing medical treatments. For some people, this approach means hope that they can eventually become parents if medical treatments should fail; for others, information about adoption may well inform their decisions about the medical treatments so that they do not come to adoption when they are completely emotionally and financially depleted.

9. What is the role of the physician/infertility specialist in adoption?

The physician/infertility specialist is an important and influential authority figure in the lives of patients. Many physicians do not see it as their place to advise patients about important decisions such as when to consider adoption or when to end infertility treatment, and most are understandably reluctant to do so. Many patients, however, not only expect this type of guidance from their doctors but also want their doctor's help. Health care professionals should take a more active role in routinely helping patients consider all options to family-building, including adoption and third-party reproduction options as well as helping patients (who are often in denial) become more realistic about their chances of conception. Doctors can also be helpful in referring patients for counseling and to support groups such as RESOLVE, the National Infertility Association.

10. What is the role of the infertility counselor in adoption?

The infertility counselor's role is to help people who are struggling with infertility work through the emotional challenges and the decision-making process of how to proceed through the labyrinth of choices involved in trying to build a family. It is the counselor's role to help people become aware of the different options open to them and to help them begin to figure out which path feels right to them. This process involves helping people explore all options, including adoption. The infertility counselor can play a vital role in helping people resolve or work through their infertility sufficiently to move toward adoption (among other options) with eagerness, enthusiasm, and hope.

11. What happens if one partner in a couple wants to adopt and the other does not?

The answer depends on how close the couple is to active pursuit of adoption. If this disparity occurs earlier in the process, it is a more *typical* stage of a couple's journey toward adoption; it is rare that both partners decide at exactly the same time. If the couple is actively trying to adopt, however, this disparity becomes a real problem and an indication that the couple is not yet ready to adopt. Because couples include two individuals, it is not surprising that each will be at a different point with regard to such an important decision. Usually, but not always (although there is a lack of definitive research in this area), the woman arrives at this decision first. An adequate amount of time is necessary to explore adoption. For couples that have ongoing difficulty in coming to an agreement, counseling with a professional experienced in infertility and adoption is recommended.

12. How does adoption address the problem of infertility?

Adoption does not address the problem of infertility per se, although it does address the problem of wanting to become a parent and being unable to have a child biologically. It is important to allow time and emotional healing from the losses of infertility before approaching adoption as well as to gain some understanding and appreciation of the differences involved in becoming an adoptive family. It is also important to begin to understand how the experience of infertility and its accompanying losses affects the individual/couple and how it will affect their relationship with the adopted child. One of the foremost adoption experts, sociologist H. David Kirk, encourages adoptive parents to become closer to their adopted children through recognizing their common losses.

13. Describe some of the most common fears and concerns about adoption.
   1. The birthmother will come and take the child away.
   2. The couple will be unable to adopt because they are too old or do not have enough money or the adoption criteria will be too strict.
   3. All adopted children are "damaged" or experience more emotional difficulties.
   4. The adoptive parents will be unable to talk with their child about adoption.
   5. Adopted children will search for their birthparents and then "abandon" their adoptive parents.
   6. Adopted children will not be accepted by their families and society.
   For the most part, these concerns are based in fear rather than reality. Issues of loss and fear of rejection and abandonment run through these concerns and are also very much the legacy of the experience of infertility. Counseling can help to address these issues (see question 33).

14. What are the similarities and differences between adopting a child and having a child through assisted reproduction?
   Similarities
   1. Both are alternative routes to family-building that originate from infertility.
   2. Both involve third parties, professionals, and financial costs.
   3. Both involve some social stigma.
   4. Both include delicate decisions about how to treat information (whether and how to disclose).
   Differences
   1. The nature of roles, rights, and regulations are far more defined in the area of adoption.
   2. The focus of the professionals: adoption experts focus on "the best interests of the child," whereas assisted reproduction professionals focus on the needs of adults.
   3. The degree of openness: adoption is usually more open than assisted reproduction.

15. When does someone decide to adopt?
   For some people, the decision to adopt was made early in life or was based on moral or religious reasons. For those who decide to adopt as a result of infertility ("traditional adopters"), the decision is often made either when they have no choice but to end medical treatments or when they decide that "enough is enough." For traditional adopters, adoption always starts as a "second choice" (or even, with the different-third party reproductive methods available today, as a "third" or "fourth choice"), and the challenge is to arrive at a point where this family building method is not seen as "second best." This point is reached when people educate themselves about adoption and when they become comfortable with the differences of adoptive parenting. Many adoptive parents view adoption as adding to and expanding their identity and definition of family.

16. Is it acceptable to pursue adoption and infertility treatments at the same time?
   Although many people who undergo infertility treatments actively pursue adoption at the same time, most mental health and adoption professionals still recommend that a choice be made between the two as the real possibility of an adoption approaches. Many people undergoing infertility treatments put themselves on waiting lists of adoption agencies, and many agencies agree to actively work with such people. But for people on short waiting lists and people pursuing "independent adoption" (which can happen very quickly), it is advisable that they have ended infertility treatments. It is important to consider the needs of the child and to take time to enjoy the child and adjust to parenthood.

17. How soon after adopting should the parents return to infertility treatments?

When a couple returns to infertility treatment after adoption, the decision may or may not be related to a lack of acceptance of the adoption. People's situations are different, and sometimes new medical treatments open up possibilities that were previously unavailable. However, two issues should be carefully considered, both of which relate to the recently adopted child. When people return to infertility treatment *immediately* after adoption, the decision raises some concern that they have not given themselves enough time to get to know their child and to adjust to parenting. There is also the consideration of the spacing between siblings, and the possible meaning to the adopted child that the parents continued to pursue a biological child after adoption. This decision needs careful reflection and consideration, and a consultation with a mental health professional is often recommended.

18. What is "embryo adoption"?

Embryo adoption refers to the third-party reproductive choice of using embryos with no genetic connection to the parents. This choice is becoming increasingly common, as unused embryos are donated or created, using "donor" (egg and sperm) gametes. Although many medical doctors and some mental health professionals do not regard this procedure as a form of adoption and many patients are counseled to regard it as a form of medical treatment and to maintain secrecy, even from the child, many other mental health and adoption experts believe that this new area of reproduction (as well as the use of any "donor" gamete) is a form of "prenatal" adoption. We have learned, over the years, that biological and genetic roots are important to adoptees, and it seems likely that there is much in common between these two family-building routes, which share many psychosocial issues.

19. How long does it take to adopt?

Adoption can take anywhere from a few months to years. The time frame depends on the different decisions that potential adoptive parents make, such as the type of child that they are willing to adopt (e.g., newborns, available only in this country, may take much longer to adopt), the amount of information desired about the child (with international adoptions, for example, little or no information is often available), the circumstances of the potential adoptive parents (e.g., age, health history, financial status), and, to some degree, the willingness of the potential adoptive parents to become active in pursuing adoption.

20. How much does adoption cost?

Many adoption professionals estimate that the average costs in a adoption are between $15,000 and $25,000. Adoption costs vary widely, with the least expense through public agencies (the foster-care system, which may even include an adoption subsidy), and the highest expense through private agency or independent adoptions. Although the costs are often similar between domestic and international adoptions, the latter may cost less than domestic adoptions because of differences in the process and because there are more "set fees" in this approach.

21. What is a home study?

All 50 states mandate that potential adoptive parents undergo a home study before, and sometimes after, a child is placed to evaluate their fitness as future parents. The process involves interviews by a social worker in the prospective adopters' homes as well as references checks and reviews of all finances, medical, and other relevant information and fingerprinting to check for possible criminal and/or child abuse records.

22. What criteria are used to evaluate prospective adoptive parents?

Home studies ascertain whether the prospective adopters are ready and prepared to become parents. When the potential adopters have struggled with infertility, the social worker evaluates whether they have sufficiently resolved their losses to move on to embrace life as an adoptive family. In recent years, home studies have shifted from performing a purely evaluative function to providing a "parenting-readiness" opportunity. Social workers help prospective adopters explore their motivations to adopt, examine their expectations about what it means to build a family through adoption, and educate themselves about becoming an adoptive family.

23. Who can adopt?

All adults must pass home studies to be able to adopt, and there are age limitations, depending on the particular route of adoption. Otherwise, the traditional profile of the two-parent adopters under 40 years of age no longer describes all those who adopt. Today, other adopters include many single people, (the majority of whom are women), homosexuals, and lesbians. Age restrictions are less strict, depending on the approach, and financial and other restrictions vary greatly (e.g. financial subsidies are available for some public agency adoptions).

24. What is open adoption?

Open adoption is generally defined as the continued communication between the birthparent(s) and the adoptive family after the adoption has been finalized. This practice has evolved in the past 20 years, after the previous practice of "closing records" came under great criticism when both birthparents and adoptees publicly described their need for contact and as birthparents started to have more involvement in their children's placements. It is now recognized by most, if not all, adoption advocates that the option to have at least the possibility of a connection, even if it is after the adoptee becomes an adult, is important to many adoptees and birthparents. As practiced, open adoption is best described as a continuum, from the annual exchange of letters and photos between adoptive parents and birthparents through a third party on one end of the continuum to ongoing contact of the birthmother (usually) in the child's life as the child grows up (with no parenting responsibility or power). This topic is still controversial, with "experts" on both sides arguing that either "open" or "closed" adoption is "in the best interests of the child." More research and time are needed to evaluate this option.

25. What is the adoption triad?

The adoption triad refers to the three different participants in an adoption: the adopted child, the adoptive parent(s), and the birthparent(s) (usually the birth mother; a discussion of the role of birth fathers is beyond the scope of this chapter). The term was developed in response to a greater openness in adoption and a more deliberate recognition of the existence of birthparents/family.

26. Describe the different ways in which one can adopt.

There are three main avenues to adoption: domestic through a private agency or an independent adoption; international adoption; and domestic through a public agency (the foster-care system). Each approach involves important decisions, such as the age of the child (new-born, infant, toddler, or "older child"), the race/ethnicity of the child (same as or different from the prospective adoptive parents), whether the child has "special needs" (see question 30), whether the adoption will be "open" or "closed", and the level of openness in the adoption.

27. What are some of the reasons that people adopt domestically?

Among the chief reasons that people adopt domestically is the desire for a newborn (usually a Caucasian) baby. The *only* way to have a newborn baby enter a family through adoption is by domestic adoption, usually through independent adoption. Other reasons include a concern for the health of the child and a dislike of travel to another country.

28. Describe the reasons for an international adoption.

People pursue international adoptions for a variety of reasons. Sometimes the relative speed of an international adoption appeals to people, especially those who have struggled with a long history of infertility. Likewise, the relative guarantee of a child (children are usually freed for adoption before the adopters arrive) is seen by many as an advantage over the risks, for example, of independent adoption. Other adopters fear contact with birthparents and feel protected when they adopt internationally. Some people believe (incorrectly) that children from other countries will be healthier than children adopted through public agencies in this country. Other reasons to adopt internationally include an interest in that country or culture.

29. What is transracial adoption?

A transracial adoption refers to a difference between the race of the adoptive parents and the race of the adopted child. The term is usually applied to Caucasian parents who adopt an African-American children. There is a controversial history behind transracial adoption, with concerns by some mental health and adoption professionals about the possible handicap of children of color who are raised in white families in terms of developing a racial identity. There is a concern that some white parents are not sufficiently sensitive to the significance of race for black adoptees in a race-sensitive society. Recent laws passed by the federal government in 1994 and 1996 forbid racial consideration as the sole reason to deny a prospective adopter the right to adopt someone of a different race.

30. What does "special needs adoption" mean?

The term *special needs* covers a wide range and refers to children who are harder to place. The child may be nonwhite, have a disability (physical, mental, or emotional), be older, or belong to a sibling group. Children with special needs can be found in domestic adoption (the term is frequently used to describe children in the foster-care system) as well as in international adoption.

31. Explain what is involved in adopting a child with special needs.

People who adopt children with special needs do so for a variety of reasons. Those who adopt children who have problems of various kinds often do so because they have both the interest and the means. Sometimes such parents have older children and feel that they have "more to offer" and are prepared for more of a challenge; sometimes they have special expertise; sometimes they have a strong calling; and sometimes they take this route when other paths are not as available to them (e.g., single adoptive fathers). It is extremely important to gather accurate information about the child's health history as well as to be prepared to seek substantial outside help. People with idealistic views are advised to become fully acquainted with the "realities" of this approach to parenting.

32. How often do birthmothers change their minds?

Despite dramatic media coverage, the actual incidence of birth mothers/birth fathers changing their minds after their child is placed in the home of adoptive parents is quite low (less than 1%). It is extremely rare that birth parents challenge adoptions years later. The most common change of mind occurs within 48 hours before and 48 hours after giving birth, which is always a risk for those pursuing a domestic, independent, and certain domestic agency adoptions. There are also changes of mind while pursuing independent adoptions, and it is important to retain and be advised by a lawyer who is reputable and experienced in adoption. In some domestic agency adoptions, the potential adoptive parents are protected from knowing about changes of mind. The downside of this approachis that they have access to the child only after birthparent rights have been relinquished, which means that the child has to have a temporary foster-care placement.

33. How does society view adoption?

There have been radical shifts in the role of adoption in U.S. culture and society. Although adoption is becoming more normalized and more visible through increased openness and more international and transracial adoptions, societal stigma and negative stereotypes still exist. In the 1997 Benchmark Adoption Survey by the Evan B. Donaldson Institute, which examined public perceptions about adoption, results indicated that, although most Americans say that they support adoption and think that adoptive parents and their children love each other as much as those who are biologically connected, only about half of the public thought that adopting is "as good as" having a biological child.

34. Compare attachment and bonding between families formed through adoption and non-adoptive families.

Two of the most frequently asked questions about adoption are whether an adoptive parent can bond with his or her adopted child and whether an adoptive parent loves his or her child adopted child as much as they would love a biological child. The answer to both questions is yes, although it may be hard for those looking at adoptive families from the outside to understand. We know that "blended families," which include adopted and biological children, say that there is no difference in their love for the children. Sometimes there are difficulties in attachment when children are adopted, particularly when the child is older, and professional help may be necessary. Most children respond quickly and well to professional interventions and treatment.

35. Is it always necessary to tell a child that he or she is adopted?

The clear consensus in the adoption community is that it is vital to tell a child that he or she is adopted. Almost everyone recommends that this process should begin before the child has language so that the adoptive parent(s) become used to and less anxious about saying the word "adoption" and so that the child grows up familiar with hearing about it in a positive way. Children do not begin to understand what adoption means until they are 4–5 years old, when they start to understand reproduction. Children's understanding of adoption changes as they go through different developmental stages. It is important that all discussions of adoption are balanced and integrated into family's life so that there is neither an avoidance of nor an overemphasis on the topic.

36. Describe how adoptive families handle disclosure of the adoption to family, friend, and everyone else.

Mental health and adoption professionals recommend disclosing the decision to adopt to family and close friends as soon as it is made. The reason is that it takes time for people to adjust to the idea and to prepare for the arrival of the child, and adoptions can happen quite quickly. It is important for the adoptive family to have the support of their family and friends. The issue of disclosure must be handled carefully, for information shared can never be retrieved. It is important for adoptive parents to avoid telling others important information that they would like their child to hear first from them and information that they believe that their child should own and make decisions about (in terms of when and whether to share it with others).

37. Do adopted children have more psychological problems than other children?

This is a common question and fear of all those who think about adopting. Besides the fear of the "unknown," there are other reasons for this concern. In the first place, a higher proportion of adopted children are found in mental health treatment. Some people attribute this finding to handicaps of adoption, and others attribute it to the greater willingness of adoptive parents to seek help. In addition, there are documented delays when some older children are adopted; the majority of these children, however, respond well to therapeutic interventions.

38. How does being adopted affect a child?

Adoption affects all individuals differently. It is a complex subject, which is either in the foreground or the background of adoptees' lives in a fluid way, depending on the stage of development, the situation, and the personality of the adoptee. There is no definitive "one size fits all" experience. The main differences lie in the impact on the adopted child of having a second set of parents, the birth parents, and what this means to the adopted child. Lastly, although some adoptees appear to be greatly affected by being adopted, some quite painfully so, for others the experience is an integrated part of their identity, on which they do not focus to any great extent.

39. What happens if parents of adopted children also have biological children?

Adoptive families often have biological children as well as adopted children. Such families are called blended families. Some of these families already have a biological child or children before they adopt (and many have suffered from secondary infertility, which is extremely common), and some have a biological child or children after they adopt. Despite the common myth that, if a woman adopts, she will automatically conceive afterward, pregnancy after adoption occurs at the same rate as for people who do not adopt. Blended families often face more curiosity and scrutiny than families with either all biological or all adopted children, which can bring distinct challenges and difficulties (this is even more true if there are ethnic/racial differences between the siblings). Often, however, adoptive parents in blended families feel more secure in their knowledge that they love their children equally, even though they have arrived in different ways.

40. How often do children who have been adopted search for their biological parents?
Although there are no accurate statistics to answer this question, all adoption professionals agree that there has been a tremendous shift toward searching in recent years. Some of this shift, undoubtedly, has been the result of the World Wide Web, which has made many legal restrictions obsolete (such as the denial of rights for adoptees to have access to their birth records in some states).

41. What happens when adopted children find their biological/birth parents?
The results of this experience vary with the individuals involved. Sometimes it leads to an ongoing relationship between the adoptee and birthparent(s)/family, much lilke an "extended family," and sometimes there is little contact after the initial contact is made. Most authorities believe that a large part of the motivation to do a search is related to personal questions of identity for the adoptee rather than to a desire for relationship. All adoptees fantasize about asking why they were "given away." Meeting with the real birthparents (as opposed to the fantasized ones) can be a healing experience for adoptees, but not always. Sometimes the search is met with more rejection, as birthparent(s) refuse to have contact or even acknowledge that they are the birthparent(s). The most common fear of adoptive parents is that the search will lead to their rejection by the adoptee; this fear is clearly unfounded. However, the sensitivity of adoptees to the fears of their adoptive parents has caused many adoptees to wait until after their adoptive parents have died to do a search. Many believe that this protection of the adoptive parents costs the adoptee, who often discovers that his or her birthparents have also died; therefore, the chance to make contact is lost.

42. Are adopted children happy?
Most adopted children grow up to be healthy, well-adjusted, and just as happy as most other people—contrary to media bias, which often presents adopted children as troubled and unhappy. Although there is little research on this subject, in 1994 the Search Institute in Minneapolis conducted an important 4-year study of 881 adopted adolescents, 1262 adoptive parents, and 78 non-adopted siblings. The results indicated that the majority of the adoptees were psychologically healthy, and strongly attached to their families.

BIBLIOGRAPHY

1. Berry M, Barth RP, Needell B: Preparation, support, and satisfaction of adoptive families in agency and independent adoptions. Child Adoles Soc Work J 13(2):157–183, 1996.
2. Brodzinsky D: Infertility and adoption adjustments: Considerations and clinical issues. In Leiblum SR (ed): Infertility: Psychological Issues and Counseling Strategies. New York, John Wiley & Sons, 1997, pp 246–262.
3. Evan B, for the Donaldson Adoption Institute: Benchmark Adoption Survey: Report on Findings. New York, Evan B. Donaldson Adoption Institute, 1997 (conducted by Princeton Survery Research Associates).
4. Flango V, Flango C: How many children were adopted in 1992. Child Welfare 75(5), 1995.
5. Freundlich M: Adoption and Ethics: Adoption and Assisted Reproduction. Washington DC, Child Welfare League of America, 2001.
6. Irwin Johnston P: Adopting After Infertility. Indianapolis, Perspectives Press, 1992.
7. Kirk HD: Shared Fate: A Theory and Method of Adoptive Relationships. Brentwood Bay, BC, Ben-Simon Publications, 1984.

8. Pertman A: Adoption Nation: How the Adoption Revolution Is Transforming America. New York, Basic Books, 2000.

9. Ruskai Melina L: Raising Adopted Children. New York, Harper Perennial, 1998.

10. Ruskai Melina L, Kaplan Roszia S: The Open Adoption Experience. New York, Harper Perennial, 1993.

11. Salzer LP: Adoption after infertility. In Infertility Counseling: A Comprehensive Handbook for Clinicians. New York, Parthenon Publishing Group, 1999.

12. Sharma AR, McGue MK, Benson PI: The emotional and behavioral adjustment of United States adopted adolescents. Part II: Age at adoption. Child Youth Serv Rev 18 (1,2):101–114, 1996.

13. U.S. Department of State: Immigrant Visas Issued to Orphans Coming to the U.S. (preliminary data), 2002. On-line at http://travel.state.gov/orphan_numbers.html.

INDEX

Page numbers in **boldface type** indicate complete chapters.